OXFORD MEDICAL PUBLICATIONS

Oxford Handbook of
Acute Medicine

Dose schedules are being continually revised and new side-effects recognized. Oxford University Press makes no representation, express or implied, that the drug dosages in this book are correct. For these reasons the reader is strongly urged to consult the pharmaceutical companies' printed instructions before administering any of the drugs recommended in this book.

Oxford Handbook of Acute Medicine

PUNIT S. RAMRAKHA

*Research Fellow and Honorary Senior Registrar,
Department of Cardiology and Clinical Pharmacology,
Imperial College School of Medicine
(Hammersmith Hospital), London, UK*

and

KEVIN P. MOORE

*Senior Lecturer and Honorary Consultant Gastroenterologist,
Royal Free Hospital School of Medicine, London, UK*

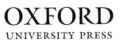
OXFORD

UNIVERSITY PRESS

OXFORD

UNIVERSITY PRESS

Great Clarendon Street, Oxford OX2 6DP

Oxford University is a department of the University of Oxford
and furthers the University's aim of excellence in research, scholarship,
and education by publishing worldwide in

Oxford New York

Athens Auckland Bangkok Bogotá Bombay Buenos Aires Calcutta
Cape Town Chennai Dar es Salaam Delhi Florence Hong Kong Istanbul
Karachi Kuala Lumpur Madrid Melbourne Mexico City Mumbai
Nairobi Paris São Paulo Shanghai Singapore Taipei Tokyo Toronto Warsaw

and associated companies in
Berlin Ibadan

Oxford is a trade mark of Oxford University Press

Published in the United States
by Oxford University Press Inc., New York

A catalogue record for this book is available from the British Library

Library of Congress Cataloging-in-Publication Data
(Data applied for)

ISBN 0 19 262682 5

Printed in Great Britain
on acid-free paper by
The Bath Press, Bath

Contents

Note: The content of individual chapters is detailed on each chapter's first page.

Contributors

Dr John Anderton
Lecturer & Hon. Senior Registrar, University of Newcastle upon Tyne, Newcastle upon Tyne

Dr Hew Beynon
Consultant Physician, Dept of Medicine, Royal Free Hospital School of Medicine, London

Dr Sarah Flint
Senior Registrar, Dept of Obstetrics and Gynaecology, Kings College Hospital, London

Dr Derek Harrington
Specialist Registrar, Cardiology, Royal Brompton National Heart Hospital, London

Dr Masud Husain
Lecturer and Hon. Senior Registrar, Dept of Clinical Neuroscience, Charing Cross Hospital, London

Dr William Lynn
Consultant in Infectious Diseases, Cameron Centre, Ealing Hospital, Southall, Middlesex

Dr Richard Marley
MRC Clinical Training Fellow, Dept of Medicine, Royal Free Hospital, London

Dr Karim Meeran
Senior Lecturer, Dept of Endocrinology, Hammersmith Hospital, London

Dr Amanda Perry
Bone Marrow Transplant Fellow, Dept of Haematology, University College Hospital, London

Dr Ian Sabroe
Senior Registrar, Dept of Respiratory Medicine, Hammersmith Hospital, London

Dr Kevin M O'Shaughnessy
Senior Lecturer and Hon.Consultant, Dept of Clinical Pharmacology, Addenbrooke's Hospital, Cambridge

Dr Sean Whittaker
Consultant Dermatologist and Hon. Senior Lecturer, Dept of Medicine, Royal Free Hospital School of Medicine, London

Artwork: **Dr Katie Darling** and **Ms Jan Foster**

Symbols and abbreviations

~	approximately
–ve	negative
+ve	positive
↓	decreased
↑	increased
↔	normal
°	degrees
A_2	aortic component of 2nd heart sound
Ab	antibody
ABPA	allergic bronchopulmonary aspergillosis
ACE	angiotensin-converting enzyme
ACTH	adrenocorticotropic hormone
ADH	antidiuretic hormone
AF	atrial fibrillation
AFB	acid-fast bacillus
AIDS	acquired immunodeficiency syndrome
Al	aluminium
ALL	acute lymphoblastic leukaemia
Alk phos	alkaline phosphatase (also ALP)
AMP	adenosine monophospate
ANA	antinuclear antibody
ANCA	anti-neutrophil cytoplasmic antibody
APTT	activated partial thromboplastin time
ARDS	adult respiratory distress syndrome
ASD	atrial septal defect
ASO	antistreptolysin O
AST	asparate transaminase
ATN	acute tubular necrosis
AV	atrioventricular
AVM	arteriovenous malformation(s)
AXR	abdominal X-ray (plain)
BAL	bronchoalveolar lavage
bd	*bis die* (twice a day)
BMJ	*British Medical Journal*
BNF	*British National Formulary*
Ca	carcinoma
CABG	coronary artery bypass graft
cAMP	cyclic AMP
CAPD	chronic ambulatory peritoneal dialysis
CCF	congestive cardac failure (ie RVF with LVF)
CHB	complete heart block
CK	creatine (phospho) kinase (also CPK)
CLL	chronic lymphocytic leukaemia
CML	chronic myeloid leukaemia
CMV	cytomegalovirus
CNS	central nervous system
COAD	chronic obstructive airways disease
CPAP	continuous positive airways pressure
CPR	cardio-pulmonary resuscitation
CRP	C-reactive protein
CRF	chronic renal failure
CSF	cerebrospinal fluid
CT	computerized tomography
CVP	central venous pressure

CVS	cardiovascular system
CXR	chest X-ray
d	day(s)
DIC	disseminated intravascular coagulation
DIP	distal interphalangeal
dl	decilitre
DM	diabetes mellitus
DU	duodenal ulcer
D&V	diarrhoea and vomiting
DVT	deep venous thrombosis
DXT	deep radiotherapy
EBV	Epstein–Barr virus
Echo	echocardiogram
EDTA	ethulene diamine tetraacetic acid (full blood count bottle)
EEG	electroencephalogram
EM	electron microscope
EMG	electromyogram
ENT	ear, nose, and throat
ESR	erythrocyte sedimentation rate
FBC	full blood count
FDP	fibrin degradation products
FEV_1	forced expiratory volume in 1st second
FFP	fresh frozen plasma
F_1O_2	partial pressure of O_2 in inspired air
FROM	full range of movements
FSH	follicle-stimulating hormone
FVC	forced vital capacity
g	gram
GA	general anaesthetic
GB	gall bladder
GFR	glomerular filtration rate
GGT	gamma glutamyl transpeptidase (also γ-GT)
GH	growth hormone
GI	gastrointestinal
GP	general practitioner
G6PD	glucose 6-phosphate dehydrogenase
GTT	glucose tolerance test
GU	genitourinary
h	hour
HAV	hepatitis A virus
Hb	haemoglobin
HBsAg	hepatitis B surface antigen
HBV	hepatitis B virus
Hct	haematocrit
HCV	hepatitis C virus
HDV	hepatitis D virus
HHT	hereditary haemorrhagic telangiectasia
HIDA	hepatic immunodiacetic virus
HIV	human immunodeficiency virus
HOCM	hypertrophic obstructive cardiomyopathy
HONK	hyperosmolar non-ketotic (diabetic coma)
HRT	hormone replacement therapy
HSV	herpes simplex virus
ICP	intracranial pressure
IDDM	insulin-dependent diabetes mellitus (compared with NIDDM: non-IDDM)
Ig	immunoglobulin

IHD	ischaemic heart disease
IM	intramuscular
IFN-α	alpha interferon
INR	international normalized ratio (prothrombin ratio)
IPPV	intermittent positive pressure ventilation
ITP	idiopathic thrombocytopenic purpura
ITU	intensive therapy unit
iu/IU	international unit
IV	intravenous
IVI	intravenous infusion
IVC	inferior vena cava
IVU	intravenous urography
JVP	jugular venous pressure
KCCT	kaolin cephalin clotting time
kg	kilogram
kPa	kilopascal
L	left
l	litre
LBBB	left bundle branch block
LDH	lactate dehydrogenase
LFT	liver function test
LH	luteinizing hormone
LMN	lower motor neurone
LP	lumbar puncture
LUQ	left upper quadrant
LVF	left ventricular failure
LVH	left ventricular hypertrophy
μg	microgram
MCV	mean cell volume
MDMA	3,4-methylene dioxymethamphetamine
mg	milligram
MI	myocardial infarction
min(s)	minute(s)
ml	millilitre
mmHg	millimetres of mercury
MND	motor neurone disease
MRI	magnetic resonance imaging
MS	multiple sclerosis (do not confuse with mitral stenosis)
MSU	midstream urine
NAD	nothing abnormal detected
NBM	nil by mouth
ND	notifiable disease
NEJM	*New England Journal of Medicine*
NG(T)	nasogastric (tube)
NIDDM	non-insulin-dependent diabetes mellitus
NMDA	*N*-methyl-D-aspartate
NR	normal range (=reference interval)
NSAID	non-steroidal anti-inflammatory drugs
N&V	nausea and/or vomiting
OCP	oral contraceptive pill
OD	*omni die* (once daily)
OGD	oesophagogastroduodenoscopy
OGTT	oral glucose tolerance test
OPD	out-patients department
OTM	*Oxford Textbook of Medicine*
P_2	pulmonary component of 2nd heart sound
$PaCO_2$	partial pressure of CO_2 in arterial blood

PAN	polyarteritis nodosa
PBC	primary biliary cirrhosis
PCR	polymerase chain reaction
PCV	packed cell volume
X PE	pulmonary embolism
PEEP	positive end-expiratory pressure
PEFR	peak expiratory flow rate
PERLA	pupils equal and reactive to light and accommodation
PID	pelvic inflammatory disease
PIP	proximal interphalangeal
PND	paroxysmal nocturnal dyspnoea
PO	*per os* (by mouth)
PR	*per rectum* (by rectum)
PPF	purified plasma fraction (albumin)
PRL	prolactin
PRN	*pro re nata* (as required)
PRV	polycythaemia rubra vera
PTH	parathyroid
PTT	prothrombin time
PUO	pyrexia of unknown origin
PV	*per vaginam* (by the vagina)
qid	*quater in die* (4 times a day)
qds	*quater die sumendus* (to be taken four times a day)
qqh	*quarta quaque hora* (every 4 hours)
R	right
RA	rheumatoid arthritis
RBBB	right bundle branch block
RBC	red blood cell
RFT	right ilia fossa
Rh	rhesus
RhF	rheumatic fever
RIF	right iliac fossa
RUQ	right upper quadrant
RVF	right ventricular failure
RVH	right ventricular hypertrophy
s/sec	second(s)
S_1, S_2	first and second heart sounds
SBE	subacute bacterial endocarditis (more correctly IE = infective endocarditis)
SC	subcutaneous
SD	standard deviation
SE	side-effect(s)
SL	sublingual
SLE	systematic lupus erythematosus
SOB	short of breath (SOBOE: on exercise)
SR	slow release
stat	*statim* (immediately; at once)
SVC	superior vena cava
SXR	skull X-ray
T°	temperature
$t_{1/2}$	biological half-life
T_3	triiodothyronine
T_4	thyroxine
TB	tuberculosis
TIA	transient ischaemic attack
tid	*ter in die* (3 times a day)
tds	*ter die sumendus* (to be taken 3 times a day)

TRH	thyroid-releasing hormone
TPR	temperature, pulse, and respirations count
TSH	thyroid-stimulating horomone
u/U	units
UC	ulcerative colitis
U&ES	urea and electrolytes
UMN	upper motor neurone
URT	upper respiratory tract
URTI	upper respiratory tract infection
USS	ultrasound scan
UTI	urinary tract infection
VDRL	venereal diseases research laboratory
VE	ventricular extrasystole
VF	ventricular fibrillation
VMA	vanilyl mandelic acid (HMMA)
V/Q	ventilation:perfusion ratio
VSD	ventriculo-septal defect
WBC	white blood cell
WCC	white cell count
wk(s)	week(s)
yr(s)	year(s)
ZN	Ziehl–Neelson

Note: other abbreviations are given in full on the pages where they occur.

Preface

As every doctor soon discovers, the management of acute medical emergencies is the most demanding and stressful aspect of medical training. Most handbooks of clinical medicine can only go into general detail about the management of medical problems and the specific advice needed to manage acutely ill patients is usually insufficient in these texts.

The aim of this handbook is to give confidence to doctors to manage acute medical problems effectively and safely, and is intended to complement the *Oxford Handbook of Clinical Medicine*. Many books on acute medicine are written by senior staff, who have not been at the frontline for some time, and certain aspects of care are assumed or overlooked. This book was written by junior doctors with first-hand experience of the practical problems and dilemmas faced in casualty.

The layout of the book reflects clinical practice: assessment, differential diagnosis, immediate management, and some aspects of long-term therapy. We have included an extensive section on practical procedures, as well as a section on pharmacotherapy to provide information on the use of certain common and unusual drugs to complement that provided in the *British National Formulary* (BNF).

Throughout the book the text commonly exceeds that required for the management of specialist problems by the generalist. We make no apology for this. This is intended to provide the doctor with an understanding of specialist interventions so that they are more conversant with what is possible and what is happening to their patient.

Acknowledgements

We would like to thank all of the contributors and particularly Masud Husain (Neurology), Bill Lynn (Infectious Diseases) and Amanda Perry (Haematology) for being prompt, comprehensive, and adhering to the format of the book. Thanks also go to Jan Foster and Katie Darling for their artwork. We would also like to thank OUP for their encouragement during the inception and writing of this book. PSR is indebted to Vandana and his parents for their support and motivation. KPM is indebted to Janet, Alice, and Thomas for their continued patience when the portable computer accompanied family holidays. Finally, we would like to acknowledge the environment at the Hammersmith Hospital where acute medicine is both interesting and fun.

PSR
KPM
October, 1997

Foreword by Professor John Ledingham

A Professor of Medicine at Edinburgh in the more leisurely days of 1862 taught that an acute illness was 'one that ran its course in 14 days'. A student courageously inclined to dispute this definition retorted that an omnibus ran from Edinburgh to Leith in 20 minutes, but that was not a definition of an omnibus. Acute in the context of this book suggests rather more urgency than was the concept in 1862! There is a need for junior doctors (and senior ones too) to have at their finger tips the essentials of management of all acute emergencies. This book will surely be a great help in achieving that aim. The authors have succeeded in producing an admirably succint and yet comprehensive account of the management of a huge variety of conditions requiring urgent treatment and have done so without being too tiresomely didactic.

Handbooks in the series from Oxford University Press are already in the pockets of most clinical students all over the world. This one is sure to be there too and will, I suspect, also be in the pockets of junior doctors and even (perhaps covertly) readily available to more senior physicians. Such a practical book as this needs to have been written by authors thoroughly and recently familiar with the whole field of acute medicine. It has been and has been done very well. I am delighted to provide a Foreword to an excellent book which really does fill an important gap.

1 Cardiovascular emergencies

Cardiorespiratory arrest   1.

Basic life support

2 Basic life support is the backbone of effective resuscitation following a cardiorespiratory arrest. The aim is to maintain adequate ventilation and circulation until the underlying cause for the arrest can be reversed. 3–4 minutes without adequate perfusion (less if the patient is hypoxic) will lead to irreversible cerebral damage. The usual scenario is an unresponsive patient who has been found by staff who then alert the cardiac arrest team. The initial assessment described below should have been performed by the person finding the patient and they should have started cardiopulmonary resuscitation (CPR). Occasionally you will be the first to discover the patient and it is important to rapidly assess the patient and begin CPR. Basic life support involves:-

AIRWAY   BREATHING   CIRCULATION

1 Assessment of the patient
- *Check whether the patient is responsive.* If not, shout for help.
- *Open the airway.* With two fingertips under the point of the chin, tilt the head up. If this fails place your fingers behind the angles of the lower jaw and apply steady pressure upwards and forwards (see figure below). Remove ill-fitting dentures and any obvious obstruction. If the patient starts breathing, roll the patient over into the recovery position and try to keep the airway open until an orophyrangeal airway can be inserted.

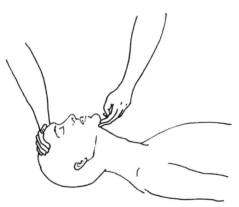

Jaw lift to open the airway

- *Watch the chest for movement* and listen and feel at the mouth for breath sounds for a few seconds.
- *Feel the carotid for a pulse*; check both sides. If the pulse is absent, shout for help and get someone to alert the cardiac arrest team.

2 Cardiopulmonary resuscitation
- *Open the airway* (tilt the chin) and blow 2 breaths into the patient. Allow the chest to fall after each breath. If there is any difficulty in inflating the chest, recheck that the mouth is clear of obstruction.

Cardiovascular emergencies

- **Start chest compressions** with the heel of your hand over the middle of the lower half of the sternum. Aim to depress the sternum about 4–5cm at a rate of approx. 80 compressions per minute.
- If you are alone, after 15 compressions, tilt the chin and give 2 further inflations, continuing in a ratio of 15:2 until help arrives.
- With 2 persons, nominate one to the breathing and the other to the compressions; give 2 full breaths after every 5–6 compressions, stopping compressions only just long enough for the breaths.

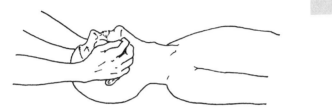

Jaw thrust (thrust the angle of the mandible upwards)

Cardiorespiratory arrest 2.

Advanced life support

4
- It is unlikely that an effective spontaneous cardiac activity will be restored by CPR without more advanced techniques (intubation for effective ventilation, drugs, defibrillation, etc.). Do not waste time. As soon as help arrives, delegate CPR to someone less experienced in advanced cardiac life support, so that you are able to continue.

- Orophryangeal (Guedel) or nasopharyngeal airways help maintain the patency of the airway by keeping the tongue out of the way. They can cause vomiting if the patient is not comatose. ET intubation is the best method of securing the airway (p812). *Do not attempt this if you are inexperienced.*

- Attach the patient to a cardiac monitor as soon as possible to determine the cardiac rhythm and treat appropriately (see table opposite).

- Establish venous access with a large bore (14–18G) cannula in a large peripheral vein. Central vein cannulation (internal jugular or subclavian) is ideal but requires more training and practice and is not for the inexperienced. If venous access fails, drugs may be given via an ET-tube into the lungs (except for bicarbonate and calcium salts). Double the doses of drugs if using this route as absorption is less efficient than iv.

Post resuscitation care

- Try to establish the events that precipitated the arrest from the history, staff and witnesses and the hospital notes of the patient. Is there an obvious cause (MI, hypoxia, hypoglycaemia, stroke, drug overdose or interaction, electrolyte abnormality, etc.)? Record the duration of the arrest in the notes with the interventions, drugs (and doses) in chronological order in the notes.

- Examine the patient to check both lung fields are being ventilated; check for ribs that may have broken during CPR. Listen for any cardiac murmurs; check the neck veins (see p 143 for causes of raised CVP and hypotension). Examine the abdomen for an aneurysm or signs of peritonism; insert a urinary catheter and consider an NG-tube if unconscious. Record the Glasgow Coma Score (p416) and perform a brief neurological assessment (see p418).

- Investigations: *ECG* [?MI, ischaemia, tall T waves ($\uparrow K^+$)]; *ABG* [mixed metabolic and respiratory acidosis is common and usually responds to adequate oxygenation and ventilation once the circulation is restored. If severe, consider bicarbonate (p716)]; *CXR* (check position of ET-tube, ?pneumothorax); *U&Es*; and *glucose.*

- After early and successful resuscitation from a primary cardiac arrest, the patient may rapidly recover completely: transfer to HDU or CCU to monitor for 12–24h. Commonly the patient is unconscious post-arrest and should be transferred to ITU for mechanical ventilation and haemodynamic monitoring and support for $\geqslant 24$ hours

- Change any venous lines that were inserted at the time of arrest for central lines inserted with sterile technique. Insert an arterial line and consider PA catheter (Swan-Ganz) if requiring inotropes.

- Remember to talk to the relatives: keep them informed of events and give a realistic (if bleak) picture of the arrest and possible outcomes.

- When appropriate consider the possibility of organ donation and do not be frightened to discuss this with the relatives. Even if discussion with the relatives is delayed, remember corneas and heart valves may be used up to 24 hours after death. Brain stem death (see p428).

Cardiovascular emergencies

Cardiorespiratory arrest
Advanced life support
Post resuscitation care **5**

Rhythms commonly associated with cardiac arrest	
• Ventricular fibrillation	page 6
• Asystole	page 8
• Electromechanical dissociation	page 10

(Cardiac output may also be lost with severe bradycardia (p68), or ventricular tachycardia (p52))

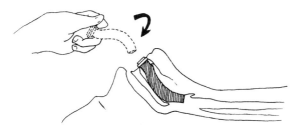

Insertion of oropharyngeal airway

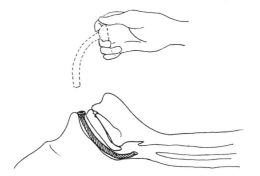

Insertion of nasopharyngeal airway

Ventricular fibrillation / Pulseless VT

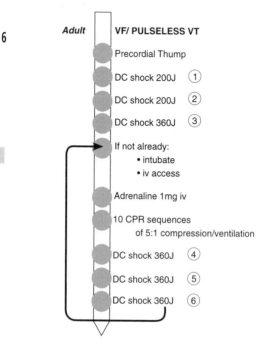

Adult   VF/ PULSELESS VT

Precordial Thump

DC shock 200J ①

DC shock 200J ②

DC shock 360J ③

If not already:
- intubate
- iv access

Adrenaline 1mg iv

10 CPR sequences
    of 5:1 compression/ventilation

DC shock 360J ④

DC shock 360J ⑤

DC shock 360J ⑥

Notes

- The priority initially is rapid defibrillation. Give the first three shocks in rapid succession checking the pulse and monitor for ~ 5s in between shocks: chest compressions between shocks is unnecessary unless the charging time is unduly prolonged.
- The interval between shocks and adrenaline should not be > 2min if the patient remains in VF. The priority now is establishing perfusion and if not already done so, intubate and establish iv access.
- Give adrenaline during every loop, approx. every 2–3mins and continue loops for as long as defibrillation is indicated.
- After three loops consider:-
  - Bicarbonate (50ml of 8.4%) after checking ABGs (see p716)
  - Anti-arrhythmic   – lignocaine 100mg iv repeated once if reqd.)
                         – bretylium 5mg/kg (see p680)
  - Changing the position of the paddles to anterior-posterior.

Ventricular fibrillation

Asystole

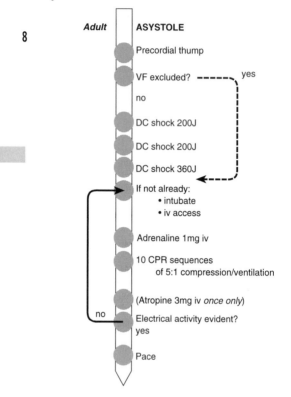

Adult   **ASYSTOLE**

Precordial thump

VF excluded? - - - - - - yes

no

DC shock 200J

DC shock 200J

DC shock 360J

If not already:
- intubate
- iv access

Adrenaline 1mg iv

10 CPR sequences
of 5:1 compression/ventilation

(Atropine 3mg iv *once only*)

no   Electrical activity evident?
yes

Pace

Notes

- Is the patient really in asystole? Check the leads and equipment and if there is any doubt treat as VF initially with DC shocks.
- External cardiac pacing (see p69) may be considered if the equipment is available. Transvenous pacing should only be tried by persons with experience.
- Further doses of atropine are unnecessary.
- After the third loop give high dose adrenaline (5mg iv).

Electromechanical dissociation (EMD)

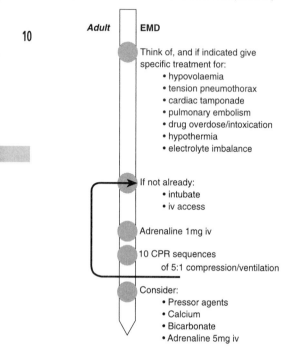

Adult **EMD**

Think of, and if indicated give specific treatment for:
- hypovolaemia
- tension pneumothorax
- cardiac tamponade
- pulmonary embolism
- drug overdose/intoxication
- hypothermia
- electrolyte imbalance

If not already:
- intubate
- iv access

Adrenaline 1mg iv

10 CPR sequences
of 5:1 compression/ventilation

Consider:
- Pressor agents
- Calcium
- Bicarbonate
- Adrenaline 5mg iv

Notes

- Search for, and treat, the underlying cause (see above).
- Hypovolaemia usually follows bleeding (trauma, leaking aneurysm, massive GI bleed, etc.) Rapidly replace volume with colloid (p210).
- If tension pneumothorax is suspected, attempt decompression with a large cannula into 2nd intercostal space, mid-clavicular line on side with reduced breath sounds and movement.
- Pericardial tamponade may be difficult to diagnose during an arrest as the 'classical' signs may be obscured by the resuscitation. If suspected, needle pericardiocentesis should be attempted by someone with experience (p788).
- Large pulmonary emboli may be broken up by chest compressions and this (with iv fluid loading) may be life-saving (see p110).
- Give calcium (10mls 10% calcium gluconate) to patients with EMD taking calcium antagonists or with ↑ K⁺ or ↓ Ca²⁺.
- Consider other pressor agents (e.g. glucagon in patients on beta-blockers (p638)), sodium bicarbonate (if acidotic). After the third loop consider high dose adrenaline (5mg iv).

Electromechanical dissociation

Myocardial infarction (MI): Assessment

Presentation

- **Chest pain** usually similar in nature to angina, but of greater severity and longer duration, not relieved by s/l GTN. Associated features include nausea and vomiting, sweating, breathlessness, and extreme distress.
- The pains may be **atypical**, epigastric, or radiate through to the back.
- Diabetics, the elderly, and hypertensives may suffer **painless infarction** ('silent' infarcts) and present with breathlessness from acute pulmonary oedema, syncope or coma from dysrhythmias, acute confusional states, diabetic hyperglycaemic crises, hypotension, or shock.

Factors associated with a poor prognosis

- Age > 70 years
- Previous MI or chronic stable angina
- Anterior MI or right ventricular infarction
- Left ventricular failure at presentation
- Hypotension (and sinus tachycardia) at presentation
- Diabetes mellitus
- Mitral regurgitation (acute)
- Ventricular septal defect

Initial management

- The referring doctor should be instructed to give asprin (300mg po if no contraindications) and **not** to give any im injections (causes a rise in total CK and risk of bleeding with thrombolysis).
- All patients with suspected MI should have continuous ECG monitoring: full resuscitation facilities should be readily available.

Immediate assessment should include:-

- **Rapid examination** to exclude hypotension, note the presence of murmurs and to identify and treat acute pulmonary oedema. RVF out of proportion to LVF suggests RV infarction (see p32).
- Secure iv *access*
- **12 lead ECG** and continuous ECG monitoring for dysrhythmias
- Give:
  - *Oxygen* (initially only 28% if history of COAD)
  - *Diamorphine 2.5–5mg iv prn for pain relief*
  - *Metoclopramide 10mg iv q8h for nausea*
  - *GTN spray 2 puffs s/l unless hypotensive*
- Take blood for:

FBC, and U&Es	Supplement K$^+$ to keep at 4–5mmol/l.
Glucose	May be ↑ acutely post MI, even in non-diabetics, and reflects a stress-catecholamine response and may resolve without treatment.
Cardiac enzymes	(see p14).
Cholesterol	Serum cholestrol and HDL remain close to baseline for 24–48 hours but fall thereafter, and take ⩾ 8 weeks to return to baseline.

- Arrange for *portable CXR* to assess cardiac size, pulmonary oedema and exclude mediastinal enlargement.
- General examination should include peripheral pulses, fundoscopy, abdominal examination for organomegaly and aortic aneurysm.

Cardiovascular emergencies

Conditions that may mimic the pain of an acute MI

Pericarditis
Dissecting aortic aneurysm
Pulmonary embolism
Oesophageal reflux, spasm or rupture
Biliary tract disease
Perforated peptic ulcer
Pancreatitis

**Conditions that may mimic the ECG changes
of an acute MI**

Left or right ventricular hypertrophy
LBBB or left ant. fascicular block
Wolff-Parkinson-White syndrome
Pericarditis or myocarditis
Cardiomyopathy (hypertrophic or dilated)
Trauma to myocardium
Cardiac tumours (primary and metastatic)
Pulmonary embolus
Pneumothorax
Intracranial haemorrhage
Hyperkalaemia
Cardiac sarcoid or amyloid
Pancreatitis

Myocardial infarction: Diagnosis

This is based on a combination of history, ECG and cardiac enzymes.

ECG changes

- **ST segment elevation** occurs within minutes and may last for up to 2 weeks. Persisting ST elevation after 1 month suggests LV aneurysm formation.

- **T wave inversion** may be immediate or delayed and generally persists after the ST elevation has resolved. T wave inversion without new Q-waves may occur with 'sub-endocardial' infarction (enzyme elevation is necessary to confirm infarction in this case).

- **Pathological Q waves** are the hallmark of transmural infarction, may take hours or days to develop and usually remain indefinitely. In the standard leads the Q wave should be $\geq$ 25% of the R wave, 0.04 seconds in duration, with negative T waves. In the precordial leads, Q waves in V4 should be > 0.4mV (4 small sq) and in V6 > 0.2mV (2 small sq), in the absence of LBBB (QRS width < 0.1s or 3 sq).

- **Non-diagnostic changes**, but ones that may be ischaemic, include new LBBB or RBBB, tachyarrhythmias, transient tall peaked T waves or T wave inversion, axis shift (left or right), or AV block.

Cardiac enzymes

CK (creatinine phosphokinase)

- Serum levels rise within 4–8 hours post MI and fall to normal within 3–4 days. The peak level occurs at about 24 hours but may be earlier (12 hours) in patients who have had reperfusion (thrombolytic or PTCA).

- False positive rates of ~ 15% occur in patients with alcohol intoxication, muscle disease or trauma, vigorous exercise, convulsions, im injections, hypothyroidism and PE.

- CK-MB isoenzyme is more specific for myocardial disease and may be elevated despite a normal total CK. However, it is present in small quantities in other tissues (skeletal muscle, tongue, diaphragm, uterus, and prostate) and trauma or surgery may cause small elevations in CK-MB.

AST (aspartate aminotransferase)

- Levels rise within 8–12 hours after onset of MI, peaks at 18–36 hours and fall to normal within 3–4 days.

- AST is less specific and may rise with most liver or skeletal muscle diseases, after im injections, and pulmonary embolism.

LDH (lactate dehydrogenase)

- Levels rise above normal 24–36 hours post MI, peak at day 4–6 and return to normal by day 10–14.

- A rise in LDH is also seen with haemolysis, pulmonary embolism, liver disease and congestion, skeletal muscle disease, megaloblastic anaemia, and a variety of neoplasms.

- Analysis of LDH isoenzymes may be useful (heart contains mainly LDH_1; skeletal muscle and liver contain LDH_4 and LDH_5).

- **HBD (hydroxybutyrate dehydrogenase)** activity is really a measure of LDH_1 isoenzyme and may be used instead of total LDH.

Troponin T

- This is a myofibrillar protein released early in the course of an MI and levels remain elevated for up to 2 weeks post MI. Elevation appears to be a specific marker for MI.

Myocardial infarction

Localization of infarcts from ECG changes	
Anterolateral	ST elevation with Q waves in V3–V6 with T wave inversion in I and aVL
Anteroseptal	Q waves in V2–V3 with ST elevation and T wave inversion
Antero-apical	Q wave in I with ST elevation. Apparent right axis deviation; sometimes with Q waves in V3–V4.
Inferior	Q waves with ST elevation and T inversion in II, III and aVF. Additional ST elevation in V4R suggests right ventricular infarction.
True posterior	Tall R waves in V1–V2 with ↓ ST in V1–V3. This can be confirmed with an oesophageal lead if available (method similar to an NG tube).

Myocardial infarction: Management

General measures

1 Control of cardiac pain

- *Diamorphine* is the drug of choice and may be repeated in doses of 2.5–5mg iv until the pain is relieved or there is evidence of toxicity (hypotension, respiratory depression). Nausea and vomiting may be treated with metoclopramide or a phenothiazine.

- *Oxygen* – hypoxaemia is frequently seen post MI due to ventilation-perfusion abnormalities secondary to LVF. In patients with refractory pulmonary oedema, positive pressure ventilation with CPAP or via formal endotracheal intubation may be necessary.

- *Nitrates* – providing the patient is not hypotensive, nitrates (sub-lingual or intravenous) may lessen pain. They need to be used cautiously in inferior MI, especially with right ventricular infarction, as venodilation may impair RV filling and precipitate hypotension. Nitrate therapy has no significant effect on mortality (ISIS-4).

2 Strategies to limit infarct size

- Beta-blockade
- ACE inhibitors
- Coronary reperfusion – Thrombolysis
  - Coronary angioplasty
  - Emergency coronary bypass grafting

Beta-blockade

Several clinical trials have demonstrated the benefits of early β-blockade in limiting infarct size and reducing mortality (e.g. ISIS-1, MIAMI, TIMI II).

- Indications: Hyperdynamic state (sinus tachycardia, ↑ bp)
  - Recurrent or persistent ischaemic pain
  - Infarct extension
  - Tachyarrhythmia refractory to Class I antiarrhythmics

- Contraindications: asthma, AV block or bradycardia, systolic bp < 95mmHg, or LVF.

- Give iv initially (metoprolol 5mg repeated at 5 minute intervals to a dose of 15mg) and, if tolerated, followed 6 hours later by 50mg po q12h. Esmolol is an ultra-short-acting iv β-blocker which may be tried if there is concern whether the patient will tolerate β-blockers (see table on p126).

ACE inhibitors

Numerous trials have now demonstrated a reduction in mortality and severe heart failure in patients with acute MI treated with ACE inhibitors (ISIS-4, GISSI-3, SAVE, AIRE, etc.). This appears to be a class effect (all ACE-I are beneficial) and treatment should be started as soon as possible, after presentation.

- Patients with large infarcts (particularly transmural anterior MI), heart failure, and impaired LV function on ECHO or MUGA, benefit the most.

- One regimen is captopril 6.25mg po on arrival, 12.5mg 2 hours later, 25mg bd 10–12 hours increasing to 50mg bd prior to discharge.

- Alternatively, lisinopril 5mg on arrival, aiming to discharge home on 10–20mg/day.

Myocardial infarction: Thrombolysis 1.

Reperfusion occurs in 50–70% of patients who receive thrombolysis within 4 hours of onset of pain (cf. ~ 20% of controls) and is marked by normalization of ST segments on ECG.

Indications for thrombolysis

- Typical history of cardiac pain within previous 24 hours and ST elevation (> 1mm in standard leads or > 2mm in V1–V6) on ECG.
- If pain started 12–24 hours previously, thrombolysis should be given for continuing pain or clinical deterioration. Initial trials suggested a benefit in all those treated up to 24 hours, but subsequent trials (EMIRAS, LATE) have suggested no benefit > 12 hours.
- Cardiac pain with LBBB on ECG.
- If ECG is equivocal on arrival, repeat in 15–30 minutes. Thrombolysis should not be given if the ECG is normal or there is isolated ST depression (exclude true posterior infarct).
- The following sub-groups of patients particularly benefit from thrombolysis:-
  - Anterior infarct
  - Marked ST elevation
  - Age > 75 years
  - Impaired LV function or LBBB, hypotensive (systolic bp < 100mmHg)
  - Patients presenting within 1 hour of onset of pain

Contraindications to thrombolysis (see p20)

These may be considered relative or absolute. In the presence of an absolute contraindication, if appropriate, PTCA should be considered. In the presence of a 'relative' contraindication the clinical state of the patient and time since onset of symptoms need to be taken into account before thrombolysis is ruled out.

Choice of thrombolytic agent

Individual units may have a specific policy.

1 *Streptokinase (SK)* is the most commonly used agent and remains the first line agent unless there is a specific contraindication.
  - The only specific contraindications to SK are known allergy or use 5 days to 1 year previously.
2 *Recombinant tissue plasminogen activator (rt-PA, alteplase)* is a fibrin-specific agent.
  - rt-PA is superior to SK in producing reperfusion but only marginally superior in reducing overall mortality.
  - This should be followed by iv heparin (see below).
  - Accelerated rt-PA should be considered for any patient with:-
    1. Large anterior MI, especially if within 4 hours of onset.
    2. Previous SK therapy or recent streptococcal infection.
    3. Hypotension (systolic bp < 100mmHg).
    4. Low risk of stroke (age < 55 years, systolic < 144mmHg).
    5. Recurrent ischaemia during hospitalization and immediate catheterization and PTCA facilities unavailable.
3 *Other agents* Anisoylated plasminogen streptokinase activator *(APSAC, anistreplase)* appears to induce a coronary patency rate similar to intracoronary SK. *Urokinase* is no longer routinely used.

Cardiovascular emergencies

Doses of thrombolytic agents

Streptokinase (SK)
- Give as 1.5 million units in 100ml normal saline iv over 1 hour.
- There is no indication for routine heparinization after SK as there is no clear mortality benefit and there is a small increase in risk of haemorrhage (see below).

Recombinant tissue plasminogen activator (rt-PA, alteplase)
- The GUSTO trial suggested the 'front-loaded' or accelerated rt-PA is the most effective dosage regimen.
- Give 15mg bolus iv then 0.75mg/kg over 30min (not to exceed 50mg), then 0.5mg/kg over 60min (not to exceed 35mg).
- This should be followed by iv heparin (see p24).

APSAC (anistreplase)
- Give as an iv bolus of 30mg over 2–5 minutes.

Myocardial infarction: Thrombolysis   2.

Contraindications to thrombolysis

- Recent CVA (6 months)
- Recent gastrointestinal haemorrhage
- Recent trauma, surgery (abdominal, neuro-, eye-, liver or kidney biopsy, dental extraction), or head injury (within 6 weeks).
- Aortic dissection or aneurysm
- LV aneurysm with mural thrombus
- Pregnancy or post-partum
- Proliferative diabetic retinopathy

Caution should be taken in patients with:-

- Prolonged cardiopulmonary resuscitation
- Uncontrolled hypertension (systolic bp > 200mmHg or diastolic bp > 110mmHg)
- Menstrual bleeding or lactation
- im injections
- Lumbar puncture within previous 1 month
- Chronic liver or renal disease
- Ulcerative colitis

Shock and advanced age are not contraindications per se.

Complications of thrombolysis

- Bleeding is seen in up to 10% of patients, mostly relatively minor at sites of vascular puncture. Local pressure is usually sufficient but occasionally transfusion may be required. In extreme cases, SK may be reversed by tranexamic acid (10mg/kg slow iv infusion).
- Hypotension during the infusion is common with SK. Lay the patient supine, if possible, slow or stop the infusion until the blood presure rises. Hypotension is not an allergic reaction and does not warrant treatment as such.
- Allergic reactions are common with SK and include a low grade fever, rash, nausea, headaches, and flushing. Give hydrocortisone 100mg iv with chlorpheniramine 10mg iv
- Intracranial haemorrhage is seen in ~ 0.3% of patients treated with SK (cf. ~ 0.6% rt-PA, ~ 0.7% APSAC).
- Reperfusion arrhythmias (most commonly a short, self-limiting run of idioventricular rhythm) may occur as the metabolites are washed out of the ischaemic tissue. If frequent and symptomatic give magnesium sulphate 8mmol in 20ml 5% dextrose over 20 minutes, repeated once after 20–30 minutes. Lignocaine (100–200mg iv bolus) or amiodarone (300mg iv over 1 hour)
- Systemic embolization may occur from lysis of thrombus within the left atrium, LV, or aortic aneurysm.

Myocardial infarction

Coronary angioplasty for acute MI

- **Primary angioplasty** can be performed safely after the onset of ischaemia and recent trials have shown a high success rate (> 93%) and shorter hospital admission with lower rates of reinfarction and recurrent ischaemia compared with patients receiving thrombolysis. Realistically however, this service cannot as yet be made availabe to the majority of patients with an MI. Thrombolysis remains the treatment of choice, but where facilities exist and if there is a contra-indication to thrombolysis, or in the setting of cardiogenic shock, primary PTCA can be life-saving.

- **Rescue angioplasty** or PTCA as an adjunct to thrombolysis, should be reserved for patients who develop ischaemia during their hospital course or at their pre-discharge stress-testing. There was no benefit in early (within 2 days) elective catheterization and PTCA after thrombolysis in the TIMI II trial.

Surgery for acute MI

Emergency surgical revascularization cannot be widely applied to patients who suffer an MI outside the hospital. However, it is useful for patients who develop acute coronary occlusion during cardiac catheterization and PTCA and in those whose coronary anatomy is known and who develop an infarct whilst waiting in hospital for their bypass operation.

Non-Q wave (sub-endocardial) infarction

- 'Q wave' or transmural infarction results from total coronary occlusion.
- Early reperfusion limits myocardial damage and the surface ECG may not develop Q waves. This has been termed 'subendocardial MI' though autopsy studies suggest pathological correlation of true sub-endocardial MI and lack of Q waves is poor (~ 50%).
- The diagnosis of non-Q wave MI depends on history and a rise in cardiac enzymes. ECG changes may be non-specific with ST depression or elevation or T inversion.

The natural history and prognosis is very different from Q wave myocardial infarction:-

- Lower in-hospital mortality (5–10%, cf. 7–15% with Q wave MI).
- Smaller infarcts initially with lower incidence of heart failure (reflection of degree of LV dysfunction).
- More frequent post infarct angina (viable myocardium with reduced blood supply).
- Higher incidence of infarct extension or early recurrent infarction (~ 40%, cf. ~ 8% with Q wave MI).
- Higher 1 year mortality (up to 65% cf. 34% with Q wave MI).

Management

Patients with non-Q wave MI require a more aggressive diagnostic approach with early search for ischaemia – both non-invasively (Holter monitoring and ST analysis or stress testing if appropriate) and invasively (coronary angiography ± PTCA or surgical revascularization).

Coronary angioplasty

Acute MI: Additional measures

1. Bed rest and continuous ECG monitoring for 24–36 hours and then transfer to the general ward if the clinical course is uncomplicated. A rehabilitation programme should be started aiming for discharge from hospital by day 7–10 if progress is satisfactory.

2. *Heparin* This remains controversial.

- iv heparin (5000 units iv bolus followed by 1000 units/hour adjusted for an APTT ratio of 1.5–2.0 times control) should be used routinely following rt-PA for 24–48 hours.
- There is no indication for 'routine' iv heparin following SK.
- Low dose sub-cutaneous heparin (5000 units s/c bd) helps prevent DVTs and should be used post SK in patients slow to mobilize.
- Higher dose s/c heparin (12,500 units bd) is thought to prevent mural thrombus but does increase the risk of intracranial bleeding.
- Generally, patients with large infarcts should receive iv heparin, as above, rather than s/c high-dose heparin.

3. *Magnesium*

- Earlier trials giving Mg^{2+} before or with thrombolytics showed some benefit in mortality. ISIS-4 showed no benefit from the routine use of iv magnesium post MI. However, Mg^{2+} was given *after* thrombolysis and the protective effect of Mg^{2+} on reperfusion injury may have been lost.
- Mg^{2+} is clearly of use in treating ventricular or atrial tachy-arrhythmias post MI.
- We suggest using Mg^{2+} in those patients not suitable for thrombolysis, prior to direct PTCA, those with 'reperfusion' arrhythmias and those who may be Mg-deficient (eg on diuretics).
- Dose: 8mmol in 20ml 5% dextrose over 20 minutes followed by 65mmol in 100ml 5% dextrose over 24 hours. Contraindications: serum $Cr > 300\mu mol/l$, 3° AV block.

4. *Calcium antagonists* are probably best avoided, especially in the presence of LV impairment. However, there are trials that have shown some benefit with either diltiazem or verapamil started after day 4–5 in patients post MI with normal LV function.

5. *Risk stratification*

- It is important to identify the sub-group of patients who have a high risk of reinfarction or sudden death and they should undergo coronary angiography, preferably prior to discharge or soon after. Those at risk are:-
  - Significant post infarct angina or unstable angina.
  - Patients with non-Q wave infarction.
  - Positive exercise test (modified Bruce protocol) with angina, > 1mm ST depression or fall in bp prior to discharge.
  - Cardiomegaly on CXR; poor LV function on ECHO or MUGA (EF < 40%).
  - Documented episodes of ventricular tachycardia.
  - Frequent episodes of silent ischaemia on Holter monitoring.

Secondary prevention

- The patient should remain on long-term aspirin (75mg od) and a beta-blocker, if there are no contraindications.
- If there is impaired LV function (LVEF < 40%) there is convincing evidence to support long-term ACE inhibition.
- Modifiable risk factors are smoking, hypertension and hyper-cholesterolaemia. There is emerging evidence that treatment with HMG CoA reductase inhibitors (eg simvastatin 20mg daily or pravastatin 40mg daily) to reduce total cholesterol to < 4.2mmol/l reduces long-term mortality in patients with documented coronary artery disease. Further data on the mechanism and whether other agents of similar class are effective is awaited.

Myocardial infarction: Complications

Complications include:
- Further chest pain.
- Fever.
- A new systolic murmur (VSD, acute MR or pericarditis; p28.
- Dysrhythmias (bradycardia, AV block, ectopics, VT; p40).
- Hypotension and shock (p32).

Further chest pain
- Chest pain post MI is not necessarily angina. Take a careful history of the character of the pain. In the absence of ECG changes with pain, and if there is doubt that it is cardiac in origin, stress-thallium imaging may aid diagnosis.
- A bruised sensation and musculoskeletal pains are common in the first 24–48 hours, especially in patients who have received CPR or repeated DC shock. Use topical agents for skin burns (silver sulphadiazine (Flamazine ®), but not if allergic to sulpha-drugs).
- *Pericarditis* presents as sharp, pleuritic, and positional chest pain, usually 1–3 days post infarct, and more commonly with full-thickness infarcts. A pericardial friction rub may be audible. ECG changes are rarely seen. Treat with high-dose aspirin (600mg po q6–8h) covered with H_2 antagonist (eg cimetidine 400mg po bd). Other NSAIDs have been associated with higher incidence of LV rupture and increased coronary vascular resistance and are probably best avoided.
- *Infarct extension* with further ST elevation should be treated with repeat thrombolysis unless there is a specific contraindication (see above). Where available, the patient should have urgent coronary angiography.
- *Post infarction angina* (angina developing within 10 days of MI) should be treated with standard medical therapy (beta-blockers, nitrates and calcium channel blockers). *Unstable angina* (angina at rest or on minimal exertion) refractory to the standard medical therapy requires urgent coronary angiography.

Fever
- Often seen and peaks 3–4 days post MI.
- Associated with elevated WCC and raised CRP.
- Other causes of fever should be considered (infection, thrombophlebitis, venous thrombosis, drug reaction, pericarditis).

A new systolic murmur
Causes:
- Ventricular septal defect (VSD)
- Mitral regurgitation (MR)
- Pericardial friction rub only audible in systole
- Long-standing murmur missed at presentation.

The absence of haemodynamic compromise does not exclude a VSD or MR: in the presence of cardiogenic shock, prompt diagnosis is essential, surgical correction may be possible.

Ventricular septal defect (VSD) post MI

- Classically seen 5–10 days post MI. Patients present with sudden deterioration, pulmonary oedema and hypotension.
- *Physical signs* are a harsh, pan-systolic murmur, maximal at the lower left sternal edge, and often pulmonary oedema.
- *Diagnosis* is usually made with echocardiography – the defect may be visualized on 2D-ECHO and colour flow doppler shows the presence of left-to-right shunt. Anterior infarction is associated with apical VSD and inferior MI with basal VSD. Failure to demonstrate a shunt on ECHO does not exclude a VSD.
- If ECHO is not available or suspicion remains high, insert a PA catheter. A step-up in oxygen saturation from RA to RV confirms the presence of a shunt, which may be calculated by:-

$$Q_p{:}Q_s = \frac{(\text{Art sat} - \text{RA sat})}{(\text{Art sat} - \text{PA sat})} \text{ where } \begin{array}{l} Q_p = \text{pulmonary blood flow} \\ Q_s = \text{systemic blood flow} \end{array}$$

Management

Hypotension and pulmonary oedema should be managed as on p32; important principles are:-
- Inotropes such as dobutamine or dopamine if severely hypotensive.
- If systolic bp > 100mmHg, cautious use of vasodilator therapy, e.g. nitroprusside, will lower the systemic vascular resistance and reduce the magnitude of the shunt. Nitrates will cause venodilatation and increase the shunt.
- If vasodilatation is not tolerated and the patient remains unstable, an intra-aortic balloon should be inserted for counterpulsation.
- Liaise with surgeons early for possible repair.
- Closure of the VSD with catheter placement of an umbrella-shaped device has been reported to stabilize critically ill patients until definitive repair is possible.

Acute mitral regurgitation post MI

- MR due to ischaemic papillary muscle dysfunction or partial rupture is seen 2–10 days post MI. Complete rupture causes torrential MR and is usually fatal.
- More commonly associated with inferior MI (posteromedial papillary muscle) than anterior MI (anterolateral papillary muscle).
- Diagnosis is by ECHO. In severe MR, PA catheterization will show a raised pressure with a large *v* wave.

Management (p104)

- Treatment with vasodilators, generally nitroprusside, should be started as early as possible once haemodynamic monitoring is available.
- Mechanical ventilation may be necessary.
- Liaise with surgeons early for possible repair.

Ventricular septal defect

Dysrhythmias after acute MI

These require treatment when they cause haemodynamic compromise or, by increasing myocardial oxygen demand, jeopardize myocardial viability.

i. *Sinus bradycardia or junctional escape rhythm (accelerated idioventricular rhythm)*

- Common, especially in the setting of inferior or posterior MI. Treat only if hypotensive, rate < 50/min, or if there is a junctional or ventricular escape rhythm.
- Give atropine in 0.6mg boluses iv (up to max. 2mg).
- When atropine is ineffective, electrical pacing is indicated. If there is significant LV impairment atrial pacing or sequential pacing is superior to simple ventricular pacing (p782–4).
- If the patient has been treated with β-blockers, consider reversing with isoprenaline (p638).

ii. *AV block and bradycardia*

- **Inferior MI**: the block may be transient, does not always require treatment, and should not delay thrombolysis. A right internal jugular sheath may be inserted prior to thrombolysis through which a pacing wire may be introduced at a later stage if necessary. Treat as above for sinus bradycardia.
- **Anterior MI**: 2° AV block, 3° block, new bifascicular block (RBBB with either LAD (S wave > R in II) or RAD (S wave > R in I)) or alternating RBBB and LBBB require prophylactic temporary pacing.

iii. *Ventricular ectopics* are associated with a poorer long-term prognosis post MI but there is no evidence that treatment alters prognosis.

- Correct P_aO_2, K^+ and Mg^{2+}.
- If ectopics continue (especially if multifocal, couplets or runs and there is a danger of R on T), give magnesium sulphate 8mmol iv (in 50ml saline over 15–20 min).
- Lignocaine 1mg/kg iv (loading dose) followed by infusion may be necessary, but only if there is haemodynamic compromise (see table p54).
- Beta-blockers may be effective, if tolerated (see table p126).

iv. *Tachyarrhythmias* Treat in the standard way (p42–66). Important principles are:-

- Arrhythmias are exacerbated by hypokalaemia, acidosis, hypoxia, hypomagnesaemia, and excessive sympathetic drive (anxiety) and these should be avoided.
- **Broad complex tachycardia** in this setting is most likely to be VT rather than SVT with aberrant conduction.
- **Ventricular tachycardia** within the first 24 hours is often precipitated by a late ventricular ectopic and is usually transient and benign. VT later in the course of MI is sustained and usually causes marked haemodynamic deterioration and has a high in-hospital mortality. It is more common in the setting of full-thickness MI with LV impairment.
- Treat as described on p52.

Hypotension and shock post MI

(see cardiogenic shock p210)

The important principles in managing hypotensive patients with myocardial infarction are:-

- If the patient is well perfused peripherally, no pharmacological intervention is required. Consider lying the patient flat with legs elevated if necessary, provided there is no pulmonary oedema.
- Try to correct any arrhythmia, hypoxia, or acidosis.
- Arrange for an urgent ECHO to exclude a mechanical cause for hypotension (e.g. mitral regurgitation, VSD, ventricular aneurysm) that may require urgent surgery.

Patients may be divided into two sub-groups

1 *Hypotension with pulmonary oedema*

- Secure central venous access – internal jugular lines are preferable if the patient may receive thrombolytic therapy.
- Commence **inotropes** (see cardiogenic shock p210).
- Further invasive haemodynamic monitoring as available

  (PA pressures and wedge pressure monitoring, arterial line).
- Ensure optimal filling pressures, guided by physical signs, PA diastolic or wedge pressure. Significant mitral regurgitation will produce large *v* waves on the wedge trace and give spuriously high estimates of LVEDP.
- Is coronary reperfuson possible, either with thrombolytic therapy or primary PTCA where available ?
- Intra-aortic balloon counterpulsation (see p796) may allow stabilization until angioplasty can be performed.

2 *Hypotension without pulmonary oedema*

This may be due to either RV infarction or hypovolaemia.

Diagnosis

- Check the JVP and right atrial pressure. This will be low in hypovolaemia and high in RV infarction.
- RV infarction on ECG is seen in the setting of inferior MI as ST elevation in right-sided chest leads (V4R-V6R).

Management

- In either case, cardiac output will be improved by cautious plasma expansion: give *100–200mls of colloid over 10 minutes* and reassess.
- Repeat once if there is some improvement in blood pressure and the patient has not developed pulmonary oedema.
- *Invasive haemodynamic monitoring* with a PA wedge catheter (Swan-Gantz) is necessary to ensure hypotension is not due to low left-sided filling pressures. Aim to keep PCWP at 12–15mmHg.
- Start *inotropes* if blood pressure remains low despite adequate filling pressures.
- Use iv nitrates and diuretics with caution as venodilatation will compromise RV and LV filling and exacerbate hypotension.

Pulmonary oedema (Treat as described on p78).

Unstable angina: Assessment

The **definition** varies from new onset angina to crescendo angina (more severe, prolonged, or more frequent pains) occurring at rest or on minimal exertion on a background of 'stable' angina. This is thought to result from a combination of coronary vasospasm and/or transient non-occlusive platelet thrombi occurring in areas of pre-existing atheromatous stenosis. Clearly there is a spectrum of severity with unstable angina falling between 'stable' exertional angina and acute MI.

Presentation

- *Chest pain* similar to angina but occurring at rest or on minimal exertion, often less severe than the presentation of an acute MI; frequent and/or prolonged episodes of pain.
- Physical examination may be normal. Look for signs of the risk factors for coronary disease. Evidence of transient LV dysfunction due to ischaemia may be present (third and fourth heart sounds, transient mitral regurgitation). Always try to exclude aortic stenosis.
- *ECG* May be normal. ST depression or elevation and T wave inversion is common and changes resolve with relief of pain.

Factors associated with a poor prognosis

Patients with the following characteristics are more likely to have a subsequent unfavourable hospital outcome (MI, death, or need for revascularization).

- Advanced age
- Angina at rest
- Angina lasting > 48 hours (intermittent or continuous)
- Angina refractory to maximum medical therapy
- ECG ST-T wave changes during pain or recovery
- 'Silent ischaemia' on Holter monitoring
- Evidence of heart failure
- History of ischaemic heart disease or previous positive ETT, or previous abnormal coronary angiogram

Initial management

1. *Stabilize the patient; relieve pain and anxiety*

- Patients with what is believed to be significant cardiac pain at rest or who have had a prolonged episode (> 1h) should be admitted irrespective of ECG or cardiac enzyme results, even if they are currently pain free.
- Strict bed rest with continuous ECG monitoring.
- Give oxygen, aspirin 300mg stat., sublingual or buccal nitrate and mild sedation if required.
- If pain persists give diamorphine 2.5–5mg iv prn with metoclopramide 10mg iv q8h.
- Take blood for U&Es, cardiac enzymes, FBC, and cholesterol. Check CXR for evidence of LVF.

2. *Confirm the diagnosis; exclude MI*

- Serial ECGs and cardiac enzymes should be carried out to exclude acute myocardial infarction. If there is a rise in cardiac enzymes without ECG ST elevation, arrange for urgent coronary angiography (see p38).
- Look for and treat factors that may be exacerbating myocardial ischaemia, e.g. infection, anaemia, thyrotoxicosis, arrhythmias, and heart failure.

Unstable angina

Unstable angina: Management 1.

Medical therapy

- *Nitrates:* iv GTN (50mg in 50ml saline at 0–10ml/h) or iv isosorbide dinitrate (0–10mg/h by infusion) may be titrated to pain, keeping systolic blood pressure > 100mmHg.

  N.B. Tolerance to continuous iv nitrates develops within 24 hours and the lowest efficacious dose should be used. Commercial GTN preparations contain alcohol at 0.01–0.14ml/mg of GTN. With continuous iv GTN the patient may receive a significant amount of alcohol (though this is seldom clinically important).

- *Anticoagulants and antiplatelet drugs:* Give a loading dose of heparin (5000 units iv) and aspirin (300mg po). Both heparin (1000U/hr aiming for APTT ratio of 2–3) and aspirin (75–325mg daily) have been shown to reduce the incidence of myocardial infarction in patients with unstable angina, and the combination is better than either alone. Newer anticoagulants (e.g. hirudin and argatroban) are still undergoing clinical trial.

- *β-blockers:* Start the patient on a short acting agent (e.g. metoprolol 25–50mg po tds) which, if tolerated, may be converted to a longer acting agent (atenolol 50mg od). Rapid β-blockade may be achieved using iv esmolol (0.5mg/kg over 1min loading dose, 50–200 µg/kg/min iv infusion – p126). Aim for HR of ~ 50–60 beats/min.

  By reducing heart rate and blood pressure, β-blockers reduce myocardial oxygen demand and thus angina. When either used alone or in combination with nitrates and/or calcium antagonists, β-blockers are effective in reducing the frequency and duration of both symptomatic and silent ischaemic episodes.

  Mild LVF is not a contraindication to β-blocker therapy as the pulmonary congestion may be secondary to LV systolic failure or reduced compliance as a consequence of ischaemia. If there is overt heart failure or β-blocker is contraindicated, start a calcium antagonist (diltiazem 60mg tds or amlodipine 5mg od).

- *Calcium antagonists:* Diltiazem 60mg po tds, titrated up to 360mg daily, aiming for a reduction in heart rate and blood pressure, is a useful adjunct to the treatment above. Amlodipine 5mg daily may be better in the setting of poor LV function.

  N.B. Calcium antagonists alone do not appear to reduce mortality or risk of MI in patients with unstable angina. However, when combined with nitrates and/or β-blockers they are effective in reducing symptomatic and silent ischaemic episodes, non-fatal MI, and need for revascularization.

- *Potassium channel openers:* Nicorandil 10–20mg bd po may be added to the 'triple' therapy in patients with refractory angina.

  This is a newer class of anti-anginals with vasodilator activity on both arterioles and venules which is extensively used in Japan, though experience in the UK is currently limited. Side-effect profile is similar to that of nitrates. Avoid in renal failure (may cause hyperkalaemia). Long-term effects on mortality and risk of MI are awaited.

- *Thrombolytic therapy:* There appears to be no role for the use of thrombolytic agents in patients with unstable angina (TIMI III).

- *Coronary angiography* is indicated for continuing angina and is discussed on p38.

Subsequent management

- When pain-free for 24 hours, stop heparin, start oral nitrates (iso-sorbide mononitrate SR. 60mg od) and wean off iv nitrates.
- If pain occurs on mobilizing, intensify medical treatment as above and consider coronary angiography if appropriate.
- If symptoms settle on medical therapy, arrange stress-testing prior to discharge to assess treatment and identify patients who need urgent cardiac catheterization. If the stress-test is negative the patient may be discharged from hospital.
- Reduce risk factors – advice on lifestyle modification, stop smoking, treat hyperlipidaemia, hypertension, and optimize diabetic control.

Unstable angina: Management 2.

Coronary angiography and intervention

Coronary arteriography helps management by allowing stratification of patients into one of the following groups:-

- Patients requiring urgent surgery – left main-stem stenosis or three-vessel disease ± impaired with no clear 'culprit' lesion which would be suitable for PTCA.
- Patients with no demonstrable coronary disease – prognosis with medical therapy is excellent in this group.
- Patients with coronary disease suitable for PTCA.
- Patients with diffuse multivessel disease and impaired LV function not suitable for PTCA or CABG.

Indications

- The patient must realize that angiography may be a prelude to angioplasty or surgical revascularization. Do not refer patients who would not accept further intervention. Advanced age per se is not a contraindication.
- Continuing angina at rest or on minimal exertion despite maximal medical therapy is an indication for ***urgent coronary angiography***.
- *Intra-aortic balloon counterpulsation* (see page 796) is useful in achieving haemodynamic stability and relief of symptoms when medical therapy has failed. It is usually initiated at the time of coronary angiography and continued until revascularization (by PTCA or CABG) is possible.
- In patients under 70 years of age whose condition has stabilized on medical therapy, refer for angiography if:
  i ECG changes during pain (exercise test prior to discharge assesses efficacy of treatment and identifies patients requiring urgent, rather than routine, coronary angiography).
  ii A positive stress-test (ideally with myocardial perfusion scanning or 2D echocardiography to identify reversible, regional myocardial ischaemia to help plan effective strategy for PTCA).
  iii Recent MI with continued pain.
- In patients over the age of 70 years, consider referral if persistent symptoms despite maximal medical therapy. Try to identify reversible ischaemia first.

Prognosis

Overall hospital mortality is ~ 1.5% (cf. ~ 15% for acute MI) and 1 year mortality is ~ 9% (cf. ~ 27% for MI). Repeat hospital admission occurs in ~ 28%. Risk of adverse events (death, MI, recurrent unstable angina) is high for the first 3–4 months. In addition to the factors noted above (p24), patients with a worse prognosis post discharge may be identified by:-

- Positive pre discharge stress-test.
- Intracoronary thrombi on angiography.
- Complex multi-vessel coronary disease
- Significant ischaemia on Holter monitoring during hospitalization

Arrhythmias: General approach

Both tachyarrhythmias and bradyarrhythmias may present with haemo-dynamic compromise. The approach to patients with arrhythmias depends upon:-

1. The effects of the rhythm on the patient.
2. The diagnosis from the ECG and rhythm.
3. Any underlying cardiac abnormality or identifiable precipitant.

The effect of the rhythm on the patient

i Patients with signs of severe haemodynamic compromise:

- Impending cardiac arrest.
- Severe pulmonary oedema.
- Shock – systolic bp < 90mmHg.
- Depressed consciousness.

Treat immediately: generally DC shock for a tachyarrhythmia or temporary pacing for a bradycardia (see p42 and 68).

ii Patients with mild-moderate compromise:

- Mild pulmonary oedema.
- Low cardiac output with cool peripheries and oliguria.
- Angina at rest.

Try to record an ECG and long rhythm strip before giving any drugs (e.g. amiodarone). This will be invaluable for long-term management. If they deteriorate, treat as above.

Diagnosing the arrhythmia

The main distinctions to make are:-

- Tachy- (> 120/min) vs brady- (< 60/min) arrhythmia.
- Narrow (≤ 120ms or 3 small sq) vs. broad QRS complex.
- Regular vs irregular rhythm.

Precipitating factors

Underlying cardiac disease

- Ischaemic heart disease
  - Acute or recent MI
  - Angina
- Mitral valve disease
- LV aneurysm
- Congenital heart disease
- Abnormalities of resting ECG
  - Pre excitation (short PR interval)
  - Long QT (congenital or aquired)

Drugs

- Anti-arrhythmics
- Sympathomimetics (β_2 agonists, cocaine)
- Antidepressants (tricyclic)
- Adenylate cyclase inhibitors (aminophylline, caffeine)
- Alcohol

Metabolic abnormalities

- ↓ or ↑ K^+
- ↓ or ↑ Ca^{2+}
- ↓ Mg^{2+}
- ↓ P_aO_2
- ↑ P_aCO_2
- Acidosis

Endocrine abnormalities

- Thyrotoxicosis
- Phaeochromocytoma

Miscellaneous

- Febrile illness
- Emotional stress
- Smoking
- Fatigue

Tachyarrhythmias (HR > 120/min)

- *History:* Previous cardiac disease, palpitations, dizziness, chest pain, symptoms of heart failure, and recent medication. Ask specifically about conditions known to be associated with certain cardiac arrhythmias (e.g. AF – alcohol, thyrotoxicosis, mitral valve disease, IHD, pericarditis; VT – previous MI, LV aneurysm).
- *Examination:* bp, heart sounds and murmurs, signs of heart failure, listen for carotid bruits.

Investigations

• 12 lead ECG & rhythm strip	• Regular vs.irregular rhythm. • Narrow vs broad QRS complex.
• Blood tests	• FBC, U&Es, glucose (urgently) • Ca^{2+}, Mg^{2+} (especially if on diuretics) • Cardiac enzymes
• Where appropriate	• Blood cultures, CRP • Thyroid function tests • Drug levels • Arterial blood gases
• Chest X-ray	• Heart size • ?signs of pulmonary oedema • Other pathology (e.g. Ca bronchus → AF, pericardial effusion → tachycardia (sinus), hypotension ± AF)

Management

Haemodynamically unstable patients

Arrhythmias causing severe haemodynamic compromise (cardiac arrest, systolic bp < 90mmHg, severe pulmonary oedema, evidence of cerebral hypoperfusion) require urgent correction, usually with DC shock. Drug therapy requires time and haemodynamic stability.

- The only exception is a patient in chronic AF with an uncontrolled ventricular rate – DC shock is unlikely to cardiovert to SR. Rate control and treatment of precipitant is first line.
- Sedate awake patients with midazolam (2.5–5mg iv) ± morphine (2.5–5mg iv) for analgesia. Beware respiratory depression and have an anaesthetist, flumazenil, and naloxone to hand.
- Formal anaesthesia with propofol is preferred, but remember the patient may not have an empty stomach and precautions should be taken to prevent aspiration (e.g. cricoid pressure, ET intubation).
- Start at 200J., synchronized shock, increasing as required (p793).
- If tachyarrhythmia recurs or is unresponsive try to correct $\downarrow P_aO_2$, $\uparrow P_aCO_2$, acidosis or $\downarrow K^+$. Give Mg^{2+} (4–8mmol iv) and shock again.
- Give specific anti-arrhythmic therapy (see p44).

Haemodynamically stable patients

- Admit and arrange for continuous ECG monitoring.
- While recording a continuous rhythm strip :-
  - Try vagotonic manoeuvres (e.g. Valsalva or carotid sinus massage). Eyeball massage is no longer recommended.
  - Give **adenosine** 6mg fast iv bolus (3mg if via central line) followed by 5ml saline flush; if no response try 12mg and then 18mg (p676).
  - If the diagnosis is made give definitive treatment (p44–66).

- *Narrow complex tachycardias* originate in the atria or AV node (i.e. supraventricular tachycardias SVT; see figure p48).
- *Irregular, narrow complex tachycardia* is most commonly AF or atrial flutter with varying AV block.
- *Broad complex tachyarrhythmias* may originate from either the ventricles (VT) or from the atria or AV node (SVT) with aberrant conduction to the ventricles (RBBB or LBBB configuration).
- If the patient has previous documented arrhythmias, compare the morphology of the current arrhythmia to old ECGs. The diagnosis of VT vs.SVT and therapy may be evident from the last admission.

Treatment options in tachyarrhythmias

Sinus tachycardia	Look for cause. Beta-blockade if anxious		
Atrial fibrillation Atrial flutter SVT (p48–66)	*Rate control (AV node)* • Adenosine • Digoxin • β-blockade • Verapamil	*Version to SR* • Disopyramide • Amiodarone • Sotalol • Flecainide • Synchronized DC shock	*Prevention* • Amiodarone • Sotalol • Quinidine • Procainamide
Junctional tachycardia (AVNRT) (p48)	• Adenosine • Digoxin • β-blockade • Flecainide • Verapamil • Synchronized DC shock • (Vagal stimulation)		
Accessory pathway tachycardias (i.e. AVRT) (p66)	*At AV Node* • Adenosine • β-blockade	*At accessory pathway* • Sotalol • Flecainide • Disopyramide • Quinidine • Amiodarone	*Termination only* Synchronized DC shock
Ventricular tachycardia (p52)	*Termination and Prevention* • Lignocaine • Flecainide • Procainamide • Disopyramide • Amiodarone • Propafenone • Magnesium • β-blockade • DC shock		*Termination only* Bretylium

Tachyarrhythmias

Broad complex tachycardia: Diagnosis

(QRS width > 120ms or > 3 small sq)

Diagnostic approach

1. *Examine the rhythm strip. Is it regular or irregular?*

Regular
- VT
- SVT or atrial flutter with bundle branch block
- Atrial flutter or SVT with pre-excitation (e.g. WPW)

Irregular
- AF, atrial flutter or multifocal atrial tachycardia with bundle branch block
- Pre-excited AF (e.g. WPW)
- Torsades de pointes (VT)

2. *Are there any features on the 12 lead ECG that help distinguish VT from SVT with aberrancy?*

Factors favouring SVT include:-

- A grossly irregular broad complex tachycardia with rates ≥ 200/min suggests AF with conduction over an accessory pathway.
- Slowing or termination by vagotonic manoeuvres.
- Evidence of atrial and ventricular coupling (e.g. with 1:2 AV block).

Diagnosis of VT

Look for:-
- Fusion or capture

- Independent atrial activity (seen in ~ 25%)

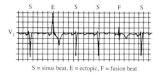

S = sinus beat, E = ectopic, F = fusion beat

- Cycle length stability (< 40ms R-R variation)
- QRS > 140 ms (3.5 small sq) especially with normal duration in SR.
- Marked left axis deviation (negative in lead II).
- QRS concordance in chest leads. If the predominant deflection of the QRS is positive this is highly suggestive of VT.
- In patients with previous LBBB or RBBB, it is difficult to distinguish VT from SVT with aberrancy. A different QRS morphology in tachycardia suggests VT. Other clues are given in the table opposite.

3. *What are the effects of adenosine?* (see p48)

The transient AV block produces one of three results:-
- *The tachycardia terminates.* This suggests an SVT with aberrancy, or right ventricular outflow tract (RVOT) tachycardia (technically a form of VT).
- *The ventricular rate slows unmasking atrial activity.* Either 'flutter' waves (atrial flutter with block or intra-atrial tachycardia) (see figure opposite), or AF. The tachycardia typically continues after a few seconds once the adenosine wears off.
- *No effect on the rhythm.* Check that the patient received a therapeutic dose of adenosine (and experienced chest tightness with the injection). Higher doses are required in patients on theophyllines. The diagnosis is most likely to be VT.

Morphological rules

For any broad complex tachycardia with 'bundle branch block' morphology, assume it is VT *unless*:-

	RBBB	LBBB
Lead V1	rSR' with R' > r RS with R > S	rS or QS with time to S wave nadir < 70 msec
Lead V6	If a Q wave is present, it must be 40 ms & < 0.2mV	R wave with no Q wave

(Sensitivity 90%, Specificity 67–85%) [1]

[1]   Griffith *et al* (1994) *Lancet* **343:** 386–388.

Narrow complex tachyarrhythmias (SVT)

These originate within the atrium or the conduction system above the bundle of His. The important distinction to make is between regular and irregular tachyarrhythmias:-

Regular

- Sinus tachycardia
- Atrial flutter (with 2:1 block)
- Atrioventricular re-entry tachycardia (AVRT) (i.e. with accessory path, e.g. WPW)
- AV nodal re-entry tachycardia (AVNRT)
- Intra-atrial re-entry tachycardia

Irregular

- Atrial fibrillation
- Atrial flutter with variable block
- Multifocal atrial tachycardia

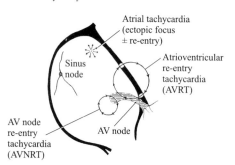

Types of supraventricular tachycardia

- Cinical features of the different arrhythmias are shown on p49.
- The diagnosis not to miss is AVRT (tachycardias involving an accessory pathway), as digoxin and verapamil are contraindicated.

Making the diagnosis

Look for atrial activity (P waves) in the ECG

- There are no P waves in AF. The baseline is chaotic (f waves).
- Atrial flutter produces 'saw-tooth' flutter waves best seen in the inferior leads and V1.
- AVNRT produces negative P waves, following the QRS complex, in inferior leads (II, III, aVF); (most commonly with PR > RP interval).
- Sinus tachycardia or sinus node re-entry produces P waves with normal morphology.
- Atrial tachycardia and AVRT have P waves different from sinus, the former with PR < RP interval, the latter with PR > RP interval.
- Multifocal atrial tachycardia (MAT) often has P waves if several different morphologies (≥ 3) with varying PP intervals and thus producing an irregular rhythm.

What are the effects of adenosine ?

- Adenosine will terminate re-entry tachycardias involving the AV node (AVNRT and AVRT). For the remainder, transient AV block will be produced but the tachycardia continues.
- The exact diagnosis may be left to an experienced cardiologist!

Differential diagnosis of supra-ventricular tachycardias

Arrhythmia	P wave configuration	Effect of adenosine (p676)	Comment
Sinus tachycardia (100-200/min)	Normal P waves	Transient AV block	
Atrial fibrillation (<200/min)	'f'-waves. Chaotic	Transient AV block	Irregular rhythm. Adenosine causes rate to slow briefly. Fast AF with broad QRS seen in AVRT (e.g. WPW)
Atrial flutter (75-175/min)	Flutter waves (saw-tooth II,III,aVF and V1)	Transient AV block	Adenosine may convert to AF
AVNRT (140-200/min)	Inverted, buried in QRS (usually not seen)	Terminates	Most common recurrent SVT in adults
AVRT (e.g. WPW or accessory pathway) (150-250/min)	Inverted, after QRS (inferior leads, RP>PR interval)	Terminates	Normal QRS if antegrade down AV node; broad QRS if antegrade down pathway
Atrial tachycardia (intra-atrial re-entry) (100-200/min)	Abnormal P wave (PR<RP) 2:1 AV block may be seen	Transient AV block	Dig toxicity, lung disease organic heart disease.
Multifocal atrial tachycardia (100-130/min)	Multiple P morphologies	Transient AV block	Assoc. with lung disease and hypoxaemia

Note: Any of these may be associated with broad QRS complexes either from pre-existing bundle branch block, or rate-related intraventricular conduction abnormality.

SVT: Management

- General approach is described on p42. If the patient is severe compromised proceed to synchronized DC shock.

- If the rhythm is obviously irregular with no discernible P waves, trea as **atrial fibrillation** (p58).

- If the rhythm is irregular with multiple P wave morphologies treat a **MAT** (multifocal atrial tachycardia – p64).

- Try measures to increase AV block:-

  - Try **vagotonic manoeuvres** (Valsalva, carotid sinus massage).

  - If unsuccessful, give **adenosine** 6mg fast iv bolus (3mg if via centra line) followed by 5ml saline flush; if no response try 12mg and ther 18mg (p678). Check that the patient received a therapeutic dose o adenosine (and experienced chest tightness with the injection) Higher doses are required in patients on theophyllines.

  - This may terminate the tachycardia (AVNRT or AVRT).

- Transient AV block will unmask AF or atrial activity. If P waves outnumber QRS complexes the diagnosis is atrial flutter or atrial tachycardia. But the arrhythmia continues.

- Treatment options available are listed in the table on p44.

- Suggested drugs for alternative diagnoses are given in the table opposite.

  - If LV function is not impaired, give a **beta-blocker** (see table p51). Make sure there are no contraindications to β-blockade. Do not give if the patient has received verapamil.

  - An alternative is **verapamil** 5–10mg iv repeated as necessary to a total dose of 20mg. Do not give if there is any possibility the rhythm is VT or if the patient is on a beta-blocker.

  - If the arrhythmia persists consider a second agent (table opposite) or synchronized DC shock.

Cardiovascular emergencies

Dosage of selected anti-arrhythmics for SVT

Drug	Dosage
Digoxin	*Loading dose:* iv 0.75–1mg in 50ml saline over 1–2 h. po 0.5mg q12h for 2 doses then 0.25mg q12h for 2 days *Maintenance dose:* 0.0625–0.25mg daily (iv or po)
Propranolol	iv 1mg over 1 min, repeated every 2min up to maximum 10mg po 10–40mg 3–4 times a day
Atenolol	iv 5–10mg by slow injection po 25–100mg daily
Sotalol	iv 20–60mg by slow injection po 80–160mg bd
Verapamil	iv 5mg over 2 min; repeated every 5min up to maximum 20mg po 40–120mg tds
Procainamide	iv 100mg over 2 min; repeated every 5min up to maximum 1g po 250mg q6h
Amiodarone	Loading dose: iv 300mg over 60min via central line followed by 900mg iv over 23 hours OR po 200mg tds x 1 week then 200mg po bd x 1 week *Maintenance dose:* 200–400mg od iv or po
Disopyramide	iv 50mg over 5min; repeated every 5min up to maximum 150mg iv 100–200mg q6h po
Flecainide	2mg/kg iv over 10min (max 150mg) or 100–200mg po bd

Ventricular tachycardia

- Defined as ≥ 3 consecutive ventricular ectopics at a rate $\geq 100/min$.
- Common early post MI (up to 40%) and, if self-limiting, without
haemodynamic compromise, does not require treatment (p30).
- Sustained VT in the setting of acute MI ($\pm$ LV dysfunction) is
associated with a poor prognosis (short- and long-term) and requires
urgent treatment.
- *Accelerated idioventricular rhythm* or 'slow VT' (rate 50–100/min)
requires treatment if hypotensive (from loss of atrial contribution)
(see p30).

Management

- If haemodynamically unstable treat as on p42.
- Correct any **electrolyte** abnormality.
- If severe **acidosis** (pH $\leq$ 7.1) give sodium bicarbonate 50ml of 8.4%
slowly iv via a central line over 20 minutes.
- Give **lignocaine** 100mg iv over 1–2 minutes (loading dose);
  - If arrhythmia persists after 5–10 minutes, repeat loading dose.
  - If arrhythmia is controlled start infusion:-
    4mg/min for 30 minutes, then
    2mg/min for 2 hours, then
    1–2mg/min for 12–24 hours.

  Increase infusion rate briefly if breakthrough occurs.
- Also give iv **magnesium sulphate** (8mmol in 50ml N saline over 15
minutes) especially if the patient was on diuretics or if there is a history
of alcohol intake (potential hypomagnesaemia). Repeat once if
necessary. Save a serum sample for analysis later.
- If this fails give **procainamide** 100mg over 2 minutes repeated at 5min
intervals until arrhythmia controlled; max 1g. Oral maintenance dose
is 250mg q6–8h.
- **Amiodarone** may be given instead of procainamide. Give 300mg
($\sim$ 5mg/kg) into a central line over 60 minutes followed by 900mg over
23 hours (see p678). The disadvantages are the side-effects and further
electrophysiological testing will need to be delayed until the patient is
fully loaded.
- Other drugs that may be used are listed in the table on p54.
- If this fails and VT persists, **synchronized DC shock** is preferred to
further anti-arrhythmics.
- **Ventricular or atrial pacing** via temporary pacing wires may be
combined with anti-arrhythmics for recurrent VT. This is generally
only effective in situations where the VT is provoked by bradycardia.
Look at the onset of runs of VT and consider if there is evidence of
heart block or sick sinus syndrome. Dual chamber temporary pacing
may improve cardiac output by restoring AV synchrony.
- **Maintenance therapy** (oral) should be started (see table p54) and
arrange Holter monitor to assess efficacy.
- If VT was secondary to myocarditis or followed acute MI, treat for 3–6
months and repeat Holter monitor on, and while withdrawing, therapy.

Investigation of ventricular tachycardia	
• ECG	Acute MI, prolonged QT interval
• CXR	Cardiomegaly, pulmonary oedema
• U&Es	Hypokalaemia, renal impairment
• Mg^{2+}, Ca^{2+}	?deficiency
• Cardiac enzymes	Small rises common after DC shock.
• ABG	?Hypoxia, acidosis
• ECHO	For LV function and to exclude structural abnormality (e.g. aneurysm)

Once acute episode is over, consider referral to cardiologist for:-

- Holter monitoring
- Exercise testing
- Coronary angiography
- VT stimulation (provocation) testing

Ventricular tachycardia: Drugs

Dosages of selected anti-arrhythmics for the acute treatment of VT
(see section 13, p673 for actions, administration, and side effects)

Drug	Dosage
Magnesium sulphate	*Loading dose* 8mmol (2g) iv over 2–15min (repeat once if necessary) *Maintenance dose* 60mmol/48ml saline at 2–3ml/hr
Lignocaine	*Loading dose* 100mg iv over 2min (repeat once if necessary) *Maintenance dose* 4mg/min for 30min 2mg/min for 2 hours 1–2mg/min for 12–24 hours
Procainamide	*Loading dose* 100mg iv over 2 min Repeat every 5min to max 1g *Maintenance dose* 2–4mg/min iv infusion 250mg q6h po
Amiodarone	*Loading dose* 300mg iv over 60min via central line followed by 900mg iv over 23 hours OR 200mg po tds x 1 week then 200mg po bd × 1 week *Maintenance dose* 200–400mg od iv or po
Disopyramide	*Loading dose* 50mg iv over 5min repeated up to maximum 150mg iv 200mg po *Maintenance dose* 2–5mg/min iv infusion 100–200mg q6h po
Flecainide	*Loading dose* 2mg/kg iv over 10min (max 150mg) *Maintenance dose* 1.5mg/kg iv over 1 hour then 100–250µg/kg/hour iv for 24 hours or 100–200mg po bd
Bretylium	*Loading dose* 5–10mg/kg (~ 500mg) iv over 10–15 min *Maintenance dose* 1–2mg/min iv infusion

Torsades de Pointes

This is an irregular polymorphic (often self-limiting) VT which appears to 'twist' about the isoelectric line. It occurs in the setting of prolongation of the QT interval (QTc > 500ms) but the relationship between degree of prolongation and risk of serious arrhythmias is unpredictable. It may present as recurrent syncope or dizziness.

Causes of prolonged QT interval

- **Drugs** Anti-arrhythmics   (quinidine, procainamide, disopyramide, amiodarone, sotalol)

    Anti-psychotics   (pimozide, thioridazine)

    Anti-histamines   (terfenadine, astemizole, esp. if prescribed drugs interact with them, e.g. ketoconazole, erythromycin)

    Anti-malarials   (esp. halofantrine)

    Organophosphate poisoning

- Electrolyte abnormalities ($\downarrow K^+$, $\downarrow Mg^{2+}$ and $\downarrow Ca^{2+}$)
- Severe bradycardia (complete heart block or sinus bradycardia)
- Intrinsic heart disease (IHD, myocarditis)
- Intracranial haemorrhage (especially sub-arachnoid)
- Congenital long QT syndromes

    Jervell, Lange-Neilsen syndrome (AR, with deafness)

    Romano-Ward syndrome (AD, normal hearing)

Note: Although amiodarone and sotalol prolong QT interval, poly-morphic VT from these drugs is rare.

$$\text{Normal QTc} = \frac{QT}{\sqrt{(RR \text{ interval})}} = \frac{0.38\text{–}0.46s}{(9\text{–}11 \text{ small squares})}$$

Management

- Give iv magnesium sulphate 8mmol as a bolus over 2–3 minutes. Repeat once if necessary and follow with an infusion (60mmol in 48ml saline at 2–3 ml/hr)
- Overdrive temporary pacing (either ventricular or atrial – p782) terminates the arrhythmia which often does not recur.
- Isoprenaline may be used while preparations are being made for pacing (p696). This accelerates the atrial rate and captures the ventricles.
- Try to correct the cause of QT prolongation.
- Consider stopping anti-arrhythmics that may prolong QT interval. Congenital long-QT syndromes should be treated with long-term propranolol.

Atrial fibrillation: Assessment

Presentation

- This may present with palpitations, chest pain, breathlessness, collapse, or hypotension. Less commonly, it may present with an embolic event (stroke, peripheral embolus) or be asymptomatic. It occurs in 10–15% of patients post MI (p30).
- Look for signs of an underlying cause (see table opposite).
- Try to establish the duration of the AF: this will determine the subsequent management (see below).

Investigations

These should be directed at looking for a precipitant and underlying heart disease. All patients should have:-

- ECG   Broad QRS if aberrant conduction; ST-T wave changes may be due to rapid rate, digoxin or underlying cardiac disease.
- CXR   Cardiomegaly, pulmonary oedema, intrathoracic precipitant, valve calcification (MS).
- U&Es   Hypokalaemia, renal impairment.
- Cardiac enzymes   ?MI. Small rise after DC shock.
- Thyroid function   Thyrotoxicosis may present as AF only.
- Drug levels   Especially if taking digoxin.
- Mg^{2+}, Ca^{2+}
- ABG   If hypoxic, shocked or ?acidotic.
- ECHO ± TOE   For LV function, valve lesions and to exclude intracardiac thrombus prior to version to SR.
- Other investigations depend on suspected precipitant.

Immediate management

Stabilize the patient

- General measures (p42) are as for any patients with an arrhythmia. Obtain venous access. Send bloods (p42) and if possible check the K^+ immediately on an ITU machine.
- Correct any **electrolyte** abnormality.
- If severe **acidosis** (pH ≤ 7.1) give sodium bicarbonate 50ml of 8.4% slowly iv over 20 minutes.
- **Carotid sinus massage (CSM)** or **iv adenosine** may help confirm the diagnosis, revealing chaotic atrial activity. In patients with a rate of 150/min always consider atrial flutter; CSM or adenosine will slow the ventricular rate and reveal flutter waves.
- Does the ECG in AF show intermittent or constant delta waves? This suggests WPW and digoxin and verapamil are contraindicated.

Further management

1 Cardiovert to sinus rhythm if appropriate.
2 Control the ventricular response rate.
3 Try to prevent further episodes of AF.

Causes of atrial fibrillation	
Underlying cardiac disease	*Separate intrathoracic pathology*
• Ischaemic heart disease	• Pneumonia
• Mitral valve disease	• Malignancy (1° or 2°)
• Hypertension	• Pulmonary embolus
• Heart failure	• Trauma
• Cardiomyopathy	*Metabolic disturbance*
• Pericarditis	• Electrolytes ($\downarrow K^+$, $\downarrow Mg^{2+}$)
• Endocarditis	• Acidosis
• Myocarditis	• Thyrotoxicosis
• Atrial myxoma	• Drugs
• Post cardiac surgery	(alcohol, sympathomimetics)

DC cardioversion for atrial fibrillation

All *hypotensive patients* should be DC cardioverted, as soon as possible, using a synchronized shock of initially 50 joules, EXCEPT:-

- Do not attempt to cardiovert patients with known chronic AF and a known progressive underlying cause (e.g. mitral stenosis, severe LV dysfunction). The chances of success are low.
- Relative contraindications to cardioversion need to be weighed against the patient's clinical condition :-
  - Hypokalaemia may be quickly corrected by giving 20mmol over 1 hour in 100 mls N saline via a central line.
  - Possible toxic levels of digoxin: ensure K^+ is 4.5–5mmol/l, give magnesium sulphate 8mmol in 50ml N saline over 15 min, cardiovert with low energies initially (e.g. 20–50 joules).
  - AF > 48 hours duration: the risk of embolism is greater. TOE may indicate the presence of a left atrial thrombus. Heparinization does not reduce the risk of embolism from pre-formed thrombus acutely.
  - Try to correct hypotension: ensure the patient is adequately filled and, if necessary, commence inotropic support.
- The procedure is detailed on p792.
- If DC shock fails initially :-
  - Give iv amiodarone 300mg over 1 hour via a central line. (Followed by iv infusion of 900mg over 23 hours).
  - Correct any hypokalaemia (aim for K^+ 4.5 – 5.0 mmol/l).
  - Attempt further DC shock.
  - If AF persists, control ventricular rate with amiodarone and digoxin and attempt further DC shock after fully loading the patient with amiodarone.

AF > 2 days duration:

- There is a 5–7% risk of systemic embolus if not anti-coagulated, and < 1.6% if on warfarin (see p794).
- If available, perform **TOE** to look for intracardiac thrombus or spontaneous contrast (a marker of very sluggish flow). If negative, DC cardioversion may be performed safely.
- **Control ventricular rate** using digoxin, beta blockers (i.e. sotalol), verapamil, or amiodarone (see below).
- Commence **heparin** and **warfarinize**.
- **Sinus rhythm may be restored** by oral amiodarone (loading then maintenance dose), sotalol (80mg bd) or quinidine (300mg po q6h).
- Discharge when stable. Consider readmission following 4–6 weeks of warfarin for DC cardioversion.

AF < 2 days duration:

- Risk of embolism with DC cardioversion is low.
- Anti-coagulate the patient iv heparin 5000 units and infusion of 1000–2000 units/hr from admission. Aim for APTT ratio of 2–2.5.
- Chemical cardioversion may be attempted (see table p51):-
  - **Flecainide** 2mg/kg over 10mins (maximum dose 150mg).
  - **Disopyramide** 50–100mg iv. Ventricular rate may increase and fibrillatory waves coarsen before reverting to sinus rhythm, so load with digoxin iv before giving this.
  - **Amiodarone** may be used (see above): iv dosing requires central line and it may take 24–48 hours for sinus rhythm to be achieved.
- **DC cardioversion** may be performed if drug therapy fails (p792).

Atrial fibrillation: Control and management

Controlling the ventricular response rate

- Check that there is no history of WPW and that no delta waves are visible on the ECG.
- **Digoxin** is the drug of choice. The patients should be given a full loading dose. The maintenance dose varies (0.0625–0.25mg od) depending on body mass, renal function, age, etc.
- Low dose **beta-blockers** (e.g. sotalol 40mg bd or atenolol 25mg od) may be added once loaded with digoxin, and the dose gradually increased. Ensure LV function is adequate and there are no contra-indications to beta-blockade.
- If LV function is poor, use **verapamil** instead (40mg po tds increasing up to 120mg tds as necessary). This is less negatively inotropic than beta-blockers but may still precipitate heart failure. Monitor response closely.
- If these measures fail, **amiodarone** may be tried instead. (Amiodarone will increase the plasma digoxin level so halve the maintenance digoxin dose).
- Other drugs that may be tried to control the ventricular rate are listed in the table on p44.
- Difficult to control ventricular rate? Consider if the diagnosis could be MAT (multifocal atrial tachycardia). Digoxin may make the arrhythmia worse (see p64).

Long-term management

- Look for causes (see table p59) and arrange an ECHO.
- Patients successfully cardioverted acutely should be commenced on prophylaxis (e.g. sotalol, amiodarone, flecainide). If subsequently considered to be at low risk, treatment may be stopped at one month.
- Patients cardioverted electively should remain on warfarin and prophylaxis for one month pending out-patient review (p794).
- Patients with *paroxysmal AF* require long-term therapy to try to maintain sinus rhythm (amiodarone, disopyramide, flecainide, or quinidine). Digoxin only controls the ventricular rate and does not prevent AF. The patients need long-term warfarin.

Atrial flutter

- This is rarely seen in the absence of underlying coronary disease, valve disease, primary myocardial disease, pericarditis, or thyrotoxicosis.
- The atrial rate is 280–320/min and atrial activity is seen as flutter waves in the inferior leads and V1 on the ECG.
- The AV node conduction is slower (most commonly 2:1 block, sometimes 3:1 or 4:1) and this determines the ventricular rate.
- Vagotonic manoeuvres and adenosine increase the AV block and reveal the flutter waves but only very rarely terminate the arrhythmia.

Management

- **DC cardioversion** is the therapy of choice in unstable patients with acute MI, critical valvular disease, or impaired LV function. Anticoagulation is not necessary and typically low energies are needed (20 joules) p793.
- **Digoxin** increases the AV block and slows the ventricular response rate (see p51 for doses). It may produce atrial fibrillation which may be treated in the standard way (p58–62).
- iv **verapamil** (2.5–5mg over 1–2 minutes repeated every 5 minutes to a maximum dose of 20mg) will slow the response rate and will restore sinus rhythm in 15–20% of patients.
- **Beta-blockade** may be tried instead of verapamil (see table p51).
- **Amiodarone** slows the flutter rate (e.g. to 100–130/min), increases the AV block (thus slowing ventricular response rate), and will restore sinus rhythm in a small number of patients.
- **Quinidine** and **procainamide** have been used to try to restore sinus rhythm. They should only be used once the rate has been controlled to avoid enhanced AV conduction and an increase in rate.

Multifocal atrial tachycardia (MAT)

- Rapid irregular rhythm that may be difficult to differentiate from atrial fibrillation.
- Most commonly occurs in patients with obstructive airways disease who may be hypoxaemic and hypercapnic.
- Characterized by at least 3 different P wave morphologies with varying PP and PR intervals.

Management

- **Treat the underlying lung disease** to improve P_aO_2 and P_aCO_2.
- Consider **verapamil** (5mg iv over 2 min; repeated every 5min up to maximum 20mg; then 40–120mg po tds) if the ventricular rate is consistently > 100/min and the patient is symptomatic.
- DC shock and digoxin are ineffective.

Accessory pathway tachycardias

- The three most common accessory pathways that produce paroxysmal tachycardias are listed below.
- During re-entry tachycardia, the delta wave is lost as the accessory pathway is only conducting retrogradely.
- AF may produce very rapid ventricular rates as the accessory path has rapid antegrade conduction (unlike the AV node). The ECG will show the delta wave in some or all the QRS complexes.

Management

- DC cardioversion should be used early if the tachycardia is poorly tolerated (see p42).
- The drug of choice is iv flecainide; iv disopyramide or beta-blocker may be given also (see table p51).
- Digoxin and verapamil should be avoided as they may accelerate conduction down the accessory pathway. Amiodarone is dangerous unless given very slowly (e.g. 300mg iv over 2–4 hours).
- Long-term control may require dual therapy (sotalol and diso-pyramide) until the pathway can be ablated.

Types of accessory pathways

1 *Kent bundle (Wolff-Parkinsin-White syndrome)*

- ECG   Short PR interval and delta wave

Type A	Positive δ wave in V1–V6 Negative in lead I (Posterior left atrial pathway)
Type B	Biphasic or negative δ wave in V1–V3 Positive in lead I (Lateral right atrial pathway)
Concealed	No δ wave visible as pathway only conducts retrogradely.

- Associated with   Ebstein's, HOCM, mitral valve prolapse

2 *Mahaim pathway (rare)*

- Pathway connects AV node to right bundle resulting in a tachycardia with LBBB morphology.

3 *James pathway (Lown-Ganong-Levine syndrome) (rare)*

- Short PR interval but no delta wave.
- Pathway connects atria to AV node, His, or fascicles.

Accessory pathway tachycardias

Bradyarrhythmias: General approach

- Ask specifically about previous cardiac disease, palpitations, black-outs, dizziness, chest pain, symptoms of heart failure, and recent drugs.

- Examine carefully, noting the bp, JVP waveform (?cannon waves), heart sounds and murmurs, and signs of heart failure.

Investigations

- 12 lead ECG & rhythm strip — Look specifically for the relationship between P waves and QRS complex.

  A long rhythm strip is sometimes necessary to detect complete heart block if atrial and ventricular rates are similar.

- Blood tests — FBC, U&Es, glucose (urgently)

  Ca^{2+}, Mg^{2+} (especially if on diuretics)

  Cardiac enzymes

- Where appropriate — Blood cultures, CRP

  Thyroid function tests

  Drug levels

  Arterial blood gases

- Chest X-ray — Heart size

  ?signs of pulmonary oedema

Management

Haemodynamically unstable patients

- Give **oxygen** via face mask if the patient is hypoxic on air.
- **Keep NBM** until definitive therapy has been started to reduce the risk of aspiration in case of cardiac arrest or when the patient lies supine for temporary wire insertion.
- Secure peripheral venous access.
- Bradyarrhythmias causing *severe* haemodynamic compromise (cardiac arrest, systolic bp < 90mmHg, severe pulmonary oedema, evidence of cerebral hypoperfusion) require *immediate treatment* and temporary pacing. (The technique is described on p782.)
- Give **atropine 1mg iv** (Min-I-Jet®) bolus; repeat if necessary up to a maximum 3mg.
- Give **isoprenaline 0.2mg iv** (Min-I-Jet®) if there is a delay in pacing and the patient remains unstable. Set up an infusion (1mg in 100ml bag N saline starting at 1ml / min).
- Set up **external pacing system**, if available, and arrange for transfer to a screening room for transvenous pacing. If fluoroscopy is not available, 'blind' transvenous pacing using a balloon-tipped pacing wire may be attempted.
- Bradycardia in shock is a poor prognostic sign (p208). Look for a source of blood loss and begin aggressive resuscitation with fluids and inotropes.

Haemodynamically stable patients

- Admit and arrange for continuous ECG monitoring.
- Keep atropine drawn up and ready in case of acute deterioration.
- Does the patient require a temporary wire immediately (see p780)?
- Refer the patient to a cardiologist.

Cardiovascular emergencies

External cardiac pacing

- In emergencies, *external cardiac pacing* may be used first but this is painful for the patient and is only a temporary measure until a more 'definitive' transvenous pacing wire can be inserted.

- External cardiac pacing is useful as a standby in patients post myocardial infarction when the risks of prophylactic transvenous pacing after thrombolysis are high.

- Haemodynamically stable patients with anterior myocardial infarction and bifascicular block, may be managed simply by application of the external pacing electrodes and having the pulse generator ready if necessary.

- Familiarize yourself with the machine in your hospital when you have some time – a cardiac arrest is not the time to read the manual for the apparatus!

Sinus bradycardia or junctional rhythm

(Heart rate < 50 /min)

Causes

- Young athletic individual
- Drugs (β-blockers, morphine)
- Hypothyroidism
- Hypothermia
- Increased vagal tone
  - vasovagal attack
  - nausea or vomiting
  - carotid sinus hypersensitivity
  - acute MI (especially inferior)
- Ischaemia or infarction of the sinus node
- Chronic degeneration of sinus or AV nodes or atria
- Cholestatic jaundice
- Raised intracranial pressure

Management

- If hypotensive or pre-syncopal treat as on p68.
- Atropine 600µg iv bolus repeating as necessary.
- Isoprenaline 0.5–10µg/min iv infusion.
- Temporary pacing.
- Avoid precipitants (see above).
- Stop any drugs that may suppress the sinus or AV nodes.
- Long-term treatment
- If all possible underlying causes removed and symptomatic brady-cardia remains, refer for permanent pacing.
- Consider Holter monitoring in patients with possible episodic brady-cardia. R-R intervals > 2.5s may require permanent pacing.

Intraventricular conduction disturbances

Common causes of bundle branch block

- Ischaemic heart disease
- Hypertensive heart disease
- Valve disease (especially aortic stenosis)
- Conduction system fibrosis (Lev and Lenegre syndromes)
- Myocarditis or endocarditis
- Cardiomyopathies
- Cor pulmonale (RBBB) (acute or chronic)
- Trauma or post cardiac surgery
- Neuromuscular disorders (myotonic dystrophy)
- Polymyositis
- See p780 for situations where temporary pacing is indicated.

Types of AV conduction block

1 First degree heart block

- Prolongation of the PR interval (> 0.22s, > 5 small sq)

2 Second degree heart block

- Mobitz type 1 (Wenckebach): progressive increase in PR interval with intermittent complete AV block (P wave not conducted).
- Mobitz type 2: the PR interval is constant but there is intermittent failure to conduct the P wave (2:1 or 3:1 block common). Often occurs in the presence of broad QRS complex.

3 Third degree (complete) heart block

- Complete AV dissociation; if the P and QRS rate are similar, a long rhythm strip or exercise (to speed up the atrial rate) will demonstrate dissociation.

Causes

- Associated with acute infarction or ischaemia
- Drugs (β-blockers, digitalis, Ca^{2+}-blockers)
- Conduction system fibrosis (Lev and Lenegre syndromes)
- Increased vagal tone
- Trauma or following cardiac surgery
- Hypothyroidism (rarely thyrotoxicosis)
- Hypothermia
- Hyperkalaemia
- Hypoxia
- Valvular disease (aortic stenosis, incompetence, endocarditis)
- Myocarditis (diphtheria, rheumatic fever, viral, Chagas' disease)
- Associated with neuromuscular disease, i.e. myotonic dystrophy
- Collagen vascular disease (SLE, RA, scleroderma)
- Cardiomyopathies (haemochromotosis, amyloidosis)
- Granulomatous disease (sarcoid)
- Congenital heart block
- Congenital heart disease (ASD, Ebstein's, PDA)

Management

- For symptomatic heart block give atropine $\pm$ isoprenaline (p68).
- See p780 for situations when temporary pacing is indicated.

Pulmonary oedema: Assessment

Presentation

- Acute breathlessness, cough, frothy blood-stained sputum.
- Collapse, cardiac arrest, or shock.

- Associated features may reflect underlying cause:-
  - Chest pain or palpitations.
  - Preceding history of dyspnoea on exertion.
  - Oliguria, haematuria suggesting acute renal failure (p296).
  - Seizures, signs of intracranial bleed (p348).

Causes

A diagnosis of pulmonary oedema or 'heart failure' is not adequate: an underlying cause must be sought and if possible treated. These may be divided into :-

- Increased pulmonary capillary pressure (hydrostatic).
- Increased pulmonary capillary permeability.
- Decreased intravascular oncotic pressure.

Often a combination of factors is involved (e.g. pneumonia, hypoxia, cardiac ischaemia); see table p76.

- The main differential diagnosis is acute exacerbation of COAD (previous history, quiet breath sounds ± wheeze, fewer crackles). It may be difficult to differentiate the two clinically.

Assessment

- Is the patient very unwell? (i.e. unable to speak, hypoxic, systolic bp < 100mmHg). Begin treatment immediately (see p78) and await investigations (CXR and ABG).
- Check the bp, examine the chest – if there is doubt as to the diagnosis, give oxygen but await CXR before giving drugs.

Urgent investigations for all patients

- ECG   Sinus tachycardia most common.
  - ?any cardiac arrhythmia (AF, SVT, VT)
  - ?evidence of acute ST change (MI or angina)
  - ?evidence of underlying heart disease (LVH, p mitrale)
- CXR   To confirm the diagnosis (heart size may be normal)
  - Exclude pneumothorax, pulmonary embolus (oligaemic lung fields), infection, effusion.
- ABG   Typically $\downarrow P_aO_2$ (but some correction with O_2 cf. PE) and $\downarrow P_aCO_2$ (hyperventilation). Pulse oximetry may be inaccurate if peripherally shut down.
- U&Es   ?pre-existing renal impairment. Regular K^+ measurements (once on iv diuretics).
- FBC   ?anaemia or leukocytosis indicating the precipitant.
- ECHO   As soon as practical for LV function, valve abnormalities, VSD or effusion.

The priorities of management are:

1 Stabilize the patient, relieve distress and begin definitive treatment.

2 Look for an underlying cause.

3 Optimize long-term therapy.

Cardiovascular emergencies

Investigations for patients with pulmonary oedema
All patients should have:- • FBC, U&Es • Serial cardiac enzymes • LFTs, albumin, total protein • ECG • CXR • ECHO (± TOE) • Arterial blood gases
Where appropriate consider:- • Septic screen (sputum, urine, blood cultures) • Holter monitor (?arrhythmias) • Coronary angiography (? ischaemic heart disease) • Right and left heart catheter (pressures, ?shunts, valve disease) • Endomyocardial biopsy (myocarditis, infiltration) • MUGA scan • Cardiopulmonary exercise test with an assessment of peak oxygen consumption

Pulmonary oedema: Causes

Look for an underlying cause for pulmonary oedema

Increased pulmonary capillary pressure (hydrostatic)	
↑ Left atrial pressure	• Mitral valve disease • Arrhythmia (e.g. AF) with pre-existing mitral valve disease • Left atrial myxoma
↑ LVEDP	• Ischaemia • Arrhythmia • Aortic valve disease • Cardiomyopathy • Uncontrolled hypertension • Pericardial constriction • Fluid overload • High output states (anaemia, thyrotoxicosis, Paget's, AV fistula, beri-beri)
↑ Pulmonary venous pressure	• Renovascular disease • L → R shunt (e.g. VSD) • Veno-occlusive disease
Neurogenic	• Intracranial haemorrhage • Cerebral oedema • Post ictal
High altitude pulmonary oedema	• See p762
Increased pulmonary capillary permeability	
Acute lung injury	• ARDS, see p188
Decreased intravascular oncotic pressure	
Hypoalbuminaemia	• ↑ losses (e.g. nephrotic syndrome, liver failure) • ↓ production (e.g. sepsis) • Dilution (e.g. crystalloid transfusion)
(Note: The critical LA pressure for hydrostatic oedema ≈ serum albumin (g/l) × 0.57)	

Pulmonary oedema: Management   1.

Stabilize the patient

- Patients with acute pulmonary oedema should be monitored and initially managed where full resuscitation facilities are available.
- Sit the patient up in bed.
- Give 60–100% oxygen by face mask.
- If the patient is severely distressed, summon the 'on-call' anaesthetist. If dyspnoea cannot be significantly improved by acute measures (below) the patient may require CPAP or mechanical ventilation.
- Connect to ECG monitor – treat any arrhythmia (p40).
- Secure venous access and send blood for urgent U&Es and FBC.
- Unless thrombolysis is indicated take an arterial blood sample for blood gases; check potassium.
- Give:
  - Diamorphine 2.5–5mg iv
  - Metoclopramide 10mg iv
  - Frusemide 40–120mg slow iv injection
- If the systolic blood pressure is $\geq$ 90mmHg and the patient does not have aortic stenosis:-
- Give sublingual GTN spray (2 puffs)
- Start iv GTN infusion 2–10mg/h, increase the infusion rate every 15–20 minutes, titrating against blood pressure (aiming to keep systolic bp ~ 100mmHg).
- Monitor pulse, bp, respiratory rate, O_2 saturation with a pulse oximeter (if an accurate reading can be obtained) and urine output.
- Repeat blood gases and K^+ if the clinical condition deteriorates or after 2h if the original sample was abnormal.
- Insert a urinary catheter to monitor urine output.

Further management

The subsequent management of the patient is aimed at ensuring adequate ventilation and gas exchange and correcting the haemodynamic disturbance that has precipitated acute pulmonary oedema.

- **Assess the patient's respiratory function**
- Does the patient require respiratory support?   p800
- **Assess the patient's haemodynamic status**
- Is the patient in shock?   p206
- **Look for an underlying cause**   p76
- **Conditions that require specific treatment**
  - Acute aortic regurgitation   p102
  - Acute mitral regurgitation   p104
  - Diastolic left ventricular dysfunction   p84
  - Fluid overload   p84
  - Renal failure   p276
  - Severe anaemia   p84
  - Hypoproteinaemia   p84

Pulmonary oedema

Pulmonary oedema: Management 2.

Assess the patient's respiratory function

- Wheeze may be caused by interstitial pulmonary oedema. If there is a history of asthma, give nebulized salbutamol (2.5–5mg). Consider commencing an aminophylline infusion. (This will 'off-load' by systemic vasodilatation as well as relieving bronchospasm (p167). This can cause dysrhythmias; ensure K^+ is 4–5mmol/l.)

- *Indications for further respiratory support include:-*
  - Patient exhaustion or continuing severe breathlessness.
  - Persistent $P_aO_2 < 8\,kPa$
  - Rising P_aCO_2
  - Persistent or worsening acidosis (pH < 7.2)

- *Continuous positive airways pressure (CPAP).* This may be tried for a co-operative patients who can protect their airway, have adequate respiratory muscle strength and who are not hypotensive. The positive pressure reduces venous return to the heart and may compromise the blood pressure and cardiac output.

- *Endotracheal intubation* and mechanical ventilation may be required, and some positive end expiratory pressure (PEEP) should be insti- tuted (p812).

- Discuss the patient with the on-call anaesthetist or chest team.

Assess the patient's haemodynamic status

Non-cardiogenic pulmonary oedema (p188) may be difficult to distin- guish from cardiogenic pulmonary oedema. If there is any doubt a PA wedge catheter should be inserted to measure PCWP, as soon as the patient is stable.

- PCWP > 18mmHg is diagnostic

- Pulmonary oedema occurs when the hydrostatic pressure within the capillary overcomes the plasma oncotic pressure and, in patients with hypoalbuminaemia, will occur at PCWP less than 15mmHg. The critical PCWP may be estimated by *serum albumin (g/l) × 0.57.* Thus a patient with a serum albumin of 15g/l will develop hydrostatic pulmonary oedema at a LA pressure of 8mmHg; a serum albumin of 30g/l will require an LA pressure of > 17mmHg.

- The gradient between PA diastolic pressure and PCWP (PAD-PCWP) is generally < 5mmHg in cardiogenic pulmonary oedema and > 5mmHg in ARDS.

- The pulse and bp are most commonly elevated due to circulating catecholamines and over activity of the renin-angiotensin system. Examination reveals sweating, cool 'shut-down' peripheries, high pulse volume (assess carotid or femoral pulses).

- Hypotension or low output states are seen in patients with valvular heart disease or VSD (i.e. 'mechanical' impairment to forward flow) or severe myocardial disease (acute myocarditis, cardiomyopathy).

Management

The general approach involves combination of diuretics, vasodilators ± inotropes if cardiac output is inadequate. The patients may be divided into two groups:-

- Patients in shock (with systolic bp < 100mmHg) – p82.
- Haemodynamically stable patients (systolic bp > 100mmHg). – p83.

Pulmonary oedema: Management   3.

Patients with systolic bp < 100mmHg

- The patient is in incipient (or overt) shock. The most common aetiology is cardiogenic shock but remember non-cardiogenic causes (e.g. ARDS, septic shock, p188).

- Insert a central line ± PA catheter (Swan-Ganz). Internal jugular lines are preferable as the risk of pneumothorax is lower.

- Insert an arterial line for monitoring bp and arterial gases.

- Check that the patient is not underfilled (mistaken diagnosis e.g. septic shock from bilateral pneumonia).

- Start on 'renal dose' dopamine infusion (2.5–5µg/kg/min). This may cause slight fall in bp if used alone (systemic vasodilatation) and should be combined with another agent (see below).

- *Is there a mechanical cause that may require emergency surgery?*

- Arrange an urgent ECHO

- Discuss (with cardiologists) all patients who have had:-
  - Recent MI and new murmur [? VSD or acute MR (p28)].
  - A prosthetic heart valve (?dehiscence, ?infection) or pre-existing aortic or mitral disease that may require surgery.

The **choice of inotropic agent** depends on the clinical condition of the patient and to some extent, the underlying diagnosis:-

- Treatment of septic shock is discussed elsewhere (p216).

- Systolic 80–100mmHg and cool, peripheries: start **dobutamine infusion** at 5µg/kg/min (p694), increasing by 2.5µg/kg/min every 10–15 minutes to a maximum of 20µg/kg/min until bp > 100mmHg.

- **Phosphodiesterase inhibitors** (enoximone or milrinone) should be considered where dobutamine fails. They may be combined with dobutamine (see p688 for dose details).

- If severely hypotensive (systolic bp < 80mmHg) give a slow iv **bolus of adrenaline** (2–5ml of 1 in 10,000 solution Min-I-Jet®, repeated if necessary).

- **Dopamine** at doses of > 2.5µg/kg/min has a pressor action in addition to direct and indirect inotropic effects and may be used at higher doses (10–20µg/kg/min) if the blood pressure remains low. However, it tends to raise the pulmonary capillary filling pressure further and should be combined with vasodilators (e.g. nitroprusside or hydralazine) once the blood pressure is restored (see below). Beware of arrhythmias at these doses.

- **Adrenaline infusion** may be preferred to high-dose dopamine (see p689 for details) as an inotrope. Once the blood pressure is restored (> 100mmHg), vasodilators such as nitroprusside or hydralazine should be added to counteract the pressor effects.

- If there is a potentially reversible cause for the pulmonary oedema and shock, consider **intra-aortic balloon counterpulsation** (p796).

- Further doses of diuretic may be given.

Cardiovascular emergencies

Pulmonary oedema

Patients with systolic bp ≥ 100mmHg

- Further doses of diuretic may be given [frusemide 40–80mg iv q3–4h or as a continuous infusion (20–80mg/hr)].
- Continue the GTN infusion, increasing the infusion rate every 15–20 minutes up to 10mg/hr, titrating against blood pressure (aiming to keep systolic bp ~ 100mmHg).
- Arteriolar vasodilators (nitroprusside or hydralazine) may be added or used instead of GTN in patients with adequate bp (see p 698 for dose). Arterial pressure should be monitored continuously, via an arterial line, to prevent inadvertent hypotension.

Long-term management

- Unless a contraindication exists, start an ACE inhibitor increasing the dose to as near the recommended maximal dose as possible.
- If ACE inhibitors are contraindicated or not tolerated, consider the use of hydralazine and isosorbide mononitrate in combination.
- If the patient is already on high doses of diuretics and ACE inhibitors consider the addition of a thiazide (bendrofluazide 2.5–5mg or metolazone 2.5–5mg) in view of the synergism with loop diuretics (NB monitor renal function and serum potassium).
- If the patient is in AF or has a poorly functioning left ventricle, consider long-term anti-coagulation.
- Patients < 60 years, who remain symptomatic despite maximal medical treatment, should be considered for cardiac transplantation.

Pulmonary oedema: Specific conditions

Diastolic LV dysfunction

- This typically occurs in elderly hypertensive patients with LV hypertrophy. There is marked hypertension, pulmonary oedema and normal or only mild LV impairment. However, there is impaired relaxation of the ventricle in diastole.
- With tachycardia, diastolic filling time shortens. As the ventricle is 'stiff' in diastole, LA pressure is increased and pulmonary oedema occurs (exacerbated by AF as filling by atrial systole is lost).
- Treatment involves control of hypertension with iv nitrates (and/or nitroprusside), calcium blockers (verapamil or nifedipine) and even selective beta-blockers (e.g. carvedilol).

Fluid overload

- Standard measures are usually effective.
- In extreme circumstances venesection may be necessary.
- Check the patient is not anaemic (Hb $\geqslant$ 10g/dl). Remove 500mls blood via a cannula in a large vein and repeat if necessary.
- If anaemic (e.g. renal failure) and acutely unwell, consider dialysis (p282).

Known (or unknown) renal failure

- Unless the patient is permanently anuric, large doses of iv frusemide may be required (up to 1g given at 4mg/min) in addition to standard treatment.
- If such treatment fails, or the patient is known to be anuric, dialysis will be required.
- In patients not known to have renal failure an underlying cause should be sought (p278).

Anaemia

- Cardiac failure may be worsened or precipitated by the presence of significant anaemia. Symptoms may be improved in the long term by correcting this anaemia.
- Generally, transfusion is unnecessary with Hb > 9g/dl unless there is a risk of an acute bleed. Treatment of pulmonary oedema will result in haemoconcentration and a 'rise' in the Hb.
- If the anaemia is thought to be exacerbating pulmonary oedema, ensure that an adequate diuresis is obtained prior to transfusion. Give slow transfusion (3–4h per unit) of packed cells, with iv frusemide 20–40mg before each unit.

Hypoproteinaemia

- The critical LA pressure at which hydrostatic pulmonary oedema occurs is influenced by the serum albumin and approximates to (serum albumin concentration (g/l) $\times$ 0.57 – see p80.
- Treatment involves diuretics, cautious albumin replacement, spironolactone (if there is secondary hyperaldosteronism), and treatment of the underlying cause for hypoproteinaemia.

Pulmonary oedema

Infective endocarditis: Presentation

Infective endocarditis (IE) may present insidiously and be mistaken for a variety of other disorders such as collagen diseases or cerebrovascular disease. Patients may present with:-

- ***Symptoms and signs of the infection*** This includes malaise, anorexia, weight loss, fever, rigors, and night sweats. Long-standing infection produces anaemia, clubbing, and splenomegaly.
- ***Cardiac manifestations of the infection*** Congestive cardiac failure, palpitations, tachycardia, new murmur, pericarditis, or AV block.
- ***Symptoms and signs due to immune complex deposition***
  - Skin :   Splinter haemorrhages, petechiae

    Osler's nodes [small tender nodules (pulp infarcts) on hands and feet]

    Janeway lesions (non tender haemorrhagic areas on the palms and soles)
  - Eye: Roth spots (oval retinal haemorrhages with a pale centre located near the optic disc) Conjunctival splinter haemorrhages

    Retinal flame haemorrhages
  - Renal: Microscopic haematuria or glomerulonephritis
  - Cerebral: Toxic encephalopathy
  - Musculoskeletal: Arthralgia or arthritis
- ***Complications of the infection***
- ***Local effects***
- Valve destruction results in a new or changing murmur. This may result in progressive heart failure and pulmonary oedema.
- A new harsh pan-systolic murmur and acute deterioration may be due to perforation of the interventricular septum or rupture of a sinus of Valsalva aneurysm into the right ventricle.
- High degree AV block (2–4% of IE) occurs with intracardiac extension of infection into the interventricular septum (e.g. from aortic valve endocarditis).
- Intracardiac abscess may be seen with any valve infection (25–50% of aortic endocarditis, 1–5% of mitral but rarely with tricuspid) but is most common in prosthetic valve endocarditis.
- ***Embolic events***
  - Septic emboli are seen in 20–45% of patients and may involve any circulation [brain, limbs, coronary, kidney, or spleen; pulmonary emboli with tricuspid endocarditis (p96)].
  - 40–45% of patients who have had an embolic event will have another.
  - The risk depends on the organism (most common with G-ve infections, *Staph. aureus* or *candida*) and the presence and size of vegetations (emboli in 30% of patients with no vegetation on ECHO cf. 40% with vegetations < 5mm, and 65% with vegetations > 5mm).
- Ask specifically for a history of dental work, infections, surgery, iv drug use or instrumentation, which may have led to a bacteraemia.
- Examine for any potential sources of infection, especially teeth or skin lesions.
- Risk factors for endocarditis are shown in the table opposite.

Risk factors for infective endocarditis

1 Cardiac abnormalities[2]

• *High risk*	Prosthetic valves
	Previous bacterial endocarditis
	Aortic valve disease
	Mitral regurgitation
	Cyanotic congenital heart lesions
	Uncorrected L→ R shunts (except ASD)
• *Moderate risk*	MVP with regurgitation or leaflet thickening
	Isolated mitral stenosis
	Tricuspid valve disease
	Pulmonary stenosis
	Hypertrophic cardiomyopathy
	Mural thrombus (e.g. post infarct)
• *Low / no risk*	Isolated ASD
	Ischaemic heart disease ± previous CABG
	Surgically corrected L→ R shunt with no residual shunt
	MVP with thin leaflets and no regurgitation
	Calcification of mitral annulus
	Permanent pacemakers
	Atrial myxoma

2 Other predisposing factors
- Arterial prostheses or arteriovenous fistulae.
- Recurrent bacteraemia (e.g. iv drug-users, severe periodontal disease, colon carcinoma).
- Condition predisposing to infections (e.g. diabetes, renal failure, alcoholism, immunosuppression).
- Recent central line.

In many case no obvious risk factor is identifiable.

[2] Michel PL & Acar J (1995) *Eur Heart J.* **16** (*Suppl B*): 2–6.

Infective endocarditis: Investigations

Microbiology	
50–60%	Streptococci (esp. *Strep. viridans* group)
10%	Enterococci
25%	Staphylococci
	S. *aureus* = coagulase +ve
	S. *epidermidis* = coagulase -ve
5–10%	Culture negative
<1%	Gram negative bacilli
<1%	Multiple organisms
<1%	Diptheroids
<1%	Fungi

(See p96 for IE on prosthetic valves and in iv drug-users)

Investigations

- **Blood cultures** — Take 3–4 sets of cultures from different sites at least an hour apart and inoculate at least 5 mls/bottle for the optimal pick-up rate. Ask for prolonged (fungal) cultures.

- **FBC** — May show normochromic, normocytic anaemia (exclude haematinic deficiency), neutrophil leukocytosis and perhaps thrombocytopenia.

- **U&Es** — May be deranged. (This should be monitored throughout treatment.)

- **LFTs** — May be deranged, especially with an increase in ALP and γ-GT.

- **ESR/CRP** — Acute phase reaction.

- **Urinalysis** — Microscopic haematuria ± proteinuria.

- **Immunology** — Serum Igs ↑ (polyclonal), complement ↓.

- **ECG** — May have changes associated with any underlying cause. There may be AV block or conduction defects; rarely (embolic) acute MI.

- **CXR** — May be normal. Look for pulmonary oedema or multiple infected or infarcted areas from septic emboli (tricuspid endocarditis).

- **ECHO** — Transthoracic echo may confirm the presence of valve lesions and/or demonstrate vegetations if > 2mm in size. TOE is more sensitive for aortic root and mitral leaflet involvement. A normal ECHO does not exclude the diagnosis.

- **Dentition** — All patients should have an OPG (orthopentamogram – a panoramic dental X-ray) and a dental opinion.

- **Swabs** — Any potential sites of infection (skin lesions).

- **V/Q scan** — In cases where right-sided endocarditis is suspected this may show multiple mismatched defects

- **Save serum for:-** *Aspergillus* precipitins
  Candida antibodies (rise in titre)
  Q fever complement fixation test
  Chlamydia complement fixation test
  Brucella agglutinins

Infective endocarditis: Antibiotics

'Blind' treatment for endocarditis

- Infective endocarditis is usually a clinical diagnosis and must be considered in any patient with a typical history, fever and a murmur with no other explanation. Often antibiotics need to be started before the culture results are available. Be guided by the clinical setting (see table below[3]).

Presentation	Choice of antibiotic
Gradual onset (weeks)	Benzyl penicillin + Gentamicin
Acute onset (days) or history of skin trauma	Flucloxacillin + Gentamicin
Recent valve prosthesis (possible MRSA, diptheroid *Klebsiella*, corynebacterium or nosocomial staphylococci	Vancomycin + Gentamicin + Rifampicin
iv drug-user	Vancomycin

Suggested antibiotic doses are:	
Benzyl penicillin	4MU (2.4g) q4h iv
Flucloxacillin	2g q6h iv
Vancomycin	15mg/kg q12h iv over 60 min, guided by levels
Gentamicin	3mg/kg divided in 1–3 doses guided by levels
Rifampicin	300mg q12h po
Ciprofloxacin	300mg q12h iv for 1 week, then 750mg q12h po for 3 weeks

- Identification of an organism is invaluable for further management and blood cultures should be taken with meticulous attention to detail.
- Antibiotics should be administered iv, preferably via a tunnelled central (Hickman) line.
- If an organism is isolated, antibiotic therapy may be modified when sensitivities are known.
- Suggested antibiotic combinations are shown in the table above; however, individual units may have specific policies; patients should be discussed with your local microbiologist.

---

3 Oakley CM (1995) *Eur Heart J* **16**(*suppl. B*): 90–93.

Infective endocarditis

Duration of treatment

• This is controversial with a trend toward shorter courses.
The following are suggestions only.[4,5]

• Viridans streptococci
    Benzyl penicillin only (4 weeks)
    Vancomycin or teicoplanin (4 weeks)
    Penicillin + aminoglycoside (2 weeks)

• Group B, C, G streptococci
    Penicillin (4 weeks) + aminoglycoside (2 weeks)
    Vancomycin (4 weeks) + aminoglycoside (2 weeks)

• Group A streptococci
    Penicillin (4 weeks)
    Vancomycin (4 weeks)

• Extracardiac infection from septic emboli
    Penicillin (4 weeks) + aminoglycoside (2 weeks)
    Vancomycin (4 weeks) + aminoglycoside (2 weeks)

• *Staphylococcus aureus* and coagulase negative staphylococci
    Left-sided endocarditis:-
      Flucloxacillin (4–6 weeks) + aminoglycoside (2 weeks)
      If MRSA: Vancomycin + rifampicin (6 weeks)
      ± aminoglycoside (2 weeks)
    Right-sided endocarditis:-
      Flucloxacillin (2 weeks) + aminoglycoside (2 weeks)
      Ciprofloxacin (4 weeks) + rifampicin (3 weeks)
      If MRSA – Vancomycin (4 weeks) + rifampicin (4 weeks)

• Fungi
    Amphotericin B iv to a total dose of 2.5–3g.

---

4   Francioli P (1995) *Eur Heart J* **16**(*suppl. B*)**:** 75–79.
5   Bille J (1995) *Eur Heart J* **16**(*suppl. B*)**:** 80–83.

Infective endocarditis

Monitoring treatment

Clinically

- Signs of continued infection, persistent pyrexia and the persistence of systemic symptoms.
- Persistent fever may be due to drug resistance, concomitant infection (central line, urine, chest, septic emboli to lungs or abdomen) or allergy (?eosinophilia, ?leukopenia, ?proteinuria: common with penicillin but may be due to any antibiotic; consider changing or stopping antibiotics for 2–3 days).
- Changes in any cardiac murmurs or signs of cardiac failure
- The development of any new embolic phenomena
- Inspect venous access sites daily. Change peripheral cannulae every 3–4 days.

ECHO

- Regular (weekly) transthoracic echocardiograms may identify clinically silent, but progressive, valve destruction, the development of intra-cardiac abscesses or vegetations.
- The tips of long-standing central lines may develop sterile fibrinous 'fronds' which may be visible on TOE: change the line and send the tip for culture.
- 'Vegetations' need not be due to infection (see table p95).

ECG

- Looking specifically for AV block or conduction abnormalities suggesting intracardiac extension of the infection.

Microbiology

- Repeated blood cultures (especially if there is continued fever).
- Regular aminoglycoside and vancomycin levels (ensuring the absence of toxic levels and the presence of therapeutic levels). Gentamicin ototoxicity may develop with prolonged use even in the absence of toxic levels.
- Back titration to ensure that minimum inhibitory and bactericidal concentrations are being achieved.

Laboratory indices

- Regular (daily) urinalysis
- Regular U&Es and liver function (and Mg^{2+} if on aminoglycosides)
- Regular CRP (ESR every 2 weeks)
- FBC – rising Hb and falling WCC suggests successful treatment; watch for beta-lactam-associated neutropenia.
- Serum magnesium (if on gentamicin).
- The duration of treatment varies depending on the severity of infection and the infecting organism (see table p91). iv therapy is usually for at least 2 weeks, and total antibiotic therapy for 4–6 weeks.
- If the patient is well following this period, antibiotic treatment may be stopped, and, provided no surgery is indicated (p98), the patient may be discharged and followed up in out-patient clinic.
- Patients should be advised of the need for endocarditis prophylaxis in the future (see table p100).
- Patients with valvular damage following infection should be followed long term; patients with ventricular septal defects should be considered for closure.

Culture negative endocarditis

Causes of culture negative endocarditis[2]
• Previous antibiotic therapy
• Fastidious organism Nutritionally deficient variants of *Strep. viridans* *Brucella, Neisseria, Legionella* *Nocardia* Mycobacteria The HACEK group of oropharyngeal flora Cell wall deficient bacteria and anaerobes
• Cell dependent organisms *Chlamydia*, rickettsiae *(Coxiella)*
• Fungi

(HACEK = Haemophilus, Acintobacillus, Cardiobacterium, Eikenella and Kingella sp.)

- The commonest reason for persistently negative blood cultures is prior antibiotic therapy.
- If the clinical response to the antibiotics is good these should be continued.
- For a persisting fever:-
- Withhold antibiotics if not already started.
- Consider other investigations for a 'PUO', see p230.
- If the clinical suspicion of IE is high, it warrants further investigation:
- Repeated physical examination for any new signs.
- Regular ECHO and TOE. 'Vegetations' need not be due to infection (see table opposite).
- Repeated blood cultures, especially when the temperature is raised.
- Consider unusual causes of endocarditis:-
  - **Q–fever** *(Coxiella burnetii)*: Complement fixation tests identify antibodies to phase 1 and 2 antigens. Phase 2 antigens raised in the acute illness, phase 1 antigens raised in chronic illnesses such as endocarditis. Treat with indefinite (life-long) oral doxycycline ± co-trimoxazole, rifampicin or quinolone (see p250).
  - **Chlamydia psittaci:** Commonly there is a history of exposure to birds and there may be an associated atypical pneumonia. Diagnosis is confirmed using complement fixation tests to detect raised antibody titres.
  - **Brucellosis**: Blood cultures may be positive though organisms may take up to 8 weeks to grow. Serology usually confirms the diagnosis.
  - **Fungi**: *Candida*, may be cultured. The detection of antibodies may be helpful though levels may be raised in normals. The detection of a rising titre is of more use. Other fungal infections (e.g. histoplasmosis, aspergillosis) are rare but may be diagnosed with culture or serology though these are commonly negative. Antigen assays may be positive, or the organism may be isolated from biopsy material. Treatment is with amphotericin B ± flucytosine. Prosthetic valves must be removed. Mortality is > 50%.

Causes of 'vegetations' on ECHO[2]

- Infective endocarditis
- Sterile thrombotic vegetations
  Libman Sacks endocarditis (SLE)
  Primary anti-phospholipid syndrome
  Marantic endocarditis (adenocarcinoma)
- Myxomatous degeneration of valve (commonly mitral)
- Ruptured mitral chordae
- Exuberant rheumatic vegetations (black Africans)
- Thrombus ('pannus') on a prosthetic valve
- A stitch or residual calcium after valve replacement

---

[2] Michel PL & Acar J (1995) *Eur Heart J.* **16** (*Suppl B*): 2–6.

Right-sided endocarditis

- Always consider this diagnosis in iv drug-users (or patients with venous access).
- Endocarditis on endocardial, permanent pacemaker leads is rare but recognized.
- Patients most commonly have staphylococcal infection and are unwell, requiring immediate treatment and often early surgery.
- The lesions may be sterilized with iv antibiotics. Surgery may be required for :-
  - Resistant organisms (*Staph. aureus*, *Pseudomonas*, *Candida* and infection with multiple organisms).
  - Increasing vegetation size in spite of therapy.
  - Infections on pacemaker leads (surgical removal of lead and repair or excision of tricuspid valve).

Prosthetic valve endocarditis (PVE)

- Conventionally divided into early (< 2 months post operatively) and late (> 2 months post operatively).

Early prosthetic valve endocarditis:

- Most commonly due to staphylococci, Gram negative bacilli, diptheroids or fungi.
- Generally, infection has begun either per operatively or in the immediate post operative period.
- Often a highly destructive, fulminant infection with valve dehiscence, abscess formation and rapid haemodynamic deterioration.
- Discuss with the surgeons early: they commonly require re-operation. Mortality is high (45–75%).

Late prosthetic valve endocarditis:

- The pathogenesis is different: abnormal flow around the prosthetic valve ring produces microthrombi and non-bacterial thrombotic vegetations (NBTV) which may be infected during transient bacteraemia. The source is commonly dental or urological sepsis or from in-dwelling venous lines.
- Common organisms are coagulase negative staphylococci, *Staph. aureus, Strep. viridans* or enterococci.
- Frequently needs surgical intervention and this carries a high mortality, but less than for early PVE.
- It may be possible to sterilize infections on bioprostheses with iv antibiotics only. Surgery may then be deferred.

Right-sided endocarditis

Surgery for infective endocarditis

- *Discuss early with the regional cardiothoracic centre: immediate intervention may be appropriate.*

Indications

Surgical intervention may be necessary either during active infection or later because of degree of valve destruction. Optimal timing depends on a number of factors:-

  1 Haemodynamic tolerance of lesion.
  2 Outcome of the infection.
  3 Presence of complications.

1 *Haemodynamic tolerance*

- *If the patient is haemodynamically stable,* surgery may be delayed until after the antibiotic course is completed. The final management depends on the valve affected, the degree of destruction and its effect on ventricular function. Severe aortic and mitral regurgitation usually require surgery; tricuspid regurgitation, if well tolerated, is managed medically.

- *Decompensation* (severe congestive cardiac failure or low cardiac output syndrome with functional renal failure) may respond to surgery but the mortality is high.

- *'Metastable'* patients who have been successfully treated after an episode of acute decompensation should be considered for early operation after 2–3 weeks antibiotic therapy.

2 *Outcome of infection*

- *Persistence or relapse of infection* (clinical and laboratory indices) despite appropriate antibiotics at an adequate dose may either be due to a resistant organism or an abscess (paravalvular, extracardiac).

  Consider valve replacement if no extracardiac focus found.

- *The organism* may influence the decision: consider early surgery for fungal endocarditis or prosthetic endocarditis with *E. coli* or *Staph. aureus.*

3 *The presence of complications*

Urgent surgery indications
• High degree AV block.
• Perforation of intraventricular septum.
• Rupture of an aneurysm of the sinus of Valsalva into the RV.
• Intracardiac abscess.
• Recurrent septic emboli
• Prosthetic endocarditis especially when associated with an unstable prosthesis.

Surgery for infective endocarditis

Endocarditis prophylaxis[6]

Procedures that require antibiotic prophylaxis	
Dental	• All procedures
Upper respiratory tract	• Tonsillectomy, adenoidectomy
Gastrointestinal	• Oesophageal dilatation or laser therapy • Oesophageal surgery • Sclerosis of oesophageal varicies • ERCP • Abdominal surgery • Barium enema • Sigmoidoscopy ± biopsy
Urological	• Instrumentation of ureter or kidney • Biopsy or surgery of prostate or bladder
Procedures for which the risk of IE is controversial	
Upper respiratory tract	• Bronchoscopy • Endotracheal intubation
Gastrointestinal	• Upper GI endoscopy ± biopsy
Genital	• Vaginal hysterectomy or delivery

- The table on p87 shows cardiac conditions at risk of IE. High and moderate risk requires prophylaxis; 'low' risk does not.
- The regimen may be modified depending on the 'degree of risk' (both patient and procedure related) as in the table below.

Antibiotic prophylaxis

Minimal regimen		
	1h before	**6h after**
No penicillin allergy	Amoxycillin 3g po	No 2nd dose
Allergy to penicillin	Clindamycin 300–600mg po	No 2nd dose
Flexible modifications depending on the 'degree of risk' • Additional doses after procedure • Additional aminoglycosides • Parenteral administration		
Maximal regimen		
	1h before	**6h after**
No penicillin allergy	Amoxycillin 2g iv + Gentamicin 1.5mg/kg im/iv	1–1.5g po No 2nd dose
Allergy to penicillin	Vancomycin 1g iv over 1 hr + Gentamicin 1.5mg/kg im/iv	1g iv at 12h No 2nd dose

[6] The following is one regime (after Leport C *et al* (1995) *Eur Heart J* **16** (*suppl. B*): 126–131). Refer to your local policy.

Acute aortic regurgitation

Presentation

- Sudden, severe aortic regurgitation presents as ***cardiogenic shock and acute pulmonary oedema***.
- The haemodynamic changes are markedly different from those seen in chronic AR: the previous normal sized LV results in a smaller effective forward flow and higher LVEDP for the same degree of aortic regurgitation.
- Patients often extremely unwell, tachycardic, peripherally shut down, may have pulmonary oedema. Unlike chronic AR, pulse pressure may be near normal.
- If available, ask for a history of previous valvular heart disease, hypertension, features of Marfan's syndrome, and risk factors for infective endocarditis (p87).
- Physical signs of severe AR include: quiet aortic closure sound (S2); an ejection systolic murmur over aortic valve (turbulent flow); high pitched and short early diastolic murmur (AR); quiet S1 (premature closure of the mitral valve).
- Examine specifically for signs of an underlying cause (see below).
- Where there is no obvious underlying cause (e.g. acute MI), assume infective endocarditis until proven otherwise.

Diagnosis Transthoracic and/or transoesophageal ECHO.

Causes

- Infective endocarditis
- Ascending aortic dissection
- Collagen vascular disorders (e.g. Marfan's)
- Connective tissue diseases (large and medium vessel arteritis)
- Trauma
- Dehiscence of a prosthetic valve

Management

- Definitive treatment is aortic valve replacement: the patient's clinical condition will determine the urgency (and mortality). Liaise early with local cardiologists and cardiothoracic surgeons.

General measures (see p78)

- Admit the patient to intensive care or medical HDU.
- Give oxygen, begin treating any pulmonary oedema with diuretics.
- Monitor blood gases; mechanical ventilation may be necessary.
- Blood cultures × 3 are essential. Other investigations as on p88.
- Serial ECG: watch for developing AV block or conduction defects.

Specific measures

- These patients must be discussed with the regional cardiothoracic centre – urgent surgery may be life-saving.
- Vasodilators such as sodium nitroprusside or hydralazine may temporarily improve forward flow and relieve pulmonary oedema.
- Inotropic support with dobutamine may be necessary if hypotensive.
- All patients with haemodynamic compromise should have immediate or urgent aortic valve replacement.
- Infective endocarditis: indications for surgery are given on p98.

Acute aortic regurgitation

Acute mitral regurgitation

Presentation

- Patients most commonly present with acute breathlessness. Symptoms may be less severe, or spontaneously improve as left atrial compliance increases. There may be a history of previous murmur, angina, or myocardial infarction.

- Patients with mitral valve prostheses may describe a feeling of something giving if a tissue valves suddenly fails.

- The signs are different to those seen in chronic MR because of the presence of a non-dilated, and relatively non-compliant left atrium. Acute MR results in a large left atrial systolic pressure wave (v wave), and hence pulmonary oedema.

- Patients may be acutely unwell with tachycardia, hypotension, peripheral vasoconstriction, and pulmonary oedema with a harsh pansystolic murmur of MR.

- Later in the illness, probably because of sustained high left atrial and pulmonary venous pressures, right heart failure develops.

- Examine for signs of any underlying conditions (see table opposite).

- The important differential diagnosis is a VSD. Pulmonary artery catheterization in acute MR will exclude the presence of a left to right shunt and the pulmonary artery wedge pressure trace will demonstrate a large v wave (see p774).

- Where there is no obvious underlying cause (e.g. acute MI), assume the patient has infective endocarditis until proven otherwise.

Diagnosis: Transthoracic or transoesophageal ECHO.

Management

General measures (see p78)

- Admit the patient to intensive care or medical HDU.

- Give oxygen, begin treating any pulmonary oedema with diuretics.

- Monitor blood gases; mechanical ventilation may be necessary.

- Blood cultures × 3 are essential. Other investigations as on p88.

- If present, myocardial infarction should be treated in the standard manner (p16–32).

Specific measures

- Pulmonary oedema may be very resistant to treatment (see p78–83).

- Systemic vasodilators (e.g. sodium nitroprusside or hydralazine).

- Patients may require inotropic support (dobutamine ± adrenaline), and respiratory support (CPAP or mechanical ventilation).

- Patients who present with haemodynamic disturbance and pulmonary oedema must be considered for mitral valve replacement – discuss with a cardiologist/surgeon.

- *Infective endocarditis:* indications for surgery are given on p98.

- *Post infarct MR:* management depends upon the patients condition following resuscitation. Patients who are stabilized may have MVR deferred because of the risks of surgery in the post infarct patient. Their pre operative management should consist of diuretics and vasodilators, including ACE inhibitors if tolerated. Patients should also be advised regarding endocarditis prophylaxis (see p100).

Cardiovascular emergencies

Causes of acute mitral regurgitation

- Infective endocarditis
- Papillary muscle dysfunction or rupture (post MI, p28).
- Rupture of chordae tendinae (e.g. infection, myxomatous degeneration, SLE)
- Trauma (to leaflets, papillary muscle or chordae)
- Prosthetic valve malfunction (e.g. secondary to infection)
- Left atrial myxoma
- Acute rheumatic fever
- Collagen vascular disorders (e.g. Marfan's)
- Connective tissue diseases (large and medium vessel arteritis)

Deep vein thrombosis (DVT): Assessment

Presentation

- Most commonly asymptomatic or with minor leg discomfort or swelling only (> 65%). The main symptoms, when present, are pain and swelling of the affected leg. Breathlessness or chest pain in addition may be secondary to pulmonary embolism.

- Signs include erythema and swelling of the leg, dilated superficial veins and calf discomfort on dorsiflexion of the foot (Homan's sign). The thrombus may be palpable as a fibrous cord in the popliteal fossa. Confirm the presence of swelling (> 2cm) by measuring the limb circumference 15 cm above and 10cm below the tibial tuberosity.

- In all case of leg swelling abdominal and rectal (and pelvic in women) examination must be carried out in an attempt to exclude an abdominal cause.

Risk factors for DVT

Pro-coagulant states

Congenital	*Acquired*
Factor V_{Leiden}	Malignant disease (~ 5%)
Antithrombin III deficiency	Antiphospholipid syndrome
Protein C deficiency	Myeloproliferative disorders
Protein S deficiency	Oral contraceptive pill
	(combined OCP and 3rd generation OCP
	especially with Factor V_{Leiden} mutation)
	Nephrotic syndrome (via renal AT III losses)
	Homocystinuria
	Paroxysmal nocturnal haemoglobinuria
Venous stasis	Immobility (e.g. long journeys)
	Recent surgery
	Pelvic mass
	Pregnancy or recent childbirth
	Severe obesity
Miscellaneous	Hyperviscosity syndromes (p590)
	Previous DVT or PE
	Family history of DVT/PE

Investigations

- Doppler ultrasound of leg veins is largely replacing venography as the initial investigation of choice. It is quick, non-invasive and does not carry the risk of contrast allergy or phlebitis.
- Consider baseline investigations [FBC, U&Es, ECG, CXR, urinalysis and pulse oximetry (± ABG if abnormal)] on all patients.
- If appropriate, look for an underlying cause (see above).
  - Coagulation screen
  - Pro-coagulant screen (protein C, S, antithrombin III levels, Factor V_{Leiden} mutation, anticardiolipin antibody, Ham test, etc.)
  - Screen for malignancy – Ultrasound ± CT (abdomen and pelvis), CXR, LFTs, PSA, CEA, etc.

Note: Doppler USS can only detect thrombi that extend to the popliteal vein. Small undetectable thrombi may still propagate (~5%), and can only be detected by venography which remains the gold standard for routine clinical care.

Deep vein thrombosis

Deep vein thrombosis: (DVT) Management

- Thrombi limited to the calf have low risk of embolization and may be treated with compression stockings and sub-cutaneous heparin, 5000 U/12h until mobile to deter proximal propagation of thrombus.
- A brief period of systemic anti-coagulation with heparin may lessen the pain from below knee DVT.
- Thrombi within the thigh veins warrant full anti-coagulation with heparin, and subsequently, warfarin.

Anticoagulation

1. *Heparin*

- If the clinical suspicion of DVT is high (the presence of risk factors and absence of an alternative diagnosis increase this), start emperic anti-coagulation with heparin: this may be discontinued if subsequent investigations are negative.
- iv heparin is more effective than intermittent subcutaneous dosing[7]
- Give loading dose heparin 5000 units (~ 100 units/kg) and start an infusion of 1000–2000units/h; check APTT every 4 hours until stable aiming for an APTT between 2.5 and 3.5 times normal.
- Low molecular weight heparins are as effective as unfractionated heparin in preventing progression of DVT and PE and may allow out-patient treatment of uncomplicated DVT until warfarin therapy is established (enoxaparin 1mg/kg s.c bd[8]). (In addition to antithrombin III-mediated effects, they inhibit of thrombin formation and have direct effects on the endothelium).

2. *Warfarin*

- Always heparinize before starting warfarin. Protein C (a vit. K-dependent anti-coagulant) has a shorter half-life than the other coagulation factors and levels fall sooner resulting in a transient pro-coagulant tendency .
- If DVT is confirmed commence warfarin and maintain on heparin until INR > 2 (see p706 for a regimen).
- Anti-coagulate (INR 2–2.5) for 3 months.
- If recurrent DVT, or patient at high risk of recurrence consider life-long anti-coagulation.

Thrombolysis

- This should be considered for recurrent, extensive, proximal venous thrombosis (e.g. femoral or iliac veins), as it is more effective than anti-coagulation alone in promoting clot dissolution and produces a better clinical outcome.
- Catheter-directed thrombolytic therapy (rt-PA or SK) is superior to systemic thrombolysis.
- One approach is streptokinase 250,000U over 30 min. then 100,000U every hour for 24–72 hours (see data sheet). See p20 for contra-indications to thrombolysis.

Further management

- Women taking the combined OCP should be advised to stop this.
- If there are contraindications to anti-coagulation, consider the insertion of a caval filter to prevent PE.
- All patients should be treated with thigh-high compression stockings to try to reduce symptomatic venous distension when mobilizing.

[7] Hull RD *et al* (1986) NEJM 315: 1109.
[8] Schafer AI (1996) NEJM 334: 724.

Deep vein thrombosis

Pulmonary embolism: (PE) Assessment

Presentation

Symptoms

- Classically presents with sudden onset, pleuritic chest pain, associated with breathlessness and haemoptysis. Additional symptoms include postural dizziness or syncope.
- Massive PE may present as cardiac arrest (particularly with electro-mechanical dissociation) or shock.
- Presentation may be atypical, i.e. unexplained breathlessness or un-explained hypotension or syncope only.
- PE should be suspected in all breathless patients with risk factors for deep vein thrombosis (DVT) or with clinically proven DVT (p106). Consider right-sided endocarditis (p96).
- Recurrent PEs may present with chronic pulmonary hypertension and progressive right heart failure.

Signs

- Examination may reveal tachycardia and tachypnoea only. Look for postural hypotension (in the presence of raised JVP).
- Look for signs of raised right heart pressures and cor pulmonale (raised JVP with prominent 'a' wave, tricuspid regurgitation, para-sternal heave, right ventricular S3, loud pulmonary closure sound with wide splitting of S2, pulmonary regurgitation).
- Cyanosis suggests a large pulmonary embolism.
- Examine for a pleural rub (may be transient) or effusion.
- Examine lower limbs for obvious thrombophlebitis.
- Mild fever ($> 37.5°C$) may be present. There may be signs of co-existing COAD.

Causes

- Most frequently secondary to DVT (leg $>>$ arm; see p106).
- Other causes:

  Rarely secondary to right ventricular thrombus (post MI)

  Septic emboli (e.g. tricuspid endocarditis).

  Fat embolism (post fracture).

  Air embolism (venous lines, diving, p754).

  Amniotic fluid

  Parasites

  Neoplastic cells

  Foreign materials (e.g. venous catheters)

Prognostic features

The prognosis in patients with pulmonary emboli varies greatly, associated in part with any underlying condition. Generally, worse prognosis is associated with larger pulmonary emboli, poor prognostic indicators include:

- Hypotension
- Hypoxia
- ECG changes (other than non-specific T wave changes)

Pulmonary embolism: Investigations

- **ABG** Normal ABG do **not** exclude PE.
  $\downarrow P_aO_2$ is invariable with larger PEs. Other changes include mild respiratory alkalosis and $\downarrow P_aCO_2$ (due to tachypnoea) and metabolic acidosis ($2°$ to shock).

- **ECG** Commonly shows sinus tachycardia $\pm$ non-specific ST and T wave changes in the anterior chest leads. The classical changes of acute cor pulmonale such as $S_1Q_3T_3$, right axis deviation, or RBBB are only seen with massive PE. Less common findings include AF.

- **CXR** May be normal. Less commonly may show focal pulmonary oligaemia, a raised hemidiaphragm, small pleural effusion, wedge-shaped shadows based on the pleura, sub-segmental atelectasis, or dilated proximal pulmonary arteries.

- **Blood tests** There is no specific test. *FBC* may show neutrophil leukocytosis; mildly elevated *CK, AST, LDH* and *bilirubin* may be seen. Analysis of *FDPs* (D-dimers) shows some promise in predicting PE .

- **ECHO/TOE** To exclude other causes of hypotension and raised right-sided pressures (e.g. tamponade, RV infarction, p209). In PE it will show RV dilatation and global hypokinesis; doppler may show tricuspid and pulmonary regurgitation and allow estimation of RV systolic pressure. Rarely, the thrombus in the pulmonary artery may be visible.

Ventilation/perfusion lung scanning

A perfusion lung scan (with iv Technetium-99 labelled albumin) should be performed in all suspected cases of PE. A ventilation scan (inhaled Xenon-133) in conjunction increases the specificity by assessing whether the defects in the ventilation and perfusion scans 'match' or 'mismatch'. Pre-existing lung disease makes interpretation difficult.
- A normal perfusion scan rules out significant sized PE.
- Abnormal scans are reported as low, medium, or high probability.
  - A high probability scan establishes the diagnosis of PE.
  - A low probability scan with a low clinical suspicion of PE should prompt a search for another cause for the patient's symptoms.
  - If the clinical suspicion of PE is high and the scan is of low or medium probability, proceed to pulmonary angiography.

Pulmonary angiography

- This is the 'gold standard' investigation. It is indicated in patients with a high clinical suspicion of PE and a non-diagnostic lung scan. Look for sharp cut-off of vessels or obvious filling defects.
- If there is an obvious filling defect, the catheter, or a guide wire passed through the catheter, may be used to poke at the embolus to disrupt it and force it further distally into the pulmonary vasculature.
- After angiography, the catheter may be used to give thrombolysis directly into the affected pulmonary artery (see p116).
- The contrast can cause systemic vasodilatation and haemodynamic collapse in hypotensive patients.

CT scanning

- This may demonstrate thrombus within the proximal pulmonary arteries and may be a useful alternative investigation in patients who are too unstable for pulmonary angiography. It may also be used for follow-up imaging after thrombolysis or embolectomy.

Investigations for an underlying cause for PEs

- Ultrasound deep veins of legs
- USS abdomen and pelvis (?occult malignancy / pelvic mass)
- CT abdomen / pelvis
- Screen for inherited pro-coagulant tendency
  (protein C, S, antithrombin III, Factor V_{Leiden})
- Autoimmune screen (anticardiolipin antibody, ANA)
- Biopsy of suspicious lymph nodes / masses
- Blood cultures

Pulmonary embolism: Management

Immediate management

Stabilize the patient

- Unless an alternative diagnosis is made the patient should be treated as for a pulmonary embolus until this can excluded.
- Monitor cardiac rhythm, pulse, bp, respiration rate every 15 minutes with continuous pulse oximetry and cardiac monitor. Ensure full resuscitation facilities are available.
- Give maximal inspired oxygen via face mask to correct hypoxia; mechanical ventilation may be necessary if the patient is tiring; beware of cardiovascular collapse when sedation is given for endotracheal intubation.
- Obtain venous access and start iv fluids (crystalloid or colloid).
- Give iv heparin 5000–10,000U loading dose and start an infusion of 1500–2000 U/h adjusting to achieve an APTT > 1.5 times normal.

Cardiac arrest (see p1–10)

- Massive PE may present as cardiac arrest with electromechanical dissociation (EMD). Exclude the other causes of EMD (see p10).
- Chest compressions may help break-up the thrombus and allow it to progress more distally, thereby restoring some cardiac output.
- If clinical suspicion of PE is high and there is no absolute contraindication to thrombolysis, give rt-PA (0.6mg/kg/15 min, max. 50mg iv bolus, followed by heparin).[9]
- If cardiac output returns, consider inserting a PA catheter to try to mechanically disrupt the embolus.

Hypotension

The acute increase in pulmonary vascular resistance results in right ventricular dilatation and pressure overload which mechanically impairs LV filling and function. Patients require a higher than normal right-sided filling pressure but may be worsened by fluid overload.

- Insert an internal jugular sheath (in case a PA line is necessary) and central line prior to anti-coagulation. This can be used to insert monitoring or angiography catheters if necessary.
- If hypotensive give colloid (e.g. 500ml *Haemacell* ® stat).
- If hypotension persists invasive monitoring and/or inotropic support is required; the JVP is a poor indicator of the left-sided filling pressures in such cases. Adrenaline is the inotrope of choice.
- Femorofemoral cardiopulmonary bypass may be used to support the circulation until thrombolysis or surgical embolectomy can be performed (see p116–118).
- Pulmonary angiography in a hypotensive patient is hazardous as the contrast may cause systemic vasodilatation and cardiovascular collapse.

Analgesia

- Patients may respond to oral NSAIDs. Avoid im injections (anticoagulation and possible thrombolysis).
- Opiate analgesia: use with caution. The vasodilatation caused by these drugs may precipitate or worsen hypotension. Give small doses (1–2mg diamorphine iv) slowly. Hypotension should respond to iv colloid.

---

[9] Bottiger, BW *et al* (1994) *Resuscitation* **28(1):** 45–54.

Pulmonary embolism: Specific therapy

Anti-coagulation

Heparin enhances the inhibitory effects of antithrombin III on thrombin and Factor Xa over 1000-fold and improves the outcome in patients with PE. For reasons that are not clear, patients with DVT and PE have a higher heparin requirement, and shorter heparin half-life compared with patients with DVT.

- The dosage is empiric; the following is one approach:-
- Uncomplicated suspected PE, treat with a loading dose (100U/kg) of heparin and subsequently maintain on an iv heparin infusion of 1000U/h. Check the APTT every 4 hours until stable at 2–3 times normal, increasing the infusion by 200U/h if subtherapeutic.
- If hypoxic or hypotensive, increase the loading dose to 10,000 units and start with an infusion of 1500U/h.
- Patients with anticardiolipin antibodies (lupus anti-coagulant) have a prolonged APTT even before heparin is commenced. Contact your local haematologist for advice; it is more appropriate to monitor heparin levels or the ACT (activated clotting time) where available.
- Low molecular weight heparins have been used in the treatment of patients with DVT but as yet there are no trials in the treatment of acute or chronic PE.
- If appropriate, take blood for protein C, protein S, antithrombin III *before* starting warfarin (see table p113).
- Start warfarin as soon as the diagnosis is confirmed and aim for an INR of 2–2.5.
- Duration of therapy depends on underlying aetiology. If predisposing factors are transient, we recommend anti-coagulation for a minimum of 6 months. Otherwise, indefinite anti-coagulation with warfarin.

Thrombolytic therapy

- Thrombolysis can rapidly improve the haemodynamic and angio-graphic changes in patients with PE, especially those who present with hypotension or acute right ventricular dysfunction.
- Patients who are hypotensive and/or hypoxic at presentation, with a high clinical suspicion of thromboembolic PE should be treated with, oxygen, iv colloid and loaded with heparin (as above). If haemo-dynamic disturbance persists, consider stopping the heparin and giving thrombolysis.
- If possible, the diagnosis should be confirmed with lung scanning or pulmonary angiography. In extreme circumstances, when there is a high clinical suspicion of PE in a critically ill patient, thrombolysis may be given empirically: CPR is not a contraindication to thrombolysis.
- The choice of thrombolytic agent is also unclear. Streptokinase, uro-kinase and rt-PA, given either as a bolus or continuous infusion, either through a peripheral vein or via PA catheter, have all been shown to be effective, though studies suggest that rt-PA is more effective in improving the haemodynamic changes, and is safer than urokinase.[10]
- Timing: some authorities advocate thrombolysis up to 2 weeks from the acute event.[11]

---

[10] Goldhaber, SZ *et al* (1988) *Lancet* **2:** 293.
[11] Goldhaber SZ. (1995) *Chest* **107** (1 Suppl): 45S-51S.

Dosages of thrombolytic drugs for pulmonary embolism	
Streptokinase	250,000 units over 30 minutes followed by 100,000units/h infusion for 24 hours
Urokinase	4400units/kg over 10 minutes followed by 4400units/kg/h infusion for 12–24 hours.
rt-PA	100mg / 2 hours (or 0.6mg/kg/15 min, max. 50mg), followed by iv heparin infusion.

(See p20 for contraindications to thrombolysis)

Pulmonary embolism: Specialist therapy

Pulmonary embolectomy

- In patients who have contraindications to thrombolysis and are in shock requiring inotropic support, there may be a role for embolectomy if appropriate skills are on site.[12]
- Discuss with the surgeons early.
- Radiological confirmation of extent and site of embolism is preferable before thoracotomy.
- Mortality is ~ 25–30%.
- Pulmonary endarterectomy is sometimes successful in treating chronic pulmonary hypertension from recurrent PE. Refer to a specialist unit.

Inferior Vena Cava (IVC) filter

- Up to 20 % of medically treated patients will have re-embolism. If anti-coagulation is contraindicated, re-embolism occurs inspite of anti-coagulation or extensive venous thrombus that may embolize persists, IVC interruption should be considered.
- This may be performed surgically (via laparoscope or formal laparotomy) or percutaneously.
- A number of transvenous devices are available (e.g. Greenfield filter, 'Bird Nest' filter) which reduce the recurrent embolism rate to 2.5–5%. Complications include malposition of the filter, IVC or femoral vein thrombosis, and bleeding.

---

[12] Gulba DC *et al* (1994) *Lancet* **343**: 576–7.

Fat embolism

Commonly seen in patients with major trauma. There is embolization of fat and micro-aggregates of platelets, RBCs and fibrin in systemic and pulmonary circulation. Pulmonary damage may result directly from the emboli (infarction) or by a chemical pneumonitis and ARDS (see p188).

Clinical features

- There may be a history of fractures followed (24–48h later) by breathlessness, cough, haemoptysis, confusion, and rash.
- Examination reveals fever (38–39°C), widespread petechial rash (25–50%), cyanosis, and tachypnoea. There may be scattered crepitations in the chest, though examination may be normal. Changes in mental state may be the first sign, with confusion, drowsiness, seizures and coma. Examine the eyes for conjunctival and retinal haemorrhages; occasionally fat globules may be seen in the retinal vessels. Severe fat embolism may present as shock.

Investigations

- ABG   Hypoxia and a respiratory alkalosis (with low P_aCO_2) as for thromboembolic PE.
- FBC   Thrombocytopenia, acute intravascular haemolysis
- Coagulation Disseminated intravascular coagulation
- U&Es, Glc   Renal failure, hypoglycaemia
- Ca^{2+} May be low
- Urine   Microscopy for fat and dipstick for haemoglobin.
- ECG   Usually non-specific (sinus tachycardia); occasionally signs of right heart strain (see p112).
- CXR   Usually lags behind the clinical course. There may be patchy, bilateral, air space opacification. Effusions are rare.
- CT head   Consider if there is a possibility of head injury with expanding subdural or epidural bleed (p342).

Differential diagnosis

- Pulmonary thromboembolism, other causes of ARDS (p188), septic shock, hypovolaemia, cardiac or pulmonary contusion, head injury, aspiration pneumonia, transfusion reaction.

Management

- Treat respiratory failure (p178). Give oxygen (maximal via face mask; CPAP and mechanical ventilation if necessary).
- Ensure adequate circulating volume and cardiac output. CVP is not a good guide to left-sided filling pressures and a PA catheter (Swan-Ganz) should be used to guide fluid replacement. Try to keep PCWP 12–15mmHg and give diuretics if necessary. Use inotropes to support circulation as required (p192).
- Aspirin (300mg daily), heparin and Dextran 40 (500ml over 4–6h) are of some benefit in the acute stages, but may exacerbate bleeding from sites of trauma.
- High-dose steroids (methylprednisolone 30mg/kg q8h for 3 doses) have been shown to improve hypoxaemia[13] but steroids are probably most effective if given prophylactically.

---

[13] Lindeque BG *et al* (1987) *J Bone Joint Surg,* **69:** 128–131.

Hypertensive emergencies

Assessment

A number of conditions require urgent or semi-urgent lowering of blood pressure (see table opposite). For some of these disorders, the raised bp is directly responsible for acute microvascular damage (e.g. accelerated or malignant hypertension): for others, lowering the bp will reduce the complications from the underlying condition (e.g. aortic dissection). If untreated, the mortality for malignant hypertension is uniformly high (> 75% at 1 year, > 99% at 5 year).

Presentation

- Occasionally minimal symptoms only: mild headaches, nose-bleeds.
- A small group of patients present with symptoms resulting from microvascular damage resulting from the high blood pressure:-
  - Neurological symptoms: severe headache, nausea, vomiting, visual loss, focal neurological deficits, fits, confusion, coma (see below).
  - Chest pain (hypertensive heart disease or aortic dissection) and congestive cardiac failure.
  - Symptoms of renal failure: renal impairment may be chronic (secondary to long-standing hypertension) or acute (from the necrotizing vasculitis of malignant hypertension).
- Patients may present with hypertension as one manifestation of an underlying 'disease' (renovascular hypertension, chronic renal failure, CREST syndrome, phaeochromocytoma, pregnancy).
- Examination should be directed at looking for evidence of end-organ damage even if the patient is asymptomatic (heart failure, focal neurology).

Priorities in management are:-

1 Confirm the diagnosis and assess the severity.
2 Identify those patients needing specific emergency treatment.
3 Plan long-term treatment.

Diagnosis and severity

- **Ask about** previous blood pressure recordings, previous and current treatment, sympathomimetics, antidepressants, non-prescription drugs, recreational drugs.
- **Check the blood pressure** yourself, in both arms, after a period of rest and if possible on standing. Monitor the patient's blood pressure regularly while they are in A&E.
- **Examine** carefully for clinical evidence of cardiac enlargement or heart failure, peripheral pulses, renal masses or focal neurological deficit. Always examine the fundi – dilate if necessary (p129).
- **Investigations:** All patients should have:-
  - U&Es   Renal impairment and / or $\downarrow K^+$ (diffuse intra-renal ischaemia and $2°$ hyperaldosteronism)
  - FBC   Microangiopathic haemolytic anaemia with malignant HT
  - Coagulation screen DIC with malignant HT
  - ECG   ?LVH (table opposite) or acute ischaemia.
  - Chest X-ray   Cardiac enlargement
                   Aortic contour (?dissection)
                   Pulmonary oedema
  - Urinalysis   Protein and red cells ± casts

Cardiovascular emergencies

Hypertensive emergencies

- Accelerated and malignant hypertension
- Hypertensive encephalopathy
- Eclampsia and pre-eclampsia
- Intracranial haemorrhage   (p356–66)
- Phaeochromocytoma   (p470)
- Hypertension with complications
  Aortic dissection   (p132)
  Pulmonary oedema   (p78)

Voltage criteria for LVH

- Tallest R (V4–V6) + deepest S (V1–V3) > 40mm
- Tallest R (V4–V6) > 27mm
- Deepest S (V1–V3) > 30mm
- R in aVL > 13mm
- R in aVF > 20mm
- QRS complex > 0.08s (2 small sq)
- Abnormal ST depression or T inversion in V4–V6

Hypertensive emergencies

Management

A number of other conditions may present with severe hypertension (see table opposite). Other investigations to consider include:-

- 24h urine collection — Creatinine clearance
  Free catecholamines, metanephrines or vanilmandellic acid (VMA)
- ECHO — LVH, aortic dissection
- Renal USS and — Size of kidneys
  doppler renal arteries — ?renal artery stenosis
- Renal angiography — ?renal artery stenosis
- CT brain — To exclude intracranial bleed or SOL
- Drug screen — Cocaine, amphetamine, other sympathomimetics

Indications for admission

- Diastolic blood pressure persistently ≥ 120mmHg
- Retinal haemorrhages, exudates or papilloedema
- Renal impairment

Management

- The majority of patients who are alert and otherwise well may be treated with oral therapy to lower bp gradually.
- Aim to reduce the diastolic blood pressure to < 110mmHg over approximately 24 hours.
- First-line treatment should be with a β-blocker (unless contraindicated), with a thiazide diuretic, or a low-dose calcium antagonist.
- Urgent invasive monitoring (arterial line) prior to drug therapy is indicated for patients with :-
  - Evidence of hypertensive encephalopathy
  - Complications of hypertension
    (e.g. aortic dissection, acute pulmonary oedema or renal failure)
  - Treatment of underlying condition
    (e.g. glomerulonephritis, phaeochromocytoma, CREST crisis)
  - Patients with persistent diastolic bp ≥ 140mmHg
  - Eclampsia
- It is dangerous and not usually necessary to rapidly reduce the bp. It is far safer to opt for a cautious and slow reduction. *Avoid sublingual nifedipine.*

Long-term management

- Investigate as appropriate for an underlying causes (see table opposite).
- Select a treatment regime which is tolerated and effective. Tell the patient why long-term therapy is important.
- Try to reduce all cardiovascular risk factors by advising the patient to stop smoking, appropriate dietary advice (cholesterol), and aim for optimal diabetic control.
- Monitor long-term control and look for end-organ damage (regular fundoscopy, ECG, U&Es). Even poor control is better than no control.

Cardiovascular emergencies

Conditions that may present with severe hypertension

- Coarctation of the aorta
- Renal artery stenosis
- Renal failure (acute or chronic)
- Phaechromocytoma
- Primary hyperaldosteronism
- Cushing's syndrome
- Hyperparathyroidism
- Thyrotoxicosis (systolic hypertension)
- Pre-eclampsia
- Drugs: oestrogens, steroids
- Carbenoxolone, MAOs and tyramine
- Adrenal carcinoma secreting mineralocorticoids
- Acromegaly

Conditions requiring specific treatment

- Accelerated and malignant hypertension (p128)
- Hypertensive encephalopathy (p130)
- Eclampsia
- Phaeochromocytoma (p470)
- Hypertensive patients undergoing anaesthesia (p128)

Drugs for hypertensive emergencies

Drugs for the treatment of hypertensive emergencies: IV therapy

Drug	Dosage	Onset of action	Comments
Labetalol	20-80 mg iv bolus q10min 20-200 mg/min by iv infusion increasing every 15 min.	2-5 min	Drug of choice in suspected phaeochromocytoma (p472) or aortic dissection (p136). Avoid if there is LVF. May be continued orally (see below)
Nitroprusside	0.25-10 µg/kg/min iv infusion (p698)	Seconds	Drug of choice in LVF and/or encephalopathy.
GTN	1-10 mg/hr iv infusion	2-5 min	Mainly venodilatation. Useful n patients with LVF or angina.
Hydralazine	5-10 mg iv over 20 min. 50-300 µg/min iv infusion	10-15 min.	May provoke angina
Esmolol HCl	500 µg/kg/min iv loading dose 50-200 µg/kg/min iv infusion	Seconds	Short acting β-blocker also used for SVTs (p50)
Phentolamine	2-5 mg iv over 2-5 min prn	Seconds	Drug of choice in phaeochromocytoma (p472) followed by labetalol (po) when BP controlled.

Note: It is dangerous to reduce the blood pressure quickly. Aim to reduce the diastolic BP to 100-110 mmHg within 2-4 hours. Unless there are good reasons to commence iv therapy, always use oral medication.

Drugs for the treatment of hypertensive emergencies: Oral therapy

Drug	Dosage	Onset of action	Comment
Atenolol	50–100 mg po od	30–60 min	There are numerous alternative β-blockers – see BNF.
Nifedipine	10–20 mg po q8h (q12h if slow release)	15–20 min	Avoid sublingual as the fall in bp is very rapid.
Labetalol	100–400 mg po q12h	30–60 min	Use if phaeochromocytoma suspected. Safe in pregnancy.
Hydralazine	25–50 mg po q8h	20–40 min	Safe in pregnancy
Minoxidil	5–10 mg po od	30–60 min	May cause marked salt and water retention. Combine with a loop diuretic (e.g. frusemide 40–240mg daily).
Clonidine	0.2 mg po followed by 0.1 mg hourly max. 0.8 mg total for urgent therapy, or 0.05–0.1mg po q8h increasing every 2 days	30–60 min	Sedation common. Do not stop abruptly as here is a high incidence of rebound hypertensive crisis.

Note: Aim to reduce diastolic bp to 100–110 mmHg in 24 hours and normalise bp in 2–3 days.

Accelerated and malignant hypertension

These are part of a continuum of disorders characterised by hypertension (diastolic bp often > 120mmHg) and acute microvascular damage (seen best in the retina but present in all organs). It may be difficult to decide whether the acute glomerulonephritis produced the malignant hypertension or vice versa.

- Accelerated hypertension (Grade 3 retinopathy p129) may progress to malignant hypertension, with widespread necrotizing vasculitis of the arterioles (and papilloedema).
- *Presentation* is commonly with headache or visual loss and varying degrees of confusion. More severe cases present with renal failure, heart failure, microangiopathic haemolytic anaemia and DIC.

Management

- Transfer the patient to medical HDU / ITU.
- Insert an arterial line and consider central venous line if there is evidence of necrotizing vasculitis and DIC. Catheterize the bladder.
- Monitor neurological state, ECG, fluid balance.
- Those with early features may be treated successfully with oral therapy (beta-blockers, calcium channel blockers – see table opposite) aiming to lower the diastolic blood pressures to 100–110mmHg (or by 15–20mmHg) over the first 24 hours.
- Patients with late symptoms or who deteriorate should be given parenteral therapy aiming for more rapid lowering of bp.
- Give frusemide 40–80mg iv (if there is evidence of pulmonary oedema or encephalopathy).
- If there is no pulmonary oedema, give a bolus of labetalol followed by an infusion. For patients with LVF, nitroprusside or hydralazine are preferable (see table p126).
- Consult renal team for patients with acute renal failure or evidence of acute glomerulonephritis (> 2+ proteinuria, red cell casts). ARF is managed as on p276. Dopamine should be avoided or used with care as it may worsen hypertension.
- Consider giving ACE inhibitor. High circulating renin levels may not allow control of hypertension which in turn causes progressive renal failure. ACE inhibitors will block this vicious circle. There may be marked first dose hypotension, so start cautiously.
- Haemolysis and DIC should recover with control of bp.

Hypertensive patients undergoing anaesthesia

Hypertension should be adequately controlled (diastolic ≤ 100mmHg) prior to surgery to prevent massive swings during anaesthetic induction.

Phaechromocytoma (see p470)

Accelerated and malignant hypertension

Hypertensive retinopathy	
Grade 1	Tortuous retinal arteries, silver wiring
Grade 2	AV nipping
Grade 3	Flame-shaped haemorrhages and cotton wool exudates
Grade 4	Papilloedema

Hypertensive encephalopathy

Usually gradual onset and may occur in previously normotensive patients at blood pressures as low as 150/100. It is rare in patients with chronic hypertension.

Symptoms

- Headache, nausea and vomiting, confusion, Grade 3 and iv hypertensive retinopathy.
- Late features consist of focal neurological signs, fits and coma.

Diagnosis

- Exclude other causes of encephalopathy. History is helpful, cerebrovascular accidents usually being sudden in onset. If there is doubt a head CT should be obtained.
- Starting hypotensive treatment for hypertension associated with a stroke can cause extension of the stroke (p374).
- Always exclude hypoglycaemia.

Management

- The aim of treatment is to lower the diastolic pressure to 100–110mmHg (or by 10–15mmHg) within 2–4 hours.
- Transfer the patient to ITU for invasive monitoring.
- Monitor neurological state, ECG, fluid balance.
- Correct electrolyte abnormalities (K^+, Mg^{2+}, Ca^{2+}).
- Give frusemide 40–80mg iv.
- Those with early features may be treated successfully with oral therapy (beta-blockers, calcium channel blockers – see table p127).
- Patients who deteriorate should be given parenteral therapy (see p126).

Aortic dissection: Assessment

Presentation

- **Chest pain**: Classically abrupt onset of very severe chest pain, most commonly anterior chest pain radiating to the interscapular region. Usually tearing in nature and, unlike the pain of myocardial infarction, most severe at its onset. Pain felt maximally in the anterior chest is associated with ascending aortic dissection, whereas interscapular pain suggests dissection of the descending aorta.
- **Sudden death** or **shock**: Usually due to rupture or cardiac tamponade.
- **Congestive cardiac failure**: Due to acute aortic incompetence and/or myocardial infarction.
- Patients may also present with symptoms and signs of occlusion of one of the branches of the aorta. Examples include:-
  - Stroke or acute limb ischaemia – due to compression or dissection
  - Paraplegia with sensory deficits – spinal artery occlusion
  - Myocardial infarction – usually the right coronary artery
  - Renal failure and renovascular hypertension
  - Abdominal pain – coeliac axis or mesenteric artery occlusion
- Aortic dissection may be painless.
- Ask specifically about history of hypertension, previous heart murmurs or aortic valve disease and previous chest X-rays that may be useful for comparison.

Examination

- This may be normal.
- Most patients are hypertensive on presentation. Hypotension is more common in dissections of the ascending aorta (20–25%) and may be due to blood loss, acute aortic regurgitation (which may be accompanied by heart failure), or tamponade (distended neck veins, tachycardia, pulsus paradoxus).
- Pseudohypotension may be seen if flow to either or both subclavian arteries is compromised. Look for unequal blood pressure in the arms and document the presence of peripheral pulses carefully; absent or changing pulses suggests extension of the dissection.
- Auscultation may reveal aortic valve regurgitation and occasionally a pericardial friction rub. Descending aortic dissections may rupture or leak into the left pleural space and the effusion results in dullness in the left base.
- Neurological deficits may be due to carotid artery dissection or compression (hemiplegia) or spinal artery occlusion (paraplegia with sensory loss).

Associations of aortic dissection

1. Hypertension
2. Marfan's syndrome
   - arm span > height
   - pubis to sole > pubis to vertex
   - depressed sternum, scoliosis
   - high arched palate
   - upward lens dislocation
   - thoracic aortic dilatation / aortic regurgitation
   - increased urinary hydroxyproline (in some)
3. Ehlers-Danlos syndrome
4. Bicuspid aortic valve
5. Coarctation of the aorta
6. Pregnancy
7. Chest trauma
8. Iatrogenic (instrumentation of the aorta)

Aortic dissection: Investigations

- **ECG** may be normal or show non-specific changes of long-standing hypertension [LVH (see table p123), ST-T abnormalities]. Look specifically for evidence of acute MI (inferior MI is seen if the dissection compromises the right coronary artery ostium).

- **Chest X-ray** may appear normal, but with hindsight is almost always abnormal. Look for widened upper mediastinum, haziness or enlargement of the aortic knuckle, irregular aortic contour, separation (> 5mm) of intimal calcium from outer aortic contour, displacement of trachea to the right, enlarged cardiac silhouette (pericardial effusion), pleural effusion (usually on left). Compare with previous films if available.

- **Echocardiography:** *Transthoracic ECHO* may be useful in diagnosing aortic root dilatation, aortic regurgitation and pericardial effusion / tamponade. *Transoesophageal ECHO* (TOE) is probably the investigation of choice as it allows better evaluation of ascending aorta, arch and descending aorta, may identify the intimal tear at the origin of the dissection, and allows evaluation of the origins of the coronary arteries in relation to the dissection.

- **Spiral CT with contrast** allows identification of the two lumens with differential flow, detection of intimal flap, and pleural or pericardial fluid. However, it cannot demonstrate disruption of the aortic valve which may be associated with ascending aortic dissection.

- **Angiography** using the femoral or axillary approach may demonstrate the altered flow in the two lumens, aortic valve incompetence, involvement of the branches, and the site of the intimal tear. It has largely been superseded by CT and TOE.

- **MRI** angiography is as yet experimental only, and the design of the tube does not allow easy assess to the patient in the event of emergency. Newer designs and sequences are being devised.

Differential diagnosis

- The chest pain may be mistaken for acute MI and acute MI may complicate aortic dissection. Always look for other signs of dissection (see above), as thrombolysis will be fatal.

- Severe chest pain and collapse may also be due to pulmonary embolism, spontaneous pneumothorax, acute pancreatitis and penetrating duodenal ulcer.

- Pulse deficits without back ache should suggest other diagnoses: atherosclerotic peripheral vascular disease, arterial embolism, Takayasu's arteritis, etc.

- Acute cardiac tamponade with chest pain is also seen in acute viral or idiopathic pericarditis and acute myocardial infarction with external rupture.

Aortic dissection

DeBakey classification

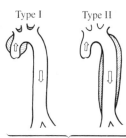

Stanford classification

Type A

Type B

Aortic dissection: Management

Stabilize the patient

- If the diagnosis is suspected, transfer the patient to an area where full resuscitation facilities are readily available.

- Secure **venous access** with large bore cannulas (e.g. Grey venflon).
- **Take blood** for FBC, U&Es and cross-match (10 units).
- When the diagnosis is confirmed or in cases with cardiovascular complications, **transfer to ITU**, insert an **arterial line** (radial unless the subclavian artery is compromised, when a femoral line is preferred), **central venous line**, and **urinary catheter**.

Plan the definitive treatment

This depends on the type of dissection (see figure p135) and its effects on the patient. General principles are:-

    a. Patients with involvement of the ascending aorta should have surgical repair.

    b. Patients with dissection limited to the descending aorta may be managed medically with aggressive blood pressure control.

Indications for surgery

1 Involvement of the ascending aorta.
2 External rupture (haemopericardium, haemothorax, effusions).
3 Arterial compromise (limb ischaemia, renal failure, stroke).
4 Contraindications to medical therapy (AR, LVF).
5 Progression (continued pain, expansion of haematoma on further imaging, loss of pulses, pericardial rub or aortic insufficiency).

The aim of surgical therapy is to replace the ascending aorta, thereby preventing retrograde dissection and cardiac tamponade, the main cause of death. The aortic valve may need reconstruction and resuspension unless it is structurally abnormal (bicuspid or Marfan's).

Principles of medical management

1 In all but those patients who are hypotensive, initial management is aimed at reducing systemic blood pressure and myocardial contractility. The goal is to stop spread of the intramural haematoma and to prevent rupture and the best guide is control of pain. Strict bed rest in a quiet room is essential.

2 *Control blood pressure:* (Reduce systolic bp to 100–120mmHg).
- Start on an iv beta-blocker (if no contraindications) aiming to reduce the heart rate to 60–70 / min (see table opposite).
- Once this is achieved, if the blood pressure remains high, add a vasodilator such as sodium nitroprusside (see table opposite). Vasodilators in the absence of β-blockade may increase myocardial contractility and the rate of rise of pressure (dP/dt) and theoretically may promote extension of the dissection.
- In patients with aortic regurgitation and congestive cardiac failure, myocardial depressants should not be given. Aim to control blood pressure with vasodilators only.

3 *Hypotension* may be due to haemorrhage or cardiac tamponade.
- Resuscitate with rapid intravenous volume (ideally colloid or blood, but crystalloid may be used also). A pulmonary artery wedge catheter (Swan-Ganz) should be used to monitor the wedge pressure and guide fluid replacement.
- If there are signs of aortic regurgitation or tamponade, arrange for an urgent ECHO and discuss with the surgeons.

4 *Long-term treatment* must involve strict blood pressure control.

Medical therapy of aortic dissection

- **Beta-blockade** (Aim for HR ≤ 60–70/min)

Labetalol	20–80mg slow iv injection over 10min
	then 20–200mg/h iv, increasing every 15 min
	100–400mg po q12h
Atenolol	5–10mg slow iv injection
	then 50mg po after 15min and at 12 hours,
	then 100mg po daily
Propranolol	0.5mg iv (test dose), then 1mg every 2–5 min.
	up to max 10mg; repeat every 2–3h.
	10–40mg po 3–4 times daily

- When HR 60–70 /min, (or if β-blocker contraindicated), add

Nitroprusside	0.25–10µg/kg/min iv infusion (p698)
Hydralazine	5–10mg iv over 20 minutes
	50–300µg/min iv infusion
	25–50mg po q8h
GTN	1–10mg/h iv infusion
Nifedipine	10–20mg po q8h (or q12h if slow release)

Prognosis

- The mortality for untreated aortic dissection is roughly 20–30% at 24 hours and 65–75% at two weeks.

- For dissections confined to the descending aorta, short-term survival is better (up to 80%) but ~ 30–50% will have progression of dissection despite aggressive medical therapy and require surgery.

- Operative mortality is of the order of 10–25% and depends on the condition of the patient pre-operatively. Post operative 5-year actuarial survival of up to 75% may be expected.

Acute pericarditis: Assessment

Presentation

- Typically presents as *central chest pain* – often pleuritic – relieved by sitting forward. Often associated with breathlessness.
- Other symptoms (e.g. fever, cough, arthralgia, rash) may reflect the underlying disease (see below).
- A *pericardial friction rub* is pathognomonic. This may be positional and transient and may be confused with the murmur of tricuspid or mitral regurgitation.
- Venous pressure rises if an effusion develops. Look for signs of cardiac tamponade (p142).

Investigations

ECG
- May be normal in up to 10%.
- 'Saddle-shaped' ST segment elevation (concave upwards) with variable T inversion and depression of PR segment.
- May be difficult to distinguish from acute MI. Features suggesting pericarditis are:-
  - Concave ST elevation (vs convex).
  - All leads involved (vs a territory e.g., inferior).
  - Failure of usual ST evolution and no Q waves.
  - No AV block, BBB, or QT prolongation.
- Early repolarization (a normal variant) may be mistaken for pericarditis. In the former, ST elevation occurs in pre-cordial and rarely in V6 or the limb leads, and is unlikely to show ST depression in V1 or PR segment depression.
- Usually not helpful in diagnosing pericarditis post MI.
- The voltage drops as an effusion develops.

ECHO
- May demonstrate a pericardial collection.
- Useful to monitor LV function in case of deterioration due to associated myocarditis.

Other investigations depend on the suspected aetiology:-

All patients should have:-

- FBC and ESR
- U&Es
- Serial cardiac enzymes
- CXR (heart size, pulmonary oedema, infection)

Where appropriate:-

- Viral titres (acute + 2 weeks later)
- Blood cultures
- Autoantibody screen (ANA, anti-DNA, complement levels)
- Thyroid function tests
- Fungal precipitins (if immunosuppressed)
- Mantoux test
- Sputum culture and cytology
- Diagnostic pericardial tap (culture, cytology)

Cardiovascular emergencies

Causes of acute pericarditis

- Idiopathic
- Infection (viral, bacterial, TB and fungal)
- Acute myocardial infarction
- Dressler's syndrome, post cardiotomy syndrome
- Malignancy (e.g. breast, bronchus, lymphoma)
- Uraemia
- Autoimmune disease (e.g. SLE, RA, Wegner's, scleroderma, PAN)
- Granulomatous diseases (e.g. sarcoid)
- Hypothyroidism
- Drugs (hydralazine, procainamide, isoniazid)
- Trauma (chest trauma, iatrogenic)
- Radiotherapy

Acute pericarditis: Management

General measures

- *Bed rest.*

- *Analgesia:* Aspirin (600mg q6h po) or an NSAID (e.g. indomethacin 25–50mg q6–8h po); opiates may be necessary.
- *Steroids:* These may be used if the pain does not settle within 48 hours (e.g. prednisolone EC 40–60mg po od for up to 2 weeks, tapering down when pain settles).
- *Colchicine:* This may be helpful in preventing relapses in patients with recurrent pericarditis (1mg stat, 500µg q6h for 48h; see p600).
- *Pericardiocentesis:* This should be considered for significant effusion or if there are signs of tamponade (p142).
- *Antibiotics:* These should be given only if bacterial infection is suspected (see below).
- Oral anticoagulants should be discontinued (risk of haemo-pericardium); the patient should be given iv heparin which is easier to reverse (iv protamine) if complications arise.

Viral pericarditis

- Pathogens include Coxsackie A+B, echovirus, adenovirus, mumps, EBV, VZV, hepatitis B, and HIV.
- Usually a self-limiting illness (1–3 weeks) but 20–30% develop recurrent pericarditis.
- Complications include recurrent pericarditis (20–30%), myocarditis, dilated cardiomyopathy, pericardial effusion and tamponade and late pericardial constriction.
- Treatment is supportive (see above).

Bacterial pericarditis

- The commonest pathogens are pneumococcus, staphylococci, streptococci, Gram -ve rods, and *Neisseria* species.
- Risk factors include pre-existing pericardial effusion (e.g. uraemic pericarditis), immunosuppression (iatrogenic, lymphoma, leukaemia, HIV)
- The infection may have spread from mediastinitis, infective endocarditis, pneumonia, or sub-diaphragmatic abscess.
- Suspect in patients with high fever, night sweats, dyspnoea, and raised JVP (chest pain may be mild or absent); there may be other intrathoracic infection (e.g. pneumonia).
- If suspected, take blood cultures and start *iv flucloxacillin* (2g q6h) and *iv gentamicin* or *iv cefotaxime* (2g q8h). Adjust treatment when sensitivities known.
- Significant sized pericardial collections should be drained to dryness if possible (p788). Send fluid for Gram and ZN stain, fungal smear, and culture. Surgical drainage may be required for recurrent effusions.
- Patients with *TB pericarditis* are very prone to developing cardiac constriction. Steroids have not been shown to prevent this but they do prevent progression once constrictive symptoms develop. Surgical pericardiectomy may be required. Take advice from cardiologists and infectious diseases team.

Uraemic pericarditis

- This is an indication for urgent dialysis (p282).

Dressler's syndrome, post-cardiotomy syndrome 141

- Complicates ~ 1% of acute MI and 10–15% patients following cardiac surgery presenting 2–4 weeks later (up to 3 months later).
- Consists of recurrent pericarditis, fever, anaemia, high ESR, neutrophil leukocytosis, and pleural effusions and transient pulmonary infiltrates on CXR.
- Treat with bed rest, aspirin (600mg po q6h) or NSAID and steroids for persisting symptoms (see above).
- **Pericarditis following acute MI** (see p26).

Neoplastic pericarditis

- The 1 year survival of patients with malignant effusive pericarditis is ≤ 25%: the approach to treatment depends on the underlying malignancy and symptoms.
- Asymptomatic pericardial effusions do not require drainage: treat the underlying malignancy (± mediastinal radiotherapy).
- Drainage is indicated for cardiac tamponade.

Cardiac tamponade: Presentation

Cardiac tamponade occurs when a pericardial effusion causes haemo-dynamically significant cardiac compression. The presentation depends on the speed with which fluid accumulates within the pericardium. Acute tamponade may occur with 100–200mls in a relatively restricted peri-cardial sac; chronic pericardial collections may contain up to 1000mls of fluid without clinical tamponade.

Causes

Acute tamponade
- Cardiac trauma
- Iatrogenic
    - Post cardiac surgery
    - Post cardiac catheterization
    - Post cardiac pacing
- Aortic dissection
- Spontaneous bleed
    - Anti-coagulation
    - Uraemia
    - Thrombocytopenia
- Cardiac rupture post MI

'Sub-acute' tamponade
- Malignant disease
- Idiopathic pericarditis
    - Uraemia
- Infections
    - Bacterial
    - Tuberculosis
- Radiation
- Hypothyroidism
- Post pericardotomy
- SLE

Presentation

- Patients commonly present either with *cardiac arrest* (commonly electrical mechanical dissociation) or with *hypotension, confusion, stupor,* and *shock.*
- Patients who develop cardiac tamponade slowly are usually acutely unwell, but not *in extremis.* Their main symptoms include:-
    - Breathlessness.
    - There may be a preceding history of chest discomfort.
    - Symptoms resulting from compression of adjacent structures by a large effusion (i.e. dysphagia, cough, hoarseness, or hiccough).
    - There may be symptoms due to the underlying cause.

Important physical signs are:-

- Tachycardia
- Hypotension ($\pm$ shock see p210) with postural hypotension.
- Raised JVP (often > 10 cm) with a prominent systolic x descent and absent diastolic y descent (see figure on p143). If the top of the JVP is visible, a rise with inspiration may be seen (Kussmaul's sign).
- Auscultation may reveal diminished heart sounds; a pericardial rub may be present and suggests a small pericardial collection.
- Look for *pulsus paradoxus* (a decrease in the palpable pulse and systolic bp on inspiration). This may be so marked that the pulse and Korotkoff sounds may be completely lost during inspiration.
- Other physical signs include tachypnoea, hepatomegaly and signs of the underlying cause for the pericardial effusion.

Causes of hypotension with a raised JVP

- Cardiac tamponade
- Constrictive pericarditis
- Restrictive pericarditis
- Severe biventricular failure
- Right ventricular infarction
- Pulmonary embolism
- Tension pneumothorax
- Acute severe asthma
- Malignant SVC obstruction and sepsis
  (e.g. lymphoma)

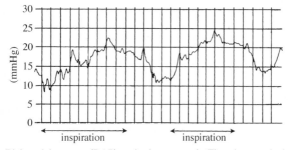

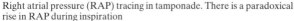

Right atrial pressure (RAP) tracing in tamponade. There is a paradoxical rise in RAP during inspiration

Cardiac tamponade: Management

Investigations

- *Chest X-ray:* The heart size may be normal (e.g. in acute haemopericardium following cardiac trauma). With slower accumulation of pericardial fluid ($> 250ml$) the cardiac silhouette will enlarge with a globular appearance. The size of the effusion is unrelated to its haemodynamic significance. Look for signs of pulmonary oedema.

- *ECG:* Usually shows a sinus tachycardia, with low voltage complexes and variable ST segment changes. With large effusions 'electrical alternans' may be present with beat-to-beat variation in the QRS morphology resulting form the movement of the heart within the pericardial effusion.

- *Echocardiography* confirms the presence of a pericardial effusion. The diagnosis of tamponade is a clinical one. ECHO signs highly suggestive of tamponade include the presence of diastolic collapse of the right atrium, ventricle, and RV outflow tract.

- If available, examine the central venous pressure trace for the characteristic exaggerated *x* descent and absent *y* descent.

Management

Following confirmation of the diagnosis:-

- While preparing for drainage of the pericardial fluid, the patient's circulation may temporarily be supported by loading with iv colloid (500–1000ml stat) and starting inotropes (i.e. Adrenaline).

- In patients with an adequate blood pressure, cautious systemic vasodilatation with hydralazine or nitroprusside, in conjunction with volume loading, may increase forward cardiac output. This is not to be recommended routinely as it may cause acute deterioration.

- Avoid intubation and positive pressure ventilation as this reduces cardiac output.

- The effusion should be urgently drained; (see p788 for pericardiocentesis).

- Surgical drainage is indicated if the effusion is secondary to trauma: there may be other injuries.

- The cause of the effusion should be established (see p142). Pericardial fluid should be sent for cytology, microbiology including TB, and, if appropriate, Hb, glucose and amylase.

Further management is of the underlying cause.

Special cases

1 *Recurrent pericardial effusion:* In some cases pericardial effusion recurs: this requires either a change in the treatment of the underlying cause or a formal surgical drainage procedure such as a pericardial window or pericardiectomy.

2 *Low pressure tamponade:* The clinical picture is altered if the patient is hypovolaemic, classically from dehydration. The JVP is not raised, right atrial pressure is normal and tamponade occurs even with small volumes of pericardial fluid.
   - The patient may respond well to iv fluids.
   - If there is a significant pericardial collection this should be drained.

Cardiac tamponade

Congenital heart disease in adults 1.

Complications

Extracardiac complications

- *Polycythaemia:* Chronic hypoxia stimulates erythropoietin production and erythrocytosis. The 'ideal' Hb level is ~ 17–18g/dl; some centres advocate venesection to control the haematocrit and prevent hyperviscosity syndrome (p590). Follow local guidelines. Generally consider phlebotomy only if moderate or severe symptoms of hyperviscosity are present and haematocrit > 65%: replace with simultaneous infusion of saline or salt-free dextran. Avoid abrupt changes in circulating volume.

- *Renal disease and gout:* Hypoxia affects glomerular and tubular function resulting in proteinuria, reduced urate excretion, increased urate reabsorption and reduced creatinine clearance. Try to avoid dehydration, diuretics, dyes (radiographic contrast) and dialysis (rapid fluid shifts). Acute gout may be treated with colchicine (p600). NSAIDs may be used with caution (see below).

- *Sepsis:* Patients are more prone to infection. Skin acne is common with poor healing of scars. Skin stitches for operative procedures should be left in for 7–10 days longer than normal. Dental hygiene is very important due to the risk of endocarditis (see p100 for antibiotic prophylaxis regimen). Any site of sepsis may result in cerebral abscesses from metastatic infection or septic emboli.

- *Thrombosis and bleeding:* Abnormal platelet function, coagulation abnormalities, polycythaemia and dehydration or oral contraceptives may result in spontaneous arterial ± venous thromboses and haemorrhagic complications (e.g. petechiae, epistaxes, haemoptyses).

- *Primary pulmonary problems* include infection, infarction and haemorrhage from ruptured arterioles or capillaries. Management is discussed on p148.

- *Stroke:* CVA is usually associated with embolic events, injudicious phlebotomy or the use of aspirin, which exacerbates the intrinsic coagulation defects and spontaneous thrombosis.

- *Complications secondary to drugs, investigations, surgery:* Avoid abrupt changes in blood pressure or systemic resistance (see above). Contrast agents may provoke systemic vasodilatation and cause acute decompensation; they may also precipitate renal failure. Before noncardiac surgery, try to optimize haematocrit and haemostasis by controlled phlebotomy and replacement with dextran, high-flow oxygen before and after surgery, precautions with iv lines (see below).

Cardiac complications

- *Congestive cardiac failure:* This may be due to *valve dysfunction* (calcification of an abnormal valve or secondary to supra- or subvalvular fibrosis and stenosis), *ventricular dysfunction* (hypertrophy, fibrosis and failure) or *pulmonary arteriolar disease* and shunt reversal. Treat as usual taking special care not to dehydrate the patient or precipitate acute changes in blood pressure (see p148).

- *Endocarditis:* The risk depends on the cardiac lesion and the pathogen. See table p87. The recommended antibiotic prophylaxis regimen is given on p100. The patients should be advised on careful skin care (e.g. acne) to prevent local infections that may 'metastasize' to heart or brain.

- *Arrhythmias:* Treat in the standard way (p40–72).

Congenital heart disease

Congenital defects with survival to adulthood	
Common	**Rarer**
• Bicuspid aortic valve	• Dextrocardia (situs solitus or invertus)
• Coarctation of the aorta	• Congenital complete heart block
• Pulmonary stenosis	• Congenitally corrected transposition
• Ostium secundum ASD	• Ebstein's anomaly
• Patent ductus arteriosus	• Coronary or pulmonary AV fistulas
	• Aneurysm of Sinus of Valsalva

Congenital defects with good prognosis after surgery

• Ventricular septal defect

• Fallot's tetralogy

Causes of cyanosis in adults with congenital heart disease

- 'Eisenmenger reaction' – R → L shunt through VSD, ASD or patent foramen ovale with pulmonary hypertension. (Pulmonary hypertension may be secondary to pulmonary vascular disease, pulmonary artery stenosis or banding, pulmonary valve stenosis, tricuspid atresia).

- Abnormal connection – transpositions, IVC or SVC to left atrium, total anomalous pulmonary venous drainage.

- Pulmonary AV fistulae.

Congenital heart disease in adults   2.

Management
General measures

- Contact and take advice from the cardiologist normally involved in the patient's care.
- iv lines are potentially very hazardous due to the risk of systemic embolization (air and particulate matter). Use an air-filter if available. Remove iv cannulae if there are any local signs of thrombophlebitis.
- Avoid sudden changes in circulating volume (e.g. vomiting diarrhoea, haemorrhage, venesection, vasovagal attacks). Any acute fall in SVR may precipitate intense cyanosis and death; an acute rise in SVR may abruptly reduce systemic blood flow and cause collapse.
- Monitor for neurological signs and symptoms from cerebral thrombo-embolism or septic embolism.

Specific measures

- **Haemoptysis** is common; most episodes are self-limiting and pre-cipitated by infection; differentiation from pulmonary embolism may be difficult. Try to keep the patient calm. Give high-flow oxygen by mask. If there is clinical suspicion of infection (fever, sputum prod-uction, leukocytosis, raised CRP, etc.) start antibiotics (p156). VQ scan may help in the diagnosis of pulmonary embolism (p110) but is often equivocal. Avoid aspirin and NSAIDs as these exacerbate the intrinsic platelet abnormalities. There is anecdotal evidence for the use of low-dose iv heparin, Dextran 40 (500ml iv infusion q4–6h), ancrod (Arvin® – reduces plasma fibrinogen by cleaving fibrin), or low-dose warfarin therapy for reducing thrombotic tendency in these patients. Severe pulmonary haemorrhage may respond to aprotinin or tranexamic acid.
- **Breathlessness** may be due to pulmonary oedema or hypoxia (in-creased shunt) secondary to chest infection or pulmonary infarction. Do not give large doses of diuretics or nitrates as this will drop systemic pressures and may precipitate acute collapse. Compare chest X-ray to previous films to try to assess if there is radiological evidence of pulmonary oedema. The JVP in patients with cyanotic CHD is typically high and should not be used as a sole marker of heart failure; they need a higher filling pressure to maintain pulmonary blood flow. Give high-flow oxygen by mask. Start antibiotics if there is a clinical suspicion of infection (p156). Give oral diuretics if there is evidence of pulmonary oedema or severe right heart failure; monitor haematocrit and renal function closely for signs of over-diuresis.
- **Effort syncope** should prompt a search for arrhythmias (Holter monitor for VT), severe valve disease or signs of overt heart failure. Treat as above.
- **Chest pain** may be secondary to pulmonary embolism or infarction (spontaneous thrombosis), pneumonia, ischaemic heart disease, or musculoskeletal causes. It requires careful evaluation and VQ scan if there is a strong possibility of PE.

2 Respiratory emergencies

Acute pneumonia: Assessment

Presentation

- Classically: Cough (productive or non-productive), fever, breathlessness, chest pain, abnormal CXR.
- All of these may be absent, particularly in the elderly, where confusion may be main symptom.
- Prodromal symptoms of coryza, headache, muscle aches, particularly with atypical pneumonias.
- Immunocompromised patients may present with agitation, fever, tachypnoea, decreased routine oximetry readings. CXR abnormalities may be subtle.
- Patients with right-sided endocarditis (e.g. iv drug-users) may present with haemoptysis, fever, patchy consolidation ± cavitation.

Markers of severe pneumonia

- Tachypnoea ≥ 30 / minute
- Diastolic bp ≤ 60mmHg
- Age ≥ 60 years
- Confusion
- Multi-lobar involvement
- Atrial fibrillation
- Hypoxia $P_aO_2 \leq 8$kPa on air
- Albumin < 35g/l
- WCC ≤ 4 or $\geq 20 \times 10^9$/l
- Bacteraemia
- Serum urea > 7mmol/l
- Underlying disease (cancer, ischaemic heart disease, etc.).

Patients with 2 or more of these features should be admitted to ITU or HDU and observed carefully for any signs of deterioration.

Management

General resuscitation and investigations

- Check the '*ABC*' (airway, breathing and circulation). Treat shock if present (p206).
- *Secure venous access:* If there are signs of dehydration, start iv crystalloids; examine regularly for signs of fluid overload.
- Check *ABG*: Correct hypoxia ($P_aO_2 \leq 10$kPa) with *oxygen*, at least 35%. If hypoxia fails to correct or there is hypercapnoea ($P_aCO_2 \geq 6$kPa) the patient is likely to require ventilation.
- Arrange for *urgent CXR*.
- *Culture blood and sputum:* Urgent sputum microscopy with Gram-stain is occasionally useful but should not be relied upon routinely.
- *Pain relief:* Paracetamol or a NSAID usually suffice. Morphine may be required; respiratory depression is unlikely to be a problem if the P_aCO_2 is low or normal, and it may be reversed with naloxone.

Indications for intensive care

- Shock (systolic bp < 90mmHg or 40mmHg fall from baseline, oliguria, signs of cerebral hypoperfusion) not responding to therapy.
- Respiratory failure ($P_aO_2 \leq 8$kPa $\pm P_aCO_2 \geq 6$kPa).
- Significant acidosis (pH ≤ 7.25, base excess < -8).
- Progressive exhaustion.

Who may be discharged from A&E ?

- Have a low threshold for admission.
- If patient is young, well, no markers of severe pneumonia, with a single lobe involved on CXR and no complications (e.g. cavitation or effusion) then consider discharge from A&E. Arrange for early out-patient review (2–3 days).

Acute pneumonia

Causes of acute pneumonia
(Causative organism not identified in 20–40% of cases)

Community-acquired
- Strep. pneumoniae (60%)
- H. influenzae (5%)
- Staph. aureus (< 5%) (more if influenza epidemic)
- Gram -ve bacteria/anaerobes (commoner with aspiration and in immunocompromised patients)
- Viruses: herpes zoster, influenza, parainfluenza,
- Tuberculosis

Hospital-acquired
- Predominantly Gram-negative enteric species
- Pseudomonas aeruginosa if mechanically ventilated
- Anaerobes

'Atypicals'
- Mycoplasma pneumoniae (< 20%) (more during epidemics)
- Legionella pneumophila (< 5%)
- *Chlamydia* species
- Coxiella burnetii (rare)

Immunocompromised
- All the above
- Also PCP, viral and fungal causes (see p256)

Acute pneumonia: Investigations

Investigations

All patients should have:

154
- Arterial blood gases (on air and oxygen)
- FBC, U&Es, liver function tests
- ESR, CRP
- ECG
- Chest X-ray (see figure below)
- Blood cultures
- Sputum culture, Gram stain, ZN stain, cytology
- Serology (acute and convalescent)
- Cold agglutinins (Mycoplasma day 7–14)
- RMAT (*Legionella* antigen test)

Diffuse infiltrates

Acute
  PCP
  Vital (e.g. CMV)
  Drug reaction
    Cyclophosphamide
    bleomycin
    busulfan
  Alveolar haemorrhage

Chronic
  TB or atypical
  mycobacteria
  Fungi
  Lymphangitis
  carcinomatosa
  Drug (Amiodarone)

Cavitation

Fungi
Anaerobic infection
Staph. aureus
Tuberculosis
Gram-ve bacteria
Malignancy

Pleural effusion (see p198)
  Reactive (sterile)
  Tuberculosis
  Empyema

Focal infiltrates

Acute
  Pneumococcus
  Staphylococci
  Legionella
  Klebsiella
  Gram negatives
  Mycoplasma
  [Pulmonary embolus]

Chronic
  Tuberculosis
  Fungi
  [Malignancy]

Patterns of shadowing on CXR in pneumonia

Where appropriate consider:
- Bronchoscopy (± BAL)
- ECHO (?right heart endocarditis p96)
- VQ scan
- Transbronchial or open lung biopsy
- Aspiration of pleural fluid for MC& S
- Viral titres

Acute pneumonia: Management

Treatment

- 'Blind' treatment should be started as soon as appropriate cultures have been sent (see table opposite). Modify therapy in the light of subsequent investigations or positive cultures.
- Start on iv therapy for at least 48 hours; adjust according to clinical condition and response (see table opposite).
- Consider treatment with salbutamol (2.5–5mg nebulized q4–6h) ± aminophylline (p167) to relieve bronchospasm, 'loosen secretions' and improve mucocilliary action.
- Continue iv fluids as necessary to keep the patient well hydrated.
- *Monitor response to therapy with:-*
  - FBC, CRP.
  - Pulse oximetry or blood gases.
  - CXR at day 3–5 (sooner if deteriorating).
- Total duration of therapy usually 10 days.
- Follow-up CXR 4–6 weeks after discharge mandatory, to exclude an underlying endobronchial lesion.

Choice of antibiotics

In severely ill patients, the history may point to a likely pathogen:-

Previous COAD	*S. pneumoniae*, *H. influenzae*, *B. catarrhalis*
Alcoholism	*S. pneumoniae*, *S. aureus*, *H. influenzae*, *Klebsiella*, TB
Recent 'flu'	*S. aureus*, *S. pneumoniae*, *H. influenzae*
Risk of aspiration	Anaerobes, Gram -ve bacteria
Contact with birds	*C. psittaci*
'Typical' onset	*S. pneumoniae*, *S. aureus*, *H. influenzae*, *Legionella*, Gram -ve bacteria
Sub-acute onset	Mycoplasma, *Legionella*, *C. burnetti* (Q fever, abattoir workers)
Haemoptysis	Streptococci, *S. aureus*, lung abscess, necrotizing Gram -ve bacteria, invasive aspergillosis
Diarrhoea, abdominal pain	*Legionella*
Pharyngitis/obits media	Mycoplasma Anaemia/Cold agglutinins
Risk factors for HIV	*S. pneumoniae*, *H. influenzae*, CMV, PCP, *Cryptococcus*
Hospital acquired	Gram -ve bacteria, *S. aureus*
Neutropenia	*P. aeruginosa*, Gram -ve bacteria, *Aspergillus*
Drug addicts	*S. aureus*, *Candida*

'Blind' treatment of Pneumonia[†]

Community-acquired pneumonia ± 'atypical' features	Cefuroxime (or Amoxycillin) + Erythromycin
Hospital-acquired pneumonia	Cefotaxime (or Ceftazidime) ± Metronidazole
Post influenza pneumonia (*Staph. aureus* possible)	Cefuroxime + Erythromycin + Flucloxacillin (or Vancomycin)
Aspiration pneumonia	Cefuroxime + Metronidazole or Benzyl penicillin + Gentamicin + Metronidazole
Patient with risk factors for HIV	Cefuroxime + Co-trimoxazole
Severe pneumonia	Cefotaxime + Flucloxacillin

[†] In patients with a good history of **penicillin allergy** (anaphylaxis, urticaria) alternatives include erythromycin, rifampicin; alternatives for flucloxacillin include vancomycin and teicoplanin – consult BNF for dosages.

Suggested antibiotic dosages

Amoxycillin	500mg – 1g iv tds
Benzyl penicillin	1.2–2.4g iv qds
Cefuroxime	750mg – 1.5g iv tds
Cefotaxime	1–2g iv tds
Ceftazidime	1–2g iv tds
Co-amoxiclav	1.2g iv tds
Co-trimoxazole	5mg/kg q6h of trimethoprim component
Erythromycin	500mg-1g iv (or po) qds
Flucloxacillin	1–2g iv qds
Gentamicin	loading dose (100–120mg iv) then 2.5mg/kg q8–12h guided by levels
Metronidazole	500mg iv tds
Vancomycin	1g iv bd guided by levels

Note: iv erythromycin causes severe phlebitis. Use central line if available or change to oral preparation after 2–3 days. Clarithromycin is an alternative to erythromycin.

Acute pneumonia: Specific situations

Community-acquired pneumonia

- Either **cefuroxime** 750mg-1.5g iv q8h or **amoxycillin** 1g iv q8h *plus* **erythromycin** 500mg-1g po/iv q6h to cover atypicals *plus* **flucloxacillin** 1–2g iv q6h if *Staph. aureus* is suspected.
- *Penicillin allergy*: Cephalosporins are usually safe where there is a history of rashes with penicillin. If there is history of anaphylaxis consider erythromycin 1g iv qds as sole therapy, or if unwell seek respiratory/microbiological advice.

Aspiration pneumonia

- Risk factors include seizures, reduced conscious level, stroke, dysphagia, periodontal disease, 'down-and-out', general anaesthesia. Always admit.
- Clinical features include wheeze and frothy non-purulent sputum (as soon as 2–4 hours after aspiration), tachypnoea, cyanosis and respiratory distress.
- Gastric acid destroys alveoli resulting in increased capillary permeability and pulmonary oedema. Haemorrhage is common. Severe necrotizing pneumonia may result.

Treatment

- **Cefuroxime** (as above) + **Metronidazole** (500mg iv q8h)
- Amoxycillin + Metronidazole + Gentamicin

Hospital-acquired pneumonia

- Most likely organisms are enteric Gram negative ± anaerobes.
- **Treatment:** Broad spectrum cephalosporin (e.g. **cefotaxime** 2g tds iv), ± **metronidazole** (500mg iv tds). If intubated ≥ 48 hours use antipseudomonal antibiotic (e.g. **ceftazidime** 2g tds, modify dose in renal failure).

Pneumonia in the immunocompromised (see p256 also)

- All 'routine' pathogens are possible; other infections depend on the nature of immunosuppression. TB and atypical mycobacteria are more common and must be considered.
- In **AIDS** the most common opportunistic infection is *Pneumocystis carinii* (see p261). Desaturation on exercise in the presence of a normal CXR or one with a diffuse interstitial shadowing is highly suggestive of PCP. *Fungal* and *viral* pneumonitides may also occur. The CXR may be abnormal secondary to *Kaposi's sarcoma* or *lymphoma*.
- Recipients of **organ transplants** have depressed cell-mediated immunity due to anti-rejection immunosuppressive therapy (p586). Additional pathogens to which they are susceptible include *PCP*, *viruses* (e.g. CMV, RSV, *Influenza* and *Parainfluenza*, adenovirus), and *fungi* (*Aspergillus* spp., *Candida* spp.). The CXR abnormalities tend not to be specific for the pathogen.
- In general, early bronchoscopy and bronchoalveolar lavage is indicated for diagnosis, management should be discussed early with a respiratory/infectious disease/or microbiology team.

Acute pneumonia: Complications

Community-acquired pneumonia that fails to respond

- Review the diagnosis (?PE, pulmonary oedema, pulmonary vasculitis, alveolar haemorrhage, cavitation).
- Repeat CXR and arrange for CT chest to look for cavitation or empyema. Consider possible resistant organism, or underlying disease, e.g. bronchial carcinoma.
- Consider bronchoscopy to exclude TB, PCP, or an obstructing lesion.
- Review antibiotic dosages and intensify (e.g. inadequate oral erythromycin for *Mycoplasma* pneumonia)

Pleural effusion or empyema

- *Relatively common.*
- *Diagnostic tap* should be performed to exclude empyema or TB, especially if it fails to resolve or increases in size over 1–2 days, occupies more than 10% of hemithorax, or is associated with persistent fever.
- Ultrasound should be used to mark the level of the effusion prior to aspiration, as underlying collapse may cause elevation of the hemidiaphragm.
- If turbid fluid or culture/ ZN positive refer to respiratory physician, discuss with cardiothoracic surgeons (see p200).

Cavitation or abscess

- Any severe pneumonia may cavitate, but particularly *Staph. aureus*, *Klebsiella* spp., TB, aspiration pneumonia, bronchial obstruction (foreign body, tumour) or pulmonary emboli (thrombus or septic emboli, e.g. from DVT with super-added infection or tricuspid endocarditis, p96).

Treatment:

- Seek advice from respiratory team. Surgical drainage or CT-guided percutaneous aspiration may be necessary.
- **Cefuroxime** 1.5g tds iv (or **cefotaxime** 2g tds iv)
  + **flucloxacillin** 1–2g qds iv
  + **gentamicin** loading dose (100–120mg iv) then 2.5mg/kg bd iv (according to renal function and levels)
  ± **metronidazole**.
- Long-term antibiotics (4–6 weeks) likely to be required.

Other complications

- Respiratory failure   p178
- Rhabdomyolysis   p294
- DIC (especially *Legionella*)   p560

Mycoplasma pneumonia

- Disease of young adults. Low grade fever, dry cough, headache, and myalgia. Erythema multiforme may be seen in ~ 25%. ~ 5% have a meningoencephalitis.

- WCC is often normal, ESR is high, specific IgM is seen early then levels decline. ~ 50% develop cold agglutinins (also seen in measles, EBV) which may cause haemolysis. CXR usually shows reticulonodular shadowing (lower lobe > upper lobe) which takes over 6 weeks to resolve (unlike bacterial pneumonia).
- Treatment is with **erythromycin, clarithromycin or tetracycline** .

Legionella pneumonia

- Illness of middle-aged men; more severe in smokers. Incubation 2–10 days followed by high fever, rigors, headache, myalgia, dry cough, progressive respiratory distress and confusion. Abdominal pain, diarrhoea, nausea and vomiting and palpable hepatomegaly are seen in ~ 30%. Complications include pericarditis (± effusion), encephalopathy (CSF is usually normal) and rarely renal failure.
- Moderate leukocytosis ($\leq 20 \times 10^9$/l, neutrophilia, lymphopenia), hyponatraemia, deranged LFTs, proteinuria, haematuria, and myoglobinuria. Diagnosis: rise in specific IgM and IgG titres.
- CXR may show anything from diffuse patchy infiltrates to lobar or segmental changes and usually deteriorates in spite of treatment. Pleural effusions are seen in ~ 50%.
- Treatment is with **erythromycin** 1g iv q6h. Continue therapy for 14–21 days (switching to po once fever settles). Add **rifampicin** (600mg po bd) if symptoms do not settle within 72 hours.
- *Pontiac fever*: a self-limiting (2–5 days), acute, non-pneumonic *Legionella* infection with high fever, rigors, myalgia, headache and tracheobronchitis.

Psittacosis

- *Chlamydia psittaci* produces fever, cough, myalgia, and, in severe cases, delirium (psittacosis). Complications include pericarditis, myocarditis and hepatosplenomegaly. Diagnosis is by serology.
- Treat with tetracycline 500mg po qds for 2–3 weeks.

Viral pneumonia

- Clinical features resemble *Mycoplasma* pneumonia (see above). Diagnosis is by 4 × increase in specific antibody titres.
- **CMV** Commonest viral infection in AIDS and following solid organ or bone marrow transplantation, presenting as fever, dry cough, and progressive respiratory distress with hypoxia and bilateral crackles. CXR shows diffuse infiltrates; a miliary pattern is associated with rapid progression and poor outcome whereas an interstitial pattern has a better prognosis. Treat with ganciclovir 5mg/kg iv q12h for 2–3 weeks (see p588).
- **Coxsackie** and **Echovirus**. Titres often rise in 'epidemic pleurodynia' (Bornholm's disease) – a self-limiting illness with chest pain exacerbated by coughing and deep breathing, myalgia and muscle tenderness. Treatment: analgesia (paracetamol, NSAIDs).

- **Varicella** pneumonia. More common in smokers and immuno-suppressed patients. All patients with varicella pneumonitis should be treated with acyclovir 10mg/kg iv 8 hourly. **163**

Miscellaneous conditions

- *Extrinsic allergic alveolitis* may mimic viral pneumonia and present as breathlessness, dry cough, myalgia and fever with neutrophilia (eosinophils usually normal acutely) and patchy radiographic changes. There is usually a history of exposure to the allergen and serum precipitins are detectable. BAL shows predominance of mast cells and lymphocytes. Treatment is with steroids.

- Purulent sputum without organisms may be due to **allergic broncho-pulmonary aspergillosis** with eosinophils in the sputum. It typically presents with bronchospasm but continuing inflammation results in proximal bronchiectasis, upper lobe fibrosis and occasionally with lobar collapse due to impacted mucus plugs. Suspect in asthmatics with lung shadows on the CXR and peripheral eosinophilia. Skin-prick testing is usually positive and serum precipitins (and IgE) are positive. Treatment is with steroids.[1]

---

[1] Oxford Testbook of Medicine (3rd Ed) Ch. 17, p. 2734.

Acute asthma: Assessment

Presentation

- The classical triad is **wheeze**, **breathlessness**, and **cough**. Pleuritic pain may be due to diaphragmatic stretch.
- Two sub-groups of patients can be identified:-
  - Patients with gradually deteriorating asthma who present with exhaustion from the effort of breathing.
  - Patients with acute, severe bronchospasm on a background of 'brittle' asthma.
- Acute attacks may build up over minutes, hours, or days and the patients may deteriorate very rapidly and present as respiratory or cardiorespiratory arrest

Precipitants

- Exposure to known allergen or irritant (e.g. pollens, animals, dusts, cigarette smoke)
- Upper respiratory tract infection (commonly viral)
- Chest infection: viral or bacterial
- Neglect of medications: omitting regular inhaled or oral steroids, +/- overuse of β-agonists
- Emotional stress
- Cold air or exercise-induced asthma
- No clear precipitating cause can be identified in over 30% of patients.

Markers of severity

- The features of life-threatening asthma are shown in the table opposite.
- The severity of an attack may be easily underestimated. Assess:-
  1 The degree of airflow obstruction.
  2 The effect of increased work of breathing on the patient.
  3 The extent of ventilation – perfusion mismatch.
  4 Any evidence of ventilatory failure.

[Patients with marked 'morning dips' in PEFR are at risk of sudden, severe attacks]

Investigations

- **ABG**   Hypoxaemia on room air is almost invariable. In attempting to maintain alveolar ventilation initially there is hypocapnoea and respiratory alkalosis.

  $\uparrow P_aCO_2$ suggests incipient respiratory failure.

  Poorly controlled asthma over several days may be recognized by a mild 'non-anion gap' acidosis (serum bicarbonate 20–24mmol/l).

  Lactic acidosis is seen with severe asthma.

- **Pulse oximetry**   Continuous oximetry is essential.
- **Chest X-ray**   Exclude pneumothorax and to diagnose any parenchymal infection.
- **ECG**   Usually normal; in severe asthmatics signs of right heart strain may be present.
- **FBC and U&Es**   Replace K^+ as necessary.

Features of severe, life-threatening asthma

1 *Severe airflow obstruction*
   - Too breathless to complete sentences in one breath
   - Peak expiratory flow rate (PEFR) $\leq$ 200 l/min (or < 33% of patient's known best PEFR)
   - Very soft breath sounds or 'silent chest'

2 *Increased work of breathing and haemodynamic stress*
   - Respiratory rate $\geq$ 25 breaths per minute
   - Use of accessory respiratory muscles
   - Tachycardia: heart rate $\geq$ 120 beats per minute
   - Systolic bp < 100mmHg
   - Pulsus paradoxus > 10mmHg (this is an unreliable sign)

3 *Ventilation-perfusion mismatch*
   - Hypoxia (P_aO_2 < 8kPa (60mmHg) irrespective of F_iO_2)

4 *Ventilatory failure*
   - Normal (4.5–6kPa) or rising P_aCO_2 in a breathless asthmatic
   - Distress, exhaustion, confusion, obtundation and depressed level of consciousness

Admission is mandatory if ANY of the markers of severe or life-threatening asthma are present.

Acute severe asthma: Immediate therapy

Priorities are:-

1 Treat hypoxia
2 Treat bronchospasm and inflammation
3 Assess the need for intensive care
4 Treat any underlying cause if present

- Patients may deteriorate rapidly and should not be left unattended.
- Details of recent use of bronchodilators must be obtained, if possible including aerosol sympathomimetics and theophylline preparations.
- *Remain calm:* reassurance is important in reducing the patient's anxiety which may further increase respiratory effort.

Severe or life-threatening attack

1 *Initial treatment*

- Sit the patient up in bed.
- **Oxygen** – the highest percentage available, ideally at least 60% or 15l/min. CO_2 retention is not a problem.
- Give a **nebulized β_2-agonist**: either salbutamol 5mg or terbutaline 10mg, administered via oxygen and repeat up to every 30 minutes.
- Add **ipratropium bromide** 0.5mg to nebulizer with β_2-agonist if patient is over 35 years.
- Obtain iv **access.**
- Start **steroids**: 200mg of hydrocortisone intravenously. (Steroids should still be used in pregnant women as the risk of fetal anoxia from the asthma is high.)
- **Antibiotics** should be given if there is evidence of chest infection (purulent sputum, abnormal CXR, raised WCC, fever). Yellow sputum may just be due to eosinophils and a raised WCC may be due to steroids. See p157 for choice of antibiotics.
- **Adequate hydration** is essential and may help prevent mucus plugging. Ensure an intake (iv or po) of 2–3 l/day, taking care to avoid overload. Supplement potassium as required.

2 *Monitoring progress*

- Pre and post nebulizer peak flows.
- Repeated arterial blood gases 1–2 hourly or according to response especially if $S_aO_2 < 93\%$.

3 *If response to above treatment not brisk or if the patient's condition is deteriorating*

- Continue oxygen and nebulized β_2-agonist up to 1/2 hourly.
- Start an iv **salbutamol infusion**: (see table opposite)
- Start an iv **aminophylline infusion**: (see table opposite)
- **Summon anaesthetic help**

Indications for admission to intensive care unit
1 Hypoxia ($P_aO_2 < 8$kPa (60mmHg) despite F_iO_2 of 60%
2 Rising P_aCO_2 or $P_aCO_2 > 6$kPa (45mmHg)
3 Exhaustion, drowsiness or coma
4 Respiratory arrest
5 Failure to improve despite maximal therapy

Intravenous bronchodilators for asthma		
Salbutamol	*Loading dose:* 100–300μg over 10 minutes	
	Maintenance infusion 5–20μg/min.	
	(5mg in 500ml saline at 1–3ml/min)	

Side-effects: Tremor, tachycardia, hypokalaemia, hyperglycaemia common. Lactic acidosis may occur and responds within hours to reduction in salbutamol infusion rate.

Aminophylline	*Loading dose* 250mg (4–5mg/kg) iv over 20 min.
	Maintenance infusion 0.5–0.9mg/kg/h
	(250mg in 1 litre N saline at 2–4ml/kg/h)

Do NOT give the loading dose if the patient is on oral theophyllines without checking an urgent level. Halve the dose in patients with cirrhosis, CCF, or those receiving erythromycin, cimetidine or ciprofloxacin.

Monitor levels every 24 hours (aim for levels of 10–20mg/l).

Acute severe asthma: Further management

- **Adrenaline** may be given sub-cutaneously 0.1mg, repeated if necessary 2 or 3 times at 30 minute intervals. Nebulised adrenaline (0.1 – 0.3mg) is also effective. (In additional to its β_2 effects, it may cause vaso-constriction and mucosal shrinkage via α-receptors.)
- **Cautious CPAP** may help reduce the work of breathing in patients with respiratory muscle fatigue but may not increase the functional residual capacity further. Ideally a device such as the BiPAP with adjustable inspiratory and expiratory pressure support would be better (see p802) and may help avoid mechanical ventilation
- **Ketamine** (a dissociative anaesthetic agent) may be useful in ventil-ated patients (1–3mg/min) probably by increasing circulating catechol-amines by blocking uptake into adrenergic nerve endings.
- **Inhalational anaesthetic agents** (e.g. halothane, enflurane, isoflurane) have been reported to improve bronchospasm and may be useful when initiating ventilation.
- **Mechanical ventilation** may be life-saving but has a high risk of com-plications and an overall mortality of ~ 13%. Barotrauma is seen in ~ 14% (e.g. pneumothorax, pneumomediastinum or subcutaneous emphysema) and hypotension in ~ 38% – usually a combination of increased intrathoracic pressure, intravascular fluid depletion due to dehydration, and dilating effects of anaesthetic agents. Seek expert advice from your intensive care physician for the practical manage-ment of ventilation of the asthmatic patient.

  General principles:-
  - Adequate humidification and warming of inspired gases
  - Low frequency ventilation (6–10 breaths/min)
  - Low tidal volumes (6–10ml/kg)
  - Long expiratory phase of the cycle (I:E ratio 1:3 or longer)
  - Minimize airway pressures (aim for $< 50cmH_2O$, normal < 25)
  - Maintain $P_aO_2 > 8.0kPa$; allow P_aCO_2 to rise provided pH > 7.2
  - Adequate sedation and paralysis to overcome respiratory drive
  - Avoid opiates and atacurium (may release histamine)
  - Consider benzodiazepine, ketamine, vecuronium, isoflurane, etc.

On-going therapy

- Once improvement established continue nebulized β_2–agonist reducing this to 4–hourly and prn after 24 – 48 hours.
- Peak flow rate should be measured before and after each nebulizer. Failure to monitor and record peak flow adequately is negligent.
- Continue nebulized ipratropium bromide 6–hourly until the condition is improving.
- Continue steroids, hydrocortisone 200mg q6h iv continuing as 30–60mg od of oral prednisolone for 10–14 days.
- Monitor intravenous aminophylline levels every 24 hours.
- Monitor serum K^+ daily whilst unwell and supplement as necessary.

Acute severe asthma

Discharge after hospital admission

- The PEFR should be $\geq 75\%$ of best without significant morning dipping (dips $\leq 25\%$ of best), and with no nocturnal symptoms.
- The patient should be established on inhalers with no requirement for nebulizers for 24–48 h prior to discharge. Check inhaler technique.
- Drugs on discharge: ***Prednisolone*** po ≥ 30mg od for 1–3 weeks (plan gradual dose reduction if treatment > 14 days).

     Inhaled corticosteroids at high dose (usually 1000–1500µg beclomethasone via spacer).

     Inhaled prn β-agonist.

     Oral theophyllines if required (confirm drug levels before discharge).
- Provide PEFR meter and chart and arrange follow-up with GP (within one week) and chest clinic (within one month).

Mild-moderate asthmatic attacks

Mild asthmatic attack

No severe features, PEFR $\geq$ 75% of predicted (or of best when well).

- Administer the patient's usual bronchodilator (e.g. 2 puffs salbutamol by metered dose inhaler). Consider adding ipratropium bromide if the patient is over 35 years.
- Observe for 60 minutes. If PEFR remains $\geq$ 75% of predicted value, then discharge.
- Ensure patient is on at least 1000μg inhaled beclomethasone or equivalent per day.
- Advise the patient to get early GP follow-up, monitor PEFR, and return to hospital early if the asthma deteriorates.

Moderate asthmatic attack

No severe features, PEFR 51–75% of predicted (or of best when well)

- Administer nebulized β-agonist (salbutamol 5mg or terbutaline 10mg) and oral prednisolone 30–60mg. Add ipratropium bromide 500μg to nebulizer if over 35 years old.
- Reassess after 30 minutes. If worse or PEFR $\leq$ 50% of predicted then admit and assess as above for severe asthma.
- If PEFR 51–75% predicted then repeat nebulizer and observe for a further 60 minutes.
- The patient may be discharged from A&E if stable after 1–2 nebulizers and PEFR $\geq$ 75%.
- If after 2nd nebulizer and a further 60 minutes observation, the patient is clearly improving and PEFR $\geq$ 60%, then discharge may be considered.
- Discharge on:
  - Oral prednisolone (usual dose 30–40mg od for 7 days),
  - Inhaled corticosteroid ($\geq$ 1000μg/day inhaled beclomethasone)
  - Inhaled β-agonist.
- Advise the patient to seek GP follow-up within 48 hours and to return early to A&E if there is any deterioration
- Consider referral to chest clinic.

Sending people home from A&E

- Mild-moderate exacerbations may be fit to be discharged from A&E.
- If there are any features of severe asthma (see table p165) then admission is mandatory.
- A history of brittle asthma or previous attacks requiring mechanical ventilation is always a requirement for admission.

Acute exacerbation of COAD

Assessment

Presentation

- Progressive dyspnoea usually on background of shortness of breath on exercise, morning cough, wheeze.
- Respiratory failure without dyspnoea ('blue bloaters').
- Wheeze unrelieved or partially relieved by inhalers.
- Increased production of purulent sputum (infective exacerbation).
- Positive smoking history (if not, then late-onset asthma is likely).
- Confusion/ impaired consciousness (exhaustion, CO_2 retention).

Causes

- *Infective exacerbation:* typically *H. influenzae*, *S. pneumoniae*, occasionally *S. viridans*, *Branhamella catarrhalis*, *Mycoplasma*, *Legionella*, or viral.
- *Exposure to known allergen:* illness may be in spectrum with asthma with bronchospasm
- *Pneumothorax* (see p184, differentiate from large bullae).
- *Expansion of large bullae*
- *Sputum retention* with lobar or segmental collapse: following surgery, trauma, sedation, and uncontrolled O_2 administration
- *Left ventricular failure*
- *Pulmonary embolism*
- *Neglect of regular medications*

Investigations

All patients should have:-

- U&Es   Look for dehydration, renal failure. Monitor K^+.
- FBC   Look for leukocytosis or anaemia (patients with COAD often have secondary polycythaemia)
- ABG   To assess degree of respiratory failure and pH.
- Septic screen   Sputum should be sent for culture. Blood cultures, if febrile or CXR changes suggest pneumonia.
- Peak flows   Ask what is normal for patient.
- Chest X-ray   Focal changes suggest pneumonia (see p154)
- ECG   Myocardial ischaemia or arrhythmia

Assessment of severity

- Potential background of fixed airflow obstruction makes absolute markers of severity less easy to determine. In the absence of a smoking history or in the presence of a long history of asthma then assess severity and treat as for acute asthma (p166). See table p165 for markers of severity.
- Try to assess the functional capacity *when well* from patient, relatives, and previous hospital notes, e.g. distance walked on flat, stairs climbed without stopping, frequency of attacks, previous admissions, ever ventilated?, concurrent illnesses (heart disease, renal impairment, liver impairment), etc.

Management

1. Treat hypoxia and respiratory failure
2. Relieve bronchial obstruction and bronchospasm
3. Determine and treat cause of exacerbation

Acute exacerbation of COAD

Acute exacerbation of COAD

Management

1 Treat hypoxia and respiratory failure

- **Commence oxygen therapy** Administer oxygen via ventimask, as nasal cannulae give an unreliable percentage of inspired oxygen depending on patients' tidal volume and respiratory rate.
  - If 'pink puffer' – (thin, not cyanosed, pursed-lip breathing, no signs of CO_2 retention) then commence 35–40% oxygen.
  - If 'blue bloater' – (signs CO_2 retention, obese, cyanosed) commence 28% oxygen until blood gas results known.

- **Arterial blood gases**
  - If patient is not retaining CO_2 ($P_aCO_2 < 6kPa$) and is hypoxic ($P_aO_2 < 10kPa$) then give oxygen 28–40%. Repeat ABGs 30 min later (sooner if consciousness level deteriorates) to ensure correction of hypoxia and exclude rising P_aCO_2.
  - If CO_2 retention is present then use 24–28% oxygen and repeat blood gases after 15–30 minutes. Aim to keep $P_aO_2 \geqslant 8kPa$ and $P_aCO_2 \leqslant 7.5kPa$, but these limits may not be achievable. Balance hypoxia (which may be fatal) against consciousness level and respiratory effort.

- **Mechanical ventilation** This is the treatment of choice for respiratory failure (see p804). For patients in whom immediate ventilation is either impractical or contraindicated (because of poor respiratory reserve), a respiratory stimulant may be tried.

- **Respiratory stimulants** May be used for patients in whom mechanical ventilation is contraindicated. This measure is rarely successful for more than a few hours and rarely influences prognosis. Doxapram is no substitute for ventilation in an appropriate patient (e.g. Bromptonpac or BiPAP, see p802).

Doxapram infusion for respiratory failure

- Doxapram hydrochloride (*Dopram*®) 500ml bottle contains 2mg/ml in 5% glucose.
- Start infusion at 1ml/min (2mg/min). Increase infusion by 0.2–0.4ml/min steps every hour, to max. 2ml/min, until improvement is established.
- Monitor ABG and respiratory rate hourly.
- Side-effects include agitation and confusion, tachycardia, hypertension, sweating, nausea, and vomiting.

An alternative regime for post operative respiratory depression or to temporize until mechanical ventilation is established:-

- Slow iv bolus (over 30s–1min) 1.5mg/kg, repeated at hourly intervals, guided by response.

---

2 Treat bronchospasm and obstruction

- Patients with COAD may have relatively fixed bronchospasm, but where the patient is very unwell then consider iv aminophylline and/or iv β-agonists as for severe asthma (p167).
- *Nebulized β-agonists* (salbutamol 5mg or terbutaline 10mg. q4h and prn) via oxygen or air if CO_2 retaining. (If patient is very hypoxic, give 2 l/min oxygen via nasal cannulae whilst nebulizer in progress.)
- Include *nebulized ipratropium bromide* 500µg 6 hourly.
- Give *steroids:* 200mg hydrocortisone iv or 30–40mg prednisolone po.
- Urgent physiotherapy may help clearing bronchial secretions.

Acute exacerbation of COAD

Mechanical ventilation

- COAD per se is not a contraindication to ventilation in appropriately selected patients. Ventilation should be considered where respiratory failure ($P_aO_2 \leq 8kPa$) with or without hypercapnoea, particularly where failure is acute.
- Consider whether non-invasive measures such as NIPPV, Bromptonpac or BiPAP (see p802) are available and would prevent the need for formal endotracheal intubation.
- Discuss with a senior colleague prior to intubation.

In favour of ventilation

- Acute respiratory failure (normal bicarbonate, acute history).
- Relatively young patient.
- Obvious remediable cause (e.g. pneumonia).
- Good recent exercise tolerance and quality of life.
- Not previously known to retain CO_2 when well.

Against ventilation

- Relatively old.
- Previous difficulty weaning from ventilator.
- On maximal therapy at home (home nebulizer, long-term oxygen therapy).
- Poor quality of life or poor exercise tolerance.

- Patients who are chronically hypoxic or CO_2 retainers will tolerate poor blood gases better than those patients with other causes of respiratory failure.
- When ventilating patients with COAD it is vital to remember that achieving a 'normal' P_aCO_2 and P_aO_2 may not be appropriate. In those who are chronically hypoxic or who chronically retain CO_2 (as evidenced by previous abnormal gases or a raised bicarbonate with a normal or near-normal pH) then they are unlikely to breath spontaneously or wean from the ventilator unless their blood gases are allowed to mirror what is probably their chronic state. Thus a 'blue bloater' may need a P_aCO_2 of 6–7.5kPa +/- mild hypoxia even on the ventilator to achieve successful weaning.

Treat cause of exacerbation

Infective exacerbation

- Suggested by purulent sputum or increase in sputum production.
- For lobar consolidation or bronchial pneumonia follow guidelines on p156. Otherwise treat with *amoxycillin* 500mg-1g tds po/iv; if unwell or failure to respond treat with *cefuroxime* 750mg tds iv for improved cover of resistant *Haemophilus* sp.
- Follow local protocols.

Pneumothorax (unless very small, consider aspiration ± drain, p184).

Pulmonary oedema p74.

Pulmonary embolism p110.

Acute exacerbation of COAD

Respiratory failure: Assessment

Respiratory failure is present when gas exchange becomes significantly impaired. Clinically, it is not possible to predict the P_aO_2 or P_aCO_2 and so this diagnosis relies on ABG. Respiratory failure may be divided into:-

Type 1: Hypoxia $P_aO_2 \leqslant 8kPa$ on air or oxygen with normal or low P_aCO_2 (i.e. mainly ventilation-perfusion mismatch).

Type 2: Hypoxia $P_aO_2 \leqslant 8kPa$ on air or oxygen with raised P_aCO_2 ($> 6kPa$) (i.e. predominantly alveolar hypoventilation).

In practice, both types may co-exist.

Presentation

- *Shortness of breath* is the commonest presentation. Ask about the speed of onset (sudden onset may suggest pneumothorax, pulmonary embolus, or cardiac failure).
- Respiratory failure may present without dyspnoea, particularly exacerbations of COAD in 'blue bloaters', and non-respiratory causes such as Guillain-Barré syndrome (p408) or drug overdose. Neuro-muscular respiratory failure is discussed on p398.
- *Confusion* may be the sole presentation in the elderly.

The history may point to the cause of respiratory failure.

- History of asthma/chronic bronchitis and smoking.
- Sputum production and fevers (pneumonia).
- Swollen legs due to the development of cor pulmonale (right ventricular failure) in patients with chronic lung disease.
- Haemoptysis (pneumonia, PE).
- Cardiac history including palpitations and/or chest pain.
- Try to assess the functional capacity when well, e.g. distance walked on flat, stairs climbed without stopping, frequency of attacks, previous admissions, ever ventilated?, concurrent illnesses (heart disease, renal impairment, liver impairment), etc.
- Drug and/or overdose history.
- History of DM (incl. recent polyuria/polydipsia) or renal disease.
- Neurological symptoms including painful legs and paraesthesiae (Guillain-Barré syndrome).
- Allergies.

Physical examination

- Listen to the breathing (stridor, wheeze, coarse crackles)
- Look for wheeze [airflow limitation, either localized (local obstruction] or generalized (e.g. asthma, COAD, pulmonary oedema), coarse crackles (infection or pulmonary oedema), bronchial breathing (indicates consolidation or collapse, but may also occur with fibrosis or above a pleural effusion), signs of pneumothorax (hyperesonance, decreased breath sounds), or pleural effusion (stony dull, decreased breath sounds).
- Palpate the upper chest and neck for crepitus (pneumothorax or pneumomediastinum).
- Look for signs of a DVT (swollen, hot leg ± pain, see p106).

Causes of respiratory failure	
Common	*Rarer causes*

Common
- Asthma (p164).
- Infective exacerbation of COAD, kyphoscoliosis, or pulmonary fibrosis.
- Left ventricular failure or tachyarrhythmias (p74).
- Pneumonia (p152).
- Pleural effusion (p198).
- Pneumothorax (p110).
- Pulmonary embolus (p110).
- Metabolic acidosis (renal, ketoacidosis, aspirin) (p430).
- ARDS (usually in-patient) rarely presents via A&E (p188).
- Respiratory depression via drugs e.g. opiates (p660).

Rarer causes
- Atelectasis (tumour or infection)
- Acute interstitial pneumonitis
- Airway obstruction (foreign body, tumour, epiglottitis) (p202).
- Chest trauma.
- Guillain-Barré syndrome (p408).
- Poliomyelitis.
- Anaphylaxis (p212).

Respiratory failure: Investigations

Urgent investigations

- ABG   On air immediately, or if very unwell whilst on oxygen (remember to note F_iO_2)
- Chest X-ray   (see figure below)
- ECG   Look for signs of PE (S_1 Q_3 T_3, p112), tachy-arrhythmias, or myocardial ischaemia.
- Blood tests   FBC (anaemia, leukocytosis), U&Es, glucose.
- Inspect sputum   Yellow, green, mucoid, streaky, or frank blood.
- FEV_1 and FVC   Especially for Guillain-Barré syndrome (p408).
- Septic screen   Sputum culture, blood cultures if febrile or if CXR suggests infection.

Where indicated consider:-

- Aspirin and paracetamol levels.
- Plasma and urine for toxicology.
- Urinalysis for glucose and ketones.
- Examine the CXR systematically for any abnormality.

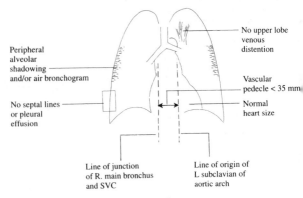

CXR in non-cardiogenic pumonary oedema
(sensitivity 80–90%: peripheral shadowing is the most reliable sign) (after Flenley DC (1971) *Lancet* I 270–3)

Chest X-ray This should be examined systematically for:-
- Pneumothorax (distinguish from large bullae).
- Consolidation (lobar or patchy, presence of an air-bronchogram due to pneumonia, see p154).
- Pulmonary oedema ('bats wing'/peri-hilar appearance, upper lobe blood diversion, Kerley-B lines in peripheral lung fields).
- Pleural effusion.
- Bronchogenic tumour.
- Oligaemia, and wedge infarcts ± small effusion (PE).
- Trauma/ rib fractures.

Respiratory failure: Management

(see p398 for neuromuscular respiratory failure)

(see p398 for neuromuscular respiratory failure)

The severity of respiratory failure depends upon response to oxygen. Failure of hypoxia to correct on 40–60% oxygen or progressive hypercapnoea implies that total respiratory failure necessitating pressure or mechanical support is present or imminent.

Poor prognostic signs on presentation include:

- Inability to speak due to dyspnoea.
- Respiratory rate (resp. rate > 40).
- Reduced peak flow $\leq$ 75% of predicted (typically < 150 in an adult).
- Tachycardia HR $\geq$ 100 or bradycardia HR $\leq$ 60.
- Exhaustion or coma (ventilatory support is required urgently).
- Stridor (this indicates upper airway obstruction, see p202).
- Pulse oximetry saturation of < 90%
- Shock (tachycardia + hypotension). May indicate tension pneumothorax (p184) or severe LVF (p74).

Hypercapnoea is the end result of many causes of respiratory failure (including asthma and pneumonia), not just COAD. Even if relatively elderly the patient may respond well to ventilation with a satisfactory final outcome depending on the disease and premorbid condition.

Management Priorities are:

1 General resuscitation and relief of hypoxia.
2 Definitive treatment of cause (see table p179).

General resuscitation (ABC)

- Ensure the airway is patent and the mouth is clear.
- If stridor is present request anaesthetic and/or ENT assistance urgently (p202).
- Sit the patient up (unless hypotensive) and administer oxygen at 60% unless there is a history of COAD (use 28% oxygen).
- Ensure that respiratory effort is adequate and effective (measure respiratory rate and assess depth of respiration), use pulse oximetry to monitor the PO_2.
- If the patient is exhausted with a failing respiratory drive, or respiratory failure is severe, call for anaesthetic assistance and consider urgent transfer to ITU.
- In comatose patients with poor respiratory effort consider drug overdose with opiates (pin-point pupils) or benzodiazepines. Give naloxone 200–400µg (2–4µg/kg) iv bolus followed by infusion depending on response (pXX) and/or iv flumazenil (200µg over 15s then 100µg at 60s intervals if required (max. total dose 1mg (2mg if on ITU)].
- Methods of respiratory support are discussed on p800.
- Secure iv access.
- Measure the bp and heart rate, look for signs of cardiac failure (raised JVP, inspiratory crackles, oedema) or the signs of pulmonary embolism (raised JVP, tachycardia, hypotension, normal breath sounds $\pm$ pleural rub).

Indications for intensive care
1. Progressive exhaustion or impaired conscious level
2. Shock not responding rapidly to initial resuscitation
3. Respiratory failure not responding rapidly to initial therapy

Pneumothorax: Assessment

Presentation

The average DGH sees approximately 25 spontaneous pneumothoraces per annum. The commonest presenting symptoms are:-

- **Breathlessness**: usually abrupt in onset. (Young, fit patients may have very little, but patients with chronic airflow limitation or asthma may present with a sudden deterioration)
- **Chest pain**: Dull, central, heavy; or there may be a pleuritic element
- Consider the diagnosis in any in-patient who is:-
  - breathless after an invasive thoracic procedure (e.g. subclavian vein cannulation).
  - increasingly hypoxic or has rising inflation pressures on mechanical ventilation.

Causes

- ***Spontaneous:*** Tall, slender men age 20–40, probably rupture of subpleural blebs at lung apices. 25% will have recurrent episodes (usually ipsilateral).
- ***Secondary to underlying disease:*** Chronic obstructive pulmonary disease, cystic fibrosis, asthma, fibrosing lung disease, sarcoidosis.
- ***Infections:*** Tuberculosis, lung abscess, *Pneumocystis carinii* pneumonia.
- ***Trauma***
- ***Iatrogenic:*** After pleural biopsy or aspiration, transbronchial biopsy, percutaneous lung biopsy, subclavian vein cannulation, mechanical ventilation with high airway pressures.

Investigations – the chest radiograph

- The classical clinical signs may not always be present.
- In the supine patient a pneumothorax may not be easy to see. Look for hyperlucency of one lung field, unusually clear heart border, or a line parallel to the chest wall (caused by retraction of the R middle lobe).
- If patient has COAD and marked bullous disease, take care that the supsected pneumothorax is not, in fact, a large, thin-walled bullus: with a pneumothorax the pleural line is usually convex to the lateral chest wall; with a bullus, the apparent pleural line is usually concave to the lateral chest wall. If there is any doubt, chest CT will be able to distinguish the two.

Assessment of severity (signs of significant pneumothorax)

- ***Tension pneumothorax*** – Mid-line shift away from pneumothorax, raised or obstructed JVP, hypotension, tachycardia, shock.
- ***Size of pneumothorax***: percentages of pneumothorax are hard to estimate; classify the size as small, moderate, or complete pneumothorax on inspiratory CXR
- Small pneumothorax: Small rim of air around lung.
- Moderate pneumothorax: Lung collapsed 50% to heart border.
- Complete pneumothorax: Airless lung, separate from diaphragm.
- ***Hypoxia*** $P_aO_2 \leqslant 10$kPa on air
- ***Severe dyspnoea***

Pneumothorax: Management

The priorities are:-

1 *Does the patient have a tension pneumothorax?*
2 Ensure adequate oxygenation.
3 Determine if the patient requires aspiration or a chest drain.
4 Treat the underlying cause if present: to prevent recurrence.

1 Who to discharge from casualty

- *Small stable spontaneous pneumothorax* (no previous episodes) without significant dyspnoea, age < 40 years and no underlying chronic lung disease.
- *Moderate or complete collapse* with no significant dyspnoea: age < 40 years and no underlying chronic lung disease, or after successful aspiration of pneumothorax on repeat CXR.
- Follow-up in chest clinic in 10–14 days with a repeat CXR.

2 Who to admit for observation

- All patients with pneumothorax secondary to trauma or with underlying lung disease even if aspiration has been successful: discharge after 24 hours if follow-up CXR shows no recurrance.
- Patients in whom aspiration has failed to re-expand the lung fully.
- Give **oxygen** (> 35% unless there is clinical evidence of chronic airflow limitation, when start with 28%, check arterial blood gases). This accelerates the reabsorption of the pneumothorax up to 4-fold. Most of the pneumothorax is N_2 (air) and supplemental O_2 decreases the partial pressure of N_2 in the blood, increasing the gradient for its reabsorption.
- Once the air-leak is sealed, the pneumothorax reabsorbs at a rate of ~ 1.25% of volume of hemithorax per day. A 15% pneumothorax will take approx 3 weeks to reabsorb. Any larger pneumothorax should be aspirated or drained, even if asymptomatic.
- If there is moderate or complete collapse with significant dyspnoea then **aspirate** the pneumothorax (see p814). Small, relatively asymptomatic pneumothoraces do not require aspiration provided there is no underlying lung disease. If the patient is well after a successful aspiration and there is minimal or no pneumothorax on CXR after 24h, the patient can be discharged; follow-up as above.
- **Insert an intercostal drain in patients with:**
  - Significant, symptomatic, residual pneumothorax post aspration.
  - Recurrent pneumothorax < 24 hours after successful aspiration.
  - Patients with haemopneumothorax.
  - All mechanically ventilated patients with a pneumothorax.
  - All patients with a pneumothorax, prior to inter-hospital transfer.

The technique for insertion of an intercostal drain is described on p 816.

- If lung has re-expanded and drain not bubbling, wait 24 hours, repeat CXR to exclude recurrence, and remove drain.
- A collapsed lung and bubbling drain suggests a persistent air-leak and suction may be required. [Use low pressure suction (5kPa) via appropriate pump or modified wall suction: discuss with the chest team].
- A collapsed lung and no bubbling suggests the drain is blocked, displaced, or clamped. If a new drain is required it should be through a new incision.

- Consider pleurodesis in patients with recurrent pneumothoraces, either chemical (talc or tetracycline) or formal thoracotomy with oversewing of apical bullae and scarification of the pleura (persistent air-leak or lung collapse after 5 days of chest drain). Consult the cardiothoracic team.

Tension pneumothorax

Usually seen in patients receiving mehanical ventilation or post CPR. The patient is usually distressed, tachypnoeic with cyanosis and profuse sweating and marked tachycardia and hypotension.
This requires immediate attention.

Management

- Do not leave the patient unattended. Give maximal inspired oxygen to reverse hypoxia.
- Insert an 18G (green) cannula (or the largest available) perpendicular to the chest wall into the 2nd intercostal space in the mid-clavicular line on the side with the pneumothorax on clinical examination (reduced breath sounds and trachea deviated away). Relief should be almost immediate. Leave the cannula in place until air ceases to rush out.
- Improvize an underwater seal using an iv line attached to the cannula and the end held under a bowl of water, until a formal intercostal drain can be set up.
- Insert a chest drain as soon as possible.
- If no air rushes out when the cannula is inserted, the patient does not have a tension pneumothorax and the cannula should be removed.

> There are **NO** indications in the standard management of a pneumothorax for clamping chest drains. If patients are to be moved, keep the drain bottle below chest height but DO NOT CLAMP.

Adult Respiratory Distress Syndrome   1.

Acute lung injury may be caused either directly or follow systemic illness (see table opposite). The lung damage and the products of activated inflammatory cells increase capillary permeability, producing non-cardiogenic pulmonary oedema. This results in hypoxia ($2°$ to V/Q mismatch and shunting), decreased lung compliance, and is usually seen in the setting of multi-organ failure. The mortality is 50–60%.

Diagnostic criteria

- History of one or more risk factors (table opposite).
- Severe defect in oxygenation:

    $P_aO_2 < 8$kPa on room air

    or $P_aO_2 < 8$kPa with $F_iO_2 > 0.4$

    or   Ratio P_aO_2 (kPa) : $F_iO_2 \leq 25$

- Radiological evidence of bilateral pulmonary infiltrates.
- Pulmonary capillary wedge pressure < 15–18mmHg with normal colloid oncotic pressure; (in patients with hypoalbuminaemia, the critical PCWP is approx. serum albumin (g/l) × 0.57, see p80).

Investigations

All patients require:

- CXR
- ABG (insert an arterial line as regular samples will be required).
- Take blood for FBC, U&Es, LFTs and albumin, coagulation, X-match, and CRP.
- Septic screen (culture blood, urine, sputum).
- Pulmonary artery catheter to measure PCWP, cardiac output, mixed venous oxygen saturation and allow calculation of haemodynamic parameters (see pXX).

Other investigations if appropriate.

- ECG.
- CT chest.
- Bronchoalveolar lavage for microbiology and cell count (?eosinophils).
- Serum for drug screen; amylase.
- Carboxyhaemoglobin estimation.

Management[1,2]

Treatment is mainly supportive.

1 Respiratory support to improve gas exchange and correct hypoxia.
2 Cardiovascular support to optimize oxygen delivery to tissues.
3 Reverse or treat the underlying cause.

[1] Kollef MH & Schuster DP (1995) *NEJM* **332:** 27–37.
[2] MacNaughton PD & Evans TE (1992) *Lancet* **339:** 469–72.

Acute respiratory distress syndrome

Disorders associated with the development of ARDS	
Direct lung injury	*Indirect (non-pulmonary) injury*

Direct lung injury

- Aspiration
  Gastric contents
  Near-drowning
- Inhalation injury
  Noxious gases
  Smoke
- Pneumonia
  Any organism
  PCP
- Pulmonary vasculitides
- Pulmonary contusion
- Drug toxicity or overdose
  Oxygen
  Opiate overdose
  Bleomycin
  Salicylates

Indirect (non-pulmonary) injury

- Shock
- Septicaemia
- Amniotic or fat embolism
- Acute pancreatitis
- Massive haemorrhage
- Multiple transfusions
- D.I.C.
- Massive burns
- Major trauma
- Head injury
  Raised ICP
  Intracranial bleed
- Cardiopulmonary bypass
- Acute liver failure

Adult Respiratory Distress Syndrome 2.

Respiratory support

Spontaneously breathing patient

- In the early stages of ARDS the hypoxia may be corrected by 40–60% inspired oxygen with CPAP (see p802).
- Peak inspiratory flow rates of ≥ 70 l/min require a tight-fitting face mask with a large reservoir bag or a high flow generator.
- If the patient is well oxygenated on $\leq 60\%$ inspired oxygen without CO_2 retention and apparently stable, then ward monitoring may be feasible but close observation (q15–30min), continuous oximetry, and regular blood gases are required.
- Indications for mechanical ventilation are:-
  - Inadequate oxygenation ($P_aO_2 < 8$ kPa on $F_iO_2 \geq 0.6$).
  - Rising or elevated P_aCO_2 (≥ 6 kPa).
  - Clinical signs of incipient respiratory failure.

Mechanical ventilation

The aims are to increase P_aO_2 while minimizing the risk of further lung injury (oxygen toxicity, barotrauma). This is the realm of the ITU physician: seek specialist advice early to prevent complications.
The general principles are:-

- Controlled mandatory ventilation (CMV) with sedation and neuromuscular blockade (to try to suppress the respiratory drive and reduce respiratory muscle oxygen requirement).
- Start with $F_iO_2 = 1.0$, tidal volume 6–10ml/kg, PEEP ≤ 5 cmH$_2$O and inspiratory flow rates ~ 60l/min. Subsequent adjustments are done to try to achieve arterial oxygen sats. of > 90% with $F_iO_2 < 0.6$ and peak airway pressures < 40–45cmH$_2$O.
- PEEP improves P_aO_2 in most patients and allows reduction of F_iO_2. Increase by 2–5 cmH2O increments every 20 min watching for haemodynamic deterioration (due to impaired venous return and decreased cardiac output). 'Optimal' PEEP is usually 10–15cmH$_2$O.
- Inverse ratio ventilation (p806) may decrease peak inflation pressures (and thus barotrauma). Inspiratory time:expiratory time ratio (I:E ratio) of between 1:1 and 4:1 may be tried.
- The ventilatory rate required to clear CO_2 and normalize pH is commonly high (20–25 breaths/minute). However, this may result in unacceptable airway pressures. Another strategy is 'permissive hypercapnoea' which, as the name suggests, is controlled hypoventilation. P_aCO_2 up to 13kPa is generally well tolerated; acidosis (pH < 7.25) may be treated with intravenous bicarbonate.
- Changing the patient's position (lateral decubitus or prone instead of supine) can improve oxygenation by improving perfusion of aerated portions of lung. Consider this in patients with non-uniform or predominantly posterior and lower lobe infiltrates.
- Inhaled nitric oxide (18 ppm) reduces pulmonary artery pressures, intrapulmonary shunting, and improves oxygenation while not affecting mean arterial pressure or cardiac output. However, studies showing an effect on mortality are awaited.
- Newer methods such as high-frequency jet ventilation, extracorporeal gas exchange (CO_2 removal $\pm$ oxygenation) and intravascular oxygenation devices (IVOX) may be of use but are currently not widely available (p808).

Acute respiratory distress syndrome

Adult Respiratory Distress Syndrome 3.

Cardiovascular support

- Invasive monitoring is mandatory [arterial line, PA catheter (Swan-Ganz) to measure cardiac outputs, and, if available, continuous mixed venous oxygen saturation].
- In order to minimize pulmonary oedema, aim to keep PCWP low (8–10mmHg) and support the circulation with inotropes if necessary.
- The role of colloids and albumin is relatively minor: the increased capillary permeability allows these molecules to equilibrate with the alveolar fluid with little increase in net plasma oncotic pressure.
- Renal failure is common and may require haemofiltration to achieve a negative fluid balance and normalize blood biochemistry.
- Oxygen consumption (VO_2) in patients with ARDS appears to be delivery dependent. The current trend is to aim for target levels of oxygen delivery (DO_2) as guided by tissue perfusion (clinically and serum lactate, pH_i from a tonometer p838). DO_2 may be increased by blood transfusion, inotropes, and vasodilators (including prostacyclin).
- Selection of appropriate inotropes and vasodilators can only be made by repeated measurements of haemodynamic parameters and calculating DO_2 and VO_2, while evaluating the effects of the various agents.
- Nutritional support must be chosen to try to avoid fluid overload. Lipid metabolism produces marginally less CO_2 than dextrose metabolism and thus favourably affects the respiratory quotient, but there is controversy as to whether lipid can exacerbate lung injury.

Treatment of sepsis

- Fever, neutrophil leukocytosis and raised inflammatory markers (CRP) are common in patients with ARDS and do not always imply sepsis. However, sepsis is a common precipitant of ARDS.
- A trial of empirical antibiotics, guided by possible pathogens, should be given early (e.g. cefotaxime). This may be modified in light of the results of appropriate cultures. Avoid nephrotoxic antibiotics.
- Enteral feeding seems to carry a lower risk of sepsis than parenteral feeding and helps maintain the integrity of the gut mucosa. Ileus is common in multi-organ failure, so entral feeding may not be possible.

Minimizing lung injury and treating the cause

- Look for a precipitant (table opposite).
- In general prevention (e.g. of aspiration of gastric acid) is more effective than trying to treat ARDS. However, there are no effective measures for prophylaxis in patients at risk (e.g. from trauma).
- *Steroids:* There is no benefit from treatment early in the disease. Treatment later (> 7–14 days from onset) (especially in patients with peripheral blood eosinophilia or eosinophils in bronchoalveolar lavage), improves prognosis.
- Give 2–4mg/kg prednisolone (or equivalent); the duration depends on the clinical response (1–3 weeks).
- Other therapies such as inhaled nitric oxide, exogenous surfactant, antioxidants (acetylcysteine), ketoconazole, NSAIDs, pentoxifylline, and anticytokine antibodies are still under investigation.

Acute respiratory distress syndrome

Causes of sudden deterioration in ARDS	
Respiratory	*Cardiovascular*
• Pneumothorax	• Arrhythmia
• Bronchial plugging	• Cardiac tamponade
• Displaced ET tube	• Myocardial infarction
• Pleural effusion (haemothorax)	• GI bleed ('stress' ulcer)
• Aspiration (e.g. NG feed)	• Septicaemia

Haemoptysis: Assessment

Presentation

- Haemoptysis is the coughing up of blood from the lungs or tracheo-bronchial tree (see table opposite).
- Massive haemoptysis is defined as $\geq$ 400mls over 3 hours or $\geq$ 600mls over 24 hours. The common causes of *massive* haemoptysis are bronchiectasis, bronchial carcinoma, infection (e.g. TB, lung abscess, or aspergilloma), or trauma.
- Often, the cause is obvious from the history. Patients with moderate-large bleeds may be able to locate the site of bleeding by a 'gurgling' or 'bubbling' within the chest. Ask specifically for smoking and drug history.
- Examine for an underlying cause (see table opposite) and to assess the haemodynamic and respiratory effects of the bleed.

Poor prognostic factors include:

- Increasing age
- Pre-existing lung or cardiac disease
- Respiratory compromise (rate, cyanosis)
- Hypoxia ($P_aO_2 \leq 10$kPa on air)
- On-going haemoptysis of large amounts of fresh blood
- Shock (postural or supine hypotension – rare)

Initial management

Stabilize the patient

- Massive haemoptysis should usually be managed at a hospital with cardiothoracic surgical back-up, and urgent transfer should be considered if this is not available.
- Give high inspired oxygen.
- Place patient in the recovery position, with the bleeding lung down (if it is known which side the bleeding is from) to try to keep the unaffected lung free of blood.
- If aspiration of blood is threatened, get anaesthetic help urgently; anaesthetize, intubate, and ventilate. A double-lumen endotracheal tube may be used to isolate the lungs but the narrow lumen may make subsequent flexible bronchoscopy difficult.
- Insert a large bore peripheral cannula, followed by a central line if indicated; internal jugular route is preferred to minimize the risk of pneumothorax.
- Support the circulation: Haemoptyses are rarely severe enough to warrant transfusion. If the patient has postural or supine hypotension use intravenous colloid (Haemaccel®, or 4.5% Albumin) until blood is available.
- Monitor the urine output, and consider a renal dose of dopamine (2.5μg/kg/min iv infusion).
- *Investigations* All patients should have the following:
  - Take blood for FBC, U&Es, coagulation studies, X-match
  - Arterial blood gases (on air and 100% oxygen)
  - ECG
  - CXR ($\pm$ lateral)
  - Sputum (microscopy and culture, cytology)
  - Flexible bronchoscopy

Common causes of haemoptysis

Lung disease
- Bronchiectasis ($\pm$ infection)
- Bronchogenic carcinoma
- Infection
  Tuberculosis
  Pneumonia
  Lung abscess
  Aspergilloma
- Bronchitis
- Trauma
- Vasculitis
- AV malformation

Cardiovascular
- Pulmonary embolus
- Left ventricular failure
- Mitral stenosis
- Congenital heart disease
  with pulmonary
  hypertension

Systemic vasculitis
- SLE
- Wegner's
- Goodpasture's
- PAN

Haemoptysis: Further management

Diagnose the source of bleeding

- *Chest X-ray* This should be examined systematically for a mass lesion ± hilar nodes, bronchiectasis (tram-line shadows), old or new tuberculosis (potential cavities for aspergillomas). Look for causes of minor haemoptysis, if this is the current problem.
- *Fibre-optic or rigid bronchoscopy* This should be performed urgently in all cases of massive haemoptysis. This is unlikely to localize the exact source, but may help localize the lung or lobe affected, to guide surgeons or radiologists. An endoscopically positioned balloon may be tried to tamponade the bleeding if massive.
- *Selective pulmonary angiography* can identify the bleeding source in 90% of patients, and, when combined with embolization, is effective in controlling bleeding in up to 90%. Multiple procedures may be necessary
- *High resolution CT chest* may help identify parenchymal lesions and peripheral endobronchial lesions.

Specific therapeutic interventions

- *Correct coagulopathy:* If the haemoptysis is relatively minor it may be sufficient to correct an excessively elevated INR to a therapeutic range (INR 1.5–2.0) with FFP (see p546). In patients with a prosthetic valve and massive haemoptysis, the clotting must be normalized as best as possible. Discuss with your local haematologists or cardiologists. Support platelets if $< 50 \times 10^9/l$.
- Consider nebulized beta-agonist and/or aminophylline as a muco-cilliary stimulant and to relieve bronchospasm.
- Patients with minor haemoptyses should be fully investigated (see above and table opposite). No cause is found in ~ 10%.
- Patients with massive haemoptyses should undergo urgent fibre-optic bronchoscopy to locate the bleeding source.
- Angiography and embolization should be considered for patients who are not candidates for surgery (e.g. due to pre-existing medical conditions, diffuse lung disease).
- Patients who continue to bleed > 600ml/day or who have an identifiable lesion (e.g. lung abscess, aspergilloma, trauma) should have definitive surgery.
- Discuss with cardiothoracic surgeons, consider transfer (ventilated if unstable) if patient fit enough.
- Infection is a common precipitant (e.g. in bronchiectasis). Consider antibiotics (e.g. co-amoxiclav 1g iv q6–8h or cefotaxime 2g iv q8h) after appropriate cultures. TB or lung parasites will require specific antimicrobial therapy.

Referral to specialist teams

- Discuss all large haemoptyses with respiratory physician or cardio-thoracic surgeons. Patients should be managed in a centre with appropriate back-up. If possible nasal source of bleeding, urgent ENT opinion.

Further investigation of haemoptysis

- Autoantibodies (ANA, ANCA, anti-GBM antibody)
- Serum for *Legionella* serology
- *Aspergillus* precipitins
- CT chest
- VQ scan
- ECHO
- Pulmonary angiogram
- Lung biopsy
- Pulmonary function tests with transfer factor

Pleural effusions

Presentation

- Dyspnoea
- Chest discomfort or sensation of heaviness
- Symptoms of malignancy: loss of appetite, weight, energy
- Symptoms of infection: fever, cough, sputum, night sweats

Severity depends on:

- Speed of onset (e.g. traumatic or post procedural)
- Haemodynamic compromise (hypotension, tachycardia)
- Hypoxia or respiratory failure
- Presence of underlying disease (e.g. heart failure, COAD)

Causes

Transudate (protein < 30 g/l)

- *Raised venous pressure*
  Cardiac failure
  Constrictive pericarditis
  Fluid overload
- *Hypoproteinaemia*
  Nephrotic syndrome
  Cirrhosis with ascites
  Protein-losing enteropathy
- *Miscellaneous*
  Hypothyroidism
  Meigs' syndrome
  Yellow nail syndrome

Exudate (protein >30 g/l)

- *Infection*
  Pneumonia
  Empyema (bacterial or TB)
  Sub-phrenic abscess
- *Malignancy*
  Primary bronchial
  Mesothelioma
  Secondary (and lymphoma)
  Lymphangitis carcinomatosa
- *Miscellaneous*
  Haemothorax (trauma, iatrogenic)
  Chylothorax (thoracic duct trauma)
  Autoimmune (RA, SLE, Dressler's)
  Pancreatitis

Management

1 If acute then stabilize the patient and insert a chest drain.
2 If effusion is chronic then reach a diagnosis and treat accordingly.

The acute massive effusion

- Give oxygen.
- *iv access:* Via a wide-bore cannula or internal jugular central line. If central access is difficult then avoid attempting unless peripheral access is clearly inadequate. Attempt to cannulate (internal jugular veins only) on the normal side. A bilateral pulmonary problem will be a disaster.
- *Take blood:* For FBC, clotting, and urgent cross-match (6 units).
- *Restore circulating volume:* If bp low or tachycardic, then give a plasma expander (Haemaccel®, 4.5% albumin, or blood) 500ml stat., according to size of effusion drained and response.
- *Insert a chest drain:* (see p816). The drain should be left unclamped and allowed to drain freely, the amount drained should be recorded.

Indications for specialist referral

- Traumatic haemothorax should always be referred to the cardio-thoracic surgeons.
- Haemothorax secondary to procedures should be referred if the patient is shocked and/or there is on-going significant blood loss requiring transfusion at a rate ≥ 1 unit every 4 hours (approx.).
- When in doubt discuss the case with the surgical team.

Diagnostic tap of pleural effusion

The chronic massive effusion

A chronic effusion will usually have accumulated over weeks or perhaps even months. History and examination may point to a malignant cause. The primary differential is TB, empyema and cirrhotic ascites with trans-diaphragmatic movement. The amount of abdominal ascites may be minimal and the effusion is usually R-sided.

Investigation

- **Diagnostic aspiration:** The chest should be scanned and marked by ultrasound prior to tapping the effusion, as underlying collapse may cause significant elevation of the hemidiaphragm.

  A sample should then be withdrawn (20ml) for:-

  - Protein ≥ 30g/l implies an exudate
         < 30g/l is usually a transudate (see above)
  - Microscopy   Turbid fluid with neutrophils implies infection
          Uniform blood-staining implies malignancy
  - Microbiology   ZN staining, and culture
  - Cytology   Primary or secondary malignancy
  - **Pleural biopsy:** should be performed if malignancy is suspected.

Management

- The fluid should be drained by repeated aspirations of 1 litre per day until dry (see p199), or by the insertion of an intercostal drain (see p816), which should be clamped and released to drain 1 litre per day. (This is the only instance when a chest drain may be clamped). Drainage of > 1 litre per day may result in reperfusion pulmonary oedema.
- If the malignant effusion reaccumulates rapidly, consider chemical or surgical pleurodesis (discuss with chest team).

Empyema

This is a serious complication of bacterial pneumonia (p160).

- To avoid long-term scarring and loculated infection the empyema requires urgent drainage by ultrasound guidance and usually the positioning of an intercostal drain. Non-operative drainage has a high failure rate due to both the potential thickness of fluid and the likelihood of loculations.
- Empyema should always be discussed with a respiratory physician or cardiothoracic surgeon.

Acute upper airway obstruction: Assessment

Presentation

- Stridor: inspiratory noise. Generated by the collapse of the extra-thoracic airway during inspiration
- Breathlessness
- Dysphagia
- Inability to swallow secretions (hunched forward, drooling)
- Cyanosis
- Collapse

Ask colleagues to call a senior anaesthetist and ENT assistance immediately while you continue your assessment.

Identify the cause (see table opposite)

- **History:** Sudden onset, something in mouth or child playing with unsafe toy (foreign body), fever (epiglottitis, diphtheria, tonsillitis), hoarse voice (epiglottitis), sore throat (infective as listed), travel (eastern Europe – diphtheria), smoker + longer history + systemic symptoms (?carcinoma), trauma.
- **Examination:** Where infective cause is suspected then examination of oropharynx must be undertaken in area where patient may be immediately intubated, with an anaesthetist standing by.
- Fever, drooling, stridor. Bull neck, lymphadenopathy, pseudomembrane over oropharynx (diphtheria). Painful swallowing + epiglottis on direct/ indirect laryngoscopy (epiglottitis).
- **Investigations:** Do not delay treatment if the patient is in distress. If the patient is relatively stable, perform a chest X-ray (foreign body), lateral neck X-ray (swollen epiglottis). FBC U&Es, blood gases.

Indications for ITU/ surgical referral

- Prior to examination of oropharynx if infective cause suspected
- Failure to maintain adequate airway or oxygenation
- Inability to swallow secretions
- Ventilatory failure ($P_aO_2 \leqslant 10$kPa, $P_aCO_2 \geqslant 6$kPa)
- Collapse
- Severe dyspnoea

Management

- If severe liaise immediately with ITU and ENT or general surgeons (potential for urgent tracheostomy)

Priorities are:

1. Stabilize the patient – ensure adequate airway
2. Identify the cause of obstruction
3. Specific treatment measures

Stabilize the patient

- Take arterial blood gases and give high percentage oxygen ($\geqslant 60$%).
- If clear cause of obstruction (foreign body, post operative thyroid surgery), then take appropriate measures to gain patent airway (see below).
- If patient is becoming increasingly exhausted or there is acute failure of ventilation then summon colleagues as above and be prepared to intubate or perform tracheostomy.

Acute upper airway obstruction

Causes of acute stridor

- Infective: acute epiglottitis, diphtheria, tonsillitis, or adenoiditis (children)
- Inhalation of foreign body
- Tumour of trachea or larynx
- Trauma
- Post operatively (thyroid surgery)

Acute upper airway obstruction: Foreign body

With total upper airway obstruction then perform Heimlich manoeuvre (stand behind patient, grip wrists across the patients upper abdomen, and tug sharply to raise intrathoracic pressure and expel foreign body). Otherwise perform chest X-ray, liase with respiratory/ ENT/ cardiothoracic teams for retrieval under direct vision.

Epiglottitis

Usually *Haemophilus influenzae* type b, also *Strep. pneumoniae*. Treat with 3rd generation cephalosporin, e.g. cefotaxime 2g tds (adults). Children more likely to require intubation, but if any concerns over airway then patient (adult or child) should be monitored on ITU after anaesthetic assessment.

Diphtheria

Uncommon in UK, occasionally seen in patients returning from abroad. Toxin-mediated problems include myocarditis and neuritis. Treat with diphtheria anti-toxin + antibiotic eradication of organism – consult microbiology.

Tumour obstruction

Unlikely to cause life-threatening obstruction without warning. Symptoms over ≥ few days. If significant stridor present then administer 200mg hydrocortisone and thereafter prednisolone 40mg od po. If laryngeal origin liaise with ENT regarding tracheostomy. Lung cancer in trachea, or extrinsic cancer eroding into the trachea, will require urgent radiotherapy (or occasionally laser or cryotherapy via bronchoscope).

3 Shock

205

Shock

Shock is conventionally defined as a condition in which the arterial pressure is inadequate to perfuse vital organs. The precise pressure at which this occurs varies from patient to patient. In the elderly, even modest falls in blood pressure may result in significant hypoperfusion of the kidneys or brain. In general, a mean arterial pressure < 60mmHg or a systolic pressure of < 90mmHg, is regarded as pathological.

Priorities are:

- **If the blood pressure is unrecordable, call the cardiac arrest team.** Begin basic life support and establish venous access.
- The cause of hypotension is often apparent. If it is not, then one can usually make a rapid clinical assessment of likely causes.
- Cardiac pump failure
- Hypovolaemia
- Systemic vasodilatation
- Anaphylaxis
- Seek specialist help early rather than late.

Differential diagnosis of shock

1 Cardiac pump failure
- Myocardial infarction (p12)
- Dissection of thoracic aorta (p132)
- Cardiac dysrhythmias (p40)
- Acute valvular regurgitation or acute VSD (p28)
- Cardiac tamponade (p142)
- Pulmonary embolus (p110)
- Tension pneumothorax (p187)
- Drug overdose (cardiac depressants, see p631–672)

2 Hypovolaemia
- Haemorrhage [GI tract (p480), aortic dissection or leaking AAA, post trauma (splenic rupture)]
- Fluid losses (diarrhoea, vomiting, polyuria, or burns)
- '3rd space' fluid losses [acute pancreatitis (p528), ascites]
- Adrenal failure (p456)

3 Systemic vasodilatation
- Septic shock (p216)
- Liver failure (p518)
- Drug overdose (calcium antagonists or other vasodilators, drugs causing multi-organ failure, e.g. paracetamol, paraquat).
- Adrenal failure (may be both hypovolaemic and vasodilated)

4 Anaphylaxis
- Recent drug therapy
- Post intravenous injection
- Food allergy (e.g. peanut)
- Insect stings (p764)

Shock: Assessment

If the bp is unrecordable then call the cardiac arrest team. Begin basic life support (Airway, Breathing, Circulation) and establish venous access.

If the cause of hypotension is not obvious, perform a rapid clinical examination looking specifically for the following:-

- Check the airway is clear of vomit or blood and give oxygen by mask or ET tube if unconsious (40–60%). Check both lungs are being ventilated (?tension pneumothorax).
- Note the respiratory rate (increased in acidaemia, pneumothorax, embolus, and cardiac failure).
- Check the cardiac rhythm and treat if abnormal (see p40–72).
- What is the pulse pressure (systolic-diastolic)? Patients with systemic vasodilatation commonly have normal systolic pressures but low diastolic pressures.
- Is the JVP elevated (see table opposite)?
- Is the bp the same in both arms (thoracic aortic dissection)?
- Are there any unusual cardiac murmurs? (Acute valvular lesion, flow murmurs may be heard in vasodilated patients).
- Is the patient cold and clammy? This suggests cardiac pump failure or hypovolaemia; however, patients with severe septic shock may also be peripherally shut down. In the latter check for fever, and palpate the forearms for the bounding pulse of proximal arterial vasodilatation.
- Is the patient warm and systemically vasodilated (feel finger pulp, and feet). Palpate the forearm muscles for bounding pulses.
- Examine the abdomen. Is there a fullness or pulsatile mass in the abdomen (ruptured aneurysm)? Is there evidence of an acute abdomen (aneurysm, pancreatitis, perforated viscus)?
- Is the patient clinically dehydrated or hypovolaemic (skin turgor, mucous membranes, postural fall in bp)?
- Is there evidence of haematemesis (blood around mouth) or melaena (PR examination)?
- Is there any evidence of urticaria, wheals, wheezing, soft tissue swelling (e.g. eyelids or lips) suggestive of anaphylaxis?
- Is conscious level impaired (cerbral hypoperfusion)?

Investigations

- **ECG**   Acute MI, arrhythmias, PE (S_1,Q_3,T_3)
- **CXR**   Pneumothorax, PE, dissection, tamponade, pleural effusion
- **Blood tests**   *U&Es* (renal impairment, adrenal failure), *FBC* (haemorrhage, ↑ or ↓ WBC in sepsis, ↓ plts in liver disease and sepsis), *glucose, clotting studies* (liver disease, DIC), *LFTs, X-match*
- **ABGs**   Acidaemia (renal, lactic, ketoacidosis)
- **Sepsis screen**   Culture blood, urine, sputum
- **Misc.**   Where appropriate consider serum lactate, ECHO (suspected tamponade, dissection, valve dysfunction), LP, USS or CT abdomen ± head

Causes of hypotension with a raised CVP

- Pulmonary embolus (p110)
- Cardiac tamponade (p142)
- Cardiogenic shock (p210)
- Fluid overload in shocked vasodilated patients
- Right ventricular infarction (p32)
- Tension pneumothorax (p187)

Shock: Management

General measures

- Check the airway is clear and give high percentage oxygen by face mask to optimize oxygen saturation. If concious level is impaired consider ET intubation and mechanical ventilation.
- Lie the patient flat and raise the feet to try to restore bp.
- Insert 2 large-bore intravenous cannulae and commence infusion of colloid (e.g. Haemaccel®) or blood. In the **absence** of a cardiac cause it is usually safe to give colloid (200–300ml over 15 minutes) until a more detailed assessment is carried out.
- Send blood for U&Es, glucose, FBC, X-match, and blood cultures.
- Insert central venous line to monitor CVP and for inotrope infusions if necessary. Insert arterial line for more accurate assessment of bp. Catheterize the bladder to monitor urine output.
- Titrate fluid replacement according to bp, CVP, and urine output. Over-enthusiastic fluid administration in patients with cadiac pump failure will precipitate pulmonary oedema with little gain in stroke volume or cardiac output (see p228).
- Persistent hypotension in spite of an adequate filling pressure is an indication for inotropic support. The choice of first-line agent varies to some extent depending upon the underlying disgnosis.
- Treat the underlying condition (see table p206) and *enlist specialist help early*.
- Ensure someone takes time to talk to the relatives to explain the patient is seriously ill and may die.

Cardiogenic shock (cardiac pump failure)

- Correct any cardiac arrhythmias (p40–72) and U&E imbalance.
- Optimize filling pressures, guided by physical signs, PCWP. Significant mitral regurgitation will produce large v waves on the wedge trace and give spuriously high estimates of LVEDP.
- *PCWP < 15mmHg* iv fluids is the initial treatment. Give colloid challenges (100–200mls) and assess response.
- *PCWP > 15mmHg* Start iv inotrope infusion. Commence low-dose dopamine (2.5µg/kg/min) and add dobutamine (5–20µg/kg/min), or adrenaline (1–10µg/min), titrating the dose according to response (see p688 for details).
- If there is a potentially reversible cause for cardiogenic shock, consider intra-aortic balloon counterpulsation (p696). It is contraindicated in patients with aortic regurgitation.

Hypovolaemic shock

- Fluid replacement is the main-stay. There is no clear evidence to favour either colloids or crystalloids and, in practice, a mixture is used. Give blood as soon as it is available to maintain $Hb \geq 10g/dl$.
- Metabolic acidosis, Na^+ and K^+ abnormalities should be treated in the usual way. Often acidosis responds to fluid replacement only.
- If the patient remains hypotensive in spite of fluids, exclude other pathology (sepsis, tamponade, tension pneumothorax, etc). Commence inotropes – adrenaline (1–10µg/min) or dobutamine (1–20µg/kg/min) with 'renal dose' dopamine (2.5µg/kg/min).
- If oliguria persists in spite of adequate resuscitation, 'renal-dose' dopamine infusion (2.5µg/kg/min) and frusemide (10–80mg iv) may be tried, followed by a bolus of aminophylline (250mg iv-check K^+ is normal before giving). There are anecdotal reports of benefit but no clear evidence that this prevents development of acute renal failure.

Anaphylaxis

Atopic individuals are particularly at risk, but it may be the feature in some patients. Precipitants include:-

- Insect bites (especially wasp and bee stings, see p764)
- Foods and food additives (e.g. peanuts, fish, eggs)
- Drugs and intravenous infusions (blood products and intravenous immunoglobulin, vaccines, antibiotics, aspirin and other NSAIDs, iron injections, heparin)

Presentation

Cutaneous features include skin redness, urticaria, conjunctival injection, and angioedema. Rhinitis, laryngeal obstruction (choking sensation, cough), bronchospasm, tachycardia, hypotension, and shock may follow.

Management

- **Secure the airway**: If respiratory obstruction is imminent, intubate and ventilate or consider emergency cricothyroidotomy (see p810). A 14 or 16G needle and insufflation with 100% O_2 can temporize until the anaesthetist arrives.
- **Give oxygen**: if there is refractory hypoxia, intubate and ventilate.
- Lie the patient flat with head-down tilt if hypotensive.
- **Give intramuscular adrenaline 0.5–1mg** (0.5–1ml of 1 in 1000 adrenaline injection) and repeat every 10 minutes according to bp and pulse. Administer this *before* searching for intravenous access so as not to waste time.
- For children below the age of 6 years the im dose of 1 in 1000 adrenaline injection is approximately = age in years / 10. (e.g. for an otherwise robust child of 3 years start with 0.3ml). For children age 6–12 years use 0.5ml of 1 in 1000 injection.
- **Intravenous adrenaline** may be required if the patient is severely ill with poor circulation. Give *slow* injection of 500 micrograms (5ml of the dilute 1 in 10 000 adrenaline injection) at 1ml/min *stopping* when a response is obtained.
- For children requiring intravenous adrenaline, give 10µg/kg (0.1ml of the dilute 1 in 10 000 adrenaline injection) by slow injection over several minutes.
- Establish venous access and start iv fluids (colloid if hypotensive). Persistent hypotension requires adrenaline infusion.
- Give iv hydrocortisone 100–300mg and chlorpheniramine 10–20mg.
- Continue H_1–antagonist (e.g. chlorpheniramine 4mg q4–6h) for at least 24–48h; longer if urticaria and pruritis persist.
- If the patient continues to deteriorate, start intravenous aminophylline infusion (see p167). Patients on beta-blockers may not respond to adrenaline injection and require iv salbutamol infusion.

Angioneurotic oedema (C1–esterase inhibitor deficiency): see p628

Shock with systemic vasodilatation

The patients should be monitored in either an ITU or HDU. Ideally, both an arterial and PA catheter for thermodilution cardiac outputs ± mixed venous oxygen saturations (Swan-Ganz line) should be inserted. A central line alone is not adequate to monitor these patients.

The aims of management are:

• Correction of underlying cause
• Optimize oxygen delivery to tissues and oxygen consumption
• Optimize organ perfusion (CNS, myocardium, and kidneys)

It is important in the management of such critically ill patients NOT to lose sight of the needs of the patient. It is easy in an ITU setting not to examine patients but to look at charts. Always examine the patient at least twice a day, and determine whether the clinical parameters match those on the ITU chart. Ask yourself twice a day:-

• Fluid requirements [what is the fluid balance, is the patient clinically dry (↓ tissur turgor) or oedematous?].
• Is the circulation adequate? Note the bp (and MAP); examine the peripheries (are they cool and shut down or warm). Is the urine output satisfactory?
• Is the gas exchange satisfactory? Watch closely for developing ARDS (p188). Examine CXR daily for deterioration which may be masked (on ABG) by adjustments of mechanical ventilation.
• Are there signs of sepsis? Is there any new focus of infection?
• What do the tests show [U&Es, LFTs, Ca^{2+}, PO_4^{3-}, Mg^{2+}, CRP, cultures (blood, urine, sputum, line tips, etc)]?
• What nutrition is the patient getting (TPN or enteral)?

Optimizing oxygen delivery to tissues and oxygen consumption

Normally tissues only extract as much oxygen as required from the circulation. However, patients with sepsis, multi-organ failure, or liver failure exhibit supply-dependent oxygen consumption i.e. manoeuvres which increase oxygen delivery and increase tissue oxygen consumption. Many such patients also have a mild degree of lactic acidosis, again suggesting 'covert' tissue hypoxia. Treatment is therefore aimed at increasing tissue oxygen delivery. Suggested parameters are given on p218. Controlled clinical trials proving that this affects outcome are few. In a recent trial dobutamine failed to improve survival; agents which do not cause vasodilatation have not been systematically studied in controlled trials as yet.

• Aim for a MAP of at least 60mmHg. Such a pressure is usually required for good renal function. If the patient remains oliguric at this MAP, then raise the MAP by 10mmHg using vasopressor agents (see below).
• *Vasopressor agents* If cardiac output is low, adrenaline should be used, and if cardiac output is high (and SVR low), then noradrenaline should be used (noradrenaline acts as a pure vasopressor agent with little/no inotropic effect) (see p696).
• Note the effects any manoeuvre has on systemic heamodynamics and oxygen metabolism. For example, infusion of noradrenaline may improve bp, but decrease oxygen extraction; increasing the PEEP on the ventilator may decrease cardiac output.
• *Fluid replacement* Expanding the circulation will only increase the cardiac output if the heart is still able to respond to a rise in filling pressure (see p228). Fluid loading in the presence of 'leaky' pulmonary capillaries carries the potential risk of deterioriatong gas exchange (see p228). If the patient is anaemic, use blood. Aim for a haemoglobin of ≥ 10–11g/dl to optimize the oxygen carrying capacity of the blood.

Sepsis syndrome and septic shock

Definitions

Bacteraemia	Positive blood cultures
Sepsis	Evidence of infection *plus* systemic response such as pyrexia or tachycardia
Sepsis syndrome	Systemic response to infection *plus* evidence of organ dysfunction: confusion, hypoxia, oliguria, metabolic acidosis
Septic shock	Sepsis syndrome *plus* hypotension refractory to volume replacement

Presentation

Depends on the site of infection, nature of the infecting organism, and the host immune response.

General symptoms: Sweats, chills, or rigors. Breathlessness. Headache. Confusion in 10–30% of patients, especially the elderly. Nausea, vomiting, or diarrhoea may occur.

Examination: Hypotension (systolic bp < 90mmHg or a 40mmHg fall from baseline), tachycardia, with peripheral vasodilatation (warm peripheries, bounding peripheral pulse, bounding pulses in forearm muscles) are the hallmarks of septic shock. Systemic vascular resistance (SVR) is reduced, and cardiac output is increased initially but myocardial suppression may occur. Other features include fever > 38°C or hypothermia < 35.6°C (immunocompromised or elderly patients may not be able to mount a febrile response); tachypnoea and hypoxia; metabolic acidosis; oliguria. Focal physical signs may help to localize the site of infection.

Investigations

Blood tests	Blood cultures, U&Es, FBC, coagulation studies, LFTs, CRP, group and save serum, lactate, ABGs
Culture	Blood, sputum, urine, line-tips, wound swabs, throat swab, CSF (if indicated)
Imaging	USS or CT abdomen and pelvis for collections

Poor prognostic features include:

- Age > 60
- Multi-organ failure
- Renal failure
- Respiratory failure (ARDS)
- Hepatic failure
- Hypothermia or leukopenia
- Hospital-acquired infection
- Disseminated intravascular coagulation
- Underlying disease (e.g. immunocompromised, poor nutritional status, malignancy)

Prognosis

The incidence of septicaemia is 7/1000 admissions to hospital. Of these 20% develop septic shock, and 70% of these die.

	Mortality
Bacteraemia	15–20%
Bacteraemia plus shock	40–60%
Shock plus ARDS	80–90%

Sepsis syndrome

Sepsis syndrome: Management   1.

Patients with established shock require invasive haemodynamic monitoring and high-dependency facilities. The treatment is mainly supportive, trying to optimize tissue oxygenation and preserve vital organ perfusion until the infection is overcome by antibiotics and host defences. Successful management requires close liaison between several different teams (physicians, anaesthetists, surgeons, microbiologists, etc)

Resuscitation

- Check the airway is clear. Give oxygen: if there is refractory hypoxia, intubate and ventilate. Treat respiratory failure, see p182.
- Insert a large-bore peripheral venous cannula to begin fluid resuscitation. Insert central line and PA catheter and arterial line.
- Volume replacement: Use colloid initially, and blood if haemoglobin is < 10g/dl. Optimize filling pressures (aim for PCWP 12–15mmHg) watching the gas exchange closely; worsening may suggest leaking from the pulmonary capillaries. If this occurs, use vasoconstricting inotropes (e.g. adrenaline) as this appears to produce less leak even though pulmonary pressures may be similar. Once the lungs are no longer 'leaky' the fluid deficit masked by the adrenaline will need to be replaced.
- Aim to keep mean arterial pressure > 60mmHg. Vasopressor agents of choice are noradrenaline or adrenaline. If cardiac output is low, adrenaline should be used, and if cardiac output is high (and SVR low), then noradrenaline should be used. Suggested starting doses are:-
  - Noradrenaline   1–12μg/minute (see p689)
  - Adrenaline   1–12μg/minute (see p689)

  Alternatives include:-
  - Dobutamine (2.5–15.0μg/kg/min). (see p689)
  - Vasopressin (24 U over 15 min; then 0.4–1 units/min iv) (see p489)
  - Enoximone (90μg/kg/min over 30 min then 5–20μg/kg/min, p696)

  Do **NOT** use dobutamine or enoximone in the absence of pump failure (dobutamine may cause further vasodilatation in patients who are already vasodilated).

Optimize haemodynamics and oxygen delivery

- Conventional management involves trying to 'normalize' the haemodynamic parameters (see below). However, it has been argued that in the setting of sepsis, as the oxygen extraction and utilization by the tissues is impaired, one should aim for 'supra-normal' circulation to improve oxygen delivery.

	Normal range	'Ideal' in sepsis
Cardiac index ($l/min/m^2$)	2.8–3.6 l/min/m^2	> 4.5 l/min/m^2
SVR index (dynes/s/cm^5)	1760–2600	> 1460
Oxygen delivery (DO_2ml/min)	520–720	> 800
Oxygen consumption (VO_2ml/min)	110–140	> 170

(See p226 for formulae for calculations)

Sepsis syndrome

Sepsis syndrome: Management 2.

Antibiotics

Antibiotic choice is dictated by the suspected site of infection and probable microbe, host factors such as age, immunosuppression and hospitalization, and local antibiotic resistance patterns. A suggested empiric regimen in patients with sepsis syndrome **and** the following source of infection is as follows:-

Pneumonia

Community-acquired	Co-amoxiclav or
	Cefotaxime + erythromycin
Hospital-acquired	Ceftazidime alone or
	Piperacillin + gentamicin

Intra-abdominal sepsis Cefotaxime + metronidazole or
Piperacillin + gentamicin ± metronidazole

Biliary tract Piperacillin + gentamicin

Urinary tract

Community-acquired	Co-amoxiclav or cefotaxime
Hospital-acquired	Ceftazidime or
	Piperacillin + gentamicin

Skin and soft tissue Co-amoxiclav or
Amoxycillin + flucloxacillin

Sore throat Flucloxacillin + benzyl penicillin

Multiple organisms
(Anaerobes, E.coli, Strep.) Vancomycin+gentamicin+metronidazole or
Clindamycin + gentamicin

Meningitis Cefotaxime or (if pen. and cef. allergic)
Vancomycin ± rifampicin

Removal of infective foci

It is essential to identify and drain focal sites, e.g. obstructed urinary tract or biliary tree, drain abscesses, and resect dead tissue.

Causes of treatment failure

- Resistant or unusual infecting organism
- Undrained abscess
- Inflammatory response (raised CRP, raised WCC) may persist despite adequate antimicrobial therapy
- Advanced disease

Sepsis syndrome

Toxic shock syndrome

- Distinct clinical illness caused by toxin producing Gram-positive bacteria, including staphylococci and streptococci.
- Infection is often localized and illness is manifest by the toxins.
- 85% of cases are female.
- Association with menstruation in females ± the use of tampons.
- May occur with any focal infections due to a toxin-producing strain, including post operative wound infections.

Clinical features

- Fever: > 38.9°C
- Rash: diffuse macular (seen in ≥ 95%), mucous membrane involvement common. Desquamation 1–2 weeks later, palms and soles (consider drug reaction in differential diagnosis).
- Hypotension: systolic < 90mmHg, or postural hypotension
- Diarrhoea frequent
- Multi-organ failure may ensue

Laboratory findings

- Normochromic normocytic anaemia (50%) and leukocytosis (> 80%)
- Renal/hepatic failure, 20–30%
- Elevated CPK is very common
- Pyuria
- CSF pleiocytosis (sterile)
- Blood cultures rarely positive
- Vaginal swabs, throat swab, and wound swabs
- Toxin-producing *Staph. aureus* in 98% of menses-associated cases

Therapy

- Limit toxin production/release
- Drain any focal collections and remove foreign bodies
- Anti-staphylococcal antibiotics (high-dose flucloxacillin or vancomycin iv)
- Supportive care as for any patient with shock (see p210)

Toxic shock syndrome

Lactic acidosis

Lactic acidosis is a metabolic acidosis due to excess production or reduced metabolism of lactic acid. It may be divided into two types, **type A** (due to tissue hypoxia) and **type B** (non-hypoxic). In clinical practice, patients presenting with lactic acidosis almost always have a combination of both types.

Presentation

Patients are usually critically ill. Clinical features include:-

- Shock (often bp < 80/40)
- Kussmaul respiration
- Tachypnoea
- Deteriorating conscious level
- Multi-organ failure including hepatic, cardiac, and renal failure
- Clinical signs of poor tissue perfusion (cold, cyanotic peripheries)

Investigations

- ABGs (pH < 7.34, severe if pH < 7.1)
- Serum electrolytes, including bicarbonate and chloride, to calculate anion gap, if lactate unavailable. Raised anion gap > 16mmol/l
  [Anion Gap = (Na + K) − (Bicarbonate + chloride)]
- FBC (anaemia, neutrophilia)
- Blood glucose
- Blood lactate level > 5mmol/l (use a fluoride tube).
- Screen for sepsis (blood cultures, CRP, MSU)
- Paracetamol level in patients with unexplained lactic acidosis.
- Spot urine (50ml) for drug screen if cause unknown.
- CXR looking for consolidation or signs of ARDS.

Assessment of severity

Severity is assessed by the blood lactate concentration, and the degree of acidaemia. This may be confounded by the presence of acute renal failure. In the early stages, the arterial pH may be normal or even raised, since elevated lactate levels in the CNS cause hyperventilation with a compensatory respiratory alkalosis. The best predictor of survival is the arterial pH. Patients presenting with a lactate of greater than 5mmol/l and a pH < 7.35 have an 80% mortality.

Management

The principle of management is diagnosis and treatment of the cause, and amelioration of the underlying pathophysiology. All patients should be managed on an intensive care unit.

- *Sepsis*: Start broad spectrum antibiotics (e.g. cefotaxime plus metronidazole, or amoxycillin, gentamicin and metronidazole)
- *Paracetamol overdose*: Give N-acetyl-cysteine (see p664).
- *Diabetic lactic acidosis*: insulin and fluids as appropriate (see p430).
- *Shock*: Commence invasive haemodynamic monitoring (Swan-Ganz line, arterial line). Treat as on p210.
- *Renal failure*: Treat by continuous haemofiltration. These patients are usually too unstable to tolerate haemodialysis. If haemodialysis is used, it is now conventional to use bicarbonate dialysis.
- *Methanol*: Infuse ethanol (competitive metabolism p656).
- *Acidaemia:* The role of bicarbonate is controversial since it may lower CSF pH, and alter the oxygen dissociation curve unfavourably. In the absence of diabetic ketoacidosis, if arterial pH is < 7.05 then give 100ml 8.4% sodium bicarbonate over 15–30 minutes and reassess.

Causes of lactic acidosis	
Type A	**Type B**
Tissue hypoperfusion (shock)	Sepsis
Severe anaemia	Renal/hepatic failure
Severe hypoxia	Diabetes mellitus (uncontrolled)
Catecholamine excess (e.g.	Malignancy (leukaemia,
phaeo or exogenous)	lymphoma)
Severe exercise	Acute pancreatitis

Drug-induced
(metformin, methanol, ethanol, salicylates, and cyanide)

Rare causes
Heriditary enzyme defects such as Glucose-6–phosphatase, and
Fructose-1,6–diphosphatase deficiency

Haemodynamic calculations

In general, most systems these days calculate all the parameters that you require, and the formulae below should not be necessary. It is important to distinguish between indexed (modified for body surface area) and non-indexed values. Indexed values are signified by the letter I. Thus cardiac output (CO) becomes CI, and systemic vascular resistance (SVR) becomes SVRI.

Mean arterial pressure (MAP)

MAP = Diastolic pressure + ⅓(Systolic-Diastolic pressure)
e.g. bp 120/60 = MAP of 60 + ⅓(120−60) = 80mmHg

R. atrial pressure	NR	1–7mmHg
R. ventr. systolic pressure	NR	15–30mmHg
R. ventr. diastolic pressure	NR	0–8mmHg
PA systolic pressure	NR	15–30mmHg
PA diastolic pressure	NR	3–12mmHg
Mean PA pressure	NR	9–16mmHg
Pulmonary capillary wedge pressure		
v wave pressure	NR	3–12mmHg
a wave pressure	NR	3–15mmHg

The v wave pressure is increased in mitral regurgitation, and therefore it is difficult or impossible to obtain a typical 'wedged' tracing.

Cardiac output (CO)   NR $4.0 – 6.2 \, l/min^{-1}$

Cardiac Index (CI)

$$CI = \frac{Cardiac \; output}{Body \; surface \; area}$$ NR 2.8–3.6 l/min/m²

Systemic vascular resistance (SVR) and SVRI

$$SVR = \frac{(MAP - RAP) \times 80}{C.O}$$ NR   800–1500 dyne/S/cm⁻⁵

$$SVRI = \frac{(MAP - RAP \times 80)}{C.I}$$ NR   1760–2600 dyne/S/cm⁻⁵/m²

Pulmonary vascular resistance (PVR)

$$PVR = \frac{Mean \; PA - PCWP}{CO}$$ NR   20–120 dyne/S/cm⁻⁵

O_2 delivery $(DO_2) = CI \times CaO_2$ NR 520–720ml/min

O_2 consumption: $(VO_2) = (CaO_2 - CvO_2) \times CI$ NR 110–140l/min

CaO_2 = oxygen content of arterial blood (measured by haemoglobinometer or derived from arterial gases)
CvO_2 = oxygen content of mixed venous blood (obtained from PA distal line).

Oxygen content = Hb (g/l) x 1.34 x oxygen sat.

Oxygen extraction ratio (OER)

OER = VO_2/DO_2 NR   0.22–0.3 (22–30%)

Appendix: Understanding circulatory failure

Intelligent manipulation of the filling pressures and inotropic support of a patient with shock or heart failure requires a basic understanding of the way in which the left and right ventricles respond to changes in filling pressure and what effect different clinical conditions have on their function. The following is a somewhat simplified approach.

The stroke volumes of the right and left ventricles are identical, but as the resistance of the pulmonary bed is much lower than that of the systemic bed, the right ventricle is able to do this at a lower filling pressure than the left ventricle. Raising the right atrial pressure with iv fluids (and so increasing the RVEDP) will increase the stroke volume of the right ventricle. This increases the LVEDP (and thus the left atrial pressure) keeping the stroke volume of both sides of the heart matched.

Sepsis, acidosis, $\uparrow K^+$, $\downarrow Ca^{2+}$, $\downarrow Na^+$, MI or ischaemia, and certain drugs (e.g. β-blockers) are known to impair myocardial function and will depress the function curve. Inotropes will improve cardiac function and generally raise the function curves.

Expanding the circulation with iv fluids becomes progressively less effective in increasing the stroke volume (and so cardiac output) as the function curves become more depressed, i.e. the increase in stroke volume per unit transfused becomes progressively less. Furthermore, it increases the risks of precipitating pulmonary oedema (see below).

Pulmonary oedema occurs when the hydrostatic pressure within the capillary overcomes the plasma oncotic pressure (the major determinant of which is the serum proteins and albumin). The critical PCWP for hydrostatic pulmonary oedema is approx.= *serum albumin (g/l)* $\times$ *0.57* (i.e. with an albumin of 40g/l, critical PCWP=22mmHg). The lungs will, of course, get 'stiffer' as the PCWP rises, and the patient may get breathless before this pressure is reached.

Thus, even in normal patients, continued iv transfusion will eventually raise the right- and left-sided filling pressures sufficiently to precipitate pulmonary oedema.

Circulation in sepsis: Sepsis produces a systemic inflammatory response that results in 'leaky' capillaries in the lungs and elsewhere, as well as hypoalbuminaemia from a combination of impaired production and loss into extravascualr spaces. Thus, patients are at risk of pulmonary oedema at lower values of PCWP. Furthermore, the cardiac function curves are depressed so that iv fluids will produce less increase in stroke volume and cardiac output. It is more prudent to support the circulation with vaso-constricting inotropes (e.g. adrenaline) than fluids alone, remembering that when the capillaries are no longer leaky, the fluid defect masked by adrenaline will need to be replaced as the adrenaline is turned down.

---

[1] Bradley RD & Treacher DF (1996), *In* Weatherall DJ, Ledingham JGG, Warrell DA (Ed) *OTM* (3rd Ed.) Chapter **16**: 2563–76; Oxford University Press, Oxford

4 Infectious diseases

Fever in a traveller

Assessment

- It is important to obtain a very accurate history of what countries were visited and the activities of the individual whilst they were there (i.e. visits to rural areas or urban travel only, camping vs luxury hotels, etc.). What drugs were taken and what were forgotten.

- Do not forget that although the patient has travelled they may have common infections such as pneumonia or pyelonephritis.

Initial investigations

All patients should have the following:-

FBC	Look for anaemia (malaria, hookworm, malabsorption, leishmaniasis), leukocytosis (bacterial infections) or leukopenia (malaria, typhoid, Dengue fever), eosinophilia (parasites), thrombocytopenia (*P. falciparum*, typhoid, and Dengue fever).
Blood films	Thick and thin films should be examined by an expert for malaria.
U&Es	Renal failure may be seen with *P. falciparum,* viral haemorrhagic fevers (p248), and bacterial sepsis
LFTs	Jaundice and abnormal liver function is seen with hepatitis A-E, malaria, leptospirosis, yellow fever, typhoid, liver abscesses, and many others.
Clotting studies	Deranged with viral haemorrhagic fevers (p248), *P. falciparum*, bacterial sepsis, viral hepatitis.
Blood cultures	Mandatory for all febrile patients.
Urinalysis	For blood and protein, and a specimen for culture.

Other investigations to consider
Serology (hepatitis A-E); CXR; USS abdomen; sputum MC&S.

Management

- The epidemiology and drug-resistance patterns of many tropical pathogens is constantly changing and expert advice can be easily obtained from local regional infectious diseases unit. The telephone numbers of the schools of tropical medicine are given on p854.

- Patients should only be sent home if there is no evidence of serious bacterial infection and malaria has been excluded.

- **Isolation:** If there is a history of travel to rural West Africa (Nigeria, Sierra Leone, or Liberia) and the patient is febrile suspect *Lassa fever* (p248). Discuss the case _immediately_ with the regional infectious diseases unit. Generally, the patient is kept on site until malaria has been excluded and, then transferred. All other patients should be nursed in a side room until a diagnosis is established.

- Clinical **rabies** is rare in the UK but should be considered in travellers with severe encephalitis and an exposure history sought, particularly because it has been transmitted to healthcare workers and transplant recipients. A more common problem is that patients quite frequently present having suffered an animal bite when travelling in an endemic area. Post bite prophylaxis can prevent rabies in almost all cases.

- **Tuberculosis** should be considered when evaluating patients from the Indian sub-continent or Africa. Of particular concern is the increase in multiply drug-resistant TB in parts of the USA and also the increasing association between TB and HIV infection that is changing the presentation patterns.

Presenting feature	Diagnosis to consider
Jaundice	Malaria, hepatitis A–E, leptospirosis, yellow fever, typhoid, liver abscess
Splenomegaly	Malaria, leishmaniasis
Hepatosplenomegaly	Malaria, schistosomiasis, typhoid, *Brucellosis, leishmaniasis*
Diarrhoea and vomiting	*E. Coli, Salmonella, Shigella, Campylobacter, Giardia, E. histolytica*, cholera, *V. parahaemolyticus*, viral gastroenteritis
Skin lesions	Erythema nodosum (TB, leprosy, fungi, post streptococcal infection), Burrows (scabies), Dermatitis (onchocerciasis), Ulcers (syphilis, leprosy, leishmaniasis), Scabs (typhus, anthrax), Erythema marginatum (Lyme disease)
Abdominal pain	With diarrhoea in dysentery; perforation of bowel (typhoid, dysentery)
Haematuria	Malaria (*P. falciparum*); viral haemorrhagic fevers (p248); schistosomiasis
Meningism/confusion	Meningococcal and other bacterial meningitis, viral encephalitis
Bleeding tendency	Meningococcaemia, haemorrhagic fevers, leptospirosis
RUQ pain, intercostal tenderness ± R pleural effusion	Amoebic liver abscess (p526)
Pleural effusion	TB, liver abscess

Malaria: Assessment

Malaria is the commonest cause of death from travel-acquired infection in the UK and should be actively excluded in all febrile patients returning

from an endemic zone.

Organism

- *Plasmodium falciparum* is the causative agent of the more severe and potentially fatal or malignant form of malaria.
- *P. vivax*, *P. ovale*, and *P. malariae* often cause chronic recurrent disease but do not have the potential to cause cerebral malaria.
- Although patients with *P. falciparum* tend to be more seriously ill there are no reliable clinical guides to distinguish each type of infection. The different forms can be distinguished by their morphology on blood smears but this may need expert interpretation and, if in doubt, therapy should be directed against *P. falciparum*.

Symptoms

- Incubation period 7–14 days but may occur as late as 1 year.
- High fever, chills, and rigors followed by sweating. Periodic fever is described but most patients do not exhibit this
- Headache is a very common symptom. If associated with impairment in consciousness, behavioural change, or seizure activity consider cerebral malaria
- Generalized flu-like symptoms, malaise, and myalgia.
- Abdominal symptoms: anorexia, pain, vomiting, and diarrhoea.

Examination

- No specific features
- Pyrexia in all cases, often up to 40°C during paroxysms.
- Relative bradycardia (in less than 50%)
- Splenomegaly in at least 50%
- Hepatomegaly is less common in acute malaria. Look for jaundice
- Hyperreflexia, increased muscle tone, and seizures suggest cerebral involvement. Focal neurological signs are uncommon

Investigations

- FBC — Significant anaemia, evidence of haemolysis, leukopenia and ↓ platelets suggest *P. falciparum*.
- Blood films — Three separate blood samples taken over several hours should be examined by an experienced individual. If in doubt treat for malaria and send the films to a reference laboratory for a definitive opinion. Thick films are more sensitive but speciation is easier with thin films, and thin films are needed to calculate the percentage of red cells infected, i.e. the parasitaemia.
- Parasitaemia — < 2% mild, 2–5% moderate, > 5% severe.
- G6PDH status — Measure in case primaquine therapy is required.
- Glucose — Hypoglycaemia may occur with *P. falciparum* or quinine therapy, especially during pregnancy.
- U&Es, LFTs — Acute renal failure and haemoglobinuria may occur in severe *P. falciparum*, elevated unconjugated bilirubin, AST, and LDH reflect haemolysis.
- Blood cultures — Even if malaria is confirmed, other infections such as typhoid may also be present.
- Head CT scan and LP — May be required in suspected cerebral malaria to exclude other pathologies.
- ABG — Metabolic acidosis indicates severe malaria.

Poor prognostic signs in malaria

- Neurological features
  (deep coma, seizures, decerebrate rigidity)
- Retinal haemorrhages
- Hypoglycaemia
- Parasitaemia > 5%
- Pulmonary oedema
- WCC > 12×10^9/l
- Hb < 7g/dl
- Coagulopathy (DIC)
- Renal failure (creatinine > 250 μM)
- Lactic acidaemia (> 6 mM)

Malaria: Management[1]

Plasmodium falciparum

General measures

- Admission is mandatory as rapid progression and death can occur within hours. Lower fever with tepid sponging and paracetamol.
- If there is evidence of *cerebral malaria* or *parasitaemia* > 2% admit to ICU. Give prophylactic phenobarbitone 3.5mg/kg im.
- In severe cases catheterize the bladder to monitor urine output and insert a CVP line to help manage fluid balance, as ARDS can easily be precipitated in these patients. Renal support may be required.
- Hourly blood glucose estimations. Regular TPR, bp, urine output.
- Cardiac monitor is required for intravenous quinine.
- In severe cases repeat blood films every 4 hours until parasitaemia clearly falling and then perform daily. Daily U&Es, FBC, bilirubin.

Antimalarial therapy

- *Chloroquine* resistance is now widespread and quinine considered first-line therapy, although some low-grade quinine resistance has been described.
- *Mefloquine* and *halofantrine* are also effective but resistance is emerging and it is best to contact a malaria expert for advice on the best regimen for the country of origin.
- *Quinine* may be given orally (600mg 8 hourly). Give iv [loading dose: 20mg/kg (max 1.4g) over 4 hours, then 8–12h later, maintenance 10mg/kg infused over 4 hours (max. 700mg) q8–12h] if parasitaemia > 2% or if evidence of cerebral malaria or vomiting until oral quinine is tolerated or for 7 days.
- Treat for 5–7 days followed by a single dose of three tablets of Fansidar® (pyrimethamine+sulfadoxine), or if Fansidar®-resistant, give tetracycline 250mg q6h for 7 days when renal function normal..

Adjunctive therapy

- Steroids are no longer recommended for cerebral malaria.
- Exchange transfusion remains somewhat controversial but may be indicated for extreme parasitaemias (> 10%). Seek specialist advice.
- Daily blood films until trophozoites cleared, repeat films at end of treatment and then weekly for one month.

Plasmodium vivax, P. ovale and P. malariae

Admission If diagnosis secure and the patient is stable, admission is not always necessary. General measures are as above.

Acute therapy

- Chloroquine remains the drug of choice with only very limited resistance reported for *P. vivax*. Never treat with chloroquine if it was used as prophylaxis. Give chloroquine: 600mg (base) stat followed by 300mg 6 hours later and 300mg daily for 2 days.
- Quinine, mefloquine and halofantrine are all effective.

Radical cure Relapse due to persistent hepatic phase occurs with *P. vivax* and *P. ovale*. Treatment is with primaquine 15mg daily for 14 days. In G6PDH deficient patients primaquine induces severe haemolysis.

Patient advice Avoid contact sports for one month because of the risk of splenic rupture.

---

[1] For advice in the UK phone 0171 387 4411 (London) or 0151 708 9393 (Liverpool).

Infections presenting with fever and rash

Infections may involve the skin by direct invasion (e.g. varicella), by bacterial toxins (e.g. scarlet fever), or via the host inflammatory responses (e.g. infection-related vasculitis). The common childhood exanthems are described in the table on p237.

Primary varicella infection (chickenpox)

The classical rash is described on p237. Atypical presentations may occur in the immunocompromised host who may have fulminant cutaneous involvement with haemorrhagic chickenpox, or conversely, can develop systemic involvement with minimal rash.

Complications

Systemic complications are rare in the immunocompetent child but more frequent in adults and the immunocompromised. In the UK chickenpox is responsible for about 20 deaths per year in otherwise healthy adults.

- *Secondary bacterial infections:* Most frequent complication, 20–50% of hospitalized adults, and responsible for approximately 50% of chickenpox-associated deaths. Skin superinfections with streptococci and staphylococci (including toxic shock syndrome) or bacterial pneumonia predominate.
- *Viral pneumonia:* Approximately 1:400 adult cases with 20% mortality. Commoner in smokers. Characterized by cough, breathlessness, and hypoxia with diffuse pneumonitis on CXR.
- *Hepatitis:* Rare except in severely immunocompromised.
- *Encephalitis:* Incidence of 0.1% in adults, 20–30% mortality.
- *Cerebellar ataxia:* ~ 1:4000 cases in children, generally self-limited.
- *Reyes syndrome:* Epidemiological association in childhood.

Management

Anti-viral and antimicrobial therapy

- *Immunocompetent children:* Antiviral therapy not indicated. Have a high index of suspicion for bacterial infection if ill enough to require hospitalization.
- *Immunocompetent adult moderately unwell:* Within first 72 hours of the onset of rash may benefit from oral acyclovir 800mg five times per day with reduction in fever and number of lesions. However, no trials have been performed to detect a reduction in complications or mortality with acyclovir.
- *Immunocompetent adult with evidence of pneumonitis:* Intensive care monitoring required. iv acyclovir 10mg/kg q8h and cefotaxime plus flucloxacillin for secondary bacterial infection.
- *Immunocompromised adult or child:* Acyclovir indicated in all cases. If mild disease and minimal immunosuppression, oral therapy with 800mg five times per day may be sufficient. In more severe immunosuppression, e.g. post transplant, ± any evidence of dissemination then treat with iv 10mg/kg q8h (adult dose).

Prophylaxis for high-risk susceptible patient

Hyperimmune immunoglobulin (VZIG) is effective in preventing varicella for 72–96 hours after exposure. VZIG should be given to all susceptible (i.e. no history of chickenpox), immunocompromised individuals as soon after exposure, to chickenpox or zoster, as possible. VZIG is indicated for pregnant women and should also be given to newborn infants whose mothers have had primary varicella within 5 days of the birth.

Rashes table

Features of the common childhood exanthems

Infection	Morphology	Distribution	Incubation	Associated features	Complications
Varicella (chickenpox)	Clear vesicles on erythematous base (5-12mm), evolving into pustules that burst and crust	Lesions occur in crops.. start on trunk and spread peripherally. Mucosal involvement common	10–21d	Pyrexia 1-2 day flu-like prodrome	Bacterial infection Varicella pneumonia Encephalitis Reactivates as herpes zoster
Measles	Maculopapular, morbilliform	Starts on head and neck spreading peripherally	10–14d	Coryza, conjunctivitis, cough, lymphadenopathy. Koplik's spots in late prodrome	Otitis media, bacterial pneumonia, measles pneumonia, encephalitis (1:1000), deafness, sub-acute sclerosing panencephalitis (SSPE)
Rubella (German measles)	Pink macular	Progresses from trunk over 2-4 days, may be very mild or absent	14–21d	Lymphadenopathy especially suboccipital.	Arthritis in adults Encephalitis rare
Parvovirus (slapped cheek, erythema infectiosum, fifth disease)	Facial erythema in children. Macular or maculo-papular, morbilliform or annular	Facial rash in children (slapped cheek) Generalized in adults	5–10d	Lymphadenopathy Arthralgia	Arthritis in adults Foetal loss in pregnancy (hydrops) Anaemia in patients with haemoglobinopathies Chronic infection in immunocompromised

Herpes zoster (shingles)

Reactivation from latent virus in the sensory root ganglia. Risk increases with age and immunodeficiency. Vesicular rash developing in crops in a single dermatome, multiple dermatomes or dissemination in immuno-compromised. Suspect immunodeficiency in recurrent zoster.

Complications

These are more frequent in immunocompromised patients.

- Secondary bacterial infection.
- Post herpetic neuralgia.
- Eye complications: Keratitis occurs in 10% of patients with involvement of the trigeminal nerve (ophthalmic zoster). Rarely there may be retinal necrosis.
- Aseptic meningitis: CSF pleiocytosis is common and generally asymptomatic.
- Cerebral angiitis leading to a contralateral hemiparesis.
- Transverse myelitis: Mainly in immunocompromised patients.
- Cutaneous dissemination: In excess of 20 vesicles outside the affected dermatome suggests a high risk of systemic dissemination.
- Systemic dissemination: Lung, liver, and brain spread occurs, mainly in immunocompromised patients.

Management

- *Immunocompetent adult:* Acyclovir (800mg 5 times a day for 7 days) does not reduce the incidence of post herpetic neuralgia and only limits acute pain if within 48 hours of onset. Famicyclovir (250mg tds or 750mg od for 7 days) is an alternative to acyclovir.
- *Ophthalmic zoster:* Stain cornea with fluoroscein to detect keratitis, ophthalmology opinion vital if decreased visual acuity or any evidence of eye involvement. If keratitis present treat with topical acyclovir or trifluoridine ointment and oral acyclovir 800mg five times per day.
- *Uncomplicated zoster in immunocompromised:* Give acyclovir to prevent dissemination. Oral acyclovir (800mg five times per day) or famiciclovir (750mg od for 7 days) for patients with mild immuno-suppression (e.g. on long-term steroid therapy); iv acyclovir (10mg/kg q8h) for patients with severe immunosuppression.
- *Disseminated zoster:* Give iv acyclovir 10mg/kg q8h.

Varicella infection control

Patients with active varicella-zoster lesions should be nursed in isolation. Spread of infection is by inhalation or direct contact. Non-immune staff members should avoid treating the patient or, if that is impossible, wear a mask and gloves when in the same room.

Meningococcal infection: Assessment

Rashes

Pupuric lesions are the hallmark of meningococcal disease but several different patterns may be seen either separately or together.

Petechial: Initially 1–2mm discrete lesions, frequently on trunk, lower body and conjunctivae. Enlarge with disease progression and correlate with thrombocytopaenia and DIC, which are poor prognostic signs.

Ecchymoses: The petechial lesions coalesce and enlarge to form widespread purpura and ecchymoses, particularly on the peripheries.

Purpura fulminans: In extreme cases entire limbs or sections of the body become purpuric and then necrotic due to the combination of DIC and vascular occlusion.

Maculopapular: Non-purpuric and easily mistaken for a viral rash occurs early in some patients.

Presentation

- *Meningitis without septicaemia:* Neurological signs predominate and rash may or may not be present (see p328).
- *Meningoencephalitis:* Severe rapidly progressive neurological presentation with loss of consciousness, focal neurological signs, and evidence of meningitis.
- *Meningitis with septicaemia:* Headache, photophobia, and neck stiffness with or without focal neurological signs. Consciousness may be normal or depressed. Signs of systemic illness with fever, neutrophil leukocytosis, tachycardia, warm peripheries, and hypotension quickly develop. Rash usually present.
- *Septicaemia without meningitis:* Symptoms and signs of septicaemia. May progress from first signs to death within hours. Purpuric rash almost always develops but may be absent at presentation.
- *Bacteraemia without meningitis or sepsis:* Non-specific flu-like symptoms with or without rash. Positive blood cultures come as a surprise. Rash less often present. May develop focal spread such as septic arthritis.
- *Chronic meningococcaemia:* Low-grade fever, purpuric rash, and arthritis often confused with gonococcaemia. Sepsis and meningitis do not develop and the illness may last for weeks unless recognized.
- *Recurrent meningococcaemia:* Suspect immunocompromise, particularly complement deficiency

Antibiotics see p242.

Investigations

- *Blood cultures:* (at least 2 sets) but do not delay therapy (50% positive in patients with meningococcal meningitis)
- *Brain CT-scan* should be performed prior to lumbar puncture in all cases with depressed consciousness or focal neurological signs.
- *Lumbar puncture (LP):* Should only be performed to establish a diagnosis if there is no evidence of cerebral oedema. In a shocked patient with meningitis and a purpuric rash then the diagnosis of meningococcaemia is so likely that an LP can be avoided and the diagnosis established by blood cultures.

Opening pr.	Often elevated.
WBC	Elevated in almost 100%: median 1200 cell/μl, mainly PMN but may be mixed if partially treated.
Protein	Elevated in 90%.
Glucose	Reduced in 75–80%.
Gram-stain	Positive with a negative culture in 10–15%.
Culture	Positive in 50–80% of meningitis
Antigen testing	Positive in 50% and correlates with Gram-stain.

Differential diagnosis of purpuric rash and fever

- Gonococcaemia
- Bacterial septicaemia with DIC
- Haematologic malignancy with sepsis
- Henoch-Schönlein purpura
- In travellers consider:-
  Rocky mountain spotted fever (USA)
  Viral haemorrhagic fevers (see p248)

Meningococcal infection: Management

Antibiotic therapy

- *Treatment must be started immediately* if the diagnosis of meningo-coccal septicaemia or meningitis is suspected.
- If the patient is in A&E, take blood cultures whilst the antibiotics are being drawn up but do not wait for scans or the lumbar puncture.
- If called by a GP then instruct the GP to administer penicillin 2miu (1.2g) im/iv or a third-generation cephalosporin before effecting transfer to hospital.

All forms of invasive meningococcal disease

- Benzyl penicillin 4MU (2.4g) iv q4h. Some authors advocate an infusion of 2MU every 2 hours.

Penicillin allergy

- Cefotaxime 2g q8h or chloramphenicol 100mg/kg/day (max 4g).

Empiric therapy in meningitis without a rash until the organism known

- Cefotaxime 2g 8 hourly (see p330).

Prophylaxis

- Notify the case immediately to the local public health department
- Antibiotic prophylaxis

  Close contacts only, i.e. household, close family, institutional contacts (if from a nursing home), etc.

  Staff members only if involved in resuscitation or endotracheal intubation and suctioning without a mask on

  Adults: Ciprofloxacin 750mg as a single dose.
              or Rifampicin 600mg bd for 2 days.

  Children: Rifampicin 10mg/kg bd for 2 days.

Supportive therapy

- Intensive care monitoring is essential in any shocked patient or if significant impairment of consciousness.
- If shocked, urgent fluid replacement, aided by invasive monitoring, is essential. Supportive care for septic shock is discussed on p210.
- Treatment of DIC, the use of corticosteroids, and anti-endotoxin therapy in this group is controversial.

Prognosis

- Meningitis without shock: Mortality approximately 10%, neurological sequelae uncommon. Coma is a poor prognostic sign.
- Fulminant meningococcaemia: Mortality related to organ failure between 20–80%

Gonococcaemia

- Seen with 0.5–3.0% of cases of gonorrhoea.
- Most common cause of infectious arthritis in young adults.

Presentation

- Classic triad of fever, rash, and arthritis or tenosynovitis.
- Systemic symptoms usually mild; genital symptoms are often absent.
- Rash: Discrete papules and pustules, which may be purpuric. Usually 10–50 lesions, mainly on extremities.
- Arthritis: Asymmetrical polyarthropathy most often involving knee, ankle, elbow, or wrist with sterile effusions is seen early and often with an associated tenosynovitis. Later, one or two joints may develop septic arthritis with positive cultures.

Investigations

- Blood cultures: Positive in only 30–50%.
- Mucosal cultures: Urethra, cervix, rectum, or pharynx +ve in 80%.
- Skin pustules: Gram-negative diplococci may be seen on microscopy, but the lesions are often culture negative.
- Joint fluid: PMN leukocytosis, frequently sterile in polyarticular disease but positive in monoarticular septic arthritis.
- Syphilis serology

Differential diagnosis

- Meningococcaemia
- Infectious arthritides
- Reiter's syndrome
- Inflammatory arthritis

Therapy

- Depends on the risk of antibiotic resistance.
- Empiric therapy should be with a third-generation cephalsporin or quinolone (see below).
- If the organism is sensitive, then penicillin remains the treatment of choice.

Suitable regimens

- Benzyl penicillin 2miu (1.2g) iv 4 hourly for 72 hours followed by ampicillin 500mg qds orally for 7 days.
- Cefotaxime 1g iv 8 hourly for 7 days (or change to oral ampicillin after 3 days).
- Ciprofloxacin 750mg bd orally for 7–10 days.
  PLUS: Doxycycline 100mg bd for 7 days to cover genital chlamydia

Complications

- All rare, including endocarditis, meningitis, osteomyelitis, and septic shock.

Enteric fever (typhoid)

Presentation

- Non-specific symptoms: e.g. anorexia, myalgia, headache, malaise, fever, chills, and sweats common. Remittent temperature gradually rising during the 1st week to ~40°C with a relative bradycardia.
- Abdominal pain (30–40%), vomiting and diarrhoea (40–60%), or constipation (10–50%) may all be seen. Acute abdomen may occur in later stages with perforation of bowel. Splenomegaly in 40–60%; hepatomegaly less common 20–40%.
- Respiratory symptoms: Common, including sore throat and cough.
- Neurological manifestations, including encephalopathy, coma, meningism, and/or seizures are seen in 5–10%.
- Rose spots are 2–4 mm erythematous maculopapular lesions, blanch with pressure, and occur in crops of ~ 10 lesions on upper abdomen lasting only a few hours. Present in 10–30% and easily missed.

A fulminant, toxaemic, form occurs in about 5–10% of cases with rapid deterioration in cardiovascular, renal, hepatic, and neurological function. In other patients, onset may be quite insidious. In the first 7–10 days after infection bacteraemia occurs with seeding into the Peyer's patches of the gut, leading to ulceration and necrosis (weeks 2–3).

Investigations

- *Initial week of illness:* Normal Hb, WCC ↓ or ↑, elevated hepatic enzymes. Blood cultures positive in 80–90%.
- *2nd-3rd weeks:* ↓ Hb, ↓ WCC, and ↓ platelets due to marrow suppression. Blood cultures become negative, urine and stool cultures become positive. Marrow culture positive. Abdominal X-rays and imaging is indicated if there is abdominal pain.
- *Serology:* Unhelpful at discriminating active infection from past exposure or vaccination.

Complications (All uncommon with prompt diagnosis and therapy).

- *Toxaemia:* Acute complications include hyperpyrexia, renal and hepatic dysfunction, bone marrow failure, and myocarditis.
- *Gastrointestinal:* Late complications due to breakdown in Peyer's patches including gastrointestinal haemorrhage and perforation.
- *Metastatic infection:* Meningitis, endocarditis, osteomyelitis, liver and spleen abscess.
- *Chronic carriage:* 1–3% beyond 1 year

Management

- *Supportive care:* If toxaemic admit to intensive care, urinary catheter and CVP or Swan-Ganz line to manage fluid balance and prevent cardiovascular collapse. May need renal support.
- *Antibiotics:* Ampicillin, chloramphenicol, third generation cephalosporins, and quinolones have all been used with success but multiple drug resistance has become a problem and ampicillin can no longer be used for empirical treatment. Quinolones, e.g. ciprofloxacin, 750mg bd orally or 400mg bd iv, are currently the agents of choice but resistance has been described.
- *Steroids:* These are recommended for the severe toxaemic form and have reduced acute mortality although with a small increase in relapses. Give 60mg of prednisolone or equivalent (p459)) rapidly, tailing off over 3–5 days.
- *Surgery:* Needed for life-threatening bowel complications.
- Infection control: Notify the case to public health. Spread is faecal/oral and individuals should not prepare food until follow-up stool cultures are negative.

Teaching points

- *Salmonella typhi* and *S. paratyphi* (less severe) have a widespread distribution including Africa, South America, and Indian sub-continent.
- Incubation period is 7–21 days and it is very rare > 1 month after return from an endemic area.
- Untreated mortality 10–15%; with adequate therapy mortality is less than 1% in the UK.
- *Chronic carrier state:* Increased incidence in elderly, immunocompromised, and with gall-stones. Ampicillin (4–6g/day + probenicid 2g/day) or ciprofloxacin (750mg bd) for 6 weeks will clear 80–90% of patients, falling to 20–50% if the patient has gall-stones. With persistent carriage cholecystectomy may be needed.

Viral haemorrhagic fevers

These are occasionally encountered in the UK, presenting with fever, headache, and rash, and are frequently included in the differential diagnosis of febrile travellers. Recognition is important because the African viral haemorrhagic fevers (*Lassa* and *Ebola* virus) need special handling and transfer to a specialist facility.

Important agents of viral haemorrhagic fever in travellers

Disease	Clinical features	Outcome/management
Dengue fever (serotypes I-IV) Tropical/subtropical zones, Africa, Americas, Oceania, Asia Transmission: Mosquito-man Incubation 2–15d	*First exposure*: Dengue fever characterized by high pyrexia, headache, joint pains, maculopapular rash on trunk, ↓WCC and ↓plts *Second exposure to separate serotype*: Dengue haemorrhagic shock in 15–25% cases	Isolation not required Mortality low in non-shock cases Serological diagnosis and rapid plasma PCR for Dengue available
Lassa fever Rural districts of West Africa Transmission: Rodent-man-man Incubation 3–21d	Classically: fever, pharyngitis, retrosternal pain and proteinuria. Maculopapular rash mild or absent. CSF generally normal. Haemorrhagic complications 20–30%	Refer suspected cases to isolation facility Mortality 1–2%, rising to 15–20% in haemorrhagic cases Ribavirin effective treatment and prophylaxis Serological diagnosis, viral isolation blood and tissues in containment laboratory
Ebola virus Rural areas of Central, East, and West Africa Person-person transmission Incubation 2–21d	Fever, headache, joint pains, sore throat abdominal pain and vomiting. Haemorrhagic manifestations common 3–4 days after onset	Refer suspected cases to isolation facility Case fatality 50% Serological diagnosis, viral isolation blood and tissues in containment laboratory
Yellow fever Tropical Africa, Central and South America Mosquito-human Incubation 3–14d	Severe cases: headache, myalgia, high fever and vomiting 3–4 days. 1–2 days later symptoms return with jaundice, haemorrhage and renal failure, relative bradycardia, leukopenia, DIC and abnormal liver function	Isolation not required Case fatality 5–20% Serological diagnosis, viral isolation from blood

Rickettsial infections

These present with fever, headache, and rash and should be included in the differential diagnosis of febrile travellers. Recognition is important because the rickettsial illnesses have significant mortality if left untreated.

Imported rickettsial infections

Disease	Clinical features	Management
Epidemic typhus *Rickettsia prowazeki* World-wide in areas of poor hygiene Louse-human Incubation 5–23 days	Fever, severe headaches, maculopapular rash on trunk spreading to extremities. Complications include pneumonitis, encephalitis and myocarditis Outbreaks in overcrowded conditions	Isolation not req. Tetracycline or chloramphenicol* Untreated mortality 20%
Endemic typhus *Rickettsia typhi* North Africa, USA, SE Asia Rodent-flea-human Incubation 4–18 days	Usually mild illness, fever, headache, malaise, and maculopapular rash	Isolation not req. Tetracycline or chloramphenicol Mortality 1–2%
Scrub typhus *Rickettsia tsutugamishi* Asia, Oceania, Parts of Africa Animal-mite-human Incubation 3–21 days	Eschar at site of tick bite with painful regional lymphadenopathy, fever, headache, malaise, maculopapular rash in 60%	Isolation not req. Tetracycline or chloramphenicol
Spotted fever *Rickettsia rickettsiae* N. America Animal-tick-human Incubation 5–14 days	Fever, headache, confusion and neck stiffness, joint pains, malaise. Macular rash starts at wrists and ankles spreading to trunk, may be petechial or purpuric	Isolation not req. Tetracycline or chloramphenicol Treated mortality 4–8%, untreated 30%.

* Recommended dosages: tetracycline 500mg q6h for 7 days or chloramphenicol 500mg q6h for 7 days

Q fever

Coxiella burnetii is a disease of rural areas (reservoirs in sheep and cattle) and is transmitted by inhalation of infectious particles in dust, contact with infected carcasses (e.g. in abattoirs), and by tick bites. ***Presentation:*** Non-specific symptoms, fever, myalgia, malaise, sweats; dry cough and features of atypical pneumonia; hepatitis; PUO and splenomegaly. ***Investigations:*** Patchy CXR shadowing (lower lobes), hepatic granulomata. Complement fixation tests identify antibodies to phase 1 antigens (chronic infection – e.g. endocarditis see p94) and phase 2 antigens (acute infection). ***Treat*** with oral doxycycline (to try to prevent chronic infection) ± co-trimoxazole, rifampicin, or quinolone.

Human bites

- Superficial abrasions: Clean the wound. Re-dress the area daily.
- Give tetanus prophylaxis as needed (p414). Check Hepatitis B status and immunize if necessary (see p508). Arrange for HIV counselling (see p270 for post exposure prophylaxis)
- Have a low threshold for admission to hospital and iv antibiotic therapy: the human mouth contains a number of aerobic and anaerobic organisms that may produce aggressive necrotizing infection, particularly if the 'closed' spaces of the hand or feet are involved.
- *Antibiotic therapy*: All wounds that penetrate the dermis require antibiotics. Aerobic and anaerobic cultures should be taken prior to treatment with antibiotics. A suggested regimen is co-amoxiclav 250–500mg tds po (or iv cefuroxime and metronidazole). Consult your local microbiologists.
- *Facial bites*: Cosmetically significant bites should be referred to a plastic surgeon. Puncture wounds should be cleaned thoroughly and treated with prophylactic antibiotics (see above). Patients should be instructed to re-open the wound and express any purulent or bloody material 3–4 times a day for the first few days.
- *Hand bites*: Should be referred to the orthopaedic team; exploration is recommended. Clean the wound thoroughly. Give the first dose of antibiotics iv and subsequent doses po unless there are signs of systemic upset.

Non-human mammalian bites

- General management is as for human bites (see above); clean the wound, swab for aerobic and anaerobic culture, tetanus prophylaxis as needed, and prophylactic antibiotics as above. Rabies prophylaxis should be considered in all cases if the bite occurred outside the UK.
- ***Rabies*** is transmitted by infected saliva inoculated through the skin or by inhalation of aerosolized virus (from infected bats). Presenting features are a viral prodrome followed by parasthesiae and fasciculations. Agitation, confusion, muscle spasms, localized paralysis, and brainstem dysfunction follow. There is no effective treatment once symptoms appear; prevention is essential. Contact Virus Reference Laboratory, Colindale, London NW9 5HT. Tel: 0181 200 4400.
- ***Rabies vaccine*** should be given prophylactically (in the deltoid) to those at risk of bites from infected animals (vets, animal handlers, field workers).
- For patients who have been previously immunized and who have been bitten by a potentially infected animal, give 2 reinforcing doses of the vaccine (day 0 and day 3–7). Rabies immunoglobulin is not needed.
- For previously unimmunized patients with potential exposure, a full course of injections should be started as soon as possible (day 0, 3, 7, 14, 30, and 90) and ***specific rabies immunoglobulin*** of human origin 50% should be infiltrated around the wound and 50% given intramuscularly (day 0). The course of injections can be stopped if it is proven that the patient is not at risk.
- Staff attending to an infected patient should be offered immunization (4 intradermal doses of 0.1ml of vaccine at differing sites on the same day).

5 Infections in the HIV-positive patient

Infections in the HIV-positive patient

Patients infected with the human immunodeficiency virus (HIV) and those with the acquired immunodeficiency syndrome (AIDS) are at risk of many opportunistic infections and other problems during the course of their illness. Most of these are relatively indolent in their presentation and can be investigated electively. Pulmonary and neurological infections are common and require very different management to immuno-competent individuals.

General principles

- Unusual opportunistic infections are seen.
- Common infections may have an atypical presentation.
- Multiple pathogens may occur simultaneously or sequentially.
- Relapse is common.
- Close liaison with the microbiology laboratory is essential in detecting unusual organisms.
- Common diseases may still affect HIV-positive individuals.

Factors influencing the presentation of infections

Degree and nature of immunosuppression

- The normal CD4 count is 600–1500 $\times$ 10^{6}cells/l and gradually falls during the progression of HIV infection.
- The CD4 count is used as a guide to the individual patients' sus-ceptibility to certain infections [e.g. *Pneumocystis pneumonia* (PCP) is less likely with CD4 counts > 200/μl and invasive atypical mycobacterial infections are rarely seen with counts > 100/μl – see figure opposite)
- Other factors such as therapy-induced neutropenia may alter the spectrum of pathogens encountered.

Past history: Recurrence of previously treated infections is common.

Concomitant medication: Risk of neutropenia, effect of prophylactic antimicrobials.

Travel and ethnic origin: Many infections in HIV are reactivation of latent pathogens and this alters the spectrum of disease seen. For example, in Central America and parts of the USA disseminated histoplasmosis is a common infection but this is not seen in UK patients unless they have travelled to an endemic area.

Other medical problems: Specific situations predispose to certain infections; for example, staphylococcal infections in intravenous drug-users or line sepsis in patients with central venous catheters.

HIV testing without consent

As a general principle full, informed consent should be obtained for HIV testing. However, there are a few circumstances where testing is justified because it will lead to a change in therapy or if negative will avoid unnecessary and potentially toxic treatment.

- Testing of organ transplantation donors.
- Patients with confusion or dementia where HIV encephalopathy is clinically suspected but the patient unable to give consent.
- Severely ill patients presenting as an emergency and requiring intensive supportive care and too ill to give consent, where no clear diagnosis has been made, and there are sufficient grounds to suspect HIV infection.

Infections in the HIV-positive patient

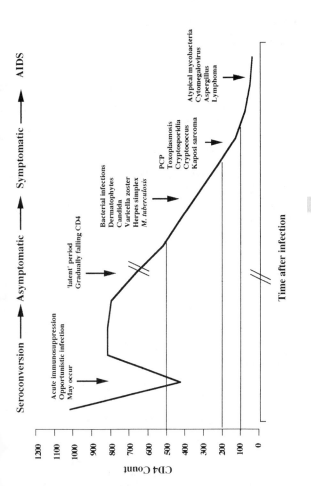

Pneumonia in HIV-positive patients

Assessment

Presentation (Symptoms are often indolent and slowly progressive).

- ***Cough/sputum:*** Purulent sputum suggests a bacterial or mycobacterial cause. Haemoptysis suggestive of mycobacterial or fungal infection or Kaposi's sarcoma (KS).
- ***Breathlessness:*** Gradually progressive exertional dyspnoea is characteristic of PCP. If sudden onset, consider pneumothorax, pulmonary oedema, or pulmonary embolism.
- ***Chest pain:*** Often absent. Pleuritic pain suggests bacterial aetiology or aspergillosis in the neutropenic host, pulmonary KS, pneumothorax, or pulmonary embolism.
- ***Fever/sweats:*** Non-specific symptom-immunocompromised patients with severe pneumonia may be afebrile.
- ***General examination:*** Look for cyanosis, anaemia, tachycardia, laboured respiration. Candidiasis, oral hairy leukoplakia, scars of Herpes zoster suggest significant immunosuppression. Look for other skin lesions, e.g. cutaneous cryptococcus or KS, cytomegalovirus (CMV) retinitis, and new lymphadenopathy.
- ***Chest examination:*** Bacterial pneumonia may present with classical signs of lobar consolidation or widespread crackles from diffuse involvement of both lungs. In pneumonitis due to PCP or respiratory viruses, chest examination may be entirely normal or there may be rather coarse inspiratory crackles.

Investigations

- ***FBC:*** Bacterial infection generally produces neutrophil leukocytosis. Leukopenia in bacterial pneumonia is a poor prognostic sign. Neutropenia may be the result of the disease or drug therapy and is important in deciding on empirical therapy.
- ***CD4 count:*** Helps to predict the type of opportunistic pathogens (see figure on p255) but may be unreliable during acute infection.
- ***U&Es:*** ↓ Na$^+$ or renal impairment are poor prognostic signs.
- ***LFTs:*** Abnormalities suggest disseminated disease or 2nd pathology.
- ***LDH:*** Elevated in most cases of PCP but non-specific.
- ***ABGs:*** ↓ P_aO_2 may be seen in any pneumonic process and arterial oxygen saturations should be monitored as a guide to severity. Hypoxia is most characteristic of PCP and may be present with a relatively normal chest X ray (CXR).
- ***Exercise oxygen saturation:*** Pulse oximetry during walking should be measured in all patients with normal resting saturations. Significant desaturation in the absence of chronic lung disease is very suggestive of a diffuse pneumonitis such as PCP.
- ***Lung function tests:*** If available these may be useful since impaired gas transfer (KCO) has the same significance as oxygen desaturation.
- ***Blood cultures:*** At least two sets prior to starting antibiotics. Consider mycobacterial and CMV cultures in patients with CD4 < 200/μl.
- ***Serology:*** For legionella, mycoplasma, and other atypical pathogens.
- ***Sputum:*** Gram-stain, and culture (low yield for PCP). Smear and culture for mycobacteria in all cases (dual infection is common).
- ***Induced sputum:*** Nebulize saline via a small particle ultrasonic nebulizer (arrange with an experienced physiotherapist). This produces a deep alveolar sputum specimen and can be assessed for PCP and other pathogens. If properly performed then the sensitivity for PCP is 85–90% compared with bronchoscopy.

.

Pneumonia in HIV-positive patients

Invasive investigations

- **Bronchoscopy:** See figure opposite. Specimens should be transported immediately to the relevant laboratories. Microscopy and culture for bacteria, mycobacteria, and fungi. Direct immunofluorescence and culture for CMV and respiratory viruses. Staining for PCP by immunofluorescence or silver stains. (PCP cannot be cultured.)
- **Pleural aspiration:** Cell count, protein, microscopy, and culture of all significant effusions.
- **Lung biopsy:** Transbronchial, percutaneous, or open lung biopsy may be required to establish the diagnosis. Expert advice should be sought in patients failing to respond to empirical therapy.
- **Radiology:** CXR is required in all cases and is used to direct initial therapy. Common patterns are given in the table below. Other radiology, such as chest CT, is performed as needed.

Chest X-ray patterns in HIV-associated disease

X-ray finding	Disease processs
Normal	• PCP, viral pneumonitis if hypoxic on exercise
Focal infiltrate	• Bacterial (*S. pneumoniae*, *H. influenzae*) • Mycobacteria (TB or MAI) • PCP (apical on nebulized pentamidine) • Fungal (cryptococcus, histoplasmosis, aspergillus, candida) • *Rhodococcus equi* or nocardia (rare) • Pulmonary Kaposi's sarcoma or lymphoma
Cavitating	• Bacterial (staphylococcal, anaerobes) • Mycobacteria, nocardia, fungi • PCP may produce thin-walled cysts (pneumatocoeles)
Pneumothorax	• PCP: occasionally when pneumatocoele ruptures • Tuberculosis
Diffuse infiltrate	• PCP, classical presentation • Respiratory viruses (RSV, adenovirus, parainfluenza) • Cytomegalovirus (often difficult to decide whether pathogenic role) • Miliary tuberculosis • Fungal (cryptococcus, histoplasmosis, candida) • Toxoplasmosis • Lipoid interstitial pneumonitis
Pleural effusion	• Bacterial, mainly *S. pneumoniae* • Mycobacteria, mainly TB • Heart failure • Lymphoma
Mediastinal lymphadenopathy	• Not a feature of HIV-related lymphadenopathy • Mycobacteria, fungal infection • Lymphoma and Kaposi's sarcoma

PCP: *Pneumocystis carinii* pneumonia, TB: tuberculosis, MAI: mycobacterium avium intracellulare, RSV: respiratory syncytial virus.

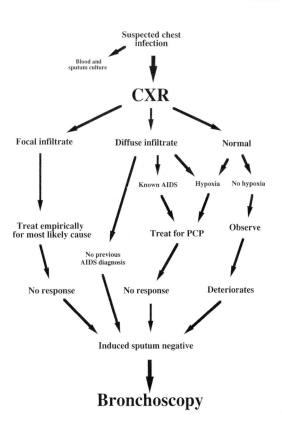

Pneumonia in HIV-positive patients

Treatment

General measures

- Monitor pulse, bp, and temperature regularly.
- Pulse oximetry should be used with supplemental oxygen as needed to maintain arterial oxygen saturation greater than 90%.

Assisted ventilation

Being HIV-positive is not in itself a contraindication to intensive therapy and ventilation when appropriate. Most acute respiratory infections in this group are potentially reversible and the decision to ventilate is based more on the overall stage of disease and prognosis plus the views of the patient and their family. It is important that this issue is considered in all patients at the time of admission so that difficult decisions do not need to be made in an emergency.

Antibiotic therapy

Empirical therapy is directed at bacterial infections and PCP unless the initial investigations strongly suggest other diagnoses. Modify treatment in the light of clinical course and/or results of investigations.

CD4 count > 200/µl, (Low probability of PCP)

- Pneumococcus and *H. influenzae* need to be considered plus atypical infections.
- Treat with co-amoxiclav (1.2g q6–8h iv) or cefuroxime (750mg-1.5g tds iv) + erythromycin (500mg qds po/iv).

CD4 count < 200/µl, (High probability of PCP)

- Still need to cover bacteria until the diagnosis is confirmed. Co-trimoxazole has good activity against most relevant bacterial pathogens and therefore high-dose co-trimoxazole (5mg/kg of the trimethoprim component q6h) is sufficient plus erythromycin (0.5–1g qds po/iv) for atypical pathogens.
- If alternative anti-PCP agents are used then co-amoxiclav (1.2g q6–8h iv) or cefuroxime (750mg-1.5g tds iv) should be included.

Hospital-acquired pneumonia

- Increased risk of enteric Gram-negative bacilli such as *E. coli*.
- Third generation cephalosporin such a cefotaxime or a quinolone such as ciprofloxacin.

Intravenous drug-user

- At risk of Gram-negative and staphylococcal infections.
- Cefotaxime (1–2g q8h iv) plus flucloxacillin (1–2g q6h iv). Add in atypical or anti-PCP treatment as indicated.

Neutropenic patient

- Increased risk of *Pseudomonas* and fungal infections.
- Ceftazidime (1–2g q8h iv) alone, piperacillin (4g q6h iv) plus gentamicin (2mg/kg iv loading dose then 3mg/kg iv in divided doses, guided by levels) or ciprofloxacin (500mg-1g po bd) plus amoxycillin (2g iv tds iv). Add in atypical or anti-PCP treatment as indicated.
- Consider amphotericin B if fails to respond.

Treatment of *Pneumocystis carinii* pneumonia

First-line therapy
- Co-trimoxazole remains the drug of choice given orally unless there are problems with absorption. Co-trimoxazole 5mg/kg of the trimethoprim component every 6 hours.
- Corticosteroids have been shown to reduce the morbidity/mortality of PCP and should be given to all cases. Prednisolone 40mg/day for five days. Then stop if no longer hypoxic or taper off over 10–21 days if hypoxia persists.

Second-line therapy
- There are various alternatives with none being clearly superior. All should be given with prednisolone as above.
- Trimethoprim 5mg/kg 6 hourly plus dapsone 100mg/day.
- Clindamycin 600mg 6 hourly plus primaquine 30mg/day.
- Pentamidine 4mg/kg/day iv. Other agents include atovaquone, trimetrexate, or dimethylfluoro-ornithine.

Neurological conditions in HIV +ve patients

Assessment

Opportunistic infections, malignancies, and the direct effects of HIV can all cause disease of the central or peripheral nervous system. The presenting features of different conditions are often quite varied and non-specific and tend to involve the same diagnostic approach and investigations. The most frequently encountered diseases are outlined on p268–269.

History and key symptoms

- **Headache:** Ask for symptoms suggestive of elevated intracranial pressure such as nausea, early morning headache, increase in intensity with coughing. Need to distinguish from facial pain due to dental or sinus disease or the prodrome of varicella zoster.

- **Meningeal symptoms:** May be absent even in cases of overt meningitis due to the reduced inflammatory response.

- **Specific symptoms:** Ask about radicular or muscle pains, bladder, and bowel symptoms that might suggest spinal cord involvement and sensory symptoms.

- **Cognitive impairment:** Ask about memory, concentration, ability to cope at work and home. Often the history from a friend or relative is more informative.

- **Psychiatric disturbances:** Opportunistic infections and HIV encephalopathy may present with depressive or frankly psychotic manifestations.

Examination

- **General examination:** Check carefully for rashes to suggest disseminated infection such as herpetic lesions. Percuss the sinuses for evidence of sinusitis, examine the ears carefully and check for neck stiffness.

- **Neurological examination:** Examine for cranial nerve lesions, focal motor deficits, reflexes, sensory loss, and cerebellar signs. Fundoscopy looking for papilloedema and for retinitis, if necessary with dilated pupils after first recording the pupillary reflexes. Assess consciousness level and test cognitive function with mental test scoring, serial sevens, and memory testing.

Investigations

General investigations

- Results of baseline CD4 count, *Toxoplasma* and syphilis serologies are helpful.

- Full blood count, electrolytes, and liver function tests may point to other abnormalities but rarely provide the diagnosis.

- Blood cultures for bacteria, fungi, mycobacteria, and CMV should be performed in all patients with neurological illness and CD4 of less than $200/\mu l$. Serum cryptococcal antigen and syphilis serology should be sent in all cases. Stool urine and throat culture for viruses.

Specific investigations

- These are discussed on p264.

Neurological conditions in HIV +ve patients

Investigations

- *General investigations* are discussed on p262.
- *Toxoplasma serology:* 90% of patients with CNS toxoplasmosis have positive *Toxoplasma* serology and therefore a positive result identifies patients at risk of disease reactivation. Serology is not helpful in diagnosing acute reactivation as the antibody titre does not reflect disease activity.
- *Skull X-ray:* Only useful for diagnosing sinusitis or cranial osteomyelitis.
- *Head CT scan:* Not as sensitive as magnetic resonance imaging (MRI) but more widely available. All patients with new symptoms should be scanned, including contrast. Space occupying lesions can be present without papilloedema and in the absence of focal signs, and therefore CT is a necessary prelude to lumbar puncture in this group of patients.
- *MRI:* Investigation of choice if there is no diagnosis after CT scanning. More sensitive for the detection of *Toxoplasma* cysts, the lesions of progressive multifocal leukoencephalopathy (PML) and HIV encephalopathy. Also the best modality for spinal cord and nerve root imaging.
- *Lumbar puncture:*
  - Cerebrospinal fluid (CSF) should be examined in all unexplained neurological syndromes: CT scan all patients before LP.
  - Send CSF (~ 20ml) for:-
    - Differential cell count
    - Protein and glucose (with simultaneous plasma glucose)
    - Bacterial, fungal, and mycobacterial culture
    - Gram-stain and TB staining (auramine fluorescence or Ziehl-Nielssen)
    - India ink stain for cryptococcus plus cryptococcal antigen
    - Syphilis serology (VDRL and TPHA)
    - Viral culture and PCR for herpes viruses including CMV
    - Serology and PCR for JC virus (cause of PML)
    - Cytology if cell count elevated
  - In patients with advanced AIDS there may be little inflammatory response and no cells in the CSF despite meningeal involvement. Therefore, normal CSF microscopy does not rule out infection and full culture should be performed in all cases.
  - In addition, minor elevation in CSF protein and cell count (usually 10–20 mononuclear cells) are common in HIV-infected individuals without overt neurological disease.
- *EEG:* Useful to confirm seizure activity but non-specific in HIV encephalopathy and opportunistic infections. Classical herpes simplex (HSV) encephalitis is rare in AIDS.
- *Brain biopsy:* Used for the diagnosis of focal lesions that fail to respond to empirical therapy.

Specific neurological conditions

Unconscious patient with HIV

- Many possible causes, including trauma, intracerebral haemorrhage in patients with HIV-related thrombocytopenia, infection, HIV encephalopathy, and drugs.
- Management is as on p304–310.

Seizures

- Increased incidence in patients with HIV infection, with about 50% having no definable underlying infective cause.
- All new seizures should be investigated with contrast CT scan and lumbar puncture. If these are normal then treat with anticonvulsant medication in standard way after two or more seizures (see p372).
- If cognitive impairment is present then treat as for HIV encephalopathy.

Intracerebral space occupying lesion

- Very wide differential diagnosis, including infection and malignancy (cerebral lymphoma).
- Treat empirically for toxoplasmosis with sulphadiazine (1g orally qds) and pyrimethamine (100mg od for 3 days then 50mg od – plus folinic acid 15mg od) and repeat the scan after 2 weeks. 90% of patients with toxoplasmosis will respond.
- In patients failing to respond, brain biopsy is indicated if the lesion is accessible and the general condition of the patient is suitable.
- Negative serology for toxoplasmosis and the absence of contrast enhancement makes this a less likely diagnosis.

Paraparesis

- This is a medical emergency due to the risk of permanent paralysis.
- The main differential diagnosis is between viral transverse myelitis (usually HIV, CMV, VZV, or HSV) and cord compression from infection or malignancy.
- Arrange for urgent MRI or CT myelogram to exclude compression, followed by a lumbar puncture.
- In the absence of compression or an immediate diagnosis, treat immediately with ganciclovir (5mg/kg q12h iv) to cover CMV and herpes, plus zidovudine (AZT – initially 250mg 6 hourly) for HIV myelitis.

Rapid visual deterioration

- Arrange for urgent ophthalmological assessment for retinitis, papillitis, or uveitis.
- It is important to remember that retinal detachment is a complication of CMV infection and often occurs on therapy. Therefore, *any* sudden change in visual acuity needs investigating even if the patient already has a diagnosis.

CNS Infections in HIV disease

Condition	Possible presentations	Diagnostic tests	Treatment
HIV	Encephalitis or aseptic meningitis Dementia Psychiatric presentation Seizures	Diagnosis of exclusion Brain biopsy diagnostic but not performed for this reason	AZT initially 250mg 6 hourly DDI or DDC if already on AZT
Toxoplasmosis	Space occupying lesion Seizures Confusion/encephalitic illness	90% anti-toxo antibody positive but do not discriminate active from inactive disease CT: Ring enhancing lesions Brain biopsy gold standard, perform if no response to empirical therapy	Sulphadiazine 1g orally qds Pyrimethamine 100mg od for 3 days then 50mg od. Plus folinic acid 15mg od 90% will show CT improvement within 2 weeks
Cryptococcosis	Headache +/- meningism SOL (cryptococcoma) Seizures Confusion and behavioural changes	CSF: Pleiocytosis with low glucose but may be normal in 20-30%. India ink stain, culture and cryptococcal antigen Serum cryptococcal antigen positive 95%	Intravenous amphotericin B increasing to 1mg/kg/day +/- flucytosine Fluconazole or itraconazole for maintenance therapy
Mycobacteria	Headache +/- meningism SOL (tuberculoma) Seizures Confusion and behavioural changes	CSF: Pleiocytosis with low glucose in most cases. ZN stain positive in only 10-20%. CSF culture takes 4-6 weeks	Mycobacterium tuberculosis: rifampicin/isoniazid/pyrazinamide MAI: combination of 4 or 5 drugs
Nocardia asteroides	Space occupying lesion or brain abscess	Brain biopsy/culture Often co-existing pulmonary disease	Combination therapy with at least two of: co-trimoxazole, amikacin, streptomycin, imipenem, and minocycline

Condition	Possible presentations	Diagnostic tests	Treatment
Cytomegalovirus	Encephalitis Transverse myelitis Polyradiculitis	Viral detection in CSF or neural tissue. PCR, culture, or immunohistochemistry	Ganciclovir 5mg/kg/12 hourly, or Foscarnet 90mg/kg/12 hourly
Varicella zoster	Encephalitis Transverse myelitis Polyradiculitis	Viral detection in CSF or neural tissue Culture, immunohistochemistry, or PCR	Acyclovir 30mg/kg/day Foscarnet in resistant cases
Herpes simplex	Encephalitis surprisingly rare Radiculitis	Viral detection in CSF or neural tissue Culture, immunohistochemistry, or PCR	Acyclovir 30mg/kg/day Foscarnet in resistant cases
PML (JC virus)	Dementia	CSF: Anti-JC virus antibodies PCR Brain biopsy White matter MRI/CT changes	High dose AZT, interferon, or cytosine arabinoside may slow progression
Lymphoma	Space occupying lesion Malignant meningitis Isolated nerve or spinal cord lesions	CSF cytology Brain biopsy	Cranial irradiation Chemotherapy Response poor

SOL: space occupying lesion, AZT: zidovudine, DDI: didanosine, DDC: zalcitidine, PML: progressive multifocal leukoencephalopathy

HIV-seroconversion illness

- It is important to consider this diagnosis and ask appropriate questions relating to risk factors for HIV infection.
- HIV antibody tests may be negative early in the illness but are generally positive within one month of the onset of symptoms. HIV p24 antigen, PCR or viral culture may establish the diagnosis earlier.

Features of HIV-seroconversion illness

General symptoms/signs
    Flu-like illness, fever, myalgia, and malaise
    Generalized lymphadenopathy
    Maculopapular rash
    Pharyngitis
Laboratory findings
    Lymphopenia and/or neutropenia
    Thrombocytopenia
    Elevated AST
    Initially HIV-antibody may be negative
    p24 antigen and viral culture positive
Acute immunosuppression
    CD4 may fall to less than $300/\mu l$
    Candidiasis, viral warts, varicella-zoster
    PCP and other opportunistic infections may occur
Specific syndromes
    Aseptic meningitis
    Encephalitis
    Oesophageal/oral ulceration

Post-exposure prophylaxis

- No therapy has been shown to reduce the risk of transmission of HIV after a needle-stick injury. The estimated risks of transmission calculated from USA data are:-
  - **High-risk exposure:** A needle containing known HIV positive blood pierces the skin and draws blood. Intraoperative wound drawing blood when operating on a known HIV-positive patient. Estimated risk 1:200.
  - **Low-risk exposure:** Needle was not in direct contact with patient or the patient is in a risk group but not known to be HIV infected. Splash of infected blood on to mucous membranes of eye or mouth. Estimated risk 1:1000.
  - **Very low risk:** Mucous membrane exposure with body fluid other than blood. Blood splash on to intact skin. Risk 1:1000+.

Action

- Immediately clean the wound and then contact the needle-stick advice service within the institution; generally occupational health department and/or consultant microbiology or virology staff.
- Whether to take AZT is a difficult decision but it is probably not warranted for low-risk exposures.
- The optimum dose and duration of treatment has not been defined and most centres use 250mg qds for 4–6 weeks.
- AZT may delay seroconversion and therefore serial HIV tests for 3–6 months are required.

Infections in the HIV-positive patient

Diarrhoea

Common pathogens, diagnostic tests, and therapy shown in table opposite.

Emergency management

- Assess for fluid and electrolyte status and rehydrate as necessary.
- Take blood cultures in all cases.
- Take blood for *Mycobacterium avium intracellulare* (MAI) and CMV culture in patients with CD4 count $< 200/\mu l$.
- Send stool for microscopy for parasites and acid-fast stain for cryptosporidiosis and MAI. Send 3 stool cultures. If no diagnosis established then proceed to upper and lower GI endoscopies with biopsies for microscopy and culture.

Antibiotic therapy

- Unlike immunocompetent host, antibiotics are often needed for bacterial gastroenteritis in patients with AIDS. Salmonella, in particular, tends to cause both prolonged and recurrent infection. Treat systemically unwell patients empirically with ciprofloxacin plus metronidazole whilst awaiting cultures. Systemically well patients can be observed.

Septic shock of unknown origin

This is relatively unusual in patients with AIDS and is usually due to bacterial pathogens. It should be diagnosed and treated along the same guidelines for other patient groups (see p216–220)

Heart failure

- Patients with HIV may develop acute cardiac failure due to dilated cardiomyopathy as the direct result of HIV or from opportunistic infections or lymphomatous infiltration.
- Patients presenting with signs of heart failure and cardiomegaly require emergency assessment including echocardiography to exclude valvular disease (for example, infective endocarditis in a drug-user) or tamponade from pericardial effusion.

Renal failure

- HIV infection may be associated with focal glomerulonephritis particularly in the context of intravenous heroin abuse.
- Acute renal failure may be due to direct HIV nephropathy, infection-related tubular necrosis, or be drug-induced (particularly with foscarnet).
- Prompt investigation of renal abnormalities and appropriate therapy is essential to preserve renal function.
- Management of renal failure is dealt with on p282–284.

Acute liver failure

- Acute liver failure is rare and is usually due to co-existent viral hepatitis.
- Drugs, disseminated fungal infection, and lymphomatous infiltration have also been reported to cause acute liver failure.
- Management of liver failure is dealt with on p518–524.

GI pathogens causing diarrhoea in HIV

Pathogen	Diagnostic test	Therapy/outcome
Salmonella	• Stool cultures • Blood cultures • Ciprofloxacin	• Relapse common, often requiring maintenance therapy
Shigella	• Stool culture	• Ciprofloxacin, resistance increasing Relapse rare
Campylobacter	• Stool culture	• Erythromycin or ciprofloxacin • Relapse rare
Giardiasis	• Stool microscopy • Duodenal aspirate/ biopsy	• Metronidazole • Tinidazole if relapses
Cryptosporidiosis	• Stool microscopy (acid-fast stain) • Duodenal or colonic biopsy	• No effective therapy. Paromomycin reduces cyst excretion • CD4 count < 200/μl persistence is common
Isospora	• Stool microscopy (acid-fast stain)	• Co-trimoxazole, usually curative
Microsporidiosis	• Stool microscopy (EM or toludene blue stain) • Duodenal biopsy	• Albendazole • Difficult to diagnose
Cytomegalovirus	• Intestinal biopsy • Can affect all parts of the gut	• Ganciclovir or foscarnet • Relapse common, maintenance therapy required
Atypical mycobacteria	• Stool microscopy (acid-fast stain) • Intestinal biopsy	• Multi-drug regimen • Not curative
HIV enteritis	• Exclusion of above	• May respond to anti-retroviral therapy

EM, electron microscopy

6 Renal emergencies

Acute renal failure (ARF)

Presentation

- Elevated creatinine (or urea) during biochemical screening
- Detection of oliguria by nursing staff

Occasionally the patient may present to the A&E department with:-

- Malaise, confusion, seizures, or coma
- Nausea, anorexia, or vomiting
- Oliguria or abnormal urine colour
- Haematuria (pink rather than frank blood)
- Drug overdose (e.g. paracetamol)
- Constitutional symptoms (arthralgia, rhinitis, respiratory symptoms)
- Vasculitic rash

In the majority of cases, their renal impairment can be resolved by adequate volume replacement, treatment of sepsis, and stopping nephrotoxic drugs. There are many causes of acute renal impairment, some of which, such as multi-system vasculitis or rhabdomyolysis, are important since their early diagnosis and treatment may have a profound effect on outcome (see table p278).

Assessment of severity

Patients with acute renal failure have a high mortality (~ 50%). The following history is important.

- Cause of hypovolaemia (D&V, diuretics, bleeding, fever).
- Cause of hypotension (hypovolaemia, drugs, shock).
- History of sepsis (e.g. UTI, fever, or hypothermia. Symptoms may be non-specific in elderly).
- Drugs (NSAIDs, ACE-I, aminoglycosides, antibiotics, amphotericin)
- Non-specific symptoms (e.g. myalgia, arthralgia), neurological signs, ophthalmological complications, sinusitis, and/or skin rashes may suggest vasculitis.
- Past history of hypertension or diabetes, prostatism, or haematuria
- Patients with diabetes or myeloma have an increased risk of contrast-induced renal impairment (avoid dehydration).
- Are there symptoms or signs of liver disease ± ascites?
- Any suggestion of bacterial endocarditis?
- Backache may suggest pelvi-ureteric obstruction. Whilst this may affect a single kidney initially the other kidney is likely to become involved. Consider aortic aneurysm.
- Cholesterol emboli (aneurysms, absent pulses, rash)
- Post partum (HELLP syndrome, HUS, fatty liver, pre-eclampsia)
- Look for signs of fluid overload (dyspnoeic with signs of pulmonary oedema, high JVP or CVP, peripheral oedema, gallop rhythm) or dehydration (postural hypotension, ↓ tissue turgor).

Poor prognostic features include:

- Age > 50 years
- Infection (esp. septicaemia)
- Burns (> 70% surface area)
- Rising urea (> 16mmol/24h)
- Oliguric for > 2 weeks
- Multi-organ failure (> 3)
- Jaundice

The main priority is to try to prevent cardiovascular collapse and death, and stabilize for transfer to a renal unit.

Acute renal failure

Urgent therapy is needed for

- Hyperkalaemia (p282)
- Pulmonary oedema (p74)
- Septicaemia and shock (p216)
- Pericarditis (p138)
- Tamponade (p142)
- Seizures (p368)

Acute renal failure: Causes

Causes of acute renal failure

Pre-renal
Hypovolaemia
Hypotension, shock (p210)
Renal artery emboli
Renal artery stenosis + ACEI
Hepatorenal syndrome

Post renal (obstructive)
Intratubular (uric acid crystals)
Ureteric
• Stones
• Retroperitoneal fibrosis / tumour
Urethral
• Prostatic hypertrophy)

Renal (parenchymal)
Vasculitis (SLE, PAN)
Glomerulonephritis
Acute tubular necrosis
• Ischaemia (e.g. hypotension)
• Septicaemia
• Toxin (myoglobin, BJ proteins)
• Drugs (e.g. gentamicin), contrast
• Prolonged pre-renal oliguria
Thrombotic microangiopathy
• Accelerated hypertension
• HUS / TTP (p562)
Scleroderma crisis
Sepsis
• Interstitial nephritis
• Drugs (NSAIDs, antibiotics)
• Infections (*Strep.*, *Staph*,
  Leptospirosis, *Brucella*, G -ve
  sepsis, *Legionella*)
Calcium, urate, oxalate overload
• Tumour lysis syndrome (p592)

Causes of immune-mediated ARF and vasculitis

• Microscopic polyangiitis
• Wegener's granulomatosis
• Churg-Strauss syndrome
• Polyarteritis nodosa
• SLE
• Rheumatoid arthritis (and
  treatment)
• Goodpasture's syndrome
• Cryoglobulinaemia
• Henoch-Schönlein purpura

• Acute proliferative
  glomerulonephitis
• Acute interstitial nephritis
• HIV
• Myeloma
• Leptospirosis (interstitial
  nephritis)
• Infective endocarditis
• IgA nephropathy (rarely)

Urgent investigations for patients in ARF.

• U&Es
• FBC and blood film
• Coagulation studies (PT, APTT, TT, fibrinogen, FDPs)
• Blood cultures
• Urine microscopy and culture
• Urine electrolytes (esp. Na^+) and osmolality
• ECG
• CXR
• USS kidneys
• Consider other investigations to aid in diagnosis (see p280)

Acute renal failure

Acute renal failure: Investigations

Blood tests

- U&Es   Urea is disproportionately raised in pre-renal uraemia, GI bleeds, catabolic states.
- Ca^{2+}, PO_4^{3-} Acidaemia increases ionized calcium concentration.
- FBC   Anaemia suggests chronic or acute on chronic renal failure. ↓ platelets – liver disease, HELLP, sepsis. with MCV, blood film (HUS, myeloma, left shift). ↓ platelets – vasculitis (e.g. Wegener's) eosinophilia – Churg-Strauss syndrome, interstitial nephritis.
- Coagulation   Abnormal in DIC, liver disease, SLE, HELLP syndrome, HUS.
- LFTs   Acute hepatitis, paracetamol overdose, cirrhosis. Alk. phosphatase often ↑ in vasculitis
- LDH / HBD   Increased in HUS
- CPK   Very high in rhabdomyolysis
- Blood cultures   Should be taken from all patients with ARF.
- Immunology   ANCA, anti-GBM, immunoglobulins, C3/C4, Rh Factor, ANA, ENA, double-stranded DNA, cryoglobulins, anti-cardiolipin antibodies
- ESR / CRP   CRP is often normal, ESR high in SLE
- Protein strip   For paraproteins (myeloma, light chain disease)
- HIV, HBsAg, HCVAb (serology required for dialysis)

Urine

- Inspect the urine yourself. Most hospitals have facilities for urine microscopy (A&E or the renal ward). If you have not done this before, contact the microbiology technician on call.
- Send a specimen to microbiology for microscopy and culture.
- *RBC casts* suggest glomerulonephritis (refer to renal physician urgently), *pigment casts* suggest myoglobinuria, *WBC casts* suggest acute pyelonephritis. *Excess eosinophils* in the urine are associated with interstitial nephritis.
- Save a specimen for Bence-Jones protein if myeloma is suspected.
- *Urine electrolytes and osmolality:* These may help but do not replace careful clinical examination, and are unreliable when diuretics have been given. They may be less reliable in the elderly when sub-clinical renal impairment may be present. See table p281.

Other investigations

- USS   All patients with ARF should have an URGENT ultrasound to exclude obstruction and to assess kidney size (small in acute-on-chronic failure).
- CXR   Look at the heart size (dilated, pericardial effusion), pulmonary vasculature (pulmonary oedema, Kerley lines), lung fields ('fluffy' shadows – oedema, haemorrhage of Goodpasture's or Wegner's, infection)
- ECG   Look for changes of hyperkalaemia (tented T waves, QRS broadening) and signs of myocardial ischaemia or pericarditis.

Urinary electrolytes and osmolality in renal failure

	Pre-renal	Renal (ATN)
Urine Na$^+$ (mmol/l)	< 20	> 40
Urine / serum creatinine	> 40	< 20
Urine osmolality (mOsm)	> 500	< 350
Urine / serum osmolality	> 1.2	< 1.2

Acute renal failure: Management

Hyperkalaemia

In general terms the absolute K^+ concentration is less important than the effect on the cardiac conducting tissue (tented T waves, broad QRS, flattened P wave), but if the K^+ is $> 7mM$ then treat urgently. If the hyperkalaemia is an unexpected isolated finding, and there are no ECG signs of hyperkalaemia, then repeat K^+ urgently.

If there are ECG changes or $K^+ > 7mM$, contact the renal team and arrange for urgent dialysis if appropriate. While this is being set up:-

- Record 12–lead ECG, attach to cardiac monitor.
- Give **10ml of 10% calcium gluconate iv**, repeated every 10–20 min. until ECG normalizes (patients may require up to 50ml). iv calcium does not lower the potassium level but reduces cardiac excitability.
- Give **nebulized salbutamol** (5–10mg) to drive K^+ intracellularly (use lower doses in patients with ischaemic heart disease).
- **50ml 50% dextrose with 10U actrapid insulin** over 15–30 min (monitor blood glucose); this should lower K^+ for several hours.
- **50–100ml 8.4% bicarbonate iv via central line over 30 min** (or 400ml 2.1% peripherally): represents a N^+ load of 50–100mmol.
- Polystyrene sulphonate resin enema (***calcium resonium®***) 30g increases gut losses of potassium. Follow with 15g po tds, with lactulose. This takes 24 hours to work.
- Monitor serum K^+ frequently to assess response to treatment.

Fluid balance

- Manage on HDU or ITU.
- Measure weight, bp (supine and sitting or upright) and pulse rate.
- Assess hydration (central skin turgor, mucous membranes, and JVP)
- Insert central venous line and measure CVP. Monitor PCWP in patients who are hypoxic or severely compromised.
- Examine fluid and weight charts, and operation notes if applicable.

If *volume depleted:-*
- If the patient has a low or normal CVP $\pm$ postural hypotension give a trial of volume expansion (500ml of colloid or N/saline) over 30min. Monitor response of urine output and venous pressure. Continue fluids until CVP is 5–10cm at mid-clavicular line.
- When adequately filled (CVP > 10 and/or PCWP > 15) reassess urine output. If oliguric or anuric, give frusemide 120mg-1g slowly iv (max. 4mg/min). Consider low dose dopamine (2–5µg/kg/min, see p689).
- If hypotension persists (mean arterial pressure $< 60mmHg$) in spite of adequate volume replacement, as indicated by a CVP of $> 10cm$, commence inotropic support (see p210).
- If anuria persists, remove the urinary catheter (source of sepsis).

If *fluid overloaded:-*
- Consider urgent haemofiltration or dialysis. Consider venesection if there is a delay for dialysis; remove 250–500mls.
- Give oxygen to maintain $S_aO_2 > 95\%$. Consider CPAP (p802).
- Start intravenous nitrates (e.g. GTN 2–10mg/h iv).
- Give frusemide 120mg-1g slowly iv (max. 4mg/min).
- Low-dose (2.5µg/kg/min) dopamine may promote diuresis (see p692).
- Paracentesis if obvious ascites is present (p822).
- Avoid opiates, although a single dose (e.g. 2.5mg diamorphine iv) may help relieve anxiety and the sensation of breathlessness.

Indications for dialysis

- Persistent hyperkalaemia ($K^+ > 7mM$)
- Fluid overload (e.g. refractory pulmonary oedema)
- Pericarditis (heralds the risk of tamponade, p138)
- Acidosis (arterial pH < 7.1, bicarbonate < 12mM)
- Symptomatic uraemia (tremor, cognitive impairment, coma, fits, urea typically > 45mM)

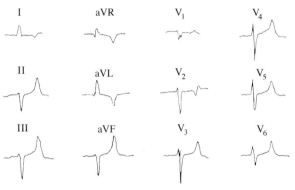

ECG changes in hyperkalaemia

Acute renal failure: Further management

Treatment of life-threatening hyperkalaemia, severe fluid overload, or dehydration take priority (p282).

Correct other abnormalities

1 **Acidaemia:** Classically produces sighing respirations (Kussmaul's breathing) and may worsen hypotension (impaired cardiac function)
   • If pH is < 7.2 give 100ml of 8.4% bicarbonate via central line over 15–30 min, (or 400ml 2.1% bicarbonate peripherally).
   • Arrange urgent dialysis.
   • Correction of acidaemia can cause symptomatic hypocalcaemia (Chvostek's, Trousseau's, fits, confusion) due to a fall in ionized Ca^{2+}: treat with iv calcium [e.g. 30ml calcium chloride over 30 min via central vein (it is irritant when given peripherally)]. If mild give oral calcium carbonate or equivalent $\pm$ alfacalcidol.

2 **Hyponatraemia:** usually dilutional (relative water excess). Management is discussed on p466.

3 **Hyperphosphataemia:** If the product of $[Ca^{2+}] \times [PO_4^{3-}]$ is > 4.0 the risk of 'metastatic' precipitation is high. Aim to lower PO_4^{3-} to 0.6–1.4 mmol/l. Give oral PO_4^{3-} binders (e.g. calcium carbonate 300–1200mg q8h po). The PO_4^{3-} usually falls with dialysis or haemofiltration.

4 **Nutrition:** There is no role for protein restriction, acutely. Institute enteral or parenteral feeding early. Insulin requirements for diabetics fall with renal impairment.

5 **Sepsis:** Common precipitant/complication of ARF. Culture blood, urine and specimens from other potential site of infection. Treat with appropriate antibiotics remembering to adjust the daily dose in view of the renal impairment. (Septic shock is covered on p216.)

Further measures

The causes of ARF are listed on p278. Most cases are multi-factorial with volume depletion or hypotension, sepsis, and drugs (e.g. injudicious use of ACE inhibitors and NSAIDs), obstruction of the urinary tract and/or pre-existing chronic renal disease. It is essential to identify treatable conditions to prevent further renal deterioration.

In practical terms it is probably simplest to divide patients into those with pre-renal, renal, and post renal acute renal failure using *clinical assessment, filling pressures* (CVP, PCWP), and *USS*. Whilst sepsis is included as a renal cause, much of the early deleterious effects (i.e. hypotension) are potentially reversible with appropriate management. The principles of further management are:-

• **Optimize fluid balance:** There is no substitute for painstaking physical examination. Careful fluid balance charts and daily weights guide replacement. Limit fluid intake to total fluid output plus 500ml/day. The most reliable sign of intravascular volume depletion is a postural drop of blood pressure.

• **Intrinsic renal disease:** Oliguria is not readily reversed by restoration of circulating volume or blood pressure, but it is important that they are optimized (CVP of 5–10cm, MAP of > 75mmHg) (see p282). If diuretics $\pm$ low-dose dopamine fail to improve urine output, established ATN is likely to be present, and the patient will require renal support.

• Patients with severe portal hypertension and ascites may have marked oliguria (as low as 250ml urine per day), and maintain a normal creatinine. Their urine is very concentrated and virtually devoid of sodium. They are usually resistant to diuretics, but may respond transiently to volume expansion. Beware of precipitating electrolyte or renal dysfunction by overdiuresis.

Renal colic and renal stones

Spasmodic pain radiating from loin to groin usually due to stones or blood clots. ~ 2–3% of population have a stone in the upper urinary tract

Presentation

- Pain: The site of the pain may vary; stones in the renal pelvis cause dull loin ache, ureteric stones produce severe colicky pain often of sudden onset radiating from loin to groin, bladder stones cause suprapubic and perineal or testicular ache and strangury.
- Haematuria (often frank) may be the only feature.
- With severe pain the patient will be restless, sweaty, pale, nauseated, and very distressed.
- Try to obtain a history of previous episodes, UTIs, fluid intake, occupation, periods of residence in hot climates, symptoms of hypercalcaemia, or family history of stone disease.
- On examination note any fever, abdominal tenderness (especially loin or subcostal), palpable kidneys. Do not miss a leaking abdominal aortic aneurysm that may be producing similar symptoms.

Investigations Acutely, the tests required are:-

- Bloods   U&Es (for renal dysfunction) and glucose, FBC (for Hb, WCC).
- Urine   Dipstick urinalysis for blood, and formal microscopy for crystals, pyuria, and bacteria. Culture for infection.
- AXR/IVU   The plain AXR film will detect > 90% of stones. ivU may show acute obstruction with dense nephrogram and delayed pyelogram in early films, dilatation below the stone if the obstruction is partial, or bladder oedema with stones at the vesico-ureteric junction.

Other investigations to determine the underlying cause of the renal colic (stone formation, papillary necrosis or clot) can usually be performed once the acute episode has been dealt with. Tests to consider include serum Ca^{2+} and urate (see p452 for investigation of hypercalcaemia) and 24h urine for Ca^{2+}, phosphate, oxalate, urate to detect a stone-forming metabolic defect.

Management of acute renal colic

- Analgesia: Diclofenac sodium 75mg im repeated after 30min. If needed pethidine 50–100mg im q4h prn with an anti-emetic.
- High fluid intake.
- Beware of infection above the stone and pyonephrosis (p300). If there is fever, bacturia, or obstruction treat empirically until culture results are known (e.g. cefuroxime 750mg iv tds) and decompress any obstruction present.
- Large-sized stones with infection or obstruction require urological management such as ureteroscopic extraction or extracorporeal shock wave lithotripsy, or surgery.

Prognosis

~ 60% of all stones will pass (half of these within 48 hours). ~ 30% will require surgical removal. The risk of stone recurrence may be reduced by dietary advice (e.g. avoid high oxalate foods such as rhubarb, spinach), a high fluid intake, controlling hypercalciuria (low calcium diet, thiazide diuretics, bran), treating the cause if hypercalcaemic (p452), urinary alkalinization (hyperuricaemia, renal tubular acidosis, cystinuria) urinary acidification to pH < 5.5 ± urease inhibitors (struvite stones), allopurinol (urate stones), or D-penicillamine (cystine stones).

Renal colic and renal stones

Causes of renal colic

- *Renal stones:* Usually divided into:-
  Radio-opaque (90%): Contain Ca^{2+} or Mg^{2+}, e.g. calcium oxalate (hypercalciuria, hypercalcaemia, dehydration, renal tubular acidosis, medullary sponge kidney, hyperoxaluria), calcium phosphate (as before and UTIs), magnesium ammonium phosphate (UTIs with urease +ve organisms, e.g. *Proteus*). Cystine stones are 'semi-opaque' due to their sulphur content.
  Lucent: (Urate or xanthine or rarely 2,8-dihydroxyadenine).

- *Renal papillary necrosis:* DM, sickle cell disease, analgesic nephropathy. Pain occurs when a papilla 'sloughs' into the ureter.

- *Blood clots* due to trauma, tumour (parenchymal or urothelial), bleeding diathesis, or polycystic kidney disease.

Haematuria

History Ask specifically about:-
- Severity of haematuria: Pink urine, frank blood, or clots?
- The timing of haematuria: Bleeding occuring at start or end of micturition suggests bladder neck, prostate, or urethral source. Blood mixed with the stream suggests a source higher in the urinary tract.
- History of trauma: Even seemingly minor trauma can cause bleeding from congenital lesions of the urinary tract.
- Unilateral loin pain: Consider calculi, tumour, cystic disease or hydronephrosis. Painless haematuria suggests neoplasm.
- Disturbance of micturition: Frequency, urgency, dysuria, hesitancy, poor stream, and dribbling suggests cystitis. Bleeding and pain at the end of the stream is typical of a bladder stone.
- Constitutional symptoms: Sore throats, arthralgia, malaise, and rash may indicate glomerulonephritis. AF is associated with renal emboli. Fever, dysuria, or abdominal pain may indicate infection. Bruising or other bleeding may indicate a bleeding diathesis.

Physical examination
- *General examination:* Hypertension (chronic or acute renal disease incl. polycystic disease), irregular pulse or heart murmurs (source of emboli), anaemia, bruising or purpura, oedema or pleural effusions.
- *Urinary tract examination:* Loin or abdominal tenderness, renal mass, pelvic mass, prostate enlargement, testes. Inspect the urine.

Investigations
- Urinalysis   Positive result seen with myoglobinuria (see p294) and haemoglobinuria; proteinuria suggests renal pathology.
- Microscopy   RBC casts or dysmorphic red cells suggest glomerular origin. WBC casts suggest pyelonephritis. Other findings include crystals (stone disease), ova (schistosomiasis), and malignant cells.
- FBC   Thrombocytopenia; anaemia (haemolysis, leukaemia); leukocytosis may indicate infection.
- U&Es   For renal function.
- Clotting   For coagulopathy.
- G&S   If post traumatic or severe.
- ASOT, C'   If glomerulonephritis is suspected. Consider measuring autoantibodies (see p280). Refer to renal team.
- Ultrasound   May diagnose polycystic disease, ureteric obstruction by stone or tumour, or gross renal abnormalities.
- IVU   May demonstrate stones, hydronephrosis, renal injury or tumour, cystic disease or urothelial tumour.
- Cystoscopy   Should be performed on all patients to exclude another cause of bleeding from the lower urinary tract.

Management
- Admit patients with:
  - Post traumatic haematuria (refer to urology).
  - Severe unexplained haematuria (incl. bleeding diathesis) esp. if there is clot retention. Insert a large (22G) triple lumen urinary catheter for continuous bladder irrigartion to wash out clots.
  - Haematuria and renal impairment (?glomerulonephritis). Arrange for urgent renal referral and biopsy.
  - Severe infection, e.g. pyelonephritis. Commence antibiotics (e.g. cefuroxime ± gentamicin) after taking appropriate cultures.
- Pain relief (pethidine 25–50mg iv with an anti-emetic); *Pro-Banthine*® (propantheline bromide) 15mg tds po relieves painful bladder spasm of haemorrhagic cystitis and clot retention (may cause urinary retention in elderly).
- Correct any bleeding diathesis (FFP ± Vit K for warfarin see p546).

Causes of haematuria	
Trauma	Blunt and penetrating injuries, iatrogenic (e.g. recent TURP, TURBT, or renal biopsy), severe exercise ('joggers haematuria'), foreign body
Stones	Renal, ureteric, or bladder.
Infections	Pyelonephritis, haemorrhagic cystitis, acute prostatitis: bacterial, TB, or parasitic (e.g. schistosomiasis)
Tumours	Urothelial, renal parenchymal, prostatic
Bleeding diatheses	Haemophilia, thrombocytopenia
Renal pathology	Glomerulonephritis, renal arterial emboli, renal vein thrombosis
Drugs	Anticoagulants, cyclophosphamide, D-penicillamine
Congenital	Polycystic disease, sickle cell disease (papillary necrosis), Alport's syndrome, hydronephrosis

N.B. *Discoloured urine may also be due to: Beetroot*, porphyria, rifampicin, co-danthramer, vegetable dyes.

Renovascular disease

Renal artery stenosis may be atherosclerotic (common in the elderly and diabetics) or fibromuscular hyperplasia (generally younger patient without vascular disease elsewhere). It should be considered in all patients presenting with:-

- Flash pulmonary oedema (sudden unexpected onset)
- Peripheral vascular disease
- Unequal kidneys on USS
- Impaired renal function in context of ACE inhibitor use
- Hypertension/arteriopathy
- Complete anuria in a patient who has previously lost a kidney

Investigations

- Ultrasound scan: To look at renal size and Doppler flow through the renal arteries.
- Isotope renogram: Done before and after giving and ACE inhibitor (captopril); GFR falls on the side with the stenosis compared to the other side. May precipitate renal infarction.
- Angiography: Probably still the gold standard. Ensure the patient is well hydrated before and maintains a good fluid intake post procedure. Although controversial, some advocate low dose dopamine ($2.5\mu g/kg/min$) peri-procedure to protect against contrast nephropathy (see p292).
- Spiral CT of kidneys and vasculature.

Management

- Optimize fluid status (see p282). There is often a fine balance between pulmonary oedema and pre-renal uraemia.
- Avoid ACE inhibitors and NSAIDs.
- Refer to a dedicated team of interventional radiologists and vascular surgeons. Generally speaking, if the kidney is > 8cm then salvage may be possible. If the kidney is small (< 8cm), then intervention is probably hazardous and without benefit.
- Treatment may be by angioplasty or bypass surgery. Remember bp control and treatment of other risk factors; the majority of patients with atheromatous renovascular disease die from their associated ischaemic heart disease.

Cholesterol embolism

Most commonly seen in arteriopaths after manipulation of vasculature (e.g. angiography) and is followed by acute renal failure. Usually silent; there is partial occlusion of small- and medium-sized arteries resulting ischaemic atrophy. More florid presentation includes widespread purpura, dusky and cyanotic peripheries with intact pedal pulses, GI bleeding, myalgia, and acute renal failure. It can be spontaneous or follow therapy with warfarin. ***Diagnosis:*** Eosinophilia, renal impairment, hypocomplementaemia, ↑ ESR, ANCA negative. Urinary sediment is usually benign; mild proteinuria may be seen. Renal biopsy shows cholesterol clefts. ***Management:*** The renal impairment is usually irreversible or only partially reversible (in contrast to ATN). Anti-coagulation is relatively contraindicated. There is no specific treatment.

Interstitial nephritis

Inflammatory cell infiltration of renal parenchyma, usually induced by drugs (NSAIDs, penicillin, cephalosporins, sulphonamides, allopurinol, rifampicin, mesalazine, interferon), some infections (e.g. *Legionella*, leptospirosis, viral), granulomatous interstitial nephritis (e.g. sarcoid). Other causes include DM, sickle cell disease, reflux nephropathy, renal transplant rejection. **Presentation:** Acute renal failure, ± fever, eosinophilia and urinary eosinophils. Precipitating cause usually precedes renal impairment by a few days to 2 weeks (very variable). **Diagnosis:** Renal biopsy. **Treatment:** Stop offending drug; steroids controversial.

Contrast nephropathy

An acute impairment of renal function which follows exposure to radiocontrast materials, for which alternative causes for the renal impairment have been excluded. Incidence in an unselected population is 2–7% but this increases to 25% if renal function is already impaired. It results from a combination of afferent arteriolar vasoconstriction, interference with tubuloglomerular feedback, tubular hypoxia, and direct nephrotoxicity of the contrast agent.

Risk factors

- Pre-existing renal disease (incidence up to 60% if $Cr > 400\mu M$)
- Proteinuria (increases risk 3–fold)
- DM (risk depends on renal function; incidence of ARF ~ 100% if $Cr > 400\mu M$)
- Congestive cardiac failure (incidence 7–8%)
- Multiple myeloma
- Pancreatitis
- Multiple contrast studies
- Dehydration
- Jaundice

Management

There is no specific treatment. Prevention is the best policy.

- Monitor U&Es, creatinine.
- Try to ensure good hydration pre-procedure (give patients who are at risk, iv fluids if they are to be kept NBM for the procedure).
- Maintain high urine output. Stop nephrotoxic drugs (esp. NSAIDs) peri-procedure.
- Some advocate low-dose dopamine ($2.5\mu g/kg/min$ via a central line) or mannitol, but there are no studies that show long-term benefit. Pre-treatment with nifedipine may be of some benefit.
- Outcome in one study: 68% regain normal renal function, 14% had partial recovery, 18% death or dialysis or transplantation.

Renal emergencies

Rhabdomyolysis

This is the development of acute renal failure secondary to extensive muscle damage and release of myoglobin.

Presentation

- Most cases occur following muscle trauma (e.g. crush syndrome) or severe physical exertion, e.g. marathon running or military training ('squat jump syndrome').
- Prolonged immobility (e.g. after drug overdose and coma) may result in pressure necrosis of the muscles.
- Symptoms include swollen tender muscles, dirty red-brown urine (like *Coca-Cola*® mixed with urine) and/or oliguria.

Investigations

U&Es	Typically $\uparrow\uparrow$ K+, $\uparrow$ creatinine:urea ratio
Ca^{2+}, PO_4^{3-}	$\uparrow\uparrow$ PO_4^{3-}, initial $\downarrow$ Ca^{2+} (as it enters damaged muscle) followed by 'rebound' $\uparrow$ Ca^{2+}.
Urate	Usually $\uparrow\uparrow$ with tissue necrosis; also $\downarrow$ excretion.
LFTs	AST very high – from skeletal muscle.
CPK	Very high (up to 1 million U/l).
ABG	Metabolic acidosis, hypoxic if here is associated acute lung injury (trauma) or infection.
Urine	The urine looks red-brown. Urinalysis is positive for blood (myoglobin tests positive), but no RBC seen on microscopy. Urinary myoglobin is diagnostic.
Misc.	FBC, glucose, blood cultures, ESR, CRP, serum for toxicology ± virology, plasma myoglobin, ECG. Serum looks clear (cf. intravascular haemolysis) as myoglobin does not bind haptoglobins and is rapidly cleared by kidneys.

Management

Patients are often febrile, dehydrated, and unwell. The priorities are:

- Hyperkalaemia needs urgent treatment (see p282).
- Rehydrate: In elderly patients or if the patient is oliguric, insert a central line and be guided by CVP. Watch for fluid overload.
- Alkaline diuresis (see p668): Alkalinization of the urine is said to enhance solubility of myoglobin. It is usually effective within the first 8 hours. Test urine regularly with pH strips to monitor treatment.
- Analgesia: Avoid NSAIDs; use opiate analgesia if required.
- Avoid frusemide: This may acidify the urine and enhance myoglobin induced tubular injury.
- Mannitol diuresis: Give 50ml of 20% mannitol slow iv bolus followed by iv infusion of 2g/h if there is a good response.
- Refer for a surgical opinion. Fasciotomies or debridement of necrotic tissue may be needed for compartment syndrome
- Avoid calcium infusion to treat hypocalcaemia: It may cause metastatic calcification in damaged muscle and cause further tissue necrosis. However, iv calcium should not be witheld for patients with life-threatening hyperkalaemia.
- Treat the underlying cause (see table opposite)
- Dialysis or haemofiltration may be necessary for the short term but full recovery of renal function is likely.

Rhabdomyolysis

Causes of rhabdomyolysis	
• Crush injury	• Hypokalaemia
• Severe exertion	• CO poisoning (p640)
• Prolonged convulsions	• Burns
• Prolonged immobility	• Diabeticketoacidosis (p430)
• Polymyositis or viral myositis	• Ecstasy abuse (p635)
• Malignant hyperpyrexia (p476)	• Snake bite (p766)
• Acute alcoholic binge	• Electric shock (p758)
• McArdle's syndrome	• Neuroleptic malignant syndrome

Hepatorenal syndrome

This is defined as the onset of renal failure in patients with severe liver disease in the absence of renal pathology. It may occur in either cirrhosis or acute liver failure. It may be characterized by a low urine sodium (< 10mM), but this is NOT a criterion in the diagnosis.

Presentation

- Renal failure is most commonly an incidental finding during biochemical screening of patients with ascites (cirrhosis), acute liver failure, or jaundice (most common in alcoholic hepatitis). Patients may rarely complain of oliguria or anuria.

There are many causes of renal failure and liver disease which are NOT synonymous with hepatorenal syndrome. These include:-

- Haemorrhage and hypotension (pre-renal failure).
- Overdiuresis (pre-renal failure)
- Nephrotoxic drugs given to patients with liver disease (e.g. gentamicin).
- Chronic viral hepatitis (HBV or HCV) causing glomerulonephritis.
- Leptospirosis (marked hyperbilirubinaemia, other liver enzymes virtually normal).
- Paracetamol overdose.
- Carbon tetrachloride or organic solvent poisoning.

Investigations

- See acute renal failure, p280.

Management

- Exclude other causes of renal failure in liver disease (see above).
- Insert a urinary catheter and monitor urine output.
- Colloid challenge (1l human albumin solution), and stop all diuretics.
- Trial of low-dose dopamine (2.5μg/kg/min, see p689).
- Broad spectrum antibiotics (e.g. cefotaxime + metronidazole, or ciprofloxacin + amoxycillin).
- If mean arterial pressure [diastolic pressure + (systolic-diastolic pressure)÷ 3] is less than 75mmHg, administer a vasopressor agent after volume expansion. The most appropriate agents are vasopressin (0.2–0.4U/min) or noradrenaline (1–10μg/min, see p689).
- If there is tense ascites, a total paracentesis will decrease the renal venous pressure and enhance renal blood flow (see p822).
- Haemofiltration or dialysis: Patients tolerate haemofiltration better than haemodialysis. There is NO value in dialysing a patient with end-stage cirrhosis and renal failure unless the patient is going to have a liver transplant. It is, however, reasonable to dialyse a patient with a reversible cause of liver failure (i.e. acute liver failure or acute alcoholic hepatitis).
- Hyperkalaemia and acidosis are rarely a problem.
- All patients should be discussed with a liver transplant centre. Hepatorenal syndrome is readily reversed by liver transplantation.

Oliguria or anuria

Oliguria is defined as urine output < 400ml/24h. Anuria implies that there is no urine output

Causes

- Obstructed urinary tract (bilateral ureteric or bladder outflow).
- Renal infarction (e.g. prolonged hypotension in patients with atherosclerotic stenosed renal arteries).
- Acute renal failure (p278).

Assessment

- Ask specifically about symptoms of prostatism, or haematuria (tumour) and backache (stones, anuerysm).
- Drug history (ACE inhibitors) as a possible cause of renal infarction, recent antibiotics, NSAIDs (interstitial nephritis).
- Recent renal angiography or angioplasty (renal infarction, contrast nephropathy).
- Constitutional symptoms suggestive of glomerulonephritis (p276).
- Has the patient previously lost a kidney?
- Measure bp (supine and sitting or upright) and pulse rate.
- Assess hydration (central skin turgor, mucous membranes, and JVP).
- Insert central line and measure CVP. Monitor PCWP in patients who are hypoxic or severely compromised (see p774).
- Examine fluid and weight charts, and operation notes if applicable.
- Arrange for urgent U&Es.

Management (see acute renal failure p282)

If patient is anuric.

- Examine for palpable bladder, enlarged prostate, or other pelvic masses. Insert urinary catheter to exclude retention.
- If the bladder is empty, an urgent ultrasound (day or night) to exclude bilateral obstruction (or obstruction of solitary functioning system). Treat bilateral hydronephrosis with urgent nephrostomies. Anterograde imaging can then determine the level of obstruction.
- If the USS is negative arrange a CT scan of the abdomen.
- If obstruction is absent (one cannot exclude acute obstruction on USS) an isotope renogram will determine whether there is renal perfusion. If there is renal perfusion, then a retrograde ureterogram will determine whether there is obstruction. Absent renal perfusion suggests renal infarction.
- Management of acute renal failure is discussed on p282. The priorities are to optimize fluid balance and treat any complications of ARF while trying to correct the underlying cause.
- If the patient is clinically dehydrated with a low or normal CVP ± postural hypotension, give a trial of volume expansion (500ml of colloid or N/saline) over 30 min. Monitor response of urine output and venous pressure. Continue fluids until CVP is 5–10cm at mid-clavicular line.
- When adequately filled (CVP > 10 and/or PCWP > 15) reassess urine output. If oliguric or anuric, give frusemide 120mg-1g slowly iv (max. 4mg/min). Consider low-dose dopamine (2.5µg/kg/min, see p689).
- If hypotension persists (mean arterial pressure < 60mmHg), in spite of adequate volume replacement, as indicated by a CVP of > 10cm commence inotropic support (see p210).
- If anuria persists, remove the urinary catheter (source of sepsis).

Acute upper urinary tract infections

Infection of the upper urinary tract may result in acute pyelonephritis, renal abscess, pyonephrosis, or perinephric abscess (see figure opposite). Beware of infection with obstruction: this leads to rapid tissue destruction unless the obstruction is relieved.

Predisposing factors

Either an ascending infection or haematogenous spread.
Organisms: *E. coli* 60%, *Proteus* 20%, *S. faecalis* 10%, *Klebsiella* 5%.

- Female (short urethra)
- Renal stones
- Bladder catheter
- Chronic liver disease
- Structural abnormality of renal tract
- Pregnancy
- Diabetes mellitus
- Intravenous drug abuse
- Infective endocarditis

Presentation

- Classical symptoms are loin pain, fever, and rigors.
- Non-specific symptoms may predominate, e.g. nausea, vomiting, anorexia, malaise, confusion, or weakness.
- Up to 75% have preceding lower urinary tract symptoms (frequency, dysuria). There may be associated haematuria.
- Severe, bilateral pyelonephritis or acute-on-chronic pyelonephritis may result in acute renal failure.
- A preceding history of intermittent loin pain may imply intermittent obstruction with pyonephrosis. Renal parenchymal abscesses are seen with iv drug use, endocarditis, or skin infections.
- Ask specifically about any predisposing factors (see above).
- Signs include fever, abdominal or loin tenderness, a palpable mass in the loin, and, with severe infection, scoliosis concave towards the affected side, hypotension, and shock (septicaemia).
- The symptoms and signs may be difficult to distinguish from pneumonia (pleuritic pain and shallow breathing on affected side) or other causes of an acute abdomen (e.g. cholecystitis, diverticulitis).

Investigations

- **Urine** Urinalysis commonly shows blood and protein. White cells, bacteria, WBC casts may be seen on microscopy. Culture may be negative in infections confined to the renal cortex (e.g. abscess).
- **Bloods** All patients should have U&Es (for renal dysfunction-dehydration, acute-on-chronic failure), glucose, FBC (anaemia, leukocytosis), and blood cultures.
- **AXR** Stones, soft tissue mass, or loss of psoas line on affected side.
- **USS** To exclude obstruction and delineate renal and perirenal collections. Arrange CT if surgery is planned.

Management

- Stabilize the patient: Resuscitate severely ill patients with iv fluids ± inotropes (see p208–10), guided by CVP and bp.
- Give iv antibiotics, e.g. cefuroxime 750mg tds, and modify treatment in light of results of cultures. Continue antibiotics for total 7–14 days.
- Fluid balance: Maintain high fluid intake (e.g. 3 litres/24h). Monitor fluid balance and urine output carefully for the first 48–72 hours.
- Analgesia: Try NSAID if renal function is normal (e.g. diclofenac sodium 75mg im). Alternatively try im pethidine 50–75mg q3h prn.
- Pyonephrosis, renal, or perinephric abscess: Requires urgent decompression and drainage via a percutaneous nephrostomy under USS or CT guidance. Formal surgical drainage may be required: contact the urologists. Remember to save a sample for MC&S.
- Once the patient has improved, investigate for any underlying cause. IVU, DMSA, and DTPA scans will determine the anatomy, extent of renal damage, and how much function remains.

Acute upper urinary tract infections

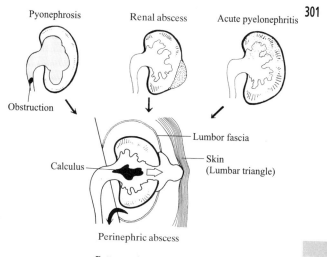

Pyonephrosis

Obstruction

Renal abscess

Acute pyelonephritis

Calculus

Lumbor fascia

Skin
(Lumbar triangle)

Perinephric abscess

Patterns of renal infections

302

7 Neurological emergencies

Coma: Assessment

Presentation

Coma is a 'state of *unarousable unresponsiveness*'.

- *No evidence of arousal:* There is no spontaneous eye opening, comprehensible speech, or voluntary limb movement.
- *Unresponsive* to external stimuli and surrounding environment, although abnormal postures may be adopted, eyes may open or grunts may be elicited in response to pain.
- *Involuntary movements*, e.g. seizures or myoclonic jerks, may occur.
- *Glasgow Coma Scale* (p416) is a useful way of assessing and monitoring level of consciousness.
- *Signs of brain shift* (p422) may accompany decreasing level of consciousness.

Causes

For practical purposes, it is best to divide these into:

- Metabolic
- Toxic
- Ineffective
- Structural lesions with or without
- Focal brainstem signs
- Lateralizing cerebral signs
- Meningeal irritation

In general, toxic and metabolic causes usually do not produce focal signs (except rarely with hypoglycaemia, liver, or renal failure), whereas infections and structural lesions do. Meningism offers a very useful clue about the cause of coma (see below).

1. Coma without focal/lateralizing neurological signs

- Anoxia/hypoperfusion
- Metabolic: e.g. hypo-/hyperglycaemia, acidosis/alkalosis, hypo- or hypernatraemia, hypercalcaemia, hepatic, or renal failure
- Intoxications: e.g. alcohol, opiates, benzodiazepines, tricyclics, neuroleptics, lithium, barbiturates, carbon monoxide
- Endocrine: hypothyroidism
- Hypo-or hyperthermia
- Epilepsy
- Hypertensive encephalopathy

2. Coma with focal/lateralizing neurological signs (due to brainstem or cerebral dysfunction)

- Vascular: cerebral haemorrhage or infarction
- Supra- or infratentorial space occupying lesion: tumour, haematoma, abscess. In order to produce coma these either have to be within the brainstem or compress it by producing brain shift (p422).

3. Coma with meningism

- Meningitis, encephalitis
- Subarachnoid haemorrhage

Assessment of severity

- Glasgow Coma Scale (p416)
- Signs of brain shift (p422–4)

Coma: Immediate management

Priorities are:

1. Stabilize the patient (airway, breathing, circulation). Give oxygen.
2. Consider giving thiamine, extrose, naloxone, or flumazenil.
3. Examine patient. Is there meningism? Establish Glasgow Coma Scale score. Is there evidence of brainstem failure? Are there focal or lateralizing signs?
4. Plan for further investigations.
5. Observe for signs of deterioration and attempt to reverse them.

Stabilize the patient

- *Open the airway* by laying the patient on their side. Note the pattern of *breathing* (see signs of brain shift, p422). If there is apnoea, laboured, or disturbed breathing, intubation and ventilation should be considered. Measure arterial blood gases.

- *Support the circulation.* Correct hypotension with colloid and/or inotropes. If prolonged therapy is required, both require careful and frequent monitoring of central venous pressure and/or pulmonary artery wedge pressure. Search for any occult source of bleeding, e.g. intra-abdominal.

- *Treat seizures* with usual drugs (p370) but beware over-sedation and hypotension.

- Take blood for *glucose, U&Es, calcium, liver enzymes, albumin, clotting screen, FBC, toxicology* (including urgent paracetamol and salicylate levels). Urine should be saved for *toxicology screen*.

Give thiamine, dextrose, naloxone, or flumazenil

- Check BM stix. There is a good argument for giving 50ml of 50% *dextrose* immediately for presumed hypoglycaemia because this will usually not cause any harm.

- The only concern is that glucose may precipitate Wernicke's encephalopathy in malnourished individuals. Some clinicians therefore favour giving a bolus of *thiamine* 1–2mg/kg iv beforehand.

- *Naloxone* should be given only if opiate intoxication is likely (small pupils) and the patient is in coma or has a markedly reduced respiratory rate. In adults, naloxone 0.8–2.0mg iv should be given at intervals of 2–3 minutes to a maximum of 10mg.

- *Flumazenil* should only be administered if benzodiazepine intoxication is likely; it is contraindicated in epileptics who have received prolonged benzodiazepine therapy. In adults, flumazenil 200 micrograms should be given over 15 seconds; further 100 microgram boluses may be given at 1 minute intervals (usual dose is 300–600 micrograms; maximum total dose outside intensive care setting is 1mg).

- Both naloxone and flumazenil may be given as intravenous infusions if drowsiness recurs but intensive care monitoring is advisable.

Coma: Diagnostic clues from examination

History If available; the assessment may be made easier. Even if the history is not extensive, a witness may help to establish whether coma commenced suddenly (suggestive of a vascular event) or whether there was a gradual decline in level of consciousness over hours or even days. Irrespective of whether a history is available, an enormous amount may be learned from a rapid but thorough examination.

General examination[1,2] should establish:

- *Core temperature:* A fever usually indicates infection but sometimes results from diencephalic lesions. Hypothermia is often forgotten as a cause for coma; the possibility of myxoedema should be considered.

- *Heart rate and rhythm:* May indicate a dysrhythmia as the reason for poor cerebral perfusion.

- *Blood pressure:* Prolonged hypotension of any cause will lead to anoxia and ischaemia. Apart from a cardiac cause, occult bleeding, a cause of sepsis, and drug intoxication need to be considered.

- *Respiratory pattern:* Shallow, slow breathing should alert the examiner to the possibility of drug intoxication, e.g. opiates. Deep, rapid Kussmaul breathing suggests acidosis. Brainstem compromise can cause distinctive patterns of breathing (p420).

- *Breath:* Alcohol, ketones, hepatic, or uraemic foetor?

- *Skin:* There may be signs to trauma to the head. Bruising over the scalp or mastoids, blood in the nostrils, or external auditory meatus raises the possibility of a basal skull fracture. A rash suggests the possibility of meningitis. There may be signs of chronic liver disease or the sallow discoloration of uraemia. Intravenous drug abuse may be suggested by needle tracks.

- *Heart:* Occasionally, bacterial endocarditis or vasculitides associated with heart murmurs present with coma.

- *Abdomen:* Apart from seeking for enlargement of organs which may give clues to the cause of coma, it is important not to miss an acute intra-abdominal event such as perforation of a viscus or a leaking aortic aneurysm.

- *Fundi:* Papilloedema indicates raised intracranial pressure but its absence does *not* exclude that possibility. Subhyaloid haemorrhages are pathognomonic of subarachnoid haemorrhage but are rare. Changes of diabetic or hypertensive retinopathy suggest the possibility of encephalopathy secondary to these conditions.

Is there meningism?

- Neck stiffness should be assessed only if it is certain that there has been no trauma to the cervical spine. Increased stiffness is a reasonably good indicator of meningeal irritation, either because of inflammation or infiltrative processes affecting the meninges, or because of the presence of blood. Meningism at once raises the possibility of meningitis, encephalitis, or subarachnoid haemorrhage.

Assess the Glasgow Coma Score: This may reveal brainstem dysfunction or lateralizing signs. When testing the motor response, decorticate or decerebrate posturing may become evident (p417). If there is a change in these signs, it may indicate brain shift (p422).

---

[1] Plum F & Posner JB (1980) *The Diagnosis of Stupor and Coma*, 3rd edition; FA Davis, Philadelphia.
[2] Bates (1993) *J Neurol Neurosurg Psychiat* **56**: 589–598.

Look for evidence of brainstem dysfunction? (see p418 for details).

Test and observe:

- *Pupillary response*
- *Corneal reflex*
- *Resting position of eyes*
- *Spontaneous eye movements*
- *Oculocephalic response/Doll's head manoeuvre* (if no C-spine injury)
- *Oculovestibular response/caloric stimulation*
- *Swallowing*
- *Respiratory pattern*
- There will be evidence of brainstem failure either because there is structural damage (intrinsic lesion of extrinsic compression due to brain shift, p422) or because of metabolic coma such as drug intoxication with diffuse, usually reversible, dysfunction.
- If there is focal brainstem dysfunction the cause is most likely structural or intrinsic brainstem disease.
- If there is rostrocaudal progression of brainstem signs consider a herniation syndrome (p422).
- If there appears to be diffuse brainstem dysfunction, it may not be easy to distinguish between structural and metabolic aetiologies. The most important clue is that in metabolic coma, irrespective of their size, the pupils continue to react except in very few exceptional cases (atropine, scopolamine, or glutethimide intoxication will depress brainstem function and produce pupillary abnormalities).

Are there lateralizing signs?

Testing or brainstem reflexes, assessing the GCS, and general examination may reveal facial asymmetry, and differences in muscle tone, reflexes, and plantar responses between the two sides. All these features point towards the possibility of a structural lesion, although, occasionally, metabolic coma is associated with focal neurological signs.

Coma: Management

Plans for further investigations

The history, physical examination, and/or laboratory studies may allow the physician to make the diagnosis. Often, however, a specific diagnosis cannot be reached so rapidly. The practical approach is to divide patients according to the following scheme.

Brainstem function intact

- Urgent CT head scan. This will reveal one of the following:-
  - Operable lesions (e.g. subdural haematoma, subarachnoid, or intra-cerebral haemorrhage); refer as appropriate.
  - Inoperable lesions (e.g. bilateral cortical infarcts); treatment is supportive.
  - Normal; a lumbar puncture should be performed. CSF analysis may suggest an infective process (e.g. meningitis, encephalitis) (p328). If the CSF is normal, the most likely diagnosis is a metabolic coma.

Brainstem function not intact

- Consider whether there are signs of brain shift (p422).
- If a herniation syndrome appears to be progressing rapidly, mannitol should be given, hyperventilation commenced, and a surgeon contacted urgently (see p348).
- If the tempo of events is not so rapid, mannitol may be given and an urgent CT scan arranged.
- Even if the brainstem signs appear to be non-progressive, a CT scan should be arranged to exclude the possibility of an operable posterior fossa mass or haemorrhage (e.g. cerebellar haemorrhage).
- If the CT is normal, a lumbar puncture should be performed to exclude infection. If this too is normal the diagnostic possibilities are intrinsic brainstem disease not detected by CT, metabolic coma, or possibly infection, e.g. encephalitis, without leukocytic response.
- MRI scanning is more sensitive in detecting intrinsic brainstem pathology.
- Lumbar puncture should be repeated the next day if there is no improvement in the patient's condition. Otherwise, treatment is supportive.

Monitoring progress

- This requires regular observations of vital signs and neurological state (including GCS score).
- An important cause of deterioration in structural brain lesions is brain shift leading to herniation syndromes (p422). The emergency treatment of raised intracranial pressure is discussed on p350.
- Other reasons for deterioration are electrolyte or metabolic changes, hypovolaemia, or fluid overload. Plasma electrolytes and fluid balance need to be regularly assessed to avoid such problems.

Prognosis

In coma due to head injury, prognosis is clearly related to GCS score. Patients scoring 8 or less have a very poor prognosis. In non-traumatic coma, GCS alone is not a very good predictor. Patients with drug intoxications, may have very low scores on admission but, in general, have good outcomes. Assessment of prognosis in non-traumatic coma is aided by simple features of the examination. For example, if after 24 hours it is still not possible to elicit pupillary responses, corneal reflexes, and oculovestibular response, survival is extremely unlikely.[3]

---

[3] Levy *et al.* (1981) *Arch Int Med* **94**: 293–301.

Limb weakness: Assessment

History

The history should establish if there has been:-

- Sudden onset or gradual progression
- Weakness or incoordination
- Upper limb or facial weakness
- Asymmetrical or symmetrical weakness
- Associated sensory symptoms, e.g. paraesthesiae or numbness
- Difficulty with swallowing, speech, micturition, or defecation
- Back or neck pain
- Systemic symptoms, e.g. malaise, fever, vomiting, arthralgia
- Recent trauma
- Previous medical history, e.g. hypertension, ischaemic heart disease, stroke, diabetes, connective tissue diseases
- Drug history, e.g. phenytoin, isoniazid, vincristine, metronidazole

Examination

- *What is the pattern of weakness?* Some common patterns, together with associated features, are illustrated on p314–5[4]. This should help to localize the level of the lesion in the nervous system.
- *Is the weakness upper or lower motor neurone/combination?*
- *If upper motor neurone, is it pyramidal?* i.e. extensor more than flexor weakness in upper limbs; flexor greater than extensor weakness in lower limbs.
- *Is there fatiguable weakness with repetitive effort?* As in myasthenia.
- *Are there any involuntary movements?* Tremor, myoclonic jerks, or fits may be noted.
- *What is the gait like?* This is important to test if at all possible. It may demonstrate, for example, a hemiplegic gait, ataxia (cerebellar or sensory), a waddling (myopathic) gait, steppage (lower motor neurone) gait, festinating movements of the Parkinsonian patient.
- *Is there any sensory loss? Where? Is there a 'sensory level'?* Sensory changes are often the most difficult to elicit. Do not forget to test all modalities or to test the back of the legs up to the anal sphincter.
- *What modalities of sensation are lost?* Dorsal column loss produces a 'discriminatory' loss with impaired two-point discrimination, joint-position and vibration loss and sensory ataxia. Spinothalamic loss usually produces a lack of awareness of pain and temperature.

The history and examination should help to localize the lesion and, together with the patient's age, give an indication of the likely pathological process involved (p314–5).[4]

Investigations

The initial investigation of choice depends upon the likely diagnosis. Investigations to consider are given in the table opposite.

---

[4] Adapted from Lindsay KW, Bone I & Callander R (1991) *Neurology & Neurosurgery Illustrated* (2nd ed.) pp.191–194; Churchill Livingstone, London (with permission)

Limb weakness

Diagnoses not to miss
- Spinal cord compression   p404
- Guillian-Barré Syndrome   p408
- Subdural haematoma   p360
- Stroke   p374

Diagnoses to consider
- Demyelination (multiple sclerosis, post infectious, etc)
- Malignancy (carcinomatous meningitis, intracranial mass)
- Syringomyelia
- Motor neurone disease
- Vitamin deficiency (sub-acute combined degeneration-B_{12})
- Peripheral neuropathy (toxic, DM, autoimmune, amyloid, etc)
- TB, syphilis

Investigations to consider

- Blood tests: FBC, U&Es, LFTs, ESR, CRP, Prostate-specific antigen, B_{12}/folate, protein strip, syphilis serology
- CT/MRI scan
- Spinal X-rays
- Myelography
- CSF analysis: Protein, cells, oligoclonal bands
- Visual evoked potentials
- Electromyograpy (EMG)
- Nerve conduction studies (NCS)
- Tensilon test
- Muscle biopsy

Limb weakness: Localizing the lesion

Monoplegia	Lesion site	Other features
• Arm only	Contralateral cortex	• Visual field defect • Dysphasia (dominant hemisphere lesion) • Cortical sensory loss (↓JPS and 2-point discrimination)
• Leg only	Contralateral cortex	• With ipsilateral sensory deficit
	Ipsilateral spinal lesions	• Contralateral pain and temperature loss • JPS lost on same side

Hemiplegia	Lesion site	Other features
	Contralateral hemisphere	• UMN VII involvement • Impaired consciousness • Visual field defect • Dysphasia (if dominant hemisphere lesion)
	Contralateral internal capsule	• UMN VII involvement • Alert • No dysphasia (even with a dominant hemisphere lesion)
	Contralateral mid-brain lesion	• Contralateral IIIrd palsy • Impaired upgaze
	Contralateral Cortex	• VII unaffected • Visual field defect • Dysphasia (if dominant hemisphere lesion) • ↓JPS and 2-point discrimination
	Contralateral Medullary	• Ipsilateral pain and temperature loss • Contralateral Horner's syndrome • Contralateral palatal and tongue weakness
	Ipsilateral spinal lesion	• Pain and temperature loss in contralateral leg • Ipsilateral loss of JPS • Ipsilateral Horner's
	Contralateral pons	• LMN face involvement on opposite side to weak limbs • Conjugate gaze deviation towards weak side

Limb weakness

Hemiplegia	Lesion site	Other features
	Medullary lesion	• Palatal and tongue weakness on the side of arm weakness

Paraplegia	Lesion site	Other features
	Mid-line cortical lesion	• Cortical sensor loss (↓JPS and 2-point discrimination) • 'Frontal' incontinence • Normal pain and temperature
	Thoracic spine	• 'Sensory level' • Acute urinary retention or hesitancy of micturition

Tetraplegia	Lesion site	Other features
	Pontine lesion	• 'Locked-in' syndrome – only vertical eye movements possible
	Cervical spine lesion	• No cranial nerve lesion • High lesions (C1–3) require ventilation • Lesions at C4 have intact diaphragmatic breathing.
	Medullary lesion	• No palatal, tongue movement or speech but intact facial movements

Combined UMN and LMN signs		
		• The LMN signs point to the level of the lesion • Two lesions (e.g. cervical and lumbar spondylosis) may produce mixed signs in limbs

LMN limb weakness (unilateral or bilateral)		
		• Nerve root distribution? • Plexopathy? • Peripheral nerve distribution (Mono- vs Polyneuropathy) • Presence of reflexes suggests a myopathy (cf. neuropathy) • Specific distribution seen in e.g. fascioscapulohumoral dystrophy • Fatiguability suggests neuro-muscular junction disease

Acute dizziness or vertigo: Assessment

History Determine whether:-

- *There is true vertigo*, i.e. a hallucination that either the patient or his environment is rotating.
- *Symptoms started acutely*, are progressively worsening, or are transient (see p390).
- *Symptoms worse with certain postures*. Vertigo is worse with certain head positions in benign position vertigo and some cases of central nystagmus (see below). Postural hypotension is a common cause of dizziness. It is frequently caused by drugs; uncommonly it is due to autonomic failure. Neck movements in cervical spondylosis or carotid sinus hypersensitivity may also lead to dizziness.
- *There is associated tinnitus* (as in Ménière's disease).
- *Hearing loss* is present in Ménière's disease, cerebellopontine angle lesions, e.g. acoustic neuromas.
- *Ear discharge* may occur with middle ear disease.
- *Associated focal neurological symptoms*, e.g unilateral weakness, clumsiness, paraesthesiae, or numbness.
- *Headache* which may be of sudden onset in intracerebral haemorrhage but may be progressive and associated with other features of raised ICP in mass lesions such as an acoustic neuroma.
- *Any recent head injury?*
- Systemic symptoms, e.g. weakness and lethargy in anaemia.
- *Previous medical/psychiatric history*, e.g. hypertension, ischaemic heart disease, diabetes, risk factors for stroke or TIAs (p390), episodes of neurological disturbance, panic attacks, and anxiety.
- *Drug history* is pertinent to both true vertigo (e.g. phenytoin, gentamicin, frusemide) and dizziness (e.g. antihypertensives, antidepressants, drugs for Parkinsons disease, hypoglycaemics).

Examination

Ear. Is there a discharge? Is the tympanic membrane normal?

Neurological examination should discover whether there are any focal signs due to brainstem or cerebellar disease (p418). Non-contiguous brainstem pathology may be due to patchy demyelination.

- Do not forget to assess the corneal reflex, absence of which is one of the earliest signs of an ipsilateral acoustic neuroma.
- Observe the gait if possible; it may be ataxic.
- Examine extraocular eye movements: Is there an intranuclear ophthalmoplegia (vascular/demyelinating brainstem disease)?
- Examine carefully for **Nystagmus** (see table opposite).
- **Hallpike manoeuvre** involves positioning the patients head over one side of the bed and watching for nystagmus.
  - Benign positional vertigo: nystagmus develops after a brief delay, but it fatigues and, with repetition, adapts.
  - Central nystagmus: no initial delay, fatigueability, or adaptation.
- **Fundoscopy** may reveal papilloedema (suggestive of intracranial space occupying lesion) or optic atrophy (which occurs with previous demyelination in multiple sclerosis).

General examination: Measure bp (lying and standing). Postural hypotension is a common cause of dizziness.

Classification of nystagmus

- *First degree* nystagmus occurs only when the eyes are deviated to one side. If it occurs in the mid-line position as well it is *second degree*. Nystagmus in all directions of gaze is termed *third degree*.
- *Vestibular nystagmus* is due to dysfunction of the labyrinth or vestibular nerve. The slow phase is towards the lesion; the quick phase is away from the lesion. There may be rotary nystagmus.
- *Central nystagmus* is due to brainstem dysfunction (vestibular nuclei or their connections); there may no vertigo associated with this form of nystagmus. The nystagmus may be horizontal, vertical, or rotatory; sometimes it is present in one eye only. The quick phase is determined by direction of gaze – it is multidirectional.
- *Positional nystagmus* may occur in benign positional vertigo but with repeated testing it adapts. It may also occur with posterior fossa, e.g. cerebellar, lesions (quick phase tends to be towards the lesion) in which there is no adaptation.

Acute dizziness or vertigo: Management

Investigations

These depend upon the likely diagnosis.

- Cerebellopontine angle lesions such as acoustic neuroma may be imaged by *CT with contrast*, but, in general, posterior fossa and brainstem disease is better appraised by *MRI scanning*.
- *Pure tone audiometry* is also a sensitive means of detecting sensorineural loss.
- *Cervical spine films* may reveal degenerative disease compromising vertebral artery circulation.
- Measure **blood sugar** and **FBC** if indicated.

Approach to dizziness/vertigo

True vertigo	*Management*
Acute labyrinthitis	• Bed rest • Consider cyclizine or prochlorperazine
Benign positional vertigo	• Avoid precipitating position • Cawthorne-Cooksey exercises
Ménière's disease (sensorineural deafness and tinnitus)	• Bed rest • Consider cyclizine or prochlorperazine • Pure tone audiometry • ENT referral
Middle ear disease	• ENT referral
Brainstem/cerebellar disease (stroke, p374; demyelination; vertebrobasilar insufficiency; migraine; vasculitis)	• Consider CT/MRI
Cerebellopontine angle lesions (e.g. acoustic neuroma)	• Pure tone audiometry CT, MRI scan

Dizziness but no true vertigo	*Management*
Hypotension	• Postural, cardiac, volume loss, or autonomic failure
Anaemia	• FBC, blood film, other investigations as necessary
Hypoglycaemia	• Diabetic on hypoglycaemics or insulin, insulinoma
Hyperventilation	• Attempt to reproduce symptoms. Explain
Cervical spondylosis	• A collar may be useful, if only to act as a reminder
Carotid sinus hypersensitivity	• See p70

Acute loss of vision

History

Determine whether:

- *Visual loss is or was monocular or binocular, complete or incomplete*, e.g hemianopia, central or peripheral loss, haziness or complete obscuration of vision.
- *Loss of acuity occurred instantly* as in amaurosis fugax.
- *Period for which it lasted.*
- *There were any other associated visual symptoms*, eg scintillations ('flashing lights and shapes') occur in migraine.
- *The eye is painful ± red.*
- *Headache or facial pain* – unilateral or bilateral.
- *Associated focal neurological symptoms*, e.g. unilateral weakness, clumsiness, paraesthesiae, or numbness.
- *Any recent trauma?*
- *Systemic symptoms*, e.g. malaise, aches, and pains.
- *Previous medical history*, e.g. hypertension, ischaemic heart disease, diabetes, other risk factors for stroke or TIAs (p374), migraine, connective tissue diseases.

Examination

- *External appearance of the eye.* Is it red (p324)? Is there corneal clouding?
- *Visual acuity* should be measured for each eye with a Snellen chart. Near vision should be tested (with newsprint if necessary). If none of these are possible, the patient's acuity for counting number of fingers, or perceiving hand movement or light should be noted. Ideally, colour vision should also be examined with Ishihara plates.
- *Attempt to plot the visual fields.* (Goldman perimetry or automated perimetry e.g. Humphrey – available in ophthalmic departments.) The loss of vision may be incomplete.
- *Is there an afferent pupillary defect?* (Swinging torch test.)
- *Fundoscopy* may reveal a retinal embolus, changes of central/branch retinal artery occlusion, swollen or pale optic nerve head, papilloedema, or hypertensive changes.
- *Is the temporal artery tender?* It need not be in temporal arteritis.
- *Complete neurological examination* is necessary to discover if there are any other associated signs.
- *Listen for carotid bruits*, although they may not be present in patients with symptomatic carotid stenosis.
- *Assess heart rhythm (including ECG) and assess cardiovascular system* for possible cardiogenic source of embolus.
- *Measure bp (lying and standing) and blood sugar.* Hypotension in the presence of arteriosclerosis can lead to occipital lobe ischaemia. Hypertension and diabetes are risk factors for TIAs.

Investigations (see p376–8)

N.B. An **ESR** should be performed in any patient aged > 50 years who presents with monocular blindness and unilateral headache. It is rarely normal in temporal arteritis. If the ESR is elevated and the presentation is compatible with temporal arteritis, high dose corticosteroid therapy should be considered (initially 60mg/day orally) because the other eye is also at risk of anterior ischaemic optic neuropathy (see p620).

Approach to acute/sub-acute visual loss

1. Monocular transient loss without prominent unilateral headache

- Amaurosis fugax [see TIAs (p390)]. In the elderly this may be due to embolism. In some younger patients it is probably due to vasospasm (a diagnosis of exclusion).
- Hyperviscosity syndrome (e.g. polycythaemia, myeloma, sickle cell anaemia), hypercoagulable state, vasculitis: Blood film, protein electrophoresis, autoimmune screen, other haematological investigations as required (p590).
- Postural hypotension (may exacerbate verterbrobasilar ischaemia): Stop any exacerbating drugs. Exclude autonomic neuropathy.

2. Monocular transient loss with prominent headache

- Migraine (usually there are positive phenomena, e.g. scintillations): Observe, give analgesics/ergot derivative. Arrange neurological consultation.

3. Monocular sustained loss with red eye

- Acute glaucoma (dilated pupil and corneal clouding): Urgent ophthalmology referral.
- Acute uveitis (inflammation of iris and ciliary body with small pupil), keratitis (corneal inflammation), endophthalmitis (involvement of vitreous, uvea and retina with cellular debris/pus in anterior chamber) or ocular trauma. Urgent ophthalmic referral.

4. Monocular sustained loss without red eye

a. Central visual loss with relative afferent pupillary defect

- Optic neuritis +/− orbital pain exacerbated by eye movement. The commonest cause is demyelination but consider the possibility of mass lesions compressing the optic nerve. (Consider evoked potentials, CT orbit.)
- Anterior ischaemic optic neuropathy due to presumed atherosclerosis of posterior ciliary arteries or to temporal arteritis. (Consider steroids, perform ESR, temporal artery biopsy.)

b. Central visual loss without relative afferent pupillary defect

- Vitreous haemorrhage
- Macular disorder: macular degeneration, haemorrhage, or exudate
- Branch retinal vein/artery occlusion

c. Peripheral visual loss

- Retinal detachment
- Chorioretinitis
- Intraocular tumour
- Retinal vascular occlusion

5. Binocular sustained loss

- Field loss (e.g. quadrantopia, hemianopia, bitemporal) → CT scan.
- Hypotension (e.g. cardiac failure) leading to posterior circulation insufficiency. Dysrhythmias or vertebrobasilar insufficiency may produce transient episodes of binocular visual loss. CT scan.
- Toxic optic neuropathies (e.g. tobacco, alcohol, methanol).

Painful red eye: Assessment

History This should establish if there has been:-

- *Ocular trauma or foreign body (including contact lens) in the eye.*
- *Sudden or gradual onset of symptoms, nature, and location of pain.* Irritation, soreness, or gritty sensations may occur with conjunctivitis, but the pain is severe in acute glaucoma.
- *Diminution of visual acuity* occurs with conditions affecting the cornea (variable reduction of acuity), iris (mild reduction), and glaucoma (severe reduction of acuity).
- *Discharge (not simply lacrimation) from eyes* may be mucopurulent with bacterial and chlamydial conjunctivitis. It may be mucid and stringy with allergic conditions or dry eyes.
- *Headache or facial pain* is common with orbital cellulitis. It may precede cavernous sinus thrombosis or herpes zoster ophthalmicus.
- *Photophobia* suggests corneal involvement or iritis.
- *Systemic symptoms*, e.g. malaise and fever, may occur with orbital cellulitis and cavernous sinus thrombosis, vomiting is a feature of acute glaucoma; arthralgia and urethral discharge may occur in Reiter's syndrome or chlamydial infection.
- *Previous history.* Recurrent red eyes may occur with episcleritis, iritis, herpes simplex corneal ulcer. Ask specifically about ↑ bp, heart disease, diabetes, connective tissue diseases, and atopy.

Examination

What is red? The conjunctiva, iris, sclera, or episclera (which lies just beneath the conjunctiva and next to the sclera), eye lid, skin around orbit? Is there a visible haemorrhage, either sub-conjuctival or in the anterior chamber (hyphaema)? In conjunctivitis there is 'injection' or increased filling of existing light red vessels, with individual branches distinctly visible; the vessels can be moved with the conjunctiva over the sclera. Ciliary or circumcorneal injection refers to a blue-red discoloration, most conspicuous at the limbus (cornea-scleral border) and occurs in anterior uveitis or iritis (the anterior uvea consists of the iris and ciliary body) and keratitis (corneal inflammation). Mixed injection (conjunctival + ciliary) also occurs in uveitis.

Is there proptosis? suggesting a retro-orbital/intraorbital mass or cavernous sinus thrombosis in which it may become bilateral. *Is it pulsatile?* as in carotico-cavernous fistula, with an audible bruit. *Is there ophthalmoplegia?* This may occur with any mass lesion or cavernous sinus thrombosis.

Is visual acuity diminished? A Snellen chart should be used and near-vision tested (with newsprint if necessary). In acute glaucoma, there is marked reduction in acuity; in acute iritis or keratitis acuity is only modestly diminished; in conjunctivitis it is normal.

What is the size of the pupil? Fixed and dilated in acute glaucoma; small with reduced reaction to light in iritis; normal in conjunctivitis.

Is the red reflex normal? If it is, does the cornea appear normal? The red reflex may be impaired in keratitis, central corneal ulcer or oedema, anterior chamber hyphaema (blood in anterior chamber after blunt trauma), anterior uveitis, glaucoma, or endophthalmitis (involvement of vitreous, uvea and retina with cellular debris/pus in anterior chamber). *Fundoscopy* may not be possible (e.g. corneal clouding due to acute glaucoma).

Are there any anterior chamber abnormalities? In acute anterior uveitis there are exudates in the anterior chamber.

Is there a rash or vesicles on the face, nose, or eyelid? Herpes zoster can lead to conjunctivitis, iritis, corneal ulceration, and 2° glaucoma.

Painful red eye

Painful red eye: Management

With a careful history and examination, the diagnosis may become clear. *Unless you are absolutely sure of the diagnosis, discuss the patient with an ophthalmologist.*

Diagnosis of painful red eye in non-traumatic cases
With prominent ocular discharge

- Viral/bacterial conjunctivitis (watery/mucopurolent discharge, normal red reflex, normal pupil).
- Bacterial/fungal keratitis (mucopurolent discharge, opaque cornea with impaired red reflex, normal or slightly reduced pupil).
- Keratoconjunctivitis sicca or atopic response (dry eye, mucoid strands).

Without prominent discharge and normal red reflex
Normal cornea

- Episcleritis, scleritis, or sub-conjunctivial haemorrhage.
- Orbital cellulitis (skin around orbit erythematous and tender).
- Carotico-cavernous fistula (dilated conjunctival vessels, forehead veins and choroidal vessels because of 'arterialization', reduced acuity because of optic nerve ischaemia, pulsatile proptosis, and bruit).
- Cavernous sinus thrombosis [fever, acute onset painful ophthalmoplegia, conjunctival oedema and congestion, proptosis, oedema over mastoid (emissary vein) → may progress to meningitis].

Abnormal cornea

- Corneal abrasion or ulcer (N.B. herpes simplex and herpes zoster).

Without prominent discharge and impaired red reflex

- Acute glaucoma (severe pain, markedly reduced acuity, cloudy cornea, purple congestion at limbus, fixed dilated pupil, rock hard globe).
- Acute anterior uveitis (malaise, clear cornea, blue-red congestion at limbus, anterior chamber exudate, iris muddy and injected, small pupil with reduced response to light).
- Endophthalmitis (reduced acuity, eyelid swelling, conjunctival injection, anterior chamber cellular debris, vitreous clouding, retinal haemorrhages).
- Keratitis (red congestion at limbus, pupil normal or reduced in size, cornea opaque).
- Central corneal ulcer.

Acute bacterial meningitis: Assessment

Presentation

- *Headache, fever, neck stiffness, photophobia* (often over hours-days).

- *Rash.* Meningococcal meningitis is most commonly associated with a mascular rash progressing to petechiae or purpura (see p240), but other organisms may also cause a rash.

- *Confusion, psychiatric disturbance* (e.g. mania) or *altered level of consciousness.* In the elderly (especially those with diabetes mellitus or cardiopulmonary disease) and the immunocompromised or neutropenic, there may be little other than confusion.

- *Focal neurological signs* complicate meningitis in at least 15% cases. These can suggest cerebral damage (e.g. hemiparesis following venous infarction or arteritis) or indicate cranial nerve and brainstem involvement by basal exudation and inflammation (e.g. in *Listeria monocytogenes* meningitis). They can also indicate brain shift secondary to raised intracranial pressure (see p422). Consider the possibility of brain abscess or encephalitis if focal signs or seizures are prominent.[5] Papilloedema is uncommon ($< 1\%$) and should suggest an alternative diagnosis.

- *Seizures* are the presenting feature in up to 30%.

Predisposing factors

Usually none. But acute otitis media, mastoiditis, pneumonia, head injury, sickle cell disease, alcoholism, and immunocompromised states are all associated.

Causes in adults

Common	Rarer
• *Strep. pneumoniae*	• Gram-negative bacilli (in elderly)
• *Neisseria meningitidis*	• *Listeria* (in elderly)

Assessment of severity

Mortality increases as consciousness decreases ($\sim$ 55% for adults in coma). *However*, meningitis can proceed with alarming rapidity even in the most alert patients.

Management

1. Stabilize the patient (Airway, Breathing, Circulation); give oxygen.
2. Commence antibiotics. It is **not** necessary to await CSF analysis.
3. CT scan prior to lumbar puncture (this is the safest option).
4. Make a definitive diagnosis with lumbar puncture.
5. Reconsider antibiotic regimen after CSF analysis. Consider adjunctive corticosteroid therapy.
6. Arrange for contacts to have prophylaxis. Notify the Public health Service.
7. Observe for and, if necessary, treat complications.

---

[5] Anderson M (1993) *J Neurol Neurosurg Psychiat* **56:** 1243–1258.

Acute bacterial meningitis

Immediate management

1. Antibiotic therapy

- In adults, one suggested regimen is iv **benzyl penicillin** 2.4g (4 MU) every 4h and **cefotaxime** 2g q8h. If the individual is allergic to penicillin, consider iv **erythromycin** 1g q6h and **chloramphenicol** 100mg/kg/day in divided doses (max. 4g). Discuss the case with your microbiologist.

- *Blood cultures* should be taken but it is dangerous to withhold intravenous antibiotics until these are taken or lumbar puncture is performed. Most organisms will be diagnosed from blood cultures.

- Meningococcal infections are discussed on p242.

2. CT scan

- Our policy is that all patients should have a CT scan prior to lumbar puncture. Others suggest this need be performed only if there is decreased level of consciousness, focal signs, papilloedema (very unusual in meningitis) or signs suggesting impending cerebral herniation (p422). You should discuss the patient with a senior member of your team.

3. Lumbar puncture

- *Measure opening pressure.* CSF pressure is often raised (> 14 cm CSF) in meningitis and there are only a few reports of cerebral herniation (coning) following the procedure. If the pressure is raised the patient must be observed closely at no less than 15-minute intervals. A CT scan is required, if it has not already been performed, to exclude a complication of meningitis or a space occupying lesion, e.g. cerebral abscess.

- *Analysis of CSF* (see table opposite)

- CSF WCC   bacterial meningitis characteristically demonstrates a high (usually $> 1000/mm^3$) WCC with neutrophillis predominance. A low CSF WCC ($0–20/mm^3$) with high bacterial count on Gram-stain is associated with a poor prognosis.

- CSF glucose   usually reduced (CSF:blood glucose ratio < 0.31 in $\sim 70\%$) but may be normal.

- CSF protein   usually elevated (> 1.0g/l).

- Gram-stain   is positive in 60–90% but may not be if there has been a significant delay between starting antibiotics and lumbar puncture. Similarly, the yield of CSF culture falls to $< 50\%$ from 70–85%.

This CSF profile may also occur with viral and tuberculous meningitis in the early phase, but repeat CSF analysis shows transformation to a lymphocytic predominance. Patients with a CSF profile characteristic of bacterial meningitis should be treated as if they had this condition until proven otherwise.

CSF composition in meningitis

	Bacterial	Viral	TB meningitis
Appearance	Turbid	Clear	Clear
Cells (mm^3)	5-2000	5-500	5-1000
Main cell type	Neutrophil	Lymphocyte	Lymphocyte
Glucose (mM)	Very low	Normal	Low
Protein (g/l)	Often > 1.0	0.5 –0.9	Often > 1.0
Other tests	Gram-stain	PCR	Ziehl-Neesen
	Bacterial antigen		Fluorescent test
			PCR

(See p846 for reference intervals for CSF analysis)

Acute bacterial meningitis

Continuing therapy

Reconsider antibiotics? Adjunctive steroids?

- *CSF lymphocytosis.* If the CSF pleocytosis is predominantly lymphocytic the diagnosis is unlikely to be bacterial meningitis. This is discussed further on p336.

- *CSF polymorphs* $> 50,000/mm^3$ suggests possibility of cerebral abscess. A CT brain scan should be performed.

- *Gram-negative bacilli on CSF Gram-stain.* Cefotaxime may not be adequate therapy. A third generation cephalosporin in combination with gentamicin may need to be administered. Intrathecal treatment may be required and the source of infection needs to be discovered. Discuss the case with your microbiologist.

- *Adjunctive corticosteroid therapy* has been shown to reduce the incidence of deafness and neurological sequelae in children and many neurologists now favour its use to reduce inflammation. In patients with raised ICP, stupor, or impaired mental status, give 10 mg dexamethasone iv loading dose, followed by 4–6mg po q6h.

Prophylaxis for contacts should be given immediately

- *Public Health Services* should be notified of any case of bacterial meningitis. They will be able to give advice on current prophylactic treatment and vaccination (possible with some strains of meningococcus); they will also assist in contact tracing. Patients with meningococcus are infectious and can spread organisms to others. Liaise with your local microbiologists.

- *Prophylaxis* should be given as soon as the diagnosis of bacterial meningitis is suspected. In the UK, for adult contacts, rifampicin 600mg bd for 2 days is recommended. The alternative for adults is ciprofloxacin 750mg as a single dose. (For children older than 1 year: 10mg/kg bd for 2 days; for children 3 months–1 year: 5mg/kg bd for 2 days).

Acute bacterial meningitis

Complications and their treatment

- *Raised intracranial pressure* may respond to steroids and, as discussed above, some neurologists give this routinely to reduce inflammatory reaction. In the acute situation, if there is evidence of brain shift of impending transtentorial herniation (p422) mannitol should be given 1 g/kg over 10–15 minutes (~ 250ml of 20% of solution for an average adult) and elevate the head of the bed to 30° (see p344). Oral glycerol has also been shown to be effective in some small trials.

- *Hydrocephalus* may require an intraventricular shunt and should be discussed urgently with neurologists. It can occur because of thickened meninges obstructing CSF flow or because of the adherence of the inflamed lining of the aqueduct of Sylvius or fourth ventricular outflow. Papilloedema may not be present.

- *Seizures* should be treated as seizures of any other aetiology (see p370).

- *Persistent pyrexia* suggests that there may be an occult source of infection. The patient should be carefully re-examined (including oral cavity and ears).

- *Focal neurological deficit* may occur because of arteritis or venous infarction or space occupying lesion, e.g. subdural empyema. Inflammatory reaction at the base of the skull may lead to cranial nerve palsies. A CT scan should be requested if it has not already been performed. Anti-coagulation is not of benefit for treatment of thromboses.

- *Subdural empyema* is a rare complication. Focal signs, seizures, and papilloedema suggest the diagnosis. It requires urgent surgical drainage.

- *Disseminated intravascular coagulation* is an ominous sign. Platelet and fresh frozen plasma may be required. The use of heparin should be discussed with a haematologist and neurologist.

- *Syndrome of inappropriate ADH* may occur. Fluid balance and electrolytes need to be checked regularly (p446).

Meningitis with lymphocytic CSF

Presentation

- Viral meningitis may be indistinguishable on clinical grounds from acute early bacterial meningitis but it is usually self-limiting.
- TB meningitis is usually preceded by a history of malaise and systemic illness for days-weeks before meningeal features develop. However, it may present very acutely. TB meningitis may be associated with basal archnoditis, vasculitis, and infarction leading to focal neurological signs, e.g. cranial nerve palsies, and obstructive hydrocephalus with papilloedema.
- Cryptococcal or syphilitic meningitis in the immunocompromised present with features indistinguishable from TB meningitis.

Causes

Viral

- Coxsackie
- Echo
- Mumps
- Herpes simplex type 1
- Varicella zoster
- HIV
- Lymphocytic choriomeningitis virus

Non-viral

- TB
- Cryptococcus
- Leptospirosis
- Lyme disease
- Syphilis
- Brucellosis
- Parameningeal infection with a CSF reaction

CSF findings

The CSF usually demonstrates a lymphocytosis (see table) but the CSF in viral meningitis may initially demonstrate predominantly neutrophils. It is important not to dismiss the possibility of TB meningitis if CSF glucose is normal; it may be in ~ 20% of cases and the tuberculin test may also be negative initially in a similar percentage.

Treatment regimens

- ***Viral meningitis:*** Usually supportive treatment only.
- ***TB meningitis:*** Pyrazinamide 30mg/kg/day and isoniazid 10mg/kg/day (up to a max of 600mg/day) achieve best CSF penetration. Give pyridoxine 10mg daily as prophylaxis against isoniazid neuropathy. For the first 3 months, add rifampicin (450mg/day if wt. < 50 kg or 600mg/day if wt > 50 kg) and ethambutol (25mg/kg/day). Thereafter, for the next 7–10 months give isoniazid (at a lower dose of 300mg/day) and rifampicin.
- There are several other regimens in use for *M. tuberculosis* meningitis; *M. avium intracellulare* requires a different combination of drugs.[6] **Corticosteroids** are often prescribed if there are focal signs, raised intracranial pressure, or very high levels of CSF protein (see adjunctive therapy for acute bacterial meningitis, p332).
- ***Cryptococcal meningitis:*** Several regimens are used. Amphotericin B 0.6–1.0mg/kg/day alone or at a lower dose of 0.5mg/kg/day in conjunction with flucytosine 150mg/kg/day for 6 weeks appears effective. Fluconazole (400mg/day initially, then 200–400mg/day for 6–8 weeks) is an alternative which appears to be as effective in AIDS.

---

[6] Berger JR (1994) *Curr Opin Neurol* **7**: 191–200.

Acute viral encephalitis   1.

Presentation
- *Change in personality.*
- *Confusion, psychiatric disturbance, or altered level of consciousness.*
- *Headache, fever, and some neck stiffens.* Meningism is usually not prominent: some individuals have a meningo-encephalitis.
- *Focal neurological signs.* Hemiparesis or memory loss (usually indicative of temporal lobe involvement) is not uncommon.
- *Seizures* are common; some are complex partial in nature.
- *Raised intracranial pressure* and signs of brain shift (p422).
- *Predisposing factors:* immunocompromised patient.

Management
1 *Antibiotic therapy*
If there is any suspicion that the illness is meningitis, start antibiotics (p330). It is not necessary to await CSF analysis.

2 *Specific antiviral therapies*
Acyclovir has dramatically reduced mortality and morbidity in HSV encephalitis. Most clinicians therefore give it in suspected encephalitis without waiting for confirmation that the pathogen is herpes simplex.
- *Acyclovir* 10mg/kg iv (infused over 60 mins) every 8h (reduced dose in renal insufficiency) is given for 10–14 days.
- *Ganciclovir:* 2.5–5.0mg/kg iv (infused over 60 mins) every 8h should be given if cytomegalovirus is a possible pathogen (more likely in renal transplant patients or those with AIDS). Treatment is usually for 14–28 days depending upon response.

3 *CT scan: Our policy is to do a CT scan on all patients prior to LP*
- In a patient with focal neurological signs, focal seizures, or signs of brain shift, a CT scan must be arranged urgently and performed prior to LP. CT may not demonstrate any abnormalities. In herpes simplex encephalitis there may be low attenuation areas, particularly in the temporal lobes, with surrounding oedema.

4 *Lumbar puncture*
- *Measure opening pressure.* CSF pressure may be raised (> 14cm CSF) in which case the patient must be observed closely at 15 minute intervals. A CT scan is required to exclude a space occupying lesion, e.g. cerebral abscess.
- *Analysis of CSF* usually reveals a lymphocytic leukocytosis (usually 5–500/mm³) in viral encephalitis, but it may be entirely normal. Increasingly, polymerase chain reaction (PCR) is being used to amplify viral DNA and CSF should be saved for this analysis. Other causes of a lymphocytic picture in the CSF are discussed on p336. CSF protein is only mildly elevated and glucose is normal.

5 *Further investigations*
- *Serology:* Save serum for viral titres (IgM and IgG). If infectious mononucleosis is suspected a monospot test should be performed.
- *EEG:* Should be arranged even in those without seizures. There may be generalized slowing and, in herpes simplex encephalitis, there may be bursts of periodic high voltage slow wave complexes over temporal cortex.
- *Brain biopsy:* Some clinicians in the USA have advocated this procedure in order to make a definitive diagnosis. In the UK this is performed less frequently.[7]

---

[7]   Whitley RJ (1990) *NEJM* **323**: 242–250.

Complications   339

Neurological observations should be made regularly. Two complications may require urgent treatment.

- ***Raised intracranial pressure*** secondary to cerebral oedema may require treatment with dexamethasone (see intracranial space occupying lesion p354). There is some experimental evidence that steroids may potentiate spread of herpes virus, so dexamethasone should not be given prophylactically without a specific indication. In the acute situation, if there is evidence of brain shift, mannitol may be used (see raised intracranial pressure p348).

- ***Seizures*** may be difficult to control but are treated as seizures of any other aetiology.

Causes in UK

- Herpes simplex
- Varicella zoster
- Coxsackie
- Cytomegalovirus (in immunocopromised)
- Mumps
- Epstein-Barr virus
- Echo virus

Head injury: Presentation

- Varies from transient 'stunning' for a few seconds, to coma.
- A fraction of patients who attend A&E need be admitted for observation. (Indications for admission are given on p345.)

In the alert patient, determine:

- ***Circumstances surrounding injury.*** Was it caused by endogenous factors, e.g. loss of consciousness whilst driving? Or exogenous factors, e.g. another driver? Was there extracranial trauma?
- ***Period of loss of consciousness.*** This relates to severity of diffuse brain damage.
- ***Period of post traumatic amnesia.*** The period of permanent memory loss after injury also reflects degree of damage. (N.B. Period of retrograde amnesia or memory loss for events prior to injury does not correlate with severity of brain damage.)
- ***Headache/vomiting.*** Common after head injury but if they persist raised intracranial pressure should be considered (p348).
- ***Glasgow Coma Scale score.***
- ***Skull fracture present?***
- ***Neurological signs.*** Are there any focal neurological signs?
- ***Extracranial injury.*** Is there evidence of occult blood loss?

The drowsy or unconscious patient needs:

- Urgent assistance from senior A&E staff and anaesthetists.
- ***Protection of airway.*** The patient who has a deteriorating level of consciousness or is in coma should be intubated because hypocarbia and adequate oxygenation are effective means of reducing intracranial pressure rapidly. If the patient is neurologically stable and protecting his airway, intubation may not be necessary. Assume there is a cervical spine injury until an X-ray (of all seven cervical vertebrae) demonstrates otherwise.
- ***Hyperventilation.*** The pattern of breathing should be noted (p420). If intubated, the patient should be hyperventilated to achieve a P_aCO_2 of 3.7–3.9kPa (see p350). in adults, an initial rate of ~ 12–14 breaths/min with a volume of 750–1000mls of 100% oxygen is recommended.
- ***Support of circulation.*** Hypotension should be treated initially with colloid. If persistent or severe, exclude a cardiac cause (ECG) and occult haemorrhage (e.g. intra-abdominal).
- ***Treatment of seizures*** with diazepam 5–10mg iv/rectally, which may be repeated to a maximum of 20mg. If seizures continue, consider iv lorazepam or phenytoin (p370).
- ***Rapid survey of chest, abdomen, and limbs*** looking for a flail segment or haemo/pneumothorax, possible intra-abdominal bleeding (if there are any doubts peritoneal lavage may be required), limb lacerations, and long bone fractures.
- ***Brief history*** should be obtained from ambulance crew or relatives. The patient may have lost consciousness just before the injury, e.g. due to subarachnoid haemorrhage, seizure, or hypoglycaemia. The tempo of neurological deterioration should be established.

Guidelines for performing skull X-rays and CT scans are on p342.

Symptoms following head injury

- ***Symptoms associated with minor head injury***
- Headache, dizziness, fatigue, reduced concentration, memory deficit, irritability, anxiety, insomnia, hyperacusis, photophobia, depression, and general slowed information processing.

- ***Symptoms associated with moderate – severe head injury***
  As above, but also:-
  Behavioural problems include irritability, impulsivity, egocentricity, emotional lability, impaired judgement, impatience, anxiety, depression, hyper- or hypo-sexuality, dependency, euphoria, aggressiveness, apathy, childishness, and disinhibition.
  Cognitive impairment includes deficits of memory, difficulty in abstract thinking, general slowed information processing, poor concentration, slow reaction time, impaired auditory comprehension, reduced verbal fluency, anomia, and difficulty planning or organizing.

Head injury: Assessment

Examination

Rapid neurological assessment should take only a few minutes.

- The level of consciousness must be noted with Glasgow Coma Scale (GCS) score (p416).
- Note the size, shape, and reactions of pupils to bright light.
- Resting eye position and spontaneous eye movements should be observed. If the latter are not full and the patient unresponsive, test oculocephalic and/or oculovestibular responses (p426).
- The doll's head manoeuvre should not be attempted if cervical spine injury has not been excluded.
- Test the corneal reflex (cranial nerves V and VII).
- Motor function should be assessed (see p416); any asymmetry should be noted.
- Look for features suggesting brain shift and herniation (p422).

Head and spine assessment

- The skull should be examined for a fracture. Extensive periorbital haematomas, bruising behind the ear (Battle's sign), bleeding from the ear and CSF rhinorrhoea/otorrhoea suggest a basal skull fracture. Look for facial (maxillary and mandibular) fractures.
- Only 1% of patients will have a skull fracture. This greatly increases the chances of an intracranial haematoma (from 1:1000 to 1:30 in alert patients; from 1:100 to 1:4 in confused/comatose patients). N.B. Potentially fatal injuries are not always associated with skull fracture.
- **Consider** the possibility of spinal cord trauma. 'Log-roll' the patient and examine the back for tenderness over the spinous processes, paraspinal swelling, or a gap between the spinous processes. The limbs may have been found to be flaccid and unresponsive to pain during the neurological assessment. There may be painless retention of urine.

Indications for skull X-ray
- Decreased level of consciousness
- Amnesia
- Neurological signs/symptoms
- CSF/blood from nose/ear
- Scalp bruising/swelling
- Suspected penetrating injury
- Difficulty in clinical assessment (e.g. alcohol, drugs, very young/elderly)
- Seizures
If GCS < 8/15, arrange an urgent head CT.

Things to look for on the skull X-rays

- Linear skull fracture (see above)
- Depressed skull fracture (requires elevation if depressed by more than the vault thickness)
- > 3mm shift of a calcified pineal (if present)
- Integrity of craniocervical junction
- Fluid level in sphenoid sinus

Definite indications for CT scan

- Skull fracture and persistent neurological dysfunction
- Depressed level of consciousness and/or neurological dysfunction (inc. seizures)
- Coma after resuscitation
- Suspected compound fracture of vault or base of skull (e.g. CSF leak)
- Depressed skull fracture
- Confusion/neurological disturbance persisting > 12h

Things to look for on C-spine films

- Check all seven C-spine vertebrae and C7-T1 junctions are visible
- Check alignment   – anterior and posterior of vertebral bodies
  - posterior margin of spinal canal
  - spinous processes
- A step of > 25% of vertebral body suggests facet joint dislocation
- Check contours   – outlines of vertebral bodies
  - outlines of spinous processes
- Look for avulsion fractures, wedge fractures (> 3mm height difference between anterior and posterior body height)
- Check odontoid   – open mouth and lateral views
- The distance between ant. arch C1 and odontoid should be < 3mm
- Check soft tissues   – disc spaces
  - space between anterior C3 and back of pharyngeal shadow > 5mm suggests retropharyngeal mass (e.g. abscess or haematoma from fracture of C2)

Head injury: Immediate management

- After resuscitation, **take blood** for **FBC, G&S, U&Es, arterial blood gases**, and, if the circumstances of injury are not clear or there is a suspicion of drug intoxication, **toxicology screen**.

- **Subsequent** management depends upon the pace of events and the clinical situation. > 40% comatose patients with head injury have intracranial haematomas and it is not possible to distinguish definitively between these patients and those who have diffuse brain injury and swelling on clinical examination alone.

- **Urgent CT scan.** This is the next step in most patients who have depressed level of consciousness or focal signs (see table p343). The speed with which this needs to be arranged depends upon the tempo of neurological deterioration (relative change in GCS score p416) and/or the absolute level of consciousness (GCS < 8). If CT scanning is not available at your hospital you must discuss with your regional neurosurgical centre.

- **Treatment of raised intracranial pressure** is discussed on p350; corticosteroids have no proven benefit. Discuss with your neurosurgical centre. In a rapidly deteriorating situation it may be necessary to proceed directly to surgery. You may be able to buy some time by hyperventilation (lower P_aCO_2 to 3.7–3.9 kPa), mannitol (1g/kg over 10–15 minutes or ~ 250ml of 20% solution for an average adult) and frusemide (20–40mg iv) while obtaining an urgent CT scan.

- **Surgery** may be indicated for extradural (p356), subdural (p360), possibly some intracerebral haemorrhages (p358), and complex head wounds such as compound depressed skull fractures.
  - A general rule is urgent evacuation is required of extradural haematoma which produce mid-line shift of 5mm or more and/or 25mls in calculated volume.
  - If the extradural haemorrhage is considered too small to warrant surgery on a CT scan performed within 6 h of injury, the scan should be repeated after a few hours irrespective of whether there has been a deterioration in the patient's condition.

- **Non-operative management.** Brain contusion may be evident as areas of increased or decreased density but CT is not a sensitive way to detect primary diffuse brain injury. Effacement of the cavity of the third ventricle and of the perimesencephalic cisterns suggest raised intracranial pressure but the absence of the signs is not to be taken as an indicator of normal intracranial pressure. Many centres therefore proceed to intracranial pressure monitoring (p842) although this is a controversial subject.

Indications for admission following head injury

- Confusion
- Decreased level of consciousness
- Clinical or radiological evidence of skull fracture
- Neurological signs or severe headache + vomiting
- Difficulty in assessment (e.g. alcohol, drugs, very young/elderly)
- Concurrent medical conditions (e.g. clotting disorders, diabetes)
- Poor social circumstances/living alone

N.B. Very brief loss of consciousness or post traumatic amnesia are not absolute indicators for admission but each patient needs to be assessed on their own merits.

If patients are discharged they should be sent home with

- A responsible adult who will be with them over the next 24h.
- A head injury card which describes potential signs and symptoms (e.g. undue sleepiness, headache, vomiting, or dizziness) of delayed neurological dysfunction.

Head injury: Further management

The aim of subsequent management is to minimize secondary injury to the brain other than intracranial haematomas (see table opposite).

Patients should be managed at a neurosurgical centre and if this is arranged the guidelines below should be followed for transfer.

The principles of management are:-

- ***Regular and frequent neurological observation.*** If there is deterioration consider whether there may be a secondary cause of brain injury contributing to this (see table opposite). If there are new signs of raised intracranial pressure, declining level of consciousness, or signs or transtentorial herniation (p422), the patient requires intubation and hyperventilation if this has not already been performed. Mannitol may be started or a repeat bolus may need to be given (see p350) and repeat CT scanning may be necessary.

- ***Regular monitoring of bp, blood gases, electrolytes, urinary output.*** Pre-emptive treatment of a decline in any of these may prevent neurological deterioration. Hypotension is commonly due to sedative agents and/or hypovolaemia. But fluid therapy needs to be conducted with care because overgenerous administration may exacerbate raised intracranial pressure. Monitor CVP.

- ***Prompt treatment of seizures*** (p370).

- ***Nasogastric tube*** to administer nutrition and drugs, including ranitidine 150mg bd for prophylaxis against gastric ulceration.

- ***A bowel regimen*** of stool softeners should be started.

Before transfer to Neurosurgical Unit[8]

- Assess clinically for respiratory insufficiency, shock, and internal injuries.
- Perform CXR, arterial blood gas estimation, cervical spine X-ray.
- Appropriate treatment might be to:
  - intubate (e.g. if airway obstructed or threatened)
  - ventilate (e.g. cyanosis, $P_aO_2 < 7.9$kPa, $P_aCO_2 > 5.9$kPa)
  - commence iv fluids carefully
  - give mannitol, after consultation with neurosurgeon
  - apply cervical collar or cervical traction
- Patient should be accompanied by personnel able to insert or to reposition endotracheal tube, to initiate or maintain ventilation, to administer oxygen and fluids, and to use suction.

---

[8] Mendelow AD & Teasdale G (1991) in *Clinical Neurology*, eds. Swash M
     Oxbury J Section **14**: 698

Causes of secondary brain injury[9]	
Systemic	**Intracranial**
• Hypoxaemia	• Haematoma (extradural, subdural, or intracerebral)
• Hypotension	
• Hypercarbia	• Brain swelling/oedema
• Severe hypocapnoea	• Raised ICP
• Pyrexia	• Cerebral vasospasm
• Hyponatraemia	• Epilepsy
• Anaemia	• Intracranial infection
• DIC	

[9]   Miller JD (1993) *J Neurol Neurosurg Psychiat* **56**: 440–447

Raised intracranial pressure (ICP)

Presentation

Normal ICP in adults is 0–10mmHg at rest. Treatment is required when it exceeds 15–20mmHg for > 5 minutes. Symptoms and signs suggestive of raised ICP include:

- *Headache and vomiting* worse in mornings; exacerbated by bending.
- *Focal neurological signs* may occur if there is a space occupying lesion and in some metabolic conditions (e.g. liver failure). But there may also be false localizing signs, e.g. VIth cranial nerve palsy.
- *Seizures* may occur with space occupying lesions, CNS infection, or metabolic encephalopathies associated with raised ICP.
- *Papilloedema* is not always present.
- *Impaired level of consciousness* – from mild confusion to coma.
- *Signs of brain shift*[10] may accompany decreasing level of consciousness. They are discussed with examination of brainstem function (p418).
- *Bradycardia and hypertension* (Cushing response) probably results from direct medullary compression. Its clinical value is probably overemphasized in comparison with other signs of brain shift (p422).

Causes

- Head injury → intracranial haematoma/brain swelling/contusion
- Stroke (haemorrhagic, major infarct, venous thrombosis)
- Metabolic (hepatic or renal failure, DKA, hyponatraemia, etc.)
- CNS infection (abscess, encephalitis, meningitis, malaria)
- CNS tumour
- Status epilepticus
- Hydrocephalus (of any cause)
- 'Benign' intracranial hypertension

Assessment of severity

- Glasgow Coma Scale (p416)
- Signs of brain shift and brainstem compromise (p422).

Management

1. Stabilize the patient.
2. Consider active means of reducing ICP.
3. Attempt to make a diagnosis.
4. Treat factors which may exacerbate raised ICP.
5. Observe for signs of deterioration and attempt to reverse them.
6. Consider specific therapy.

What follows is the management for stabilizing a patient presenting acutely with raised ICP and may not be appropriate for many patients with a long progressive history of deterioration.

---

[10] Plum F & Posner JB (1980) *The Diagnosis of Stupor and Coma* 3rd Edition; FA Davis, Philadelphia

Raised intracranial pressure (ICP): Immediate management

Stabilize the patient

350

- **Open the airway** by laying the patient on their side. Give oxygen. Measure **arterial blood gases.** Intubation and mechanical ventilation may be necessary because of respiratory compromise. It may also be necessary to reduce ICP by hyperventilating the patient (see below) to keep P_aCO_2 between 3.3–3.9kPa (25–30mmHg).

- **Correct hypotension.** Volume expansion with colloids or infusions of inotropes need to be conducted with careful and frequent monitoring of central venous pressure and/or pulmonary artery wedge pressure. In general, patients with raised ICP should be fluid restricted to 1.5–2.0l/day. So, if volume expansion is required it should be kept to the minimum required to restore bp.

- **Treat seizures** (p370).

- **Examine rapidly** for signs of head injury (p340). If the patient is hypotensive, examine carefully for any occult site of bleeding. If there is a rash, consider the possibility of meningococcal meningitis; take blood cultures and give antibiotics (p330).

- Take blood for **glucose** (this may be raised in diabetic ketoacidosis or hyperosmolar non-ketotic states; it may be very low in liver failure), **U&Es** (biochemical assessment of dehydration and renal function; potassium for susceptibility to dysrhythmia; hyponatraemia from inappropriate ADH or hypernatraemia from aggressive diuretic-induced dehydration), **LFTs, albumin, clotting, studies** and **ammonium** (to assess liver function), **FBC** and **blood culture**.

Measures to reduce ICP

The value of ICP monitoring is a controversial subject. Irrespective of whether or not your patient's ICP is monitored, the following interventions should be considered.

- **Elevate head of bed** to ~ 30° (once cervical spine injury has been excluded) to promote venous drainage.

- **Hyperventilation** so that P_aCO_2 is kept between 3.7–3.9kPa will promote cerebral vasoconstriction and lower cerebral blood volume: this requires intubation and paralysis. It will also lower the bp and may compromise cerebral circulation. In patients with liver failure this is no longer recommended.

- **Mannitol** 1g/kg over 10–15 minutes (~ 250ml of 20% solution for an average adult) reduces ICP within 20 minutes and its effects should last for 2–6 hours. **Frusemide** 20–40mg iv may be given with mannitol to potentiate its effect. If required, further boluses of smaller doses of mannitol (0.25–0.50g/kg) may be given every few hours. Electrolytes and serum osmolality should be monitored because a profound diuresis may result.

- **Corticosteroids** are of benefit in reducing oedema around space occupying lesions (p354) but are not helpful in the treatment of stroke or head injury. Dexamethasone is given as a loading dose of 10mg iv. It may be followed by 4–6mg q6h po/ via NG tube.

- **Fluid restriction** to 1.5–2.0 litres/day. Electrolytes must be checked frequently.

- **Cooling** to 35°C reduces cerebral ischaemia.

- **Avoid/treat hyperglycaemia** because it exacerbates ischaemia.

Raised intracranial pressure (ICP):
Further management

Attempt to make a diagnosis

Often the history makes the diagnosis obvious and, usually, raised intra-cranial pressure is a secondary diagnosis. If a history is not available, focal neurological signs or focal seizures suggest an underlying structural cerebral lesion (although such signs may occur with hepatic or renal failure). Meningism raises the possibility of subarachnoid haemorrhage or meningitis. Blood sent for analysis on admission may help to detect metabolic causes of raised ICP.

A CT scan should be performed in all patients suspected of having raised ICP before lumbar puncture is considered.

(Lumbar puncture should be discussed with a senior colleague and/or neurologist).

Treat factors which exacerbate raised ICP[11]

- *Hypoxia/hypercapnia.* Arterial blood gases need to be measured regularly.

- *Inadequate analgesia, sedation, or muscle relaxation* leads to hypertension. N.B. Hypertension should not be treated aggressively. Pain, e.g. from urine retention, may be the cause. Rapid lowering of bp may lead to 'watershed'/'border zone' cerebral infarcts.

- *Seizures* are not always easy to identify in paralysed patients.

- *Pyrexia* increases cerebral metabolism and, as a consequence, cerebral vasodilation. It also appears to increase cerebral oedema. The cause of pyrexia should be sought but paracetamol (given rectally) and active cooling should be commenced.

- *Hypovolaemia*.

- *Hyponatraemia* is usually the result of fluid overload but may be caused by a syndrome of inappropriate ADH secretion. Treat with DDAVP 1–4µg iv daily (see p446).

Consider specific therapy

- Once a diagnosis is established it may be appropriate to consider surgery in order to decompress brain or insert a ventricular shunt to drain CSF.

- Intracranial infections need to be treated with the most suitable antibiotics.

- Hyperglycaemia (ketotic/non-ketotic), liver, or renal failure have their own specific management (see relevant sections).

- Often, however, there may not be a specific intervention that is appropriate, e.g. contusion following head injury, and management is confined to optimizing a patient's condition whilst awaiting recovery.

---

[11] Pickard JD & Czosnyka M (1993) *J Neurol Neurosurg Psychiat* **56**: 845–858.

Intracranial space occupying lesion

Presentation

- *Symptoms of raised intracranial pressure.* Headache, nausea, and vomiting (see p348).
- *Papilloedema* is present in the minority of cases.
- *Focal neurological symptoms and signs.* These depend upon location of the lesion, its extent and that of surrounding cerebral oedema, and compression of long tract fibres or cranial nerves. Some lesions, particularly those in the frontal lobe, are relatively 'silent' and may produce no signs or simply change in personality.
- *Seizures.*
- *Impaired level of consciousness* ranging from confusion to coma.
- *Signs of brain shift* (p422) may be present.
- *Fever* suggests an infection. There may be a recent history of earache/discharge, toothache, foreign travel, or immune compromise.
- *Acute onset of symptoms* suggests the possibility of a vascular event, either primary or bleeding into another type of lesion, e.g. tumour.

Management

Depends upon the diagnosis. In a comatose individual with known inoperable brain metastases it is usually not appropriate to intervene. On the other hand, if a patient presents for the first time with signs suggestive of a space occupying lesion the diagnosis needs to be established.

1. Assess severity

- If comatose, protect the airway and manage as on p310.
- If there are signs of brain shift, which suggests impending transtenorial herniation (p422), give mannitol 0.5–1g/kg over 10–15 minutes (100–250ml of 20% solution for an average adult) and hyperventilate to keep P_aCO_2 between 3.7–3.9kPa. This may be followed by smaller doses of mannitol every few hours (p350).
- If the patient is alert and stable it is best to await CT scan and in the interim make regular neurological observations.

2. If the patient is **pyrexial** or the history is suggestive of **infection**, blood (sputum and urine) cultures should be sent. An urgent CT scan should be arranged for these cases; CSF analysis may be necessary but lumbar puncture should NOT be performed before the scan or discussion with neurologists/neurosurgeons.

3. If a **vascular event** is suspected a CT should also be arranged urgently because decompression may be possible.

4. Seizures should be treated. If they are recurrent, the patient may require loading with iv phenytoin (p370). Many neurosurgeons give oral phenytoin prophylactically to patients (300mg/day; therapeutic levels are not reached for at least 5 days).

5. Steroid therapy is given if it is thought that some of the symptoms/signs are due to tumour-related brain oedema. Give dexamethasone 10mg iv (loading dose), followed by 4–6mg po or ng q6h. This is a large dose of steroid (N.B. dexamethasone 20mg/day equivalent to prednisolone 130mg/day) and urine/blood glucose should be monitored. Duration of therapy is guided by response to steroid and the patient's general condition.

6. Neurosurgery/radiotherapy may be of some benefit in some individuals and this needs to be discussed with Regional Neurosurgical Centre.

Common causes if intracranial space occupying lesions	
• Cerebral tumour (1°/2°)	• Cerebral abscess
• Subdural haematoma	• Extradural haematoma
• Intracerebral haemorrhage	• Subdural empyema
• Tuberculoma	• Toxoplasmosis (immunocompromised)

Extradural haemorrhage

Presentation

There are no specific diagnostic features. Consider the diagnosis in any head-injured patient who fails to improve or continues to deteriorate.

- *Head injury* is almost invariable.
- *Skull fracture* present in over 90% of adult cases.
- *Headache and vomiting* may occur.
- *Impaired level of consciousness.* There may be an initial lucid interval following head injury but extradural haematomas may be present in patients who have been in coma continuously after the injury. Uncommonly, if the cause is a dural venous sinus tear (rather than shearing of a meningeal artery), the lucid interval may extend for several days.
- *Seizures.*
- *Contralateral hemiparesis and extensor plantar* may be elicited.
- *Signs of brain shift* (p422).

Causes

Common	Rare
• Head injury → tearing of meningeal artery (commonly middle meningeal)	• Head injury → dural sinus tear • Intracranial infection (sinuses, middle ear, orbit) • Anti-coagulants/blood dyscrasia

Assessment of severity

Bilateral extensor plantars or spasticity, extensor response to painful stimuli, and coma are severe effects of an extradural haemorrhage.

Management

Depends upon tempo of presentation.
Priorities are:-

1. Stabilize the patient: protect the airway; give oxygen, support the breathing and circulation. Assume C-spine injury till excluded.

2. Treat seizures (p370)

3. Urgent CT scan
- Haematomas with > 5mm mid-line shift on CT and/or > 25mls calculated volume require urgent evacuation.
- If the extradural haemorrhage is considered too small to warrant surgery on a CT scan performed within 6 h of injury, the scan should be repeated after a few hours, irrespective of whether there has been a deterioration in the patient's condition.

4. Closely monitor neurological state (inc. Glasgow Coma Scale)
- If the patient slips into coma and signs of tentorial herniation (p422) are progressing rapidly, give 1g/kg of 20% mannitol as a bolus and inform on-call surgeons.
- If there is evidence of brain shift, discuss with neurosurgeons: intracranial pressure should be reduced with mannitol (0.5–1.0 g/kg 20% mannitol) and hyperventilation (p350).

5. All patients must be **discussed with neurosurgeons**. Neurological impairment is potentially reversible if the extradural haematoma is treated early.

Intracerebral haemorrhage

Presentation
- *Headache, nausea, and vomiting* of sudden onset is common.
- *Focal neurological deficit:* the nature of this depends upon location of haemorrhage. Putaminal haemorrhages (~ 30% of cases) or lobar bleeds (~ 30% of cases) may lead to contralateral hemiparesis and sensory loss, visual field disturbance, dysphasia (left hemisphere), or spatial neglect (more severe with right hemisphere lesions). In other words, they may present like a middle cerebral artery infarct (p384) but often there is a greater alteration in the level of consciousness. Thalamic haemorrhages (~ 10% cases) may result in eye signs (forced down-gaze, up-gaze paralysis, or skew deviation) as well as contra-lateral sensory loss and hemiparesis. Cerebellar haemorrhage is dealt with on p388; pontine bleeds on p386.
- *Seizures* may occur.
- *Global neurological deficit* with decreasing level of consciousness progressing to coma. There may be signs of brain shift (p422).
- *Hypertension.*

Common predisposing factors
- Hypertension (40–50%)
- Anti-coagulants
- Metastatic neoplasm – bleeds may occur within
- Drug abuse (cocaine, pseudoephedrine, amphetamines)

Assessment of severity
Patients with decreasing level of consciousness, coma, and signs of brain shift (p418) have worse prognosis.

Management
Priorities are:
1 Stabilize the patient – protect the airway, give oxygen if required, support the circulation if necessary or appropriate, commence general measures for treating comatose patient (p306) if necessary. If there is evidence of raised intracranial pressure, it should be reduced (see p350).
2 Correct bleeding tendency or effects of anti-coagulants.
3 Make a definitive diagnosis with urgent CT scan. Liaise with regional neurosurgery unit early. Surgical intervention may be of benefit in some cases. Whether aggressive intervention is appropriate should be decided early.
4 If appropriate, intensive care/high dependency ward nursing observa-tions are required for the drowsy or comatose patient if they are not transferred to neurosurgical centre immediately.
5 Surgical decompression may be beneficial: usually for accessible bleeds within the posterior fossa (see cerebellar haemorrhage p388), putamen, or thalamus.
6 Hypertension is common. If systolic bp > 200 or diastolic > 120 mmHg following a haemorrhagic stroke, it probably should be treated to limit vasogenic oedema, but this is controversial.[12,13] *Sublingual* nifedipine is best avoided as it may cause a profound fall in bp. We recommend atenolol 25–50mg po if necessary.

[12] O'Connell JE & Gray C (1994) *BMJ* **308**: 1523–1524.
[13] Lavin P (1986) *Arch Int Med* 146: 66–68.

Subdural haemorrhage

Presentation

- This may present in one of two ways – acute or chronic. Both are usually the result of tearing of bridging veins (between cortical surface and venous sinuses).
- Acute haemorrhage into the subdural space follows head injury and can be impossible to distinguish on clinical grounds from extradural haemorrhage (p356).
- A chronic haematoma is also preceded in most cases by head injury but this is often so trivial that patients are unable to recollect it.
- Both types of patient may present with:-
  - *Skull fracture* (more common in acute cases).
  - *Headache.*
  - *Impaired and fluctuating level of consciousness* ranging from mild confusion, through cognitive decline (e.g. impaired memory) to coma. The diagnosis should be considered in any individual, particularly elderly, who presents with intellectual deterioration or 'dementia' of relatively recent onset.
  - *Focal neurological signs* (hemiparesis, dysphasia, hemianopia, etc).
  - *Seizures* occur in a minority of patients.
  - *Signs of brain shift* (p422) or *papilloedema.*

Common predisposing factors
- Head injury – in young or old
- Old age – cortical atrophy stretches bridging veins
- Long-standing alcohol abuse
- Anti-coagulant use

Assessment of severity
The following are severe effects of a subdural haemorrhage
- Bilateral spasticity or extensor plantars
- Extensor response to painful stimuli
- Coma

Management
Depends upon tempo of presentation.
- In suspected **chronic cases**, a CT scan is required less urgently unless there has been an acute deterioration on a background of steady neurological decline. Chronic haematomas become isodense with brain and are therefore sometimes difficult to distinguish; magnetic resonance imaging may be better.
- In **acute cases**, priorities are:
  1. Protection of airway; give oxygen; support the breathing and circulation as necessary.
  2. Liaison with neurosurgical team early.
  3. Close monitoring of neurological state (Glasgow Coma Scale).
  4. Consider methods to reduce intracranial pressure if raised (p350): If the patient slips into coma and signs of tentorial herniation (p422) are progressing rapidly, give 1g/kg of 20% mannitol as a bolus, inform on-call surgeon and arrange very urgent CT scan.
  5. Treat seizures (p370).

Subarachnoid haemorrhage: Assessment

Presentation

- *Headache*: Classically sudden and severe ('thunderclap'), radiating behind the occiput with associated neck stiffness. Less dramatic presentations are common. Consider the diagnosis in any unusually severe headache, especially if the patient does not have a previous history of headaches and is over 40 years. ~ 4% of aneurysmal bleeds occur at/after sexual intercourse, but most coital headaches are not subarachnoid haemorrhages. 10% of patients with subarachnoid bleeds are bending or lifting heavy objects at onset of symptoms.

- *Nausea, vomiting, dizziness* may be transient or protracted.

- *Impaired level of consciousness*: There may be initial transient loss of consciousness followed by variable impairment. Patients may present in coma.

- *Early focal neurological signs* may occur, especially if there has been a concomitant intracerebral haemorrhage. Third nerve palsy raises possibility of posterior communicating aneurysm.

- *Seizures* are uncommon, but subarachnoid haemorrhage in a person known to have fits suggests underlying A-V malformation.

- *Warning leak*: Up to 30% have 'minor' leaks hours or days prior to the major haemorrhage. These are often misdiagnosed as simple headaches or migraine, so a high degree of suspicion is required.

Causes

Common	Rare
• Aneurysm (70%)	• Clotting disorder/anti-coagulants
• A-V malformation (5%)	• Tumour
• No known cause in up to 20%	• Vasculitis
	• Associated with polycystic kidney disease

Assessment of severity *(prognostic features)*

- **Hunt & Hess Scale** allows grading at presentation and thereafter:

  Grade 1 Asymptomatic or minimal headache + slight neck stiffness

  Grade 2 Moderate or severe headache with neck stiffness, but no neurological deficit other than cranial nerve palsy

  Grade 3 Drowsiness with confusion or mild focal neurology

  Grade 4 Stupor with moderate to severe hemiparesis or mild decerebrate rigidity

  Grade 5 Deeply comatose with severe decerebrate rigidity

- Prognosis is best in Grade 1 (morality < 5%), worst in Grade 5 (mortality 50–70%), and intermediate in between.

- Neurological deterioration following presentation has a worse prognosis. Patients should be re-graded on the Hunt & Hess Scale.

Subarachnoid haemorrhage

Immediate management[14]

Once the diagnosis is confirmed, discuss with regional neurosurgeons. Transfer Grade 1 and 2 patients as soon as possible. Surgery will prevent rebleeding and although optimal time for operation is debated (2 days vs 7–10 days post bleed), outcome is probably improved by early transfer.

Surgery on poor prognosis patients is unrewarding; they are usually managed conservatively. However, suitability for surgery should be reassessed if their condition improves.

Stabilize the patient

- *Protect the airway* by laying the drowsy patient in the recovery position. Give oxygen.

- Consider *measures to reduce intracranial pressure* if signs suggest it is raised (p348) but avoid dehydration and hypotension.

- *Treat seizures* with usual drugs (p370) but beware over-sedation and hypotension.

- *Correct hypotension* if necessary with colloid or inotropes.

- *To avoid hypertension* the patient should be nursed in a quiet room, sedatives may be required, stool softeners should be given to avoid straining. Once the diagnosis is established, nimodipine (see below) is usually given to reduce vasospasm; it helps also to reduce blood pressure.

- *ECG monitoring* and *treat dysrhythmias* if they compromise blood pressure or threaten thromboembolism. Rarely, subarachnoid haemorrhage is associated with (neurogenic) pulmonary oedema.

- Take blood for *clotting screen* (if bleeding diathesis suspected) and *U&Es* (biochemical assessment of dehydration; potassium for susceptibility to dysrhythmia; hyponatraemia from inappropriate ADH or hypernatraemia from aggressive diuretic-induced dehydration).

Confirm the diagnosis

- *Urgent CT scanning* is required. This will clinch the diagnosis in 95% of patients scanned within 24h. Furthermore, it gives valuable information regarding possible location of aneurysm and may even demonstrate A-V malformation. It may also display concomitant intracerebral and/or intraventricular bleeds.

- *Lumbar puncture* is NOT usually required, unless CT scan is normal but the history is highly suggestive. It is important to examine the CSF for blood under these circumstances; the presenting event may be a 'warning leak'. Blood in the CSF may result from a traumatic tap. If this is the case there should be diminishing numbers of red cells in each successive tube of CSF. If the blood has been present for over 6h, the supernatant should be xanthochromic after centrifugation.

---

[14] Kopitnik TA & Samson DS (1993) *J Neurol Neurosurg Psychiat* **56**: 947–959.

Subarachnoid haemorrhage

Subarachnoid haemorrhage

Further management

Specific therapies

- *Nimodipine* is a calcium channel blocker which works preferentially on cerebral vessels to reduce vasospasm and (and consequent cerebral ischaemia).[15] It has been shown to reduce morbidity and mortality following SAH. Give 60mg po (or NG in the comatose patient) every 4h; intravenous therapy is costly and requires central venous access.

- *Antifibrinolytics* used to be introduced to prevent lysis of clot and rebleeding. They have been associated with increased thrombotic complications and are not advised at present.

Observe for deterioration. Attempt to reverse it

- *Neurological observations* should be performed regularly. If there is a deterioration, e.g. lowering of the level of consciousness, a CT scan should be performed.

- There are several possible mechanisms for deterioration.

  - *Cerebral ischaemia* is usually insidious and multifocal. It may give rise to focal and/or global neurological deterioration. Volume expansion with colloid, or induced hypertension with inotropes have been attempted but these procedures have not been properly studied.

  - *Rebleeding* may be immediately fatal or lead to apnoea. It is reported that assisted ventilation for 1h may be all that is necessary for spontaneous breathing to return to the majority of apnoeic individuals.[16] Patients who rebleed are at high risk of further bleeding and should be considered for emergency aneurysm clipping.

  - *Acute hydrocephalus* may be treated with ventricular drainage. This can lead to dramatic improvement in the patient's condition.

Refer for definitive treatment

Unless the patient has a poor prognosis (see Hunt & Hess scale, p362), they should be cared for at a neurosurgical centre. The complications listed above should be managed by clinicians experienced in treating them.

[15] Pickard JD *et al* (1989) *BMJ* **298**: 636–642.
[16] van Gijn J (1992) *Lancet* **339**: 653–655.

Status epilepticus (tonic-clonic)   1.

Presentation

Generalized tonic-clonic status epilepticus is either continuous tonic-clonic convulsions (30 minutes or longer) or convulsions so frequent that each attack begins before the previous post-ictal period ends.

Causes

- Cerebral tumour (1°/2°)
- Intracranial infection
- Hypoglycaemia
- Head injury
- Drug overdose (e.g. tricyclics)
- Drug withdrawal (e.g. alcohol)
- Hypoxia (e.g. post cardiac arrest)
- Sequela or stroke
- Electrolyte disturbance (low sodium, calcium, or magnesium)

Note: Most episodes of status do not occur in known epileptic patients.

Management

Priorities are:

1. Stabilize the patient. Give oxygen.
2. Anti-epileptic drug therapy.
3. Attempt to identify aetiology.
4. Identify and treat medical complications.
5. Initiate long-term maintenance therapy if appropriate.

Stabilize the patient

- ***Open the airway*** by laying the patient on their side in a semi-prone position with the head slightly lower to prevent aspiration. Usually, an oral airway will suffice and endotracheal intubation is rarely necessary.
- ***Give oxygen.***
- ***Correct hypotension*** with colloid if necessary. Obtain an ECG if the patient is hypotensive, CVP monitoring may be necessary.
- Take blood for ***U&Es, glucose, calcium, magnesium, liver enzymes, FBC (inc. platelets)***; if relevant, blood should also be sent for ***toxicology screen*** (if drug overdose or abuse suspected) and ***anticonvulsant levels***.
- ***Thiamine 250mg*** iv should be given if alcoholism or other malnourished states appear likely.
- If hypoglycaemia is suspected ***50mls of 50% glucose*** should be administered iv. Because glucose increases the risk of Wernicke's encephalo-pathy, thiamine 1–2mg/kg iv should be administered beforehand in any patient suspected of alcohol excess.

Anti-epileptic drug therapy

A number of agents may be used:

- Benzodiazepines (diazepam, lorazepam)
- Phenytoin
- Chlormethiazole
- Miscellaneous (general anaesthesia, paraldehyde)

Status epilepticus (tonic-clonic) 2.

Anti-epileptic drug therapy[17]

- **Diazepam** 10–20mg iv or rectally, repeated once 15 minutes later if necessary. Intravenous injection should not exceed 2–5mg/min. Diazepam is rapidly redistributed and therefore has a short duration of action. With repeated dosing, however, as peripheral lipid compartments become saturated, there is less redistribution and blood diazepam levels increase. When this happens there is a risk of sudden central nervous and respiratory depression, as well as cardiorespiratory collapse.

- If seizures continue, give **lorazepam** 0.07mg/kg iv (usually 4mg bolus which may be repeated once after 10 minutes). Because lorazepam does not accumulate in lipid stores, has strong cerebral binding, and a long duration of action, it has distinct advantages over diazepam in early status epilepticus.

- If seizures continue 30 minutes after first administration of an anti-epileptic agent, start an infusion of **phenytoin** at 15–18mg/kg at a rate of 50mg/min (e.g. 1g over 20 minutes). N.B. 5% dextrose is not compatible with phenytoin. The patient should have ECG monitoring because phenytoin may induce cardiac dysrhythmias; pulse, bp, and respiratory rate should also be monitored. iv phenytoin is relatively contraindicated in patients with known heart disease, particularly those with conduction abnormalities.

- An alternative is **chlormethiazole** given as an infusion. The drug is commonly supplied in 500ml bottles at a concentration of 8mg/ml (0.8% solution). An initial infusion of 40–100ml of 0.8% solution (i.e. 320–800mg) at a rate of 5–15ml/min is required. The infusion is continued at the minimum dose required to control seizures (usually 0.5–4ml/min; maximum 20ml/min in adults). Administration of chlormethiazole requires close supervision of the patient. Although the dose can be titrated at the bedside, saturation of lipid compartments can lead to a sudden rise in blood levels of the drug and subsequent cardiorespiratory collapse. If an infusion for > 12h is considered; it is recommended that the dose be reduced every few hours in order to minimize accumulation.

- In refractory status (seizures continuing for 60–90 minutes after initial therapy), the patient should be transferred to intensive care.
  - General anaesthesia with either **propofol** or **thiopentone** should be administered.
  - **Paraldehyde** (5–10ml im) is an alternative but requires glass syringes as it corrodes rubber and plastic.
  - **Treat raised intracranial pressure** (p348).
  - **EEG monitoring** should be commenced.
  - The anaesthetic agent should be continued for 12–24 hours after the last clinical or electrographic seizure; the dose should ten be tapered down.

If treatment is failing to control seizures consider whether:
- Initial drug dose is adequate
- Maintenance therapy has been started and is adequate
- Underlying cause of status epilepticus has been correctly identified
- Complications of status adequately treated (see below)
- Co-existing conditions have been identified (e.g. hepatic failure)
- There has been a misdiagnosis: is this 'pseudo status'?

[17] Shorvon SD (1993) *J Neurol Neurosurg Psychiat* **56**: 125–134.

Attempt to identify aetiology

- A history of previous anticonvulsant use, drug abuse/withdrawal (including alcohol), diabetes, trauma, or recent surgery (e.g. hypocalcaemia post thyroid or parathyroid surgery) is obviously helpful.

- Examine the patient for signs of head trauma, meningism, focal neurological deficit (the seizures may also have some focal characteristics), needle tracks, or insulin injection sites.

- Consider urgent CT scan if head injury may be a precipitant; a lumbar puncture may be necessary if CSF infection is likely.

- Although hypoglycaemia and hypocalcaemia should be corrected promptly, hyponatraemia should be reversed cautiously because of the possibility of precipitating pontine myelinosis.

Identify and treat medical complications of status

Treatment is required for:

- Hypoxia
- Lactic acidosis
- Hypoglycaemia
- Dysrhythmias
- Rhabdomyolysis
- Electrolyte disturbance (especially hyponatraemia, hypo/hyperkalaemia)
- Hypotension/hypertension
- Raised intracranial pressure
- Hyperpyrexia
- Pulmonary oedema
- Disseminated intravascular coagulation

These complications are managed as in other contexts.

Initiate long-term therapy (if appropriate)

Some disorders, e.g. hypoglycaemia in a diabetic taking insulin, do not require long-term anticonvulsant therapy, but rather correction of the underlying problem. Other conditions may need anticonvulsant treatment for a short while, e.g. alcohol withdrawal, or indefinitely, e.g. repeated status epilepticus in multi-infarct dementia.

- ***Phenytoin*** may be continued after intravenous loading at daily dosages of 5mg/kg (about 300mg for an average adult) either orally, via a nasogastric tube or slow intravenous infusion. Dosage should be guided by phenytoin level measurements. Plasma concentration for optimum response is 10–20mg/l (40–80μmol/l). Phenytoin is disadvantageous because it requires monitoring.

- ***Sodium valproate*** or ***carbamazepine*** is an alternative.[18] Initially, sodium valproate should be given 400–600mg/day orally in three divided doses (intravenous therapy can also be given). It should be increased by 200mg/day at 3–6 day intervals; the maintenance dose is 20–30mg/kg/day. (Usual adult dose is 1–2g/day.) Carbamazepine should be started at 100–200mg twice daily; the maintenance dose is 7–15mg/kg/day divided in 2–3 doses (200–800mg/day for adults).

---

[18] Richens A *et al.* (1994) *J Neurol Neurosurg Psychiat* **57**: 682–687.

Driving advice

In the UK, patients should inform the Driving and Vehicle Licensing Agency (Swansea). Driving licences are revoked until the patient has been free of daytime seizures for 1 year, treated or untreated. In the case of a single, first seizure, this period may be for 1 year at the discretion of the DVLA. Patients who continue to have nocturnal seizures must be free of daytime fits for 3 years. Drivers of large goods or passenger carrying vehicles usually have those licenses revoked permanently.

Stroke: Overview

Presentation

- Sudden-onset focal deficit of cerebral function is the most common presentation.
- Alternative presentations include declining levels of consciousness or global loss of brain function and coma.
- If the symptoms last for > 24 hours (or lead to death) and there is no apparent cause other than a vascular event, the diagnosis is most likely to be a stroke. If the symptoms last < 24 hours and, after adequate investigation, are presumed to be due to thrombosis or embolism, the diagnosis is a transient ischaemic attack (TIA).

Causes

- Thrombosis or embolism causing cerebral infarction (~ 80% cases)
- Primary intracerebral haemorrhage (~ 15% cases)
- Subarachnoid haemorrhage (~ 5% cases)
- Cerebral venous thrombosis (< 1%)

Risk factors

- Hypertension
- Increasing age
- Diabetes mellitus
- Cigarette smoking
- Previous stroke or TIA
- Ischaemic heart disease
- Recent myocardial infarct
- Hyperviscosity syndrome/polycythaemia
- Hypercoagulable states
- Drug abuse (e.g. cocaine, pseudoephedrine, amphetamines) → haemorrhage

- Atrial fibrillation
- Peripheral vascular disease
- Increasing plasma cholesterol
- Alcohol excess (?by increasing bp)
- Anticoagulant use → haemorrhage
- Thrombolysis → haemorrhage
- Oral contraceptive pill

Differential diagnosis

Many conditions may masquerade as a stroke:-

- Cerebral tumour (1° or 2°)
- Brain abscess
- Demyelination
- Focal migraine

- Subdural haematoma
- Todd's paresis (post seizure)
- Hypoglycaemic attack
- Encephalitis

An alternative diagnosis to stroke is more likely in:

- Patients less than 45
- Presence of seizures
- Presence of papilloedema
- Prolonged and/or discontinuous evolution of symptoms

- Absence of risk factors
- Fluctuating level of consciousness
- Pyrexia (at presentation)

In general, a stroke commences suddenly and the deficit is at its peak and established within 24 hours. If the evolution of symptoms is longer or progresses in a stuttering way over days or weeks, a space occupying lesion must be suspected. If there is a variable depression of consciousness, the diagnosis of a subdural haematoma should be entertained, and pyrexia at presentation should alert one to the possibility of a cerebral abscess. Seizures occur in 5–10% of strokes at their onset, although they are frequent sequelae. Papilloedema is not caused by an acute stroke.

Stroke: Haemorrhage or infarct?

Intracerebral haemorrhage often has an apoplectic onset with a combination of headache, neck stiffness, vomiting, and loss of consciousness of acute onset. Consciousness level can be depressed for over 24 hours, there may be bilateral extensor plantar responses, and the blood pressure is more likely to be raised 24 hours after admission. But, although features such as these have been integrated into scoring systems, it is not possible to differentiate with certainty ischaemic from haemorrhagic stroke on clinical grounds alone. A CT scan is required.

When to scan?

Some would say never; others advocate scanning all patients assumed to have strokes on admission. The answer, to some extent, depends upon local resources.

A CT scan is advisable in order to confirm the diagnosis (5–13% patients admitted with a provisional diagnosis of stroke to some centres turned out to have another cause for their deterioration).

In the UK most patients are not scanned on admission; the usual policy is to perform CT scanning at 1–2 days. The rationale is that although most large haemorrhages would be detected at admission, many cerebral infarcts would be missed because the changes detectable on CT take several hours-days to evolve.

The optimal time to detect small haemorrhages may be at 24–48h as well. This policy of waiting is currently under review, given the results of early intervention trials using tPA or aspirin.

Urgent CT scanning should be performed if:
- Diagnosis unclear (no history or history/examination suggestive of alternative diagnoses) or young patient with no risk factors for stroke.
- Signs of raised intracranial pressure (p348) and/or brain shift (p422). Strokes (see complications below), subdural or extradural haematomas, or other space occupying lesions may be the underlying cause; surgical decompression may be possible.
- It is important to distinguish immediately intracerebral haemorrhage from infarct. For example, the result may guide decision-making in how aggressively to reverse anti-coagulation.
- A cerebellar stroke is likely (p388), it is important to confirm the diagnosis. Early transfer to a Neurosurgical Unit may be beneficial if decompression of the posterior fossa is required.
- The possibility of a subarachnoid haemorrhage (p362) is entertained, it is important to confirm the diagnosis. Early treatment with nimodipine and transfer to a Neurosurgical Unit appears to be beneficial.

Stroke: Other investigations

Apart from a CT scan, there are some basic tests that most patients suspected of having a stroke should have.

- **FBC**, to detect polycythaemia, thrombocythaemia, or thrombocytopenia.
- **ESR**, to screen for vasculitis, endocarditis, hyperviscosity.
- **Electrolytes and calcium** (neurological defect may be non-vascular and caused by hyponatraemia, hypercalcaemia, or renal failure).
- **Glucose** to exclude hypoglycaemia and non-ketotic hyperglycaemia (which can mimic stroke) and diabetes mellitus (a risk factor).
- **Cholesterol** (if taken within 12–24h of stroke).
- **Syphilis serology** (low yield but treatable condition). N.B. Syphilis reagins may be positive in anticardiolipin syndrome.
- **Prothrombin time/INR** if the patient is taking warfarin.
- **ECG** to determine cardiac rhythm and exclude acute myocardial infarction.
- **Carotid doppler ultrasound** to exclude high grade (> 70%) stenosis or dissection. This should be performed in patients who would be suitable for carotid endarterectomy. A bruit need not be present!
- **Cardiac echocardiography** may demonstrate the presence of valvular disease or intracardiac clot, or may detect some rare causes of stroke such as atrial myxoma or patent foramen ovale.

Some patients, particularly young ones without common risk factors (see above), should be investigated further. Possible tests include:

- **Serum protein, electrophoresis, viscosity.** In hyperviscosity syndromes the ESR is usually raised but not always.
- **Autoantibody screen.** (Particularly for SLE.)
- **Haemostatic profile.** In haemorrhagic stroke not apparently secondary to hypertension, measurement of PT, APTT, bleeding time, and fibrin degradation products may be indicated. In cerebral infarcts, blood should be taken for protein S, C, antithrombin III, and anticardiolipin antibodies. APTT may be prolonged in anticardiolipin syndrome. Consider testing for sickle cell in black patients. Factor V_{Leiden} mutation may be an important risk factor for the development of venous thrombosis.
- **Toxicology screen** on admission sample if drug abuse (e.g. cocaine, pseudoephedrine, or amphetamines) suspected.
- **Urine tests** may detect homocystinuria (without other clinical manifestations) or porphyria. If bp is labile consider phaeochromocytoma and measure urinary metanephrines.
- **CSF analysis** may be necessary if the diagnosis of stroke is not well established, e.g. normal CT scan and no risk factors.
- **Cerebral angiography** is also reserved for cases where the diagnosis is not well established and in those in whom cerebral vasculitis or malformation is suspected.
- **Magnetic resonance imaging** may be more sensitive in detecting venous thromboses.

Stroke: Complications[19]

Cerebral complications[19]

Further neurological deterioration may be caused by:

- **Transtentorial herniation** (p422) is the commonest cause of death within the first week. It is due to raised intracranial pressure (p348) secondary to cerebral oedema. Corticosteroids do not improve outcome; mannitol and hyperventilation may be useful (p350); surgical decompression may be indicated in large haemorrhages, particularly cerebellar ones.

- **Haemorrhagic transformation** occurs in ~ 30% of ischaemic strokes (and up to ~ 70% of cardioembolic strokes). If it leads to neurological deterioration, it is usually due to a mass effect. Early thrombolysis or iv heparin may increase its incidence and is not recommended.

- **Acute hydrocephalus** due to compression of the aqueduct of Sylvius by oedema or blood may occur. Ventricular shunting may be of value.

- **Seizures** complicate ~ 10% of infarcts or haemorrhages and usually respond to monotherapy (e.g. phenytoin).

- **Inappropriate ADH secretion** occurs in 10–15% strokes. It may initiate or worsen cerebral oedema and is treated by fluid restriction.

- **Depression** occurs in ~ 50% and may require therapy if it persists.

Systemic complications

- **Aspiration** is common. Over 25% with unilateral hemispheric strokes and 65% with brainstem strokes have dysphagia or aspiration, which is often undetected at the bedside. Testing the gag reflex is not a sufficient assessment; swallowing must be observed and if there is any suspicion video-fluoroscopy may be used. Patients should generally be fed upright.

- **Infection** is a common cause of death following stroke. Pneumonia, including aspiration pneumonia, and urinary tract infections are the usual problems.

- **Fever** usually occurs as a result of infection or deep vein thrombosis. Occasionally, it is a direct result of cerebral damage.

- **Pulmonary embolus** is a preventable cause of death in patients who are bed-bound. *Subcutaneous heparin* 5000 units bd is often given prophylactically to patients after CT scan has excluded haemorrhage. However, this is controversial.

- **Hypertension** is apparent in > 80% patients on admission. Raised bp normally falls within a few days and treatment may worsen cerebral ischaemia by reducing perfusion pressure. Do not treat systolic bp < 200 or diastolic bp < 120mmHg within 3–5 days of a stroke. If bp is consistently higher than this, treatment may reduce vasogenic oedema;[20] start atenolol (25mg) or nifedipine (5–10mg bd) po/via NG tube.[21] Do not use sublingual nifedipine.

- **Pressure sores** occur easily unless patients are regularly turned.

---

[19] Oppenheimer S & Hachinski V (1992) *Lancet* **339**: 721–724.
[20] O'Connell JE & Gray C (1994) *BMJ* **308**: 1523–1524.
[21] Lavin P (1986) *Arch Int Med* **146**: 66–68.

Stroke: Secondary prevention of stroke[22]

- *Attempt to modify risk factors* (see risk factors p374). Long-term control of hypertension is important.
- *Anti-platelet drugs.* Aspirin reduces recurrence of stroke and death from other causes. It should be commenced after ischaemic stroke unless there are contraindications. The timing of therapy is controversial with some recommending treatment after 2 weeks and others immediately after CT exclusion of haemorrhage. Most clinicians in the UK prescribe 75–150mg/day of aspirin. Ticlopidine 250mg bd is an alternative which has been shown to be effective but neutropenia is an important side-effect which requires blood monitoring. "Clopidogrel (75mg od) is another novel anti-platelet agent that is better tolerated than aspirin, and more effective in reducing further ischaemic events[22a]." Dipyridamole alone has no benefit.
- *Anti-coagulants.* Warfarin reduces stroke recurrence in patients with ischaemic stroke and atrial fibrillation. It should be prescribed to achieve an INR of ~ 2.0–2.5 provided there are no contraindications, and regular checks of prothrombin time are practicable. Aspirin is less effective. Heparin iv may be given whilst loading with warfarin but there is a risk of haemorrhagic transformation of an infarct early after stroke, so most clinicians do not advocate its use unless the risk of thromboembolism is very high, e.g. atrial fibrillation and valvular heart disease. In such cases, it is best to discuss management with a senior colleague.
- *Carotid endarterectomy.* Should be considered in patients with > 70% stenosis who have had a small carotid territory stroke/TIA and/or have potential for improvement. The operation has an appreciable morbidity (including further stroke) and mortality, but appears to improve overall prognosis in selected patients.

---

[22] Marshall RS & Mohr JP (1993) *J Neurol Neurosurg Psychiat* **56**: 6–16.
[22a] CAPRIE Steering Committee (1996) *Lancet* **348**: 1329–39.

Stroke: Secondary prevention

Cerebral infarction syndromes

Anterior (carotid territory) circulation

- *Middle cerebral artery syndrome*

  - Total occlusion of the middle cerebral artery (usually embolic) leads to contralateral hemiplegia, hemianaesthesia, homonymous hemianopia, and deviations of the head and eyes towards, the side of the lesion.
  - Left-sided lesions lead to global dysphasia; right-sided ones are more likely to lead to unilateral neglect of contralateral space.
  - Branch occlusions of the middle cerebral artery are more common and lead to incomplete syndromes. For example, occlusion of upper branches leads to Broca's ('non-fluent' or expressive) dysphasia and contralateral lower face and arm weakness; lower branch occlusion, on the other hand, may cause Wernicke's ('fluent' or receptive) dysphasia.

- *Anterior cerebral artery syndrome*

  - Occlusion of this artery (often embolic) can lead to paralysis of the contralateral leg, *gegenhalten* rigidity, perseveration, grasp reflex in the opposite hand, and urinary incontinence.

Posterior circulation

- *Posterior cerebral artery syndrome*

  - Occlusion by thrombus or embolus may lead to combinations of contralateral homonymous hemianopia/upper quadrantonopia, mild contralateral hemiparesis and/or hemisensory loss, dyslexia, memory loss, ipsilateral third nerve palsy with contralateral involuntary movements, or ataxia.

Lacunar infarction

Infarcts in small penetrating vessels, often the consequence of hypertension, lead to a number of syndromes: pure motor stroke or pure sensory stroke, or pure sensorimotor stroke, ataxic hemiparesis (combined cerebellar and pyramidal signs in the same limb).

Prognostic significance[23]

The type of stroke appears to be a significant factor in a patient's prognosis.

- Total anterior circulation infarcts, i.e. infarcts in the carotid territory leading to motor and sensory deficit, hemianopia and new disturbance of higher cerebral function have the worst prognosis in terms of death or disability.
- Posterior circulation infarcts, partial anterior circulation infarcts (PACI), and lacunar infarcts have better prognoses, although patients with PACI have a high risk of recurrent stroke within 3 months.

---

[23] Bamford *et al* (1991) *Lancet* **337**: 1521–1526.

Brainstem stroke

Presentation

Sudden onset.

- *Headache*, nausea, vomiting, vertigo.
- *Weakness* – bilateral or unilateral.
- *Sensory symptoms* (e.g. paraesthesiae) may be confined to face and if unilateral, may be contralateral to weakness.
- *Ophthalmoplegia, gaze deviation, or dysconjugate eye movements.* In unilateral pontine lesions, conjugate gaze deviation is directed away from the lesion and towards the side of the hemiparesis if there is one. The reverse obtains for frontal cortical strokes.
- *Horner's syndrome.*
- *Dysarthria or dysphagia.*
- *Ataxia* which may be uni- or bilateral due to dysfunction of cerebellar connections.
- *Impaired level of consciousness* ranges from transient loss of consciousness to coma.
- *Altered pattern of respiration.*

Signs associated with brainstem dysfunction are explained on p418. They result because of damage either to the nuclei (including cranial nerve nuclei) within the brainstem, to the cranial nerves, or to the long tracts which traverse and/or decussate within the brainstem. 'Crossed signs' may occur in brainstem strokes; e.g. part of the lateral medullary/ Wallenberg's syndrome consists of loss of pain and temperature sensation from the contralateral trunk and limbs (crossed spinothalamic) and ipsilateral loss of the same sensory modalities from the face (un- crossed trigeminal tract). There are a large number of other eponymous syndromes associated with damage to particular zones within the brain- stem. Learning these is not particularly rewarding; better to concentrate on the principles of brainstem anatomy.

Causes

- Thrombosis, embolism, or haemorrhage.

Assessment of severity

- Reduced level of consciousness and coma carry worse prognosis.
- Extent of brainstem of dysfunction may be appreciated from system- atic examination of brainstem function (p418).

Management

The management is the of strokes in general (see p374–82). Conditions which require urgent intervention include:-

- Metabolic coma with brainstem depression, e.g. opiates (p660).
- Transtentorial herniation progressive brainstem compression (p422).
- Posterior fossa mass with tonsillar herniation leading to brainstem compression (p422).
- Cerebellar haemorrhage with/without brainstem compression (p388).

Cerebellar stroke

Presentation

Triad of headache, nausea/vomiting, and ataxia is the classical syndrome. But it occurs in < 50% of cases and, of course, is common in a number of other conditions. Patients present with symptoms and signs[25,26] which are often attributed to brainstem or labyrinthine causes. Always consider the possibility of a cerebellar stroke as a serious alternative diagnosis because surgical decompression can be life-saving if there is a mass effect within the posterior fossa. If the diagnosis is a possibility, ask for an urgent CT scan.

- *Headache, nausea/vomiting.* Sudden or progressive over hours-days. Location of headache varies widely.
- *Dizziness or true vertigo.* Occurs in ~ 30% of cases.
- *Visual disturbance.* Diplopia, blurred vision, or oscillopsia.
- *Gait/limb ataxia.* Most alert patients report or demonstrate this
- *Nystagmus or gaze palsy.*
- *Speech disturbance.* Dysarthria or dysphonia in ~ 50% of alert patients.
- *Loss of consciousness.* May be transient but many present in coma.
- *Hypertension.*

Predisposing factors

- Hypertension (> 50%).
- Anti-coagulants: There is a disproportionately higher risk of cerebellar haemorrhage (cf. intracerebral haemorrhage) in patients taking warfarin.
- Metastatic neoplasm.

Assessment of severity

Patients who present in coma, or subsequently develop it, will die unless they receive surgical treatment. There is debate about the prognosis of those who remain alert.

Management

Make a definitive diagnosis with urgent CT scan (Is there a haemorrhage/infarct? Is there distortion of fourth ventricle and aqueduct with dilatation of lateral ventricles?) Liaise with regional neurosurgery unit early.

Priorities are:

1 Stabilize the patient and protect the airway. See coma (p304).
2 Correct bleeding tendency or effects of anti-coagulants.
3 Intensive care/high dependency ward nursing observations if patient is not transferred to neurosurgical centre immediately.
4 Definitive surgical decompression if necessary and possible.

---

[25] Dunne JW *et al* (1987) *QJM* **64**: 739–754.
[26] Editorial (1988) *Lancet* **i**: 1031–1032.

Transient ischaemic attacks (TIAs)

Presentation

Sudden-onset focal deficit of cerebral function or monocular blindness resolving within 24 hours. The symptoms should have developed within a few seconds and if several parts of the body (e.g. face, arm, leg) are involved they should have been affected simultaneously without any 'march' or progression.

- *Symptoms of carotid TIA:* Hemiparesis, dysphasia, or transient monocular blindness (amaurosis fugax). See anterior circulation strokes (p384)

- *Symptoms of posterior circulation/vertebrobasilar TIA:* Bilateral or alternating hemiplegia or sensory symptoms, crossed motor/sensory signs (ipsilateral face, contralateral arm, trunk or leg deficit), quadriplegia. Sudden bilateral blindness. Two or more of vertigo, diplopia, dysphagia, ataxia, and drop attacks if they occur simultaneously.

- *Symptoms of uncertain arterial territory origin:* Hemianopia alone or dysarthria lone.

- *Symptoms not acceptable as TIA:* Syncope, loss of consciousness or confusion, convulsion, incontinence of urine or faeces, dizziness, focal symptoms associated with migrainous headache, scintillating scotoma.

Causes

- Thrombosis or embolism. (See p374 for risk factors.)

Differential diagnosis

Many conditions may appear at first to be a TIA, e.g.:

- Cerebral tumour (1° or 2°)
- Brain abscess
- Demyelination
- Focal migraine
- Subdural haematoma
- Todd's paresis (post seizure)
- Hypoglycaemic attack
- Encephalitis

Investigation

A CT scan should be performed as ~ 5% of patients will have an otherwise unsuspected cause (e.g. mass lesion). Otherwise, investigation is the same as for ischaemic stroke (see p378).

Management

The objective is to prevent recurrence or complete stroke. The general principles of management are those used in treating ischaemic stroke (p376–82). Perhaps the only difference lies in treatment of recurrent TIAs not controlled by aspirin. In the acute situation, if major stroke is threatened by a 'crescendo' of recurring TIAs:-

- Give high-dose aspirin (300mg/day).

- Ticlopidine is an alternative but in the UK this is dispensed only on a 'named-patient' basis. Neutropenia is an important side-effect.

- Clopidogrel 75mg od has fewer side-effects than high-dose aspirin and in trials is more effective in preventing further ischaemic events.

- Arrange urgent carotid doppler ultrasound. Discuss use of iv heparin with a Neurologist.

Transient ischaemic attacks

Confusional states and delirium   1.

Up to 10% of acute medical admissions are complicated by acute confusion or delirium. The hallmark of **acute confusional states** is disorientation in time and place, impaired short-term memory, and impaired consciousness level. Typically, the patient is drowsy with a poor attention span and slowed mentation. In **delerium**, there are, in addition, disorders of perception such as hallucinations (seeing or hearing things not there) or illusions (misinterpreting shadows seen or sounds heard) and these may produce restlessness, agitation, and hyperactivity.

The main priority is to identify the cause of any treatable or life-threatening condition. Only a small minority ($< 10\%$) of patients will have a primary neurological disorder and commonly there are multiple factors that may apply; these patients carry a good prognosis.

Assessment

- Assess the mental state: Check for disorientation and memory impairment with the mini-mental test. An anxiety state can usually be distinguished by talking to the patient. Vivid hallucinations in the absence of history of mental illness suggests alcohol withdrawal.

- Review the patient's notes and try to obtain history from friends/relatives of previous mental state or episodes of confusion. Patients with dementia are prone to confusion with intercurrent illness.

- Review the drug chart: Benzodiazepines and narcotics may cause acute confusion in the elderly. Other drugs that may be involved are steroids, NSAIDs, β-blockers, and psychotropic medications.

- Assess the patient for acute illness: exclude faecal impaction and urinary retention. Relevant investigations are listed in the table p394.

- Examine for any focal neurological signs (pupils, limb power, reflexes, and plantar responses).

- In patients with prior high alcohol intake, examine for signs of liver disease, liver 'flap', and possible Wernicke's encephalopathy (nystagmus, ataxia, VI nerve palsy).

Mini-mental examination for the elderly
1 Age
2 Time (nearest hour)
3 42 West Street: Address for recall at the end of the test (make the patient repeat the address to check)
4 Year
5 Place (Name of hospital)
6 Recognition of two people (doctor, nurse, etc.)
7 Date of birth (day and month)
8 Year of World War 1 (or 2)
9 'Who is on the throne at the moment?'
10 Count backwards from 20 to 1

Each correct answer scores 1 point. Healthy elderly people score 8

Differential diagnosis	Investigations

Systemic disorder
• Sepsis
• Alcohol withdrawal
• Metabolic disorder
  • ↓ or ↑ glc, Na or Ca
  • Vitamin deficiency
  • Endocrine disease (thyroid, adrenal cortex)
• Myocardial ischaemia
• Organ failure (renal, respiratory, liver, cardiac)
	Check urine, blood cultures, WBC, CRP
	chest X-ray
	U&Es, glc, LFTs, Ca^{2+}
	arterial gases, pH
	ECG, cardiac enzymes
	
	Consider: magnesium, amylase, porphyrins, thiamine, B_{12}, folate, TSH, free T4

Drug toxicity	Check prescribed medication serum alcohol/drug screen
CNS disorder • Dementia • CVA (esp. non-dominant parietal lobe) • Intracranial bleed (SAH, subdural) • Infection (encephalitis, meningitis) • Trauma • Malignancy ($1°$ or $2°$) • Post ictal; non-convulsive status • Cerebral vasculitis (SLE, PAN)	Consider CT scan with contrast lumbar puncture EEG blood cultures, CRP syphilis serology Lyme serology
Malignancy	Check Chest X-ray ± CT chest Serum calcium CT brain

Management

• Treat the cause. Nurse in a moderately lit room with repeated reassurance. See if a family member can stay with the patient.

• If the patient is agitated and aggressive, sedation may be necessary. Benzodiazepines may exacerbate confusion: use major tranquillizers (e.g. haloperidol 2–10mg im po or chlorpromazine 25–50mg im/po). Observe the effect on the patient for 15–20 minutes and repeat if necessary. In patients with cardiac or respiratory failure, correcting hypoxia may calm the patient by itself. Chlormethiazole is indicated for confusion due to alcohol withdrawal (see p396).

Acute alcohol withdrawal

Minor symptoms may be managed at home by the GP but often a short admission is more effective and allows observation for complications and psychosocial assessment ± rehabilitation.

Presentation

- Initial symptoms include anxiety and tremor, hyperactivity, sweating, nausea and retching, tachycardia, hypertension and mild pyrexia. These symptoms peak at 12–30 hours and subside by 48 hours.
- Generalized tonic-clonic seizures ('rum fits') may also occur during this period, but status epilepticus is unusual. Typically these do not show the EEG characteristics of epilepsy and may be precipitated by flickering lights or other photic stimulation.
- Delirium tremens ('DTs') occurs in < 5% of individuals, usually after 3–4 days of cessation of alcohol intake. It is associated with an untreated mortality of 15%. Features include:
  - Coarse tremor, agitation, confusion, delusion, and hallucinations
  - Fever (occasionally severe), sweating, tachycardia
  - Rarely lactic acidosis or ketoacidosis
  - Also look for hypoglycaemia, Wernicke-Korsakoff psychosis, subdural haematoma, and hepatic encephalopathy.

Management

1 General measures

- Nurse in a well-lit room to prevent disorientation. Rehydrate (iv fluids if necessary; avoid saline in patients with known chronic liver disease). Monitor urine output.
- Vitamin supplements: iv therapy (e.g. *Parbinex*® 2–3 pairs of amps. iv *slowly* 8 hourly; watch for signs of anaphylaxis) for 5 days or oral therapy (thiamine 100mg po bd, vitamin B tablets (compound strong) 2 tablets tds, and vitamin C 50mg po bd) for one week.
- Monitor BMs for hypoglycaemia and treat if necessary.
- Severe hypophosphataemia may complicate alcohol withdrawal and should be treated with intravenous phosphates (polyfusor phosphates) if serum phosphate is < 0.6mM (see p454).
- Exclude intercurrent infection (pneumonia, skin, urine).

2 Sedation

- Long-acting benzodiazepines such as chlordiazepoxide (*Librium*®) or diazepam (*Valium*®) are commonly used; lorazepam is not metabolized by the liver and may be used in liver disease.
- Chlormethiazole (*Hemineverin*®) may be given either as capsules, syrup, or ivi (ivi carries a high risk of respiratory depression).
- Carbamazepine is as effective as benzodiazepines but side-effects limit its use. For severe agitation, haloperidol 10mg im may be used.

3 Wernicke-Korsakoff syndrome

- Wernicke's disease comprises the triad of ophthalmoplegia (nystagmus, VI nerve palsy), ataxia (cerebellar type), and confusional state. In Korsakoff's syndrome, confusion predominates, often with overt psychosis, amnesia (antegrade and retrograde), and confabulation. Withdrawal symptoms may also occur.
- Diagnosis: reduced red-cell transketolase activity.
- Treat with iv thiamine (see above) while waiting for results.

4 *Seizures*
- Withdrawal seizures are typically self-limiting; if needed use, iv diazepam (*Diazemuls*®) 10mg over 5min (see p370).
- Treat the patient with chlordiazepoxide (rather than chlormethiazole or carbamazepine). Phenytoin is less effective but should be added if there is a history of epilepsy or recurrent seizures.

5 *Follow-up*
- Arrange referral to an alcohol dependence clinic.

Sedation regimens in delerium tremens – a guide

• *Chlordiazepoxide*	30mg q6h for 2 days
then	20mg daily (divided doses) for 2 days
then	10mg daily (divided doses) for 2 days
then	5mg daily for 2 days.

Start women on 20mg (instead of 30mg) and taper as above. Reduce the dose in liver disease, in elderly, and in slight individuals.

• *Chlormethiazole capsules* (192mg)	
Start with	3 capsules q6h for 1 day
then	2 capsules q6h for 1 day
then	2 capsules q8h for 1–2 days
then	2 capsules bd for 1–2 days
then	2 capsules at night for 1–2 days
then	stop (total treatment for not more than 9 days)

For equivalent effect, 1 capsule = ml syrup. Reduce dose if there is marked sedation or liver disease (sedation may mask hepatic encephalopathy): start with 1 capsule and observe effect.
- *Chlormethiazole infusion* (0.8% solution)
Resuscitation facilities must be to hand as there is risk of apnoea and hypotension. Use only when oral route is not practicable.
Start at 3ml (24mg)/min until the patient is just asleep (but easily rousable) then reduce the infusion rate to 0.5–1ml (4–8 mg)/min, the minimum rate at which the patient remains mildly sedated.
Monitor respiratory rate and pulse oximetry and stop infusion if respirations < 10/min or $S_aO_2 < 90\%$.

- *Carbamazepine*
As effective as benzodiazepines and no abuse potential.
Start with 200mg/day in divided doses increasing to 400mg/day over the next 2–3 days and taper off by day 8.

Neuromuscular respiratory failure

Assessment

Presentation

A number of disorders of peripheral nerve, neuromuscular junction or muscle may present with hypercapnic (type II) respiratory failure, or impending failure. There are many differences between these conditions but consider the diagnosis if there is:-

- *Limb weakness* progressing over hours or days with diminished/no reflexes but no upper motor neurone signs.
- *Muscular tenderness or pain* may be a feature.
- *Facial weakness* with/without ptosis.
- *Bulbar dysfunction* is a particularly ominous sign because it may lead to improper clearance of secretions and aspiration.
- *Paradoxical abdominal movement.* If the diaphragm is paralysed it moves passively into the thorax with the fall in intrapleural pressure produced by expansion of the ribcage in inspiration. As a result, the anterior abdominal wall also moves in (rather than out) during inspiration.
- *Dyspnoea* or *distress in supine position.* If the diaphragm is paralysed, movement of abdominal contents towards the thorax is more prominent when the patient lies flat because gravity no longer acts to counteract this passive movement. As a result, the volume of air inspired is reduced. This is a rare but important cause of orthopnoea.
- *Sensory symptoms* may be present with or without glove-and-stocking sensory loss.
- *Autonomic instability* may be a prominent feature of Guillain-Barré syndrome and may lead to cardiac arrest.
- *Pneumonia* in known neuromuscular disease.
- *Respiratory arrest.* A common pitfall is to consider the degree of respiratory distress unimpressive. Peripheral weakness in combination with an expressionless 'myopathic' facies may lead to a false sense of well-being when the patient may in fact be confronting impending respiratory arrest.

Assessment of severity

- Bulbar dysfunction results in impaired clearance of secretions.
- Forced vital capacity (measured with Wright respirometer available from anaesthetic nurse or Intensive Care Unit) < 30ml/kg causes impaired clearance of secretions. FEV_1 and peak flow *do not correlate* with degree of neuromuscular impairment.
- Forced vital capacity < 10ml/kg suggests ventilatory failure. (In adults, ventilatory support should be considered when vital capacity is less than or equal to 1 litre.)
- Arterial blood gases: Hypercapnia occurs relatively late.
- CXR to determine extent of consolidation if there is concomitant aspiration or infective pneumonia.

Neuromuscular respiratory failure

Neuromuscular respiratory failure

Investigations for neuromuscular respiratory failure
• FBC, U&Es, CPK, ESR, CRP
• Forced vital capacity
• Arterial blood gases
• Chest X-ray
• Nerve conduction studies (NCS)
• Electromyography (EMG)
• Anti-AChR antibody/Tensilont test
• CT/MRI scan for brainstem pathology
• Nerve biopsy, muscle biopsy
• Urine/plasma toxin screen (see table p401)

Management

1. Assess severity (see p178) and measure FVC frequently.
2. Consider intubation and ventilating support if FVC < 1 litre in adults. Do not use suxamethonium as a muscle relaxant. It may cause a sudden rise in potassium in patients with denervated muscles.
3. Liaise with neurologist early. Consider transfer to regional Neurology Unit if the patient is well and FVC > 15ml/kg and stable. If the patient is unwell and FVC < 15ml/kg, or falling precipitously from a higher level, intubate electively and then consider transfer. All patients should be accompanied by an anaesthetist.
4. Investigations (see table opposite). Most of these conditions will not come into the differential diagnosis but it is advised that blood be taken for virology screen and autoimmune profile, and 20mls be saved for retrospective analysis if required.
5. ECG monitoring and frequent observation of bp and pulse is required if Guillain-Barré is suspected because there is a high incidence of autonomic instability.
6. Consider specific therapies (see table opposite) and

Guillain-Barré	p408
Myasthenia gravis	p401
Botulism	p412
Heavy metal intoxication	p401
Organophosphate exposure	p401
Rhabdomyolysis	p294
Porphyria	p401

7. Subcutaneous heparin prophylaxis for deep vein thrombosis.
8. Enteral nutrition should be considered early.

Neuromuscular respiratory failure

Condition	Investigation	Specific treatment
Central nervous system disease		
Brainstem disease	• MRI scan	• Reduce ICP • Decompress
Spinal cord disease	• MRI scan	• Decompress
Peripheral neuropathies		
Guillain-Barré (GBS) (see p408)	• NCS	• IV immunoglobulin • Plasma exchange
Organophosphates	• Red cell cholinesterase • Plasma pseudo-cholinesterase	• Atropine • Pralidoxime
Heavy metals: lead, thallium, gold, arsenic	• Blood and urine levels	• Specific antidote (see p633)
Drugs (e.g. vincristine)		• Stop drug
Malignancy	• Nerve biopsy	• Cytotoxics
Vasculitis (e.g. SLE)	• Nerve biopsy	• Immuno-suppresssants
Metabiolic (porphyria)	• Urinary porphyrins	• Avoid precipitants • iv glc/haematin
Diphtheria	• Throat swab	• Antitoxin
Neuromuscular junction disease		
Myasthenia gravis	• Tensilon® test • Anti-AChR Ab	• Steroids • Plasma exchange
Anti-cholinesterase overdose	• -ve Tensilon® test	• Stop drug
Hypermagnesaemia	• Plasma Mg	• iv calcium
Botulism (see p412)		• Antitoxin
Muscle disease		
Hypokalaemia	• plasma K^+	• K^+ replacement
Hypophosphataemia	• plasma PO_4^{3-}	• PO_4^{3-} replacement
Polymyositis	• EMG • Muscle biopsy	• Steroids
Acute rhabdomyolysis (see p294)	• EMG • Muscle biopsy	• Urine alkalinization

Myasthenic crises

Presentation

- *Generalized weakness* usually worse proximally. There may be ptosis and diplopia. Reflexes and sensation are normal.
- *Dyspnoea.* The patient may not at first glance appear very distressed. An expressionless myopathic facies, together with weak muscles of respiration, may give a false sense of well-being.
- *Bulbar dysfunction* is potentially dangerous since it may lead to impaired clearance of secretions and aspiration pneumonia.
- *Exhaustion and ventilatory failure* leading to coma.

Common predisposing factors

- Infection, surgery, drugs (see table opposite). N.B. Corticosteroids used to treat myasthenia can initially lead to an acute crisis.

Assessment of severity

- Vital capacity is the most useful indicator. Arterial blood gases are not sensitive enough and demonstrate hypercarbia late.
- Bulbar dysfunction.

Cholinergic crisis

It may not be possible, on clinical evaluation, to distinguish between worsening myasthenia and excessive anticholinesterase treatment (which leads to weakness by producing depolarization block). A Tensilon® (Edrophonium) test (see opposite) is required to decide whether anticholinesterases need to be withdrawn.

Management

1. Stabilize the patient – protect the airway; intubate and ventilate if necessary. Ensure there are no electrolyte disturbances (hypokalaemia, hypocalcaemia, hypermagnesaemia) or drugs prescribed which exacerbate weakness.
2. Consider Tensilon® (Edrophonium) test (see opposite). Anticholinesterase treatment may be helpful if cholinergic crisis is excluded. If there is no effect with Tensilon®, reconsider the diagnosis (consider Eaton-Lambert syndrome). Withold all anticholinesterase medications for 72h. The Tensilon® may be repeated at intervals.
3. Immunosuppression should be supervised by a neurologist. Prednisolone 120mg/day on alternating days produces improvement after 10–12 days, but should be introduced with care in hospital because there may be initial worsening of weakness. High-dose steroids are given until remission occurs. Azathioprine (2.5mg/kg) has also been used for maintenance therapy.
4. Plasmapheresis is used to remove circulating antibody. It usually involves exchange of 50ml/kg/day over several days. The role of immunoglobulin therapy is unclear.
5. Regular anticholinesterase inhibitor therapy should be directed and optimized by a neurologist. Therapy depends upon response but one initial strategy is to commence with pyridostigmine 60mg q4h. This can be given by NG-tube or, if necessary, im neostigmine can be used instead (1mg neostigmine should be given for every 60mg pyridostigmine).

Drugs which may exacerbate myasthenia		
Antibiotics		
Gentamicin	Tetracycline	Streptomycin
Neomycin	Tobramycin	Kanamycin
Colistin	Clindamycin	Lincomycin
Cardiac drugs		
Quindine		Quinine
Proprandolol		Procainamide
Local anaesthetics		
Lignocaine		Procaine
Anticonvulsants/Psychotropic drugs		
Phenytoin		Barbiturates
Lithium		Chlorpromazine
Muscle relaxants		
Suxamethonium		Curare
Analgesics		
Pethidine		Morphine
Hormones		
Corticosteroids (initially)		Thyroxine
Others		
Magnesium salts		

Tensilon® (Edrophonium) test

1. A history of asthma or cardiac dysrhythmias are relative contra-indications. Atropine should be drawn up prior to the test in case edrophonium (an inhibitor of acetylcholinesterase) produces a severe cholinergic reaction, e.g. symptomatic bradycardia.

2. Prepare and label two 1ml syringes: one containing saline, the other 10mg of edrophonium.

3. Select a muscle to observe for the test and ask a colleague to assess its strength prior to the test.

4. Inject, in stages, the contents of either syringe, keeping both patient and colleague blinded to the contents of each syringe. Ask the observer to reassess muscle strength after the contents of each syringe have been injected.

5. Edrophonium should first be given as a bolus of 2mg (0.2ml) and untoward cholinergic effects should be observed for. If it is tolerated the remaining 0.8ml can be given 1 minute later.

6. Improvement in muscle strength following edrophonium suggests the patient is suffering a myasthenic, not cholinergic, crisis.

Spinal cord compression: Assessment

Presentation

- *Back pain* is usually the first symptom. It often starts weeks before other features and becomes progressively unremitting, keeping the patient awake at night. There may also be *radicular pain* which is misinterpreted and leads to a long and unrewarding search for the cause of chest or abdominal pain.

- *Sensory symptoms* such as paraesthesiae or a sensation of limb heaviness or pulling may then occur.

- *Sensory loss* may be apparent at a sensory level on testing. It is wise to test for pin-prick (spinothalamic function) and joint position sense/vibration sense (dorsal column function): anterior or posterior portions of the cord may be selectively compressed. 'Sacral sparing' refers to preservation of sensation in (usually) S3-S5 dermatomes; it is a relatively reliable sign of an intramedullary lesion (see causes) which initially spares laterally placed spinothalamic tract fibres sub-serving sacral sensation.

- *Weakness* is often first described as clumsiness but soon progresses to clear loss of power.

- *Sphincter dysfunction* commences as hesitancy or urgency of micturition and may progress to painless urinary retention with overflow. Constipation is another consequence of cord compression.

- *Fever* should alert one to the possibility of an infectious cause.

- *Respiratory failure* occurs with high cervical cord compression and is one cause of acute neuromuscular respiratory failure (p398).

- *Conus medullaris lesions* compress the sacral segments of the cord and lead to relatively early disturbance of micturition and constipation, impotence, reduced perianal sensation, and anal reflex; rectal and genital pain occurs later. Plantar responses are extensor.

- *Cauda equina lesion.* Lesions at or below the first lumbar vertebral body may compress the spinal nerves of the cauda equina leading to a flaccid, areflexic, often asymmetric paraparesis. Lumbosacral pain occurs early; bladder and bowel dysfunction appear relatively late. A sensory level is found in a saddle distribution up to L1 (corresponding to roots carried in cauda equina).

- *Combined conus and cauda lesions* produce a combination of lower and upper motor neurone signs.

Assessment of severity

The degree of weakness, sensory loss, and sphincter dysfunction are useful indicators of severity.

Spinal cord compression

Causes of spinal cord compression	
• Tumour	primary or metastatic
Extradural:	metastatic lung, breast, prostatic, gastrointestinal or renal carcinoma, lymphoma, myeloma
Intradural + extramedullary:	schwannoma, meningioma
Intradural + intramedullary	astrocytoma, ependymoma
• Infection	staphylococcal abscess, tuberculoma, infected dermoid
• Prolapsed intervertebral disc	(central)
• Cyst	arachnoid, syringomyelia
• Haemorrhage	
• Skeletal deformity	kyphoscoliosis, achondroplasia, spondylolisthesis

Spinal cord compression: Management

This depends upon diagnosis and the condition of the patient. In some patients known to have disseminated cancer it may not be appropriate to make any intervention apart from analgesia. In other such cases, radiotherapy – but not surgery – may be considered. In patients without such a background and presenting for the first time it is imperative to attempt to make the diagnosis swiftly and discuss with the regional Neurosurgical Centre.

1. Plain X-rays of the spine should be obtained immediately. These may show vertebral collapse, lytic lesions, or sclerosis.

2. Magnetic resonance imaging or CT myelography is the next investigation of choice. This should be arranged urgently. If facilities are not available locally, discuss with regional Neurosurgical Centre.

3. If the diagnosis is suspected to be compression from metastatic tumour, many would start treatment with very large doses of steroid (dexamethasone up to 25mg every 6h) but this should be discussed with neurosurgeons and/or oncologists. They will also advise about merits of surgical decompression vs radiotherapy alone or in combination.

4. If the cause of compression appears to be infective (fever, neutrophilia, raised CRP, etc.), blood, sputum, and urine cultures should be sent.

5. If there is bladder dysfunction, urinary catheterization may be necessary. If immobile, start prophylactic sub-cutaneous heparin (5000U tds).

6. If there is high cervical compression or if ventilation appears to be compromised, FVC and arterial blood gases should be measured. The indications for intubation (if this is appropriate) are discussed in acute neuromuscular respiratory failure (p398).

Spinal cord compression

Guillain-Barré Syndrome (GBS)

Presentation

- *Progressive weakness of more than one limb* in an individual who may recently have experienced a mild respiratory or gastrointestinal febrile illness. Weakness is as commonly proximal as distal. It is usually symmetrical but may be asymmetrical.
- *Diminished tendon reflexes/areflexia* is common.
- *Sensory symptoms.* Paraesthesiae often precede weakness. Sensory loss is not usually profound although there may be a glove-and-stocking distribution impairment of two-point discrimination, joint position, and vibration sense. If there is a sensory level, spinal cord compression (p404) should be the diagnosis until proved otherwise.
- *Limb or back pain* is a major symptom in ~ 30%.
- *Cranial nerve dysfunction* occurs in 50%. Bulbar function and muscles of mastication are affected in 30%; ocular muscles in 10% of patients.
- *Ventilatory failure.* See acute respiratory failure (p398).
- *Autonomic dysfunction* is common. Sweating, tachycardia, sudden swings of bp, dysrhythmias, and cardiac arrest. Bladder or bowel dysfunction occurs but if it is present from the outset or if it is persistent, reconsider the diagnosis.
- *Miller-Fisher variant.* Ophthalmoplegia (giving rise to diplopia), ataxia, and areflexia without significant weakness or sensory signs.

Causes

GBS probably represents an immune-mediated attack on peripheral nerves. Infections which may precede it include cytomegalovirus, *Campylobacter jejuni*, Epstein-Barr virus, hepatitis B, *Mycoplasma*, and herpes simplex virus.

Assessment of severity

Poor prognostic features on presentation include:

- Rapid onset
- Requirement for ventilation (bulbar compromise, reducing VC, respiratory failure).
- Age > 40
- Reduced amplitude of compound muscle action potential (< 10% of control) and extensive spontaneous fibrillation in distal muscles suggesting denervation. (N.B. Electrophysiological studies may be normal in early GBS.)
- Axonal variant (often with preceding *Campylobacter jejuni* infection).

A grading system has been devised to follow a patient's progress.

- Grade 1: Able to run
- Grade 2: Able to walk 5m but not to run
- Grade 3: Able to walk 5m with assistance
- Grade 4: Chair/bed-bound
- Grade 5: Ventilated

Guillain-Barré Syndrome (GBS) 2.

Management

It is important to appreciate that GBS is a diagnosis of exclusion with an extensive differential [see acute respiratory paralysis (p398)]. The pace at which alternative diagnoses need to be excluded depends upon the history and findings.

The management of the patient with GBS is that of any patient with neuromuscular failure (p398), although there are a few important specific measures.

1. **Autonomic instability** is a common feature, so ECG monitoring and frequent assessment of bp and pulse is advisable, particularly in any patient with bulbar or respiratory involvement. (N.B. Tracheal suction may lead to bradycardia or asystole.)

2. **CSF analysis** may be required. CSF protein may be normal initially but characteristically rises and peaks in 4–6 weeks.

3. **Steroids** are of no benefit in GBS.

4. The current favoured treatment is **iv immunoglobulin** 0.4g/kg for 5 days.[27] This may improve the rate of recovery faster than plasmapheresis (five 50ml/kg exchanges over a period of 14 days). Some patients receive both immunoglobulin and plasma exchange therapy. Treatment should not be commenced without prior discussion with a neurologist.

[27] Van der Meché FG and Schmitz PI (1992) *NEJM* **326**: 1123–1129.

Guillain-Barré Syndrome

Botulism

Presentation

Botulism is caused by exotoxins of *Clostridium botulinum.* there are three syndromes: food-borne, wound, and infantile. The latter 2 causes are rare and will not be discussed here. The most common form of botulism is food-borne with outbreaks usually attributed to canned food. Patients present with symptoms usually within 18 hours of ingestion of the toxin.

- *Sore throat, fatigue, dizziness, blurred vision.*
- *Nausea, vomiting, constipation.*
- *Rapidly progressive weakness* often beginning in the extraocular and/or pharyngeal muscles and descending symmetrically in severe cases to give upper and lower limb paralysis and respiratory failure (see acute respiratory failure p398).
- *Paraesthesiae* may occur but there are no sensory signs.
- *Parasympathetic dysfunction* causes a dry mouth, ileus, and dilated non-reactive pupils in an alert patient. This pupillary response may help to distinguish botulism from other neuromuscular disorders; however, in most cases the pupils remain reactive.

Wound botulism is similar, except gastrointestinal upset does not occur.

Assessment of severity

Limb weakness and ventilatory failure are indicators of severe disease. Patients with these features have a worse prognosis, as do patients over 20 years, and those who have ingested type A toxin.

Management

1. Assess severity, **measure FVC frequently** and attempt to exclude other important causes of neuromuscular failure (p398). In particular, a **Tensilon test** should be performed to exclude myasthenia gravis (p403); **nerve conduction** should be normal but it is important to exclude Guillain-Barré syndrome (p408); **electromyography** is frequently abnormal in botulism (decrement of compound muscle action potential at slow rates of repetitive stimulation of $3s^{-1}$ and facilitation of motor response at rapid rates of $50s^{-1}$). Serum and stool should be assayed for toxin and *C. botulinum*.

2. **General management** is described elsewhere (p400).

3. **Specific treatment** If botulism is suspected 10,000 units of trivalent (A, B, E) antitoxin should be administered iv immediately and at 4 hourly intervals. Approximately 20% of patients have minor allergic reactions to this and require corticosteroid and antihistamines as for anaphylaxis (p212). (For supplies outside normal working hours contact Dept. of Health Duty Officer, Tel: 0171-210-5371).

4. **Guanidine hydrochloride** (an acetylcholine agonist) may be of benefit in some patients (35–40mg/kg/day orally in divided doses).

5. Gastric lavage, emetics, cathartics, and enemas may be used with caution to accelerate elimination of toxin from the gastrointestinal tract. The first two interventions are contraindicated if bulbar weakness is present; magnesium-containing cathartics should not be used as there is a risk that magnesium may enhance toxin activity.

Pathophysiology of botulism

Preformed botulinum toxin is a potent presynaptic blocker of acetylcholine release at the neuromuscular junction, post ganglionic parasympathetic terminals, and autonomic ganglia. There are 6 antigenically distinct toxins (A–F) but only A, B, and E appear to be associated with human illness.

Tetanus

Presentation

Tetanus is caused by the effects of exotoxins produced by *Clostridium tetani*. It occurs after *C. tetani* spores have gained access to tissues. The wound may be very trivial and in 20% of cases there is no history or evidence of injury. Incubation of spores may take weeks but most patients present within 15 days with:

- *Pain and stiffness of jaw.*
- *Rigidity and difficulty in opening mouth* – trismus or 'lockjaw'.
- *Generalized rigidity of facial muscles* leading to the classical risus sardonicus or clenched teeth expression.
- *Rigidity of body musculature* leading to neck retraction and spinal extension.
- *Reflex spasms* are painful spasms elicited by stimuli such as pressure or noise. These usually occur 1–3 days after the initial symptoms and are potentially very dangerous since they may endanger respiration and precipitate cardiorespiratory collapse.
- *Convulsive seizures.*
- *Autonomic dysfunction* with both sympathetic (sweating, hypertension, tachycardia, dysrhythmias, hyperpyrexia) and parasympathetic (bradycardia, asystole) involvement.

Cause

Exotoxin blocks inhibitory pathways within the central nervous system.

Assessment of severity

Rapidly progressing features and the onset of spasms signify worse disease and prognosis.

Management

1. **Assess severity.** In severe spasms/respiratory failure, ventilation will be required. Otherwise patients should be nursed in a quiet, dark room (to reduce reflex spasms) under close observation. Sedation with diazepam may be necessary but beware of respiratory depression.

2. **General management** as discussed on p400.

3. **Specific treatment.** Human hyperimmune globulin 3000–10,000 units iv or im should be given to neutralize circulating toxin. This will not ameliorate existing symptoms but will prevent further binding of toxin to CNS. Penicillin iv (1.2g qds), or tetracycline 500mg qds, should be prescribed to treat *C. tetani*.

4. **Wound care and debridement as appropriate.** Swabs should be sent for culture but often do not grow the organism.

5. **Prophylaxis in patients who have previously been immunized.**

   For any wound, give a booster dose of tetanus toxoid if the patient has not received a booster in the last 10 years.

   If the wound appears dirty and infected, or the patient has never been immunized/cannot recall/unable to give history, give human antitoxin (250 units im) in addition to toxoid.

Glasgow Coma Scale (GCS)

Developed to assess depth and duration of impaired consciousness in a standard fashion. The total is out of 15 (see table opposite); the worst possible score is 3 (which even the dead can achieve). The scale has a high rate of inter-observer agreement and GCS score is one useful way of monitoring consciousness level.

Eye opening

- If spontaneous, indicates brainstem arousal mechanisms are probably intact, but the patient need not be aware of his surroundings.
- Eye opening to speech is not necessarily a response to a verbal command to open the eyes; any verbal approach, e.g. calling the name of the patient, may elicit this.
- Eye opening to pain is best tested by using a stimulus in the limbs because supra-orbital or styloid process pressure can lead to grimacing with eye closure.

Verbal responsiveness

- An orientated patient knows who he is, where he is, and why he is there; he can recollect the month and year.
- A confused patient will converse but his responses indicate varying degrees of disorientation and confusion.
- An individual with inappropriate speech cannot sustain a conversation; his utterances are exclamatory or random and may consist of shouting or swearing.
- Incomprehensible speech does not consist of any recognizable words but involves moaning and groaning.

Motor response (see figure opposite)

- Patients who obey commands show the best possible motor response but be careful not to misinterpret postural adjustments or the grasp reflex.
- If there is no response to command, a painful stimulus may be applied initially by applying pressure to the fingernail bed. If this elicits flexion at the elbow, pressure may be applied to the styloid process, supra-orbital ridge, and trunk to see if there is localization.
- If pain at the nail bed elicits a rapid withdrawal with flexion of the elbow and adduction at the shoulder it is scored 4.
- If, instead, it produces a slower flexion of the elbow with adduction at the shoulder, it is considered an *abnormal flexion response* (sometimes called *decorticate posturing*).
- If pain elicits extension of the elbow, adduction, and internal rotation of the shoulder with pronation of the forearm this is noted as an *extensor response* (sometimes called *decerebrate posturing*).

Prognosis

The GCS is a valuable tool in predicting likely outcome from coma, *but it has limitations* and should not be the only factor used to assess prognosis. Patients with GCS 3–8 generally have far worse prognoses than those with > 8. But the cause of coma is also an important predictor, e.g. metabolic coma (especially due to drug intoxication) generally has a better outlook than other causes, irrespective of GCS.

Glasgow Coma Scale (GCS)	
Eye opening	
Spontaneously	4
To speech	3
To painful stimulus	2
No response	1
Best verbal response	
Orientated	5
Disorientated	4
Inappropriate words	3
Incomprehensible sounds	2
No response	1
Best motor response	
Obeys verbal commands	6
Localizes painful stimuli	5
Withdrawal to pain	4
Flexion to pain	3
Extension to pain	2
No response	1

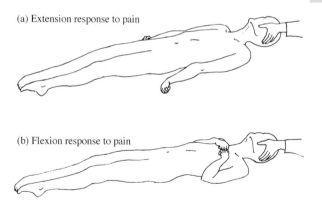

(a) Extension response to pain

(b) Flexion response to pain

Posturing in coma

Examination of brainstem function   1.

Assessment of brainstem function is vital to the management of coma (p304), raised intracranial pressure (p348), brainstem strokes (p386), and brain death (p428). It is not necessary to have a detailed knowledge of brainstem anatomy. Some simple observations reveal a great deal about function at different levels of the brainstem.

Examination of the eyes

- **Pupillary reactions** The size of the pupils and their reactions to bright light should be assessed. This tests the pathway from each eye (IInd cranial nerve) through the superior colliculus (midbrain), its connection to the nearby Edinger-Westphal IIIrd nerve nucleus (also in the mid-brain), and efferent parasympathetic outflow of the IIIrd nerve. The pupillary reflex is consensual, so light in one eye should elicit constriction of both pupils. Thus, observations of the pupillary response can interrogate brainstem function at the level of the mid-brain.

- **Corneal reflex** This tests the integrity of the afferent pathway which runs in the Vth nerve through to the VIIth nerve nucleus (pons), and the efferent pathway in the VIIth nerve. The corneal reflex is also a consensual reflex. This reflex allows one to interrogate brainstem function from the pons down to the spinal trigeminal nucleus.

- **Resting eye position** may give a useful clue to asymmetric brainstem dysfunction. If the eyes are dysconjugate there must be a disorder of the nuclei of the IIIrd, IVth, or VIth nerves, their connections, or the nerves themselves. Note the IIIrd and IVth nuclei are located in the mid-brain, whereas the VIth nucleus is located in the pons.

- **Spontaneous eye movements**
- If there are spontaneous, fast (saccadic) horizontal and vertical conjugate eye movements, the brainstem mechanism for generating saccades is intact and there is no need to test for the oculocephalic or oculovstibular response because:
- Horizontal saccades require the integrity of the paramedian pontine reticular formation (pons), IIIrd nerve nucleus. VIth nerve nucleus, and the medial longitudinal fasciculus connecting these.
- Vertical saccades require the dorsal mid-brain to be intact.
- Dysconjugate eye movements raise the possibility of unilateral damage to brainstem oculomotor nuclei, their connections, or cranial nerves innervating the extraocular muscles. In this case the resting position of the eyes may also be dysconjugate.
- A number of oculomotor signs associated with brainstem dysfunction have been identified; none are absolutely specific but they may provide useful clues to site of lesion.
- **Oculocephalic response** The 'doll's head manoeuvre' (p426) should be performed only if cervical injury has been excluded. Both it and caloric stimulation assess the integrity of the vestibulo-ocular reflex, which is a three neurone arc from the semicircular canals via the vestibular nuclei to the IIIrd and VIth nerve nuclei.
- **Oculovestibular response** Caloric stimulation (p426).

Examination of brainstem function   2.

The swallowing reflex

- This may be tested by injecting 10mls of water in a syringe into the mouth of the patient. Reflex swallowing requires, amongst other things, the swallowing centre in the reticular formation of the medulla, very close to the solitary nucleus, to be intact.

Respiratory pattern

- This is sometimes useful in localization but often is not.

- *Central neurogenic hyperventilation*, for example, has no localization value. It is rapid, regular deep continuous breathing at ~ 25/min which is not produced by acidosis or hypoxaemia. Its usefulness is that increasing regularity of this pattern signifies increasing depth of coma and worsening prognosis.

- *Apneustic breathing* (prolonged inspiration followed by a period of apnoea), on the other hand, implies damage to the pons, as does *cluster breathing* (closely grouped respirations followed by a period of apnoea). Damage to the medullary respiratory centres is suggested by *ataxic breathing* and *gasping breathing* (Biot's respirations). The former are characterized by a chaotic pattern of respiration; the latter consist of gasps followed by apnoeic periods of variable duration. Both are usually soon followed by respiratory arrest.

- Shallow, slow breathing may be due to medullary depression caused by drugs, e.g. opiates. *Cheyne-Stokes respiration* may be caused by bilateral deep hemispheric and basal ganglia damage but is more usually due to non-neural causes, e.g. primary cardiovascular or respiratory dysfunction.

- **Long tract signs** Finally, structural damage to the brainstem may produce long tract signs with dysfunction of descending pyramidal/ extrapyramidal tracts or ascending sensory pathways. There may be 'crossed signs' because of decussation of pathways within the brainstem.

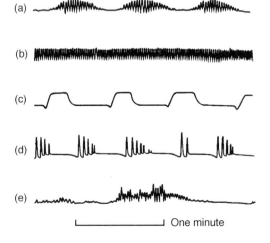

(a)

(b)

(c)

(d)

(e)

One minute

Neurological emergencies

Examination of brainstem function
The swallowing reflex
Respiratory pattern **421**

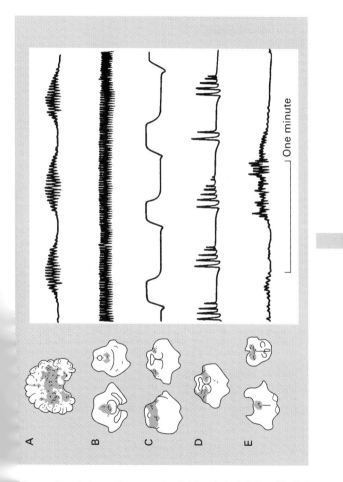

Abnormal respiratory patterns associated with pathologic lesions (shaded areas) at various levels of the brain. (a) Cheyne-Stokes respiration. (b) Central neurogenic hyperventilation. (c) Apneusis. (d) Cluster breathing (e) Ataxic breathing. (From Plum F & Posner JB (1980) *The Diagnosis of Stupor and Coma* 3rd ed; FA Davis, Philadelphia, with permission).

Examination of brainstem function 3.

Signs of brain shift[28]

Raised intracranial pressure may produce a number of distinct progressive brainstem syndromes associated with brain shift.

1. **Central herniation syndrome**
2. **Lateral (uncal) herniation syndrome**
3. **False localizing signs**
4. **Tonsillar herniation**

Assessment involves:

- Observation of respiratory pattern
- Pupillary reaction
- Oculocephalic/oculovestibular response (see p426)
- Motor response at rest or to pain (see p416)

Central herniation syndrome

- Vertical displacement of the brainstem due to a supratentorial mass.
- The first sign is not of brainstem but rather *diencephalic* impairment. The patient becomes less alert and thre may be Cheyne-Stokes breathing. The pupils are small (perhaps due to hypothalamic sympathetic dysfunction) but reactive. There may initially have been unilateral hemiplegia due to the supratentorial mass. Characteristically, in the early diencephalic stage, paratonic resistance (*gegenhalten*) develops in the contralateral limbs and both plantar responses become extensor. Eventually there is a decorticate response to pain (p416).
- *Midbrain-upper pontine* dysfunction becomes evident with fluctuations in temperature, onset of central neurogenic hyperventilation, apneustic or cluster breathing (see p420), unreactive pupils which are 'mid-position' and often irregular in shape, loss of vertical eye movements (which may be tested with the doll's head manoeuvre, p426), increasing difficulty in eliciting horizontal oculocephalic and oculovestibular responses, which may become dysconjugate (p426). Motor responses progress from decorticate (flexor) rigidity to decerebrate (extensor) rigidity in response to pain (p416).
- *Lower pontine-upper medullary* compromise is revealed by often ataxic breathing, fixed mid-position pupils, and failure to elicit oculocephalic and oculovestibular responses. The patient is flaccid at rest; painful stimuli may not elicit any motor response except occasional flexor responses in the lower limbs.
- *Medullary dysfunction* is terminal. Breathing is ataxic or gasping. The pulse rate may increase and bp drops (Cushing response). After a few gasps, breathing stops, and pupils often dilate and become fixed.

---

[28] Plum F & Posner JB (1980) *The Diagnosis of Stupor and Coma* 3rd edition FA Davis, Philadelpia

Neurological emergencies

Examination of brainstem function   4.

Lateral (uncal) herniation syndrome

- Due to lesions in the lateral middle fossa or temporal lobe pushing the medial edge of the uncus and hippocampal gyrus over the free lateral edge of the tentorium.

- The first sign is a *unilaterally dilating pupil* (due to compression of the IIIrd nerve at the tentorial hiatus) which is initially sluggish in response to light. This may soon be followed by ptosis and a complete IIIrd nerve palsy with a fixed, dilated pupil. Oculocephalic and oculovestibular responses initially reveal only the palsy, but are otherwise intact.

- *Mid-brain* compression by the herniating uncus may follow rapidly (the diencephalic stage of central herniation is bypassed). The patient becomes progressively less alert and slips into coma. The oculocephalic and oculovestibular responses cannot be elicited. A hemiplegia ipsilateral to the expanding supratentorial lesion (due to the opposite cerebral peduncle being compressed at the tentorial edge) develops and soon progresses to bilateral extensor plantar responses. As compression continues both pupils become fixed in mid-position and central neuogenic hyperventilation commences.

- The rostrocaudal progression of signs associated with central herniation then follow with decerebrate/extensor rigidity, etc. as above. Note decorticate/flexor response to pain is not usually seen in uncal herniation because the diencephalic stage is bypassed.

False localizing signs

As they expand, supratentorial lesions may distort intracranial structures and produce signs which appear to help in localizing the primary lesion but are in fact due to traction 'at a distance'. The most common of these involve cranial nerves V – VIII.

Tonsillar herniation

Sub-tenorial expanding lesions cause herniation of the cerebellar tonsils through the foramen magnum and compress the pons and mid-brain directly. A degree of upward herniation through the tentorial hiatus may also occur and lead to compression of the upper mid-brain and diencephalon. It may be difficult to distinguish these effects from those produced by supratentorial lesions. One clue is that there is usually a lack of the rostrocaudal sequence of central herniation.

Neurological emergencies

Oculocephalic and oculovestibular responses

Background

Passive rotation of the head with respect to the trunk stimulates vestibular and neck receptors. In comatose patients with intact brainstems, this leads to reflexive *slow conjugate* eye movements in the direction opposite to head rotation. The contribution of neck proprioceptors (cervico-ocular reflex) is minimal; the most important reflex pathway in the brainstem extends from the semicircular canals to the oculomotor nuclei (vestibulo-ocular reflex/VOR). Ice water irrigation of a semi-circular canal 'switches off' its contribution to this pathway and leads to unopposed function of the contralateral semicircular canal. The eyes deviate toward the irrigated semicircular canal. Both the doll's head manoeuvre and caloric tests check the integrity of the VOR; the latter is more sensitive.

1. *Oculocephalic/doll's head response*

- The doll's head manoeuvre should not be attempted if there is any possibility of cervical spine injury.
- The patient's head is first rotated laterally from one side to the other. Vertical movements may be elicited by flexion and extension of the head.
- 'Positive' responses are noted if turning of the head elicits *slow conjugate* deviation of both eyes in the direction opposite to head movement (see figure opposite).
- Because there is much confusion about what constitutes positive or negative responses, it is best simply to describe what you see.

2. *Oculovestibular/caloric response*

- Caloric testing should be performed when the oculocephalic response is abnormal or cannot be performed (e.g. spine fracture).
- The head is then raised 30° above supine and 100mls of ice water is injected into the external auditory meatus using a thin polyethylene catheter.
- A 'positive' response occurs when both eyes move toward the irrigated ear (see figure opposite). This may take up to a minute. Five minutes should elapse before the other ear is tested.

3. *Significance of results*

- If the VOR is intact, a major brainstem pathology is unlikely.
- If the horizontal VOR is absent but the vertical one is present, there may be a lesion at the level of the pons.
- If both responses are absent, there is either a major structura brainstem lesion (figure opposite) or there is a metabolic disturbanc depressing brainstem function (e.g. opiates). Check pupil size an response to light; symmetrically, reactive pupils suggests metaboli coma. Only a few drugs such as atropine, scopolamine, glutethimid depress brainstem function and produce pupillary abnormalities.
- If dysconjugate eye movements are elicited, a brainstem lesion i likely. Check to see if there is an internuclear ophthalmoplegia.
- It may not be possible to elicit a VOR using the doll's hea manoeuvre because the patient has fast, roving, saccadic ey movements. These suggest an intact brainstem.

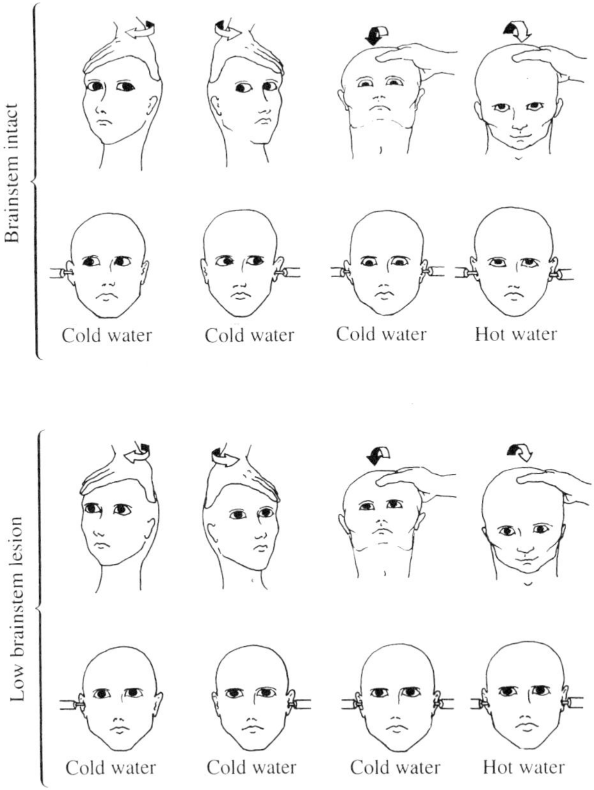

Oculocephalic responses

Brain death

This is irreversible loss of the capacity for consciousness combined with irreversible loss of the capacity to breathe. Without the brainstem, both these functions are lost. But patients with severe, irreversible brain damage who have no brainstem function may survive for weeks or months provided they have a normal circulation and are mechanically ventilated. Criteria for brain death have therefore been developed. It has been shown that patients who fulfil these, even if they are ventilated, will eventually develop cardiovascular collapse.

Preconditions

- There must be no doubt that the patient has irremediable structural brain damage which has been diagnosed with certainty. Usually this a head injury or intracranial haemorrhage, but it may be anoxia post cardiac arrest when it is not always possible immediately to be certain that brain damage is irremediable.

- The patient must be in apnoeic coma (unresponsive to noxious stimuli and on a mechanical ventiator) with no spontaneous respiratory effort.

- There must be no possibility of drug intoxication and no paralysing or anaesthetic drugs should have been administered recently. Hypothermia must be excluded as a cause of coma and the core temperature (rectal or external auditory meatus) should be $> 35°C$.

- There must be no significant metabolic, endocrine, or electrolyte disturbance either causing or contributing to coma.

Tests for confirming brain death

All brainstem reflexes must be absent:

- Pupils fixed and unresponsive to bright light. (They need not be dilated). Paralytic eye drops, ocular injury, and lesions of the IInd/IIIrd cranial nerves may pose problems in this assessment.

- Absent corneal reflexes.

- Absent vestibulo-ocular reflexes on irrigation of each ear in turn with 20ml ice-cold water.

- No motor response within the cranial nerve distribution (eye, face, head) elicited by stimulation of any somatic area (nail bed, supraorbital, and Achilles tendon pressure on each side). Purely spinal reflexes, e.g. deep tendon reflexes, may be retained.

- No reflex response to touching the pharynx (gag reflex), nor to a suction catheter passed into the trachea (cough reflex).

Apnoea

- No respiratory movements when the ventilator is disconnected and $P_a CO_2$ reaches 6.65kPa. (In order to avoid anoxia during this procedure, the patient should be ventilated with 100% oxygen for 10 minutes beforehand; during disconnection, 6l/min 100% oxygen should be delivered via a tracheal catheter. If just prior to disconnection, $P_a CO_2$ is < 3.5kPa, give 5% CO_2 in oxygen via the ventilator until this level is reached – usually within 5 minutes).

The tests must be performed by two experienced clinicians (one must be a consultant and the other a senior registrar or above) and all the above should be repeated after an interval which depends upon the clinical context.

N.B. Consider the patient a potential organ donor. Discuss with relatives and contact the transplant co-ordinator for your area. Alternatively, contact the duty officer for the UK Transplant Support Service (tel: 01179–757575).

8 Endocrine emergencies

Diabetic ketoacidosis: Assessment

Diabetic ketoacidosis (DKA) only occurs in patients with insulin-dependent diabetes (type I). It does not occur in non-insulin-dependent diabetes. Remember, patients may be prescribed insulin for poor diabetic control, and yet have non-insulin-dependent diabetes.

Clinical features include:

- Polyuria and polydipsia: patients become dehydrated over 2–3 days.
- Hyperventilation or breathlessness: the acidosis causes Kussmaul's respiration (a deep sighing respiration) and subjective dyspnoea.
- Abdominal pain: DKA may present as an 'acute abdomen'.
- Vomiting: exacerbates dehydration.
- Coma results from the fall in pH.

Investigations

- Blood glucose — This need not be high. Severe acidaemia may be present with glucose values as low as 10mM (e.g. if the patient has recently taken insulin: this, alone, is insufficient to correct the acidaemia in the presence of dehydration.)
- ABG — Assess the degree of acidaemia (pH and Bic.)
- U&Es — Corrected Na = Na + 1.6 × $\dfrac{\text{[plasma glc (mmol)-5.5]}}{5.5}$

  Assess serum K^+ and renal function. (Some creatinine assays cross-react with ketone bodies giving a falsely high creatinine.)
- Urinalysis — Ketones strongly positive. (Ketones may be present in normal individuals after a period of starvation.)
  Note: captopril can give a false positive test for urinary acetone.
- FBC — WBC may be elevated (neutrophilia): a leukaemoid reaction can occur in absence of infection.
- Septic screen — Blood and urine cultures.
- Plasma ketones — (see notes below).
- CXR — Look specifically for any infection.
- Amylase — May be high with abdominal pain ± vomiting in absence of pancreatitis.

Note

- Serum osmolality = 2 × ($Na^+ + K^+$) + urea + glucose.
- Diagnosis of DKA requires positive serum ketones and arterial pH ≤ 7.30 and/or serum bicarbonate ≤ 15mmol/l.
- The elderly patient presenting with a high glucose, relatively normal acid-base balance, and ketones in the urine does not have diabetic ketoacidosis, and may not be insulin dependent.
- Consider other causes of hyperglycaemia/acidosis e.g. aspirin overdose, and in the elderly consider lactic acidosis.
- An accurate but indirect measure of plasma ketones can be made in cases of doubt as follows. Collect 10ml blood in a heparinized tube and centrifuge. Collect the plasma (4ml approx.) and add an equal volume of saline. Using a urine ketone dipstick, a result of +++ corresponds to a plasma ketone body concentration of 5mmol/l.

Common precipitants of DKA	
• Infections	30%
• Non-compliance with treatment	20%
• Newly diagnosed diabetes	25%

Poor prognostic features in DKA
• pH < 7.0
• Oliguria
• Plasma ketone body concentration > 5mmol/l
• Serum osmolality > 320
• Newly diagnosed diabetes

Diabetic ketoacidosis: Management[1]

General measures
- Rehydration and insulin therapy are the mainstays of treatment.
- Site the iv cannula away from a major vein in the wrist. This may be required for an AV fistula in patients subsequently developing diabetic nephropathy. Start fluid replacement (see below).
- Insert a central line in patients with a history of cardiac disease/ autonomic neuropathy or the elderly (see p768).
- Consider an arterial line to monitor ABGs and potassium.
- Nil by mouth for at least 6 hours (gastroparesis is common).
- Nasogastric tube: If there is impaired consciousness level, to prevent vomiting and aspiration.
- Urinary catheter if oliguria is present or serum creatinine is high.
- Broad spectrum antibiotics if infection suspected.
- Heparin (5000U) sc tds as prophylaxis for deep vein thrombosis.
- The $t_{1/2}$ of insulin is short and continued replacement (iv or sc) is essential.

Fluid replacement
[The following should be modified for patients with cardiac disease.]
- If hypotensive and oliguric, give iv colloids ($\pm$ N saline) initially to restore bp; then:
- 1 litre N saline over the first 30 minutes then
- 1 litre N saline with potassium (see table opposite) 2 hourly for 8h then
- 1 litre N saline (with K^+, table opposite) 4 hourly until rehydrated (~ 24 hours).
- Modify this in the elderly according to CVP and clinical assessment of fluid status, aiming to restore fluid deficits in 12–24 hours.
- The use of bicarbonate is controversial. If the pH $<$ 7.0, isotonic (1.26%) sodium bicarbonate given at a maximal rate of 500ml (i.e. 75mmol) over 1 hour is safe. Faster infusion rates cause a paradoxical intracellular acidosis. Add 10–20mmoles K^+ per 500ml.
- When blood glucose is less than 12mmol/l, commence a 5% dextrose infusion and continue insulin infusion. Continued insulin is required to inhibit ketoacid production.

Potassium replacement (see table opposite)
- Total body potassium can be depleted by 1000mmoles and the plasma potassium falls rapidly as potassium shifts into the cells under the action of insulin. Use less potassium in patients with renal impairment or oliguria.

Insulin replacement (see table opposite)
Modify this regimen depending on the response to therapy.
- Aim for a fall in glc of 5mmol/l per hour (and correction of acidosis and plasma bicarbonate).
- If the glc or acidosis are not correcting, increase the insulin infusion rate accordingly.
- Keep the blood glc $>$ 10–14mmol/l for the first 24 hours or until the ketoacidosis resolves; maintain this with 5% dextrose infusion.

[1] Lebovitz HE (1996) *Lancet* **345**: 767–772.

Plasma potassium (mmol/l)	Amount of K⁺ (mmol) to add to each litre
< 3.0	40
< 4.0	30
< 5.0	20

Add 50 units of actrapid to 50ml 0.9% saline and administer by intravenous infusion. The sliding scale below is a guide.-

Blood glucose (mmol/l) (hourly)	Insulin infusion (units /hour)
0.0 – 2.0	Stop insulin – Call doctor
2.1 – 5.0	0.5
5.1 – 7.0	1
7.1 – 10.0	2
10.1 – 15.0	3
15.1 – 20.0	4
20.1 – 28.0	6
> 28.1	Call doctor

Diabetic ketoacidosis: Complications

Assessment during treatment

Remember rapid normalization of biochemistry can be detrimental in any patient. It is wiser to be cautious and sub-optimal, than enthusiastic and supra-optimal.

- Blood glucose (BM stix every hour, lab. blood glucose 4 hourly)
- Plasma K^+ every 2 hours. The main risk is hypokalaemia.
- ABGs 4 hourly, until persistent improvement or normalized.
- Plasma osmolality 4 hourly.
- Electrolytes at least daily.
- Phosphate levels should be monitored daily (see below).
- Magnesium levels should be monitored daily (see below).
- The iv insulin infusion should be continued until 4 hours after the patient is commenced on sub-cutaneous insulin.

Complications (see table opposite)

- Avoid **hypoglycaemia** from overzealous insulin replacement.
- **Cerebral oedema** may be precipitated by sudden shifts in plasma osmolality during treatment (with a failure of serum Na^+ to rise, suggesting excessive accumulation of free water). Symptoms include drowsiness, severe headache $\pm$ confusion. Treat as on p350. Give iv mannitol 1–2g/kg body weight, repeated as necessary. Mortality is ~ 70%; recovery of normal function only 7–14%.
- **Phosphate levels** fall during treatment, as it moves intracellularly with potassium. If the phosphate level falls to below 0.5mmol/l, give phosphate iv (9–18mmol/24 hours) or oral (effervescent Phosphate-Sandoz® 2 tabs tds). Excessive phosphate replacement may cause hypocalcaemia and metastatic calcification.
- **Magnesium levels** may also fall during insulin therapy. Replace if magnesium levels fall < 0.6mmol/l: give 4–8mmol (2ml of 50%) magnesium sulphate over 15–30 min in 50ml N saline, repeated as necessary.
- **Hyperchloraemic acidosis** (high anion gap acidosis in a well hydrated patient) may be seen with excessive administration of saline and increased consumption of bicarbonate. No specific treatment is required
- Tissue hypoperfusion results from dehydration and may trigger the coagulation cascade and result in **thromboembolism**. Low-dose heparin should be used for prophylaxis, esp. in elderly patients.

Complications of DKA

- Cerebral oedema
- Hypokalaemia
- Hypophosphataemia
- Hyperchloraemic acidosis
- Hypoglycaemia
- Tissue hypoperfusion / thromboembolism

Hyperosmolar non-ketotic coma (HONC)

Hyperosmolar non-ketotic coma occurs in elderly patients with non-insulin-dependent diabetes. These patients are also at increased risk of venous and arterial thromboses. The mortality is very much higher than for ketoacidotic coma.

Presentation
- A history of diabetes is not usually known, and the patient is elderly
- Insidious onset of polyuria and polydipsia
- Severe dehydration
- Impaired consciousness level: the degree correlates most with plasma osmolality. Coma is usually associated with an osmolality > 440
- Respiration is usually normal
- The patient may rarely present with a CVA, seizures or an MI

Investigations
Glucose	Usually > 40mmol/l
U&Es	Dehydration causes a greater rise in urea than creatinine [normal ratio of Cr:Ur up to 20:1 (μM:mM)]. Significant hypernatraemia may be hidden by the high glucose. The hypernatraemia may appear to worsen as the glucose falls.
ABG	Relatively normal, cf. DKA. A coexistent lactic acidosis considerably worsens the prognosis.
Plasma osm.	Calculate by $[2 \times (Na + K)) + urea + glucose)]$ Needs to be > 350mosm/kg for diagnosis
FBC	Polycythaemia and leukocytosis may indicate dehydration or infection respectively.
ECG	Look for myocardial infarction or ischaemia.
CXR	Look for signs of infection.
Urine	For urinalysis, MC&S. Remember that ketones may occur in any starved person (see p430, DKA), but the level will be below 5mM. The presence of blood and protein on urinalysis may indicate UTI.

Management: general measures
- Rehydration and insulin therapy are the mainstays of treatment. Be much more cautious in the elderly. Give oxygen if hypoxic on air.
- Avoid fluid overload: monitor central venous pressure in all patients.
- Nil by mouth for at least 6 hours and insert an NG tube in patients with impaired concious level to prevent vomiting and aspiration.
- Urinary catheter if oliguria is present, or serum creatinine is high.
- Anti-coagulate with iv heparin 12,000 units every 12 hours by infusion as prophylaxis against venous or arterial thrombosis, maintaining the KCCT (or APTT) at between 60 and 100 seconds.

Fluid replacement
- 1 litre N saline over the first 60 minutes then:
- 1 litre N saline with K^+ (see table p433) every 2h for 4h then:
- 1 litre N saline with K^+ (table p433) q6h until rehydrated (~ 48h).
- If the plasma Na is > 160mM give 0.45% saline (0.5N saline) for the first 3 litres. The Na level is artificially lowered by the high glucose level (see below) and appears to climb as the blood glucose falls.
- When blood glucose < 10mmol/l, commence a 5% dextrose infusion and consider stopping insulin therapy and starting oral hypoglycaem agents or diet alone.

Insulin regimen
- This is similar to that for diabetic ketoacidotic coma (table p433)

Hyperosmolar non-ketotic coma (HONC)

Teaching points: hyperosmolar non-ketotic coma

- Severe hyperglycaemia can cause a technical error in the measurement of Na^+ concentrations. The corrected concentration can be calculated by:-

$$\text{Corrected } Na^+ = Na^+ + 1.6 \times \frac{[\text{plasma glc (mM)} - 5.5]}{5.5}$$

- Treatment of severe hyperglycaemia causes an apparent increase in plasma Na^+ which in reality may not actually change.
- Occasionally, patients present with hyponatraemia which, based on the above, is a form of pseudohyponatraemia (see p446).

Hypoglycaemic coma: Assessment

- All unconscious patients should be assumed to be hypoglycaemic until proved otherwise. *Always* check a blood glucose using a Glucostix® (or BM stix) immediately, and *confirm* with a lab determination.
- The most common cause of coma in a patient with diabetes is hypoglycaemia due to drugs. The longer acting sulphonylureas such as chlorpropamide are more prone to do this than the shorter acting ones.
- Patients who are NOT known to have diabetes, but who are hypoglycaemic should have a laboratory blood glucose, and serum saved for insulin and C-peptide determination (insulinoma or factitious drug administration).

Presentation

Sympathetic overactivity
(glc < 3.6mmol/l)

- Tachycardia
- Palpitations
- Sweating
- Anxiety
- Pallor
- Tremor
- Cold extremities

Neuroglycopenia
(glc < 2.6mmol/l)

- Confusion
- Slurred speech
- Focal neurological defect (stroke-like syndromes)
- Coma

- Patients with well-controlled diabetes have more frequent episodes of hypoglycaemia, and can become desensitized to sympathetic activation. These patients may develop neuroglycopenia before sympathetic activation and complain of 'loss of warning'.
- β-blockers blunt the symptoms of sympathetic activation and patients taking these drugs lose the early warning of hypoglycaemia.
- Patients with poorly controlled diabetes develop sympathetic signs early, and avoid these by running a high blood glucose. They may complain of 'being hypo' when their blood sugar is normal or high. They do not require glucose.
- Patients who have diabetes following a total pancreatectomy have more frequent and severe episodes of hypoglycaemia ('brittle diabetes') because they have lost their glucagon producing (α) cells as well as their β islet cells.

Investigations

- Blood glucose (Glucostix® and lab. glucose)
- U&Es (hypoglycaemia is more common in diabetic nephropathy)
- Save serum, **prior** to giving glucose, for insulin and C-peptide levels (Send ~ 20ml blood directly to the lab for immediate centrifugation) if indicated.

Note

- A lab. glucose of less than 2.2mmol/l is defined as a severe attack.
- Coma usually occurs with blood glucose < 1.5mmol/l.
- Low C-peptide and high insulin level indicate exogenous insulin; high C-peptide and insulin level indicate endogenous insulin [e.g. surreptitious drug (sulphonylurea) ingestion or insulinoma].

Causes of hypoglycaemia

- *Drugs*
  Surreptitious insulin injection
  or oral hypoglycaemics
  Ethanol
  Salicylates
  Quinine
  Pentamidine
  Disopyramide
  β-blockers
  Prescription errors, e.g. chlorpropamide for chlorpromazine
- *Tumours*
  Insulinoma
  Retroperitoneal sarcomas
- Liver dysfunction
- Hypopituitarism
- Myxoedema

Hypoglycaemic coma: Management

Acute measures

- Remember to **take blood** prior to glucose administration (glucose, insulin, C-peptide) see p438.

- If there is a history of chronic alcohol intake or malnourishment, give iv **thiamine** 1–2mg/kg to avoid precipitating Wernicke's encephalopathy.

- If patient is conscious and co-operative, give 50g **oral glucose** or equivalent (e.g. *Lucozade®*, or milk and sugar).

- Give 50ml of **50% dextrose iv** if patient is unable to take oral fluids.

- If iv access is impossible, give 1mg of **glucagon** im. Then give the patient some oral glucose to prevent a hypoglycaemic episode later. Glucagon is ineffective in hypoglycaemia due to alcohol.

- Admit the patient if the cause is a long-acting sulphonylurea or a long-acting insulin, and commence a continuous infusion of 10% glucose (e.g. 1 litre 8 hourly) and check glucose hourly or 2 hourly.

Further management

- Patients should regain consciousness or become coherent within 10 minutes although complete cognitive recovery may lag by 30–45 minutes. Do not give further boluses of iv glucose without repeating the blood glucose. If the patient does not wake up after ~ 10 min, repeat the blood glucose and consider another cause of coma (e.g. head injury while hypoglycaemic – see p340).

- Prolonged severe hypoglycaemia (> 4h) results in permanent cerebral dysfunction.

- Patients on sulphonylureas may become hypoglycaemic following a CVA or other illness preventing adequate food intake.

- Recurrent hypoglycaemia may herald the onset of diabetic nephropathy, since this decreases insulin requirements: insulin is partly degraded by the kidney.

Liver dysfunction and recurrent hypoglycaemia

- Hypoglycaemia is common in acute liver failure, when coma may occur (as a result of liver failure rather than hypoglycaemia). Severe hypoglycaemia is rare in chronic liver disease.

- In chronic alcoholics it is advisable to administer iv thiamine (1–2mg/kg) before iv dextrose to avoid precipitating neurological damage.

- An acute ingestion of alcohol can also suppress hepatic gluconeogenesis.

- Congestive cardiac failure and septic shock are also known to cause hypoglycaemia by inhibiting hepatic gluconeogenesis.

Urgent surgery in patients with diabetes

Surgery requires patients to fast for several hours. In addition, a general anaesthetic and surgery produces significant stresses on an individual. The hormonal response to stress involves a significant rise in counter-regulatory hormones to insulin, in particular cortisol and adrenaline. For this reason, patients with diabetes undergoing surgery will require an increased dose of insulin despite their fasting state.

Type I DM (insulin dependent)

- Always try to put the patient first on the list. Inform the surgeon and anaesthetist early.
- Discontinue long-acting insulin the night before surgery if possible. If the patient has taken a long-acting insulin and requires emergency surgery, an infusion of 10% dextrose (10–100ml/h) can be used, together with an insulin sliding scale.
- Ensure iv access is available.
- When nil by mouth, start iv infusion of 5% dextrose with potassium (20mmol/litre) at 100ml/h and continue until oral intake is adequate. Remember saline requirements (~ 100–150mmol Na/24h but increases post operatively) but do not stop dextrose infusion (risk of hypo-glycaemia).
- Commence an iv insulin sliding scale (see table p443). Measure finger prick glucose hourly and adjust the insulin infusion accordingly. Aim for 7–11mmol/l.
- If close monitoring (hourly glucose measurements) is not possible and there is no risk of heart failure, an alternative is to add soluble insulin to 500ml bags of 5% dextrose (with potassium 20mmol/l) and infuse at 80–120ml/h. Adjust the amount of insulin to add to each bag from the mean blood glucose during the previous infusion using the table on p443 as a guide to requirement.
- Continue the insulin sliding scale until the second meal and restart the normal sc dose of insulin. As iv insulin has a very short half-life (3.5 min), this must be continued until the patient's sub-cutaneous insulin is being absorbed; an overlap of 4h is recommended.

Type II DM (non-insulin dependent)

- Discontinue sulphonylurea or long-acting insulin the night before surgery if possible. If the patient has taken their oral hypoglycaemic or insulin and requires emergency surgery, start an infusion of 10% dextrose (10–100ml/h) with an insulin sliding scale.
- Check a fasting glucose: if > 12mmol/l treat as above.
- If the patient's diabetes is normally managed with oral hypoglycaemic agents, these can be restarted once the patient is eating normally. The sliding scale can be tailed off 4h later.
- Diet-controlled diabetics often do not require a sliding scale at the time of surgery but may require iv insulin post operatively for a short period if blood glucose rises > 12mmol/l. This may be tailed off, when eating normally.

Urgent surgery in patients with diabetes

Add 50 units of actrapid to 50ml 0.9% saline and administer by intra- **443** venous infusion. The sliding scale below is a guide only:-

Blood glucose (mmol/l) (hourly)	Insulin infusion (units/hour)
< 2.0	Stop insulin – Call doctor
2.1 – 5.0	0.5
5.1 – 7.0	1
7.1 – 10.0	2
10.1 – 15.0	3
15.1 – 20.0	4
20.1 – 28.0	6
> 28.1	Call doctor

- Adjust the scale according to the patient's usual requirement of insulin (e.g. a patient on Mixtard® 36U/24U requires 60U/24h, i.e. 2.5U/h normally).
- If blood glucose is persistently low (< 4mmol/l) decrease all insulin infusion values by 0.5–1.0U/h.
- If blood glucose is persistently high (> 13.0mmol/l) increase all insulin infusion values by 0.5–1.0U/h.

Hyponatraemia: Assessment

Presentation

- Mild hyponatraemia is common, especially in patients taking diuretics, and is usually asymptomatic.
- Serum Na^+ ~ 120mmol/l may be associated with disturbed mental state, restlessness, confusion, and irritability. Seizures and coma prevail as the sodium approaches 110mmol/l. Mortality is high.
- Additional symptoms relate to the undelying aetiology (see below) and to the fluid status (extracellular volume ↑ or ↓).

Examination should focus on careful assessment of the ECV:-

- Evaluate the neck veins – is the JVP elevated or low?
- Supine and standing bp to look for orthostatic hypotension.
- Any signs of excess extracellular fluid (e.g. S3, oedema)?
- Skin turgor-tenting for > 1s after pinching suggests low ECV.

Investigations

- In addition to U&Es, other tests shoud be aimed at excluding other causes of hyponatraemia (see table p46).
- Measure serum osmolarity and compare it to the calculated osmolarity $[2 \times (Na^+ + K^+) + urea + glucose]$ – an **_increase in osmolar gap_** occurs with substances such as ethylene glycol, severe hyperglycaemia, mannitol, etc.
- Urine Na^+ combined with clinical assessment of fluid status may help determine the underlying cause:
  - Volume depletion from an extra-renal cause (see table p446) is normaly associated with a low urinary Na^+ (< 10mM).
  - Dehydration with a high urinary Na^+ (> 10mM) suggests inappropriate renal salt-wasting (e.g. intrinsic renal disease, adrenal insufficiency, diuretics).
  - Fluid overload with a low urine Na^+ is seen in conditions such as CCF, cirrhosis, or nephrotic syndrome, where there is sodium retention in response to poor renal perfusion ± elevated ADH.
  - Euvolaemia with a high urine Na^+ is seen with SIADH and, rarely, with severe myxoedema.
- Patients with SIADH commonly have no obvious clinical heart failure and have normal thyroid and adrenal function. Serum Na^+ (and chloride) and osmolality are decreased but the urine is inappropriately concentrated with urine Na^+ > 20mmol/l and often urine osmolality > serum osmolality (not always).

General principles

- Assessment of the patient's volume status (neck veins, orthostatic hypotension, cardiac signs of fluid overload, skin turgor) will help in both diagnosis and subsequent treatment.
- Mild asymptomatic hyponatraemia will usually respond to treatment of the underlying cause and no specific therapy is necessary.
- Correction of hyponatraemia should be gradual so as to avoid both volume overload and central pontine myelinolysis. Aim to restore th serum Na^+ to ~ 125mmol/l actively (iv fluids) and allow to rise gradually after that by treating the underlying cause.
- Seek expert help if serum Na^+ < 125mmol/l ± severely symptomatic.
- Patients with cirrhosis and ascites should be treated by water restriction before considering diuretics.

Hyponatraemia

Hyponatraemia: Management

Causes of hyponatraemia

Decreased serum osmolarity	

Decreased extracellular volume (ECV)

Renal losses (uNa > 20mmol/l)	Non-renal losses (uNa < 20mmol/l)
Diuretics	GI losses (diarrhoea, vomiting)
Addison's disease	Burns
Na-losing nephropathies	Fluid sequestration
	(e.g. peritonitis, pancreatitis)

Normal-mildly increased ECV

SIADH – Urine osm. > 100 when serum osm. low (< 260)

• CNS disorders	• Malignancy	• Pulmonary disease
Trauma	Lung (oat cell)	Pneumonia
Stroke/SAH	Pancreas	TB
Malignancy ($1°/2°$)	Lymphoma or	Lung abscess
Vasculitis (e.g. SLE)	leukaemia	Cystic fibrosis
Infection (abscess, or	Prostate	Lung vasculitis
meningo-encephalitis)	Urinary tract	

Drugs (via SIADH $\pm \uparrow$ renal sensitivity to ADH or Na > H_2O loss)

Opiates	Thioradizine	Chlorpropamide
Haloperidol	Carbamazepine	Thiazides
Amitriptyline	Clofibrate	Cyclophosphamide
Vasopressin	Oxytocin	Vincristine

Miscellaneous causes

Severe myxoedema	Psychogenic polydipsia

Markedly increased ECV

- Congestive cardiac failure
- Severe renal failure
- Cirrhosis with ascites
- Nephrotic syndrome

Normal serum osmolarity	

- Pseudo-hyponatraemia (e.g. lipaemic serum, paraprotein > 10g/dl)
- Intracellular shift of Na^+ (e.g. hyperglycaemia, ethylene glycol)

Management: specific measures

1 *Exclude pseudohyponatraemia:* Lipaemic serum may be obvious at the time of phlebotomy. Calculate the osmolar gap to chech there are no 'hidden' osmoles (p444). Always exclude the possibility of artefactual $\downarrow Na^+$ from blood taken proximal to an iv infusion.

2 *If seizures or coma:* Rapid correction may help to prevent irreversible damage. Seek expert help early. Start rapid iv infusion of normal saline (0.9%), e.g. 500ml/hour, watching carefully for fluid overload until hypertonic saline can be located. When available give 5% saline at 70mmol Na^+/hr until serum sodium > 120mmol/l.

3 *If volume deplete (dehydrated):* Start an iv infusion of normal saline (0.9% = 150mmol/l Na^+); if hypotensive give colloid in addition and insert a central venous line. Monitor fluid output: catheterize the bladder if there is renal impairment. Watch out for heart failure.

4 *If not dehydrated:* For patients with SIADH, restrict fluid intake to 800–1000ml/24h. If serum Na^+ < 125mmol/l, and not responding to fluid restriction, consider demeclocycline (250mg po tds) to induce temporary nephrogenic diabetes insipidus. Severely ill patients may respond to frusemide and hypertonic saline. Seek expert help.

Hyponatraemia

Hypernatraemia

Abnormalities in serum sodium are usually associated with changes in serum osmolality and extracellular volume (ECV). The way to determine the cause of abnormal serum Na^+ is by:

1 Careful assessment of the ECV [evaluation of neck veins, supine and standing bp, any cardiac signs of fluid overload (e.g. S3, oedema), and skin turgor], in association with,

2 Measuring the serum ($\pm$ urine) osmolality. [Serum osmolality may be estimated by $[2 \times (Na^+ + K^+) + urea + glucose]$ but this is inaccurate when there are other osmoles (e.g. ketones, ethanol, methanol, ethylene glycol, renal failure) that contribute].

Serum $Na^+ > 145mmol/l$ is always associated with hyperosmolarity.

Causes of hypernatraemia

Normal or $\downarrow$ extraellular volume (excessive Na and H_2O loss)
- *Renal losses* (urinary osm inappropriately low)
  - Diabetes insipidus (central or nephrogenic)
  - Osmotic diureses with water replacement only (e.g. DM)
- *Non-renal losses* (urinary osm > 400 mEq/l)
  - Hypotonic GI losses (e.g. diarrhoea) esp. if only H_2O replaced
  - Cutaneous losses (burns with excessive water replacement, heat shock, sweating, and high fever)
  - Chest infections with prolonged hyperventilation

Increased extracellular volume (usually 'iatrogenic')
- Concentrated $NaHCO_3$
- Concentrated infant formula
- Conn's syndrome (hypertension, hypokalaemia, alkalosis)

Presentation

- Symptoms often relate to severe volume depletion: weakness, malaise, fatigue altered mental status, confusion, delirium, or coma.
- Assess hydration status: resting or postural hypotension, tissue turgor.

Management

- If there is symptomatic hypotension, start fluid replacement with 0.9% saline iv at a rate determined by the patient's condition. This is hypotonic (as compared to the patient's current state) and will restore the circulating volume as well as lower the serum sodium.
- If the patient is haemodynamically stable encourage oral fluids.
- Once euvolaemic, the total body water deficit (in litres):

$$= [0.6 \times \text{ideal body wt (kg)}] \times \left[1 - \frac{140}{[\text{Patient's Na}^+]}\right]$$

This is the theoretical amount of 'free-water' required to restore the serum sodium to normal.

- Give half over the first 18–24 hours (as 5% dextrose iv if symptomatic or serum $Na^+ > 160mM$) and the remainder over the next 1–2 days. Too aggressive rehydration may result in cerebral oedema and seizures.
- Monitor electrolytes 4–6 hourly.

Acute hypocalcaemia

Presentation
- Abnormal neurological sensations and neuromuscular excitability
- Numbness around the mouth and paraesthesiae of the distal limbs
- Hyperreflexia
- Carpopedal spasm
- Tetanic contractions (may include laryngospasm)
- Generalized seizures
- Hypotension, bradycardias, arrhythmias, and CCF
- Chvostek's sign is elicited by tapping the facial nerve just anterior to the ear, causing ipsilateral contraction of the facial muscles. (Positive in 10% of normals)
- Trousseau's sign is elicited by inflating a blood pressure cuff for 3–5 minutes 10–20mmHg above the level of systolic blood pressure. This causes limb ischaemia, unmasks latent neuromuscular hyper-excitability and carpal spasm is observed.

Causes
- Renal failure (associated hyperphosphataemia)
- Vitamin D deficiency or abnormal vitamin D hydroxylation
- Hypoparathyroidism (primary, secondary, or post surgical)
- Pseudohypoparathyroidism
- Severe Mg^{2+} deficiency ($\downarrow$ PTH secretion and resistance to PTH)
- Acute complexing or sequestration of calcium [acute pancreatitis, rhabdomyolysis, alkalosis (e.g. hyperventilation)]

Investigations
- Plasma calcium (and albumin) and phosphate
- Plasma magnesium
- U&Es
- ECG (prolonged QT interval)
- Plasma PTH level
- SXR (intracranial calcification, esp. hypoparathyroidism)

Management
- The aim of **acute** management is to ameliorate the acute manifestations of hypocalcaemia, and not necessarily to return the calcium to normal.
- For frank tetany, 10ml of 10% calcium gluconate (2.25mmol) can be given by slow iv injection over 5 minutes. iv calcium should never be given faster than this because of the risk of arrhythmia.
- If necessary give a constant infusion of Ca^{2+}, upto 0.05mmol/kg/hour.
- Post parathyroidectomy, mild hypocalcaemia normally ensues, requiring observation only. In patients who have parathyroid bone disease however, 'hungry bones' may cause profound hypocalcaemia shortly after the parathyroids are removed. This may cause a severe and prolonged hypocalcaemia requiring prolonged (several days) treatment.
- Chronic hypocalcaemia is best managed with oral calcium together with either vitamin D, or, if the cause is hypoparathyroidism or an abnormality in vitamin D metabolism, a form of activated (hydroxylated) vitamin D such as alfacalcidol or calcitriol.

Hypercalcaemia

- The free (ionic) plasma Ca^{2+} concentration is dependent on both arterial pH (↑ during acidaemia) and the plasma albumin.
- Ionized Ca^{2+} = Measured Ca^{2+} + [40 − serum albumin(g/l)] × 0.02. (e.g. if measured Ca^{2+} = 2.10 mM and albumin = 30 g/l, the corrected Ca^{2+} = 2.10 = [(40−30) × 0.02] = 2.30 mM).

Presentation

- Routine biochemical screen in an asymptomatic patient
- Gastrointestinal features: abdominal pain (may be severe), nausea, vomiting, constipation.
- Polyuria, polydipsia, or dehydration.
- Tiredness, weakness, anorexia, and malaise
- Depression, weight loss
- Renal calculi and renal failure
- Severe hypercalcaemia may cause confusion, delirium, or coma.
- Sudden cardiac arrest

Urgent treatment is required if:

- Calcium > 3.5mmol/l
- Clouding of consciousness or confusion is present
- Hypotension
- Severe abdominal pain
- Severe dehydration causing pre-renal failure

Management

- Rehydrate patient with iv **N saline** (0.9%). Aim for about 3–6 litres in 24 hours depending on fluid status (CVP), urine output, and cardiac function.
- If patient does not pass urine for 4h, pass a urinary catheter and a central venous line to monitor CVP.
- Once patient is rehydrated, continue N saline infusion and add **frusemide** 40–120mg every 4 hours. Continue monitoring CVP carefully to prevent either fluid overload or dehydration.
- Monitor electrolytes, especially K^+ and Mg^{2+} which may fall rapidly with rehydration and frusemide. Replace K^+ (20–40mmol/l of saline) and Mg^{2+} (up to 2mmol/l saline) intravenously.
- If this fails to reduce plasma Ca^{2+} adequately (Ca^{2+} still > 2.8mM) then the following measures should be considered:
  - **Steroids** (prednisolone 30–60mg po od). Most effective in hypercalcaemia due to sarcoidosis, myeloma, or vitamin D intoxication.
  - **Salmon calcitonin** 400 IU q8h. This has a rapid onset of action (within hours) but its effect lasts only 2–3 days (tachyphylaxis).
  - **Disodium pamidronate** is a diphosphonate which binds to hydroxyapatite in bone and inhibits osteoclast activity, thereby causing a fall in plasma Ca^{2+}. Administer 30–90mg iv over 4–6 hours. (As a general rule give 30mg over 4h if Ca^{2+} is < 3mM, 60mg over 8h if Ca^{2+} is 3–4mM, and 90mg over 24h if Ca^{2+} is > 4mM.) Ca^{2+} levels begin to fall after 48 hours and remain suppressed for up to 14 days.
- *Familial benign hypocalciuric hypercalcaemia*: ↑ Ca^{2+}, N 24h urinary Ca^{2+}. This causes few symptoms (mild fatigue or lethargy). The PTH may be raised but the patients do not respond to parathyroidectomy.

Causes of hypercalcaemia

- Primary (or tertiary) hyperparathyroidism
- Malignancy
  - Humoral hypercalcaemia
  - Local osteolytic hypercalcaemia (e.g. myeloma, metastases)
- Hyperthyroidism
- Granulomatous disorders (sarcoidosis)
- Drug related
  - Vitamin D intoxication
  - 'Milk-alkali' syndrome
  - Thiazide diuretics
  - Lithium
- Immobilization (Paget's disease)
- Benign familial hypocalciuric hypercalcaemia
- HTLV-1 infection may present with severe hypercalcaemia
- Phaeochromocytoma (part of MEN type II)

Investigations for hypercalcaemia

- Plasma Ca^{2+}, PO_4^{3-} and Mg^{2+}
- U&Es
- LFTs
- CXR
- Plasma PTH level
- 24h urinary Ca^{2+}
- Urinary cAMP

Hypophosphataemia

Total body phosphorus is approximately 23 moles, of which 80% is in bone, 9% in muscle, and the rest in the viscera and extracellular fluid. Plasma phosphate is normally 0.8–1.4mmol/l. Hypophosphataemia is common, and often unrecognized by clinicians. Most intracellular phosphate is present as creatine phosphate or adenine phosphates (e.g. ATP), and in RBC the predominant species is 2,3–diphosphoglycerate. Hypophosphataemia does not necessarily indicate phosphate deficiency; similarly, phosphate deficiency may be associated with normal or high plasma phosphate concentrations.

Causes of hypophosphataemia	
Modest (0.4–0.6mmol/l)	**Severe (< 0.4mmol/l)**
• Decreased dietary intake	• Respiratory alkalosis
• Vitamin D deficiency	• Treatment of diabetic ketoacidosis
• Chronic liver disease	• Alcohol withdrawal (esp. with ketoacidosis)
• Hyperparathyroidism	
• Decreased absorption (vit. D deficiency, steatorrhoea, phosphate binding antacids)	• Acute liver failure
	• Hyperalimentaion (i.e. feeding after starvation)
• Hungry bones syndrome (post parathyroidectomy, acute leukaemia)	• Ventilation of chronic severe respiratory failure
• Lymphoma or the leukaemias	• Neuroleptic malignant syndrome
• Hyperaldosteronism	
• Diuretics	
• Steroid therapy	

Presentation

- Most cases of severe hypophosphataemia occur in very sick patients (often in an ITU). Occasionally seen in asymptomatic patients.
- Coincident magnesium deficiency may exacerbate phosphate depletion and vice versa.
- Modest hypophosphataemia has no effect, but warrants investigation. Severe hypophosphataemia (< 0.4mmol/l) may cause symptoms and requires treatment.

Manifestations of severe hypophosphataemia	
• Myopathy (involving skeletal muscle and diaphragm)	• CNS dysfunction (encephalopathy, irritability, seizures, paraesthesiae, coma)
• Rhabdomyolysis	
• Cardiomyopathy	• Respiratory failure
• Erythrocyte dysfunction	• Reduced platelet half-life
• Leukocyte dysfunction	• Mineral mobilization
• Metabolic acidosis	

Treatment

- Phosphate repletion should generally be reserved for patients with sustained hypophosphataemia. Give oral effervescent *Phosphate Sandoz®* 2 tabs tds; or potassium phosphate iv (9–18mmol/24h).
- Excessive phosphate replacement may cause hypocalcaemia and metastatic calcification; monitor Ca^{2+}, PO_4^{3-}, K^+, and other electrolytes closely.

Addisonian crisis: Assessment

Adrenocortical insufficiency may be sub-clinical for days or months in otherwise well individuals. Stress, such as infection, trauma, or surgery, may precipitate an Addisonian crisis with cardiovascular collapse and death if the condition is not suspected. Crises may also occur in patients with known Addison's disease on replacement hydrocortisone if they fail to increase their steroid dose with infections.

Presentation
- Hypotension and cardiovascular collapse (shock).
- Faintness, particularly on standing (postural hypotension).
- Nausea and vomiting.
- Hyponatraemia.
- Dehydration (thirst may not be apparent because of the low sodium).
- Diarrhoea in 20% of cases.
- Symptoms of precipitant [fever, night sweats (infection); flank pain (haemorrhagic adrenal infarction); etc]. Note signs/symptoms of other endocrinopathies.
- Non-specific symptoms – weight loss, fatigue, weakness, myalgia, anorexia.
- Hyperpigmentation suggests chronic hypoadrenalism.
- Psychiatric features are common and include asthenia, depression, apathy, and confusion. (Treatment with glucocorticoids reverses most psychiatric features.)

Causes
(See table opposite)
Malignant secondaries are present in the adrenals of a high percentage of patients with lung cancer, breast tumours, and malignant melanomas. Adrenal failure will only occur when over 90% of the gland is replaced by metastases.
Adrenal haemorrhage may complicate sepsis, traumatic shock, coagulopathies, and ischaemic disorders.
- Severe stress substantially increases the arterial blood supply to the adrenals. However, the adrenal gland has only one or two veins, making it vulnerable to venous thrombosis. Raised catecholamine levels also increase platelet aggregation.
- The clinical presentation of adrenal haemorrhage is often vague and indolent (except the Waterhouse-Friderichsen syndrome).
- Blood tests: a precipitous drop in haemoglobin, hyponatraemia, hyperkalaemia, acidosis, uraemia, and neutrophilia.
- The *Waterhouse-Friderichsen syndrome* is the association of bilateral adrenal haemorrhage with fulminant meningo-coccaemia. Adrenal haemorrhage is also seen with other Gram-negative endotoxaemias such as *Diplococcus pneumoniae*, *Haemophilus influenzae* B and DF-2 bacillus infections.

Hypopituitarism As there is no mineralocorticoid deficiency, the salt and water loss and shock are less profound than in primary Addison's disease.
Drugs Rifampicin, phenytoin, and phenobarbitone accelerate the metabolism of cortisol and may precipitate Addisonian crisis in partially compromised individuals, or in those on a fixed replacement dose. Most adrenal crises precipitated by rifampicin occur within 2 weeks of initiating therapy.

Recognized causes of an Addisonian crisis

- Autoimmune adrenalitis
- Tuberculosis of the adrenals
- Malignant secondaries in the adrenal glands
- Adrenal haemorrhage
- Hypopituitarism
- Drugs   Metyrapone (inhibits 11–hydroxylase)
  - Aminoglutethimide
  - Ketoconazole
  - Etomidate
  - Rifampicin, phenytoin, and phenobarbitone

Addisonian crisis: Management

Investigations

- U&Es — Hyponatraemia and hyperkalaemia (rarely greater than 6.0mM), with Na:K ratio < 21:1; dehydration
- FBC — Anaemia (normal MCV); moderate neutropenia ± relative eosinophilia / lymphocytosis
- Glucose — Hypoglycaemia
- Calcium — May be high (but corrected Ca^{2+} usually normal)
- Serum cortisol — (Save for routine assay) Baseline < 400nmol/l. Should be > 1000nmol/l in 'sick' patients
- ABG — Metabolic acidosis, respiratory failure, low bicarbonate
- Urine — MC&S for infection; urinary Na excretion often high in spite of hypovolaemia
- CXR — Previous TB, bronchial carcinoma
- AXR — ? Adrenal calcification

Management

- Treatment may be required before the diagnosis is confirmed.
- General measures include oxygen, continuous ECG monitoring, CVP monitoring, urinary catheter (for fluid balance), and broad spectrum antibiotics (e.g. cefotaxime) for underlying infection.
- **Treat shock** (p210): Give iv N saline or colloid (PPF or Haemaccel®) for hypotension: 1 litre stat. then hourly depending on response and clinical signs. Inotropic support may be necessary.
- Give iv **50% dextrose** (50ml) if hypoglycaemic.
- If adrenal crisis is suspected, the patient needs glucocorticoids urgently: use **dexamethasone** 8mg iv which will not interfere with the cortisol assay of a short Synacthen® test. This single extra dose can do little harm and may be life-saving.
- **Short Synacthen® test** (omit if the patient is known to have Addison's disease): Take baseline blood sample (serum) and administer tetracosactrin (Synacthen®) 250µg im or iv. Take further samples at 30 and 60 min for cortisol assay.
- Continue steroid treatment as iv **hydrocortisone** (200mg stat.), then 100mg tds. Change to oral steroids after 72h when the patient has stabilized.
- **Fludrocortisone** (100µg daily orally) when stabilised on oral replacement doses of hydrocortisone.

Prevention

- Patients on long-term steroid therapy and/or known adrenocortical failure should be instructed to increase steroid intake for predictable stresses (e.g. elective surgery, acute illnesses with fever > 38°).
- For mild illnesses, if not vomiting, double the oral dose. Vomiting requires iv/im therapy (hydrocortisone 50mg tds).
- For minor operations or procedures (e.g. cystoscopy) give hydrocortisone 100mg iv/im as a single dose before the procedure.
- More serious illnesses require hydrocortisone 100mg q6–8h iv/im until recovered, or for at least 72 hours.
- Double replacement doses if on 'enzyme-inducing drugs'.

Equivalent doses of glucocorticoids[2]	
Drug	Equivalent dose (mg)
Dexamethasone	0.75
Methylprednisolone	4
Triamcinolone	4
Prednisolone	5
Hydrocortisone	20
Cortisone acetate	25

British National Formulary (1995) Pharmaceutical Press, Royal Pharmaceutical Society of Great Britain, London; **30**: Section 6.3.2.

Myxoedema coma

A common precipitant of coma is the use of sedatives, and subsequent hypothermia, in elderly patients with undiagnosed hypothyroidism.

Presentation
- Altered mental status: disorientation, lethargy, frank psychosis.
- Coma (symmetrical, slow-relaxing reflexes; ~ 25% have seizures).
- Hypothermia (see p748).
- Bradycardia.
- Respiratory failure with CO_2 retention.
- Hypoglycaemia.

Investigations
U&Es	Hyponatraemia is common.
Glucose	Hypoglycaemia may occur.
FBC	Normocytic or macrocytic anaemia ($\pm$ coexistent pernicious anaemia).
Raised CPK	Often with a clinical myopathy.
Thyroid function	T4 and TSH
Cortisol	To exclude coexistent Addison's disease, i.e. Schmidt's syndrome.
ABG	Hypoventilation with $\uparrow P_aCO_2$, $\downarrow P_aO_2$ and metabolic acidosis.
Septic screen	Blood and urine cultures.
ECG	Small complexes with prolonged QT interval.

Poor prognostic indicators
- *Hypotension.* Myxoedematous patients are usually hypertensive. Hypotension indicates possible coexistent blood loss. Response to inotropes is poor as patients are usually maximally vasoconstricted.
- *Hypoventilation.* This is the commonest cause of death in patients with myxoedema coma. The hypoxia responds poorly to oxygen therapy which tends to exacerbate hypercapnoea.

Management
- Transfer the patient to an intensive care unit.
- Mechanical ventilation should be instituted for respiratory failure.
- Central venous access. Hypothyroid patients are usually hypertensive and hypovolaemic since chronic myxoedema is compensated for by rising catecholamines.
- Broad spectrum antimicrobials (e.g. cefotaxime). Bacterial infection i a common precipitant of myxoedema coma.
- Hypothermia should be treated as on p748: a space blanket is usuall sufficient. Rapid external warming can cause inappropriate vasc dilatation and cardiovascular collapse.
- Hydrocortisone (100mg iv tds) until Addison's is excluded.
- Institute replacement therapy before confirming the diagnosis. If th patient is euthyroid, no harm is done by a few doses of thyroxine.
- Ideally, give 5–20µg iv (slow bolus) tri-iodothyronine (T3) daily f three days and then 25µg oral T4 daily. T3 is preferable due to its sho half-life and its effect disappears 24–48h after it is stopped.
- If T3 is unavailable use T4 25–50µg po or via NG-tube daily.
- Although rapid changes are undesirable, myxoedema coma has a extremely high mortality if inadequately treated. Thyroid replaceme therapy may precipitate cardiac ischaemia, and needs to be cautious.

Precipitants of myxoedema coma
• Drugs, including sedatives and tranquillizers
• Infection
• Cerebrovascular accident
• Trauma

Thyrotoxic crisis: Assessment

The term thyrotoxic crisis refers to a constellation of symptoms and signs which together imply a poor prognosis. Thyroid function tests provide no discrimination between simple thyrotoxicosis and thyrotoxic crisis. If the diagnosis has not been made, look for clues such as a goitre, or exophthalmic Graves disease. The presentation may be confused with sepsis or malignant hyperthermia.

Presentation

Cardiovascular symptoms
- Palpitations
- Tachycardia/tachyarrhythmias
- Cardiac failure/oedema

CNS symptoms
- Anxiety/agitation
- Violent outbursts
- Psychosis/delirium
- Fitting/coma

Gastrointestinal symptoms
- Diarrhoea
- Vomiting
- Jaundice

General symptoms
- Fever
- Hyperventilation
- Sweating
- Polyuria

Precipitants of thyrotoxic crisis
- Thyroid surgery/general surgery
- Withdrawal of antithyroid drug therapy/radio-iodine therapy
- Thyroid palpation
- Iodinated contrast dyes
- Infection
- Cerebrovascular accident/pulmonary embolism
- Parturition
- Diabetic ketoacidosis
- Trauma or emotional stress

Investigations
- Thyroid function tests (most labs can perform either an urgent TSH or an urgent free T4)
- U&Es (?dehydration)
- Calcium (may be elevated)
- Glucose (may be low)
- FBC
- Liver function tests (?jaundice)
- Blood and urine cultures
- CXR (?pulmonary oedema or evidence of infection)
- ECG (rate,?atrial fibrillation)

Assessment of severity
- The table opposite is a guide for the assessment of a thyrotoxic crisis.
- Rarely, patients may present with an apathetic thyroid storm, and lapse into coma with few other signs of thyrotoxicosis.

Assessment of severity of a thyrotoxic crisis

Temp (°C)	Pulse	Cardiac failure	CNS effects	GI symptoms	Score
Apyrexial	< 90	Absent	Normal	Normal	0
> 37.2	> 90	Ankle oedema	–	–	5
> 37.8	> 110	Basal creps.	Agitation	Diarrhoea, vomiting	10
> 38.3	> 120	Pulmonary oedema	–	–	15
> 38.9	> 130		Delirium	Unexplained jaundice	20
> 39.4	> 140		–	–	25
> 40			Coma, seizure	–	30

- Add the scores for each column.
- Add an extra 10 points if atrial fibrillation is present.
- Add 10 points if there is a definable precipitant.
- A total score of over 45 indicates thyroid crisis; a score of 25–44 indicates impending crisis.

Thyrotoxic crisis: Management

Patients with a thyrotoxic crisis or impending crisis (score > 25, see p463)

- Admit the patient to intensive care.

- **Fluid balance:** CVP monitoring is essential to avoid precipitating or worsening cardiac failure. In patients with arrhythmias, the CVP will not accurately reflect left-sided pressures and PCWP monitoring with a pulmonary artery catheter should be considered. Gastrointestinal and insensible (pyrexia and excessive sweating) fluid losses may exceed 5 litres/day and must be replaced.

- Fever should be treated with **paracetamol** and aggressive **peripheral cooling techniques** such as ethanol washes, ice packs, and cooling blankets. Do not use salicylates which will displace T4 from TBG and can therefore worsen the storm.

- **Beta-block** the patient with propranolol 60mg q4h po or 1mg iv (repeated every 10–20 min as necessary) with cardiac monitoring. Propranolol inhibits peripheral T4 → T3 conversion. Fever, tachycardia, and tremor should respond immediately.

  If β-blockade is contraindicated (e.g. asthma), guanethidine (30–40mg po 6 hourly) can be used. Note that rate-dependent heart failure (pulse > 140) caused by a thyrotoxic crisis is improved by β-blockade. It is important to ascertain that the patient does not have a past history of cardiac failure, which may be worsened by β-blockade.

- **Treat precipitating factors** such as infection (cefuroxime 750mg iv tds).

- High-dose **antithyroid drugs**. Propylthiouracil (1g loading dose then 200–300mg q4h po/NG) is more effective than carbimazole (20mg 4 hourly), at it inhibits peripheral T4 → T3 conversion.

- **Hydrocortisone** 300mg iv stat., then 100mg 6 hourly. This inhibits conversion of T4 to T3.

- Once organification of iodine has been blocked by antithyroid drugs, iodine can be used to inhibit thyroxine release from thyroid gland. **Lugol's iodine** contains 5% iodine and 10% potassium iodide in water. Give 1ml every 6 hours. *Do not give Lugol's iodine until at least one hour after the antithyroid drugs have been given.* Any iodine given prior to antithyroid medication may increase thyroid hormone stores. Continue iodine containing preparations for a maximum of two weeks. (Lithium is an alternative to iodine in allergic patients.)

- **Monitor glucose** levels 4 hourly and administer glucose 5–10% as required. Hepatic glycogen stores are readily depleted during thyroid storm.

- Physical removal of circulating thyroxine with plasmapheresis has been described. This should be reserved for cases that do not respond to all the above measures. Dantrolene has been used successfully to control hyperthermia in thyrotoxic crisis (see p476).

Continuing treatment

- Response to treatment is gauged clinically and by serum T3 levels.
- Stop iodine/potassium iodide/lithium and β-blockers when controlled.
- Consider definitive treatment (e.g. surgery or radioactive iodine).
- Treat atrial fibrillation in the usual way (p62). Higher doses of digoxin may be required as its metabolism is increased. Amiodarone inhibit peripheral T4 → T3 conversion.

Pituitary apoplexy

Presentation

Pituitary infarction may be *silent*. Apoplexy implies the presence of symptoms. The clinical manifestations may be due to leakage of blood/necrotic tissue into the subarachnoid space, or rapid expansion of a suprasellar mass and pressure on local structures. This may be the presenting symptom of the pituitary tumour.

- Headache occurs in 75% of cases (sudden onset; variable intensity).
- Visual disturbance (optic tract compression usually resulting in bitemporal hemianopia).
- Ocular palsy (40%) causing diplopia. Unilateral or bilateral.
- Nausea/vomiting.
- Meningism (common).
- Hemiparesis or, rarely, seizures.
- Fever, anosmia, CSF rhinorrhoea, hypothalamic dysfunction (disturbed sympathetic autoregulation with abnormal bp control, respiration, and cardiac rhythm) are all described, but are rare.
- Altered mental state, lethargy, delirium, or coma.
- Symptoms of preceding pituitary tumour.
- Acute hypopituitarism.

Clinically, pituitary apoplexy may be very difficult to distinguish from subarachnoid haemorrhage, bacterial meningitis, mid-brain infarction (basilar artery occlusion), or cavernous sinus thrombosis. Transient neurological symptoms are common in the preceding few days.

The clinical course is variable. Headache and mild visual disturbance may develop slowly and persist for several weeks. In its most fulminant form, apoplexy may cause blindness, haemodynamic instability, coma and death. Residual endocrine disturbance (pan-hypopituitarism) invariably occurs.

Investigations

- U&Es   Hyper- or hyponatraemia may occur.
- Endocrine tests   Clotted blood for cortisol, thyroid function, prolactin, GH, and the gonadotrophic hormones.
- CT scan   Pituitary 'cuts', with administration of iv contrast, will reveal a tumour mass (or haemorrhage) within 24–48 hours.
- MRI scan   This will not replace CT scanning in the acute setting due to its inability to detect fresh bleeding, although it is especially useful in the sub-acute setting (4 days-1 month).

Management

- Stabilize the patient (Airway, Breathing, Circulation).
- Hydrocortisone 100mg iv should be given if the diagnosis is suspected after the blood samples above have been collected.
- Monitor U&Es and urine output for evidence of diabetes insipidus.
- ***Neurosurgical decompression*** via a transsphenoidal route is the definitive treatment. Obtundation and visual deterioration are absolute indications for neurosurgery. Patients without confusion or visual disturbance generally do well without surgery.
- Assess pituitary function once the acute apoplexy has resolved and treat as necessary. A TSH in the normal range may be inappropriate if the T4 is low in pituitary disease, but this may occur in the sick euthyroid state characteristic of many seriously ill patients.

Pituitary apoplexy

Causes of apoplexy in patients with pituitary adenomas

- Spontaneous haemorrhage (no obvious precipitant – the commonest)
- Anti-coagulant therapy
- Head trauma
- Radiation therapy
- Drugs (e.g. bromocriptine or oestrogen)
- Following tests of pituitary function

Hypopituitary coma

Hypopituitarism does not become evident until 75% of the adeno-hypophysis is destroyed, and at least 90% destruction is required for total loss of pituitary secretion. Complete loss of hormone secretion can rapidly become life-threatening and requires immediate therapy. In a mild or incomplete form, hypopituitarism can remain unsuspected for years.

Presentation

History
In the absence of stress, patients with severe hypopituitarism may have few symptoms or signs. A general anaesthetic or infection may precipitate hypoglycaemia and coma, due to the combination of a lack of GH, cortisol, and thyroxine, all of which have a counter-regulatory effect on insulin. Clues from the history include:-

- Known pituitary adenoma
- Recent difficult delivery: Pituitary infarction following post partum haemorrhage and vascular collapse is still the commonest cause of hypopituitarism. Features include failure of lactation (deficiency of prolactin ± oxytocin), failure of menstruation (lack of gonado-trophins), non-specific features [e.g. tiredness, weakness, loss of body hair and loss of libido (due to ACTH deficiency, hypothyroidism, and gonadotrophin deficiency)].
- Men may give a history of impotence, lethargy, and loss of body hair. Women report loss of menstruation.

Examination
- Examination of the comatose patient is discussed on p304–9.
- Examine specifically for secondary sexual characteristics and physical signs of myxoedema.
- Consider other causes for coma (p304).

Investigations
- General investigations for patients in coma are discussed on p310.
- Take blood for baseline cortisol, ACTH, thyroid function, LH, FSH, prolactin, and GH.
- Short Synacthen® test must be performed to test for adrenocortical reserve (p458).
- LHRH and TRH can be performed at the same time as the short Synacthen® test.
- Defer formal pituitary function testing until the patient is stable.
- CT scan of pituitary (tumour or empty sella).
- MRI scan may give additional information.

Management
- General measures are as for any patient in coma (p306).
- Give iv colloids ± saline to restore bp if the patient is in shock.
- Give glucose if the patient is hypoglycaemic.
- Hydrocortisone 100mg iv should be administered if the diagnosis is suspected and continued (100mg iv tds – see p458).
- Start tri-iodothyronine (10µg bd) *after* hydrocortisone is started.
- Investigate and treat any precipitating intercurrent infection.
- If the patient fails to improve, consider other causes for coma (see p304).

Causes of pan-hypopituitarism

- Destruction of the pituitary gland by primary or metastatic tumour.
- Pituitary apoplexy (p466)
- Post pituitary surgery or radiotherapy
- Ischaemic necrosis (post partum haemorrhage, eclampsia, temporal arteritis, arteriosclerosis)
- Primary empty sella syndrome

Phaeochromocytomas: Assessment

- Phaeochromocytomas are catecholamine-producing tumours derived from chromaffin cells, usually involving one or more adrenal glands. ~10% are bilateral, 10% are extra-adrenal [usually around the sympathetic chain (paragangliomas)], and ~10% are malignant. They usually secrete adrenaline (AD) or noradrenaline (NA). A small proportion secrete dopamine (DA), when hypotension may occur.
- Most are diagnosed during routine screening of hypertensive patients (they are found in only 0.1% of hypertensives). Pure AD-producing tumours may mimic septic shock due to AD-induced peripheral vasodilatation (β_2-receptors).

Presentation

- Hypertension (mild to severe sustained ± uncontrolled paroxysmal, hypertensive episodes)
- Anxiety attacks, tremor, sweating, palpitations, and tachycardia
- Cold extremities, pallor
- Cardiac arrhythmias including atrial and ventricular fibrillation
- Hypertensive crises may be precipitated by β-blockers, tricyclic antidepressants, metoclopramide, and naloxone
- Unexplained lactic acidosis

Investigations

There are no tests which will diagnose a phaeochromocytoma acutely. Investigations are listed in the table opposite.

- Hypertensive patients with ↑ glucose and ↓ K^+ may have a phaeochromocytoma, but these are both common features of treated hypertension (e.g. thiazides), or may indicate other endocrinopathies (e.g. Cushing's, Conn's, secretory adrenal carcinoma).
- **Urinary vanillyl mandelic acid** (VMA) levels (a catecholamine metabolite) are not specific since several dietary substances, including vanilla essence can give a false +ve test result. 15% of patients with essential hypertension have a false +ve VMA. **Urinary catecholamines** (AD, NA, and DA) are more specific. Urine collections must be completed before pentolinium or clonidine tests since withdrawal of these compounds can give a false +ve result.
- **Plasma catecholamines** require a heparinized sample and need to be taken directly to the lab. (on ice) for centrifugation.
- **Pentolinium suppression test.** Take two baseline samples as above, then give 2.5mg pentolinium iv, and take blood again at 10 and 30 minutes. Plasma catecholamines decrease in normal subjects following ganglion blockade with pentolinium. If the response is borderline and no hypotension occurs, then repeat with 5mg pentolinium.
- **Clonidine suppression test.** An alternative to the pentolinium suppression test employs clonidine. Following two baseline samples give 0.3mg clonidine orally, and take blood hourly for three hours. Again, if raised catecholamines are due to anxiety they will suppress into the normal range with clonidine. Raised catecholamines from phaeochromocytoma will not be affected by clonidine.
- **CT and MRI** are useful to localize the tumour.
- **MIBG scan.** MIBG (^{131}I-metaiodobenzylguanidine) is taken up selectively by adrenal tissue. Useful for localization of tumour or secondaries.
- **Selective venous sampling** may be necessary to localize extra-adrenal tumours.

Investigations for suspected phaeochromocytomas

- U&Es ($\downarrow K^+$, $\uparrow$ urea)
- Glucose ($\uparrow$)
- Urinary catecholamines (AD, NA, and DA)
- Plasma catecholamines (AD, NA, and DA)
- Pentolinium suppression test
- Clonidine suppression test
- CT or MRI scan of adrenals
- MIBG scan

Phaeochromocytomas: Management

Patients are usually volume depleted at presentation, and should be rehydrated prior to initiation of α-blockade, otherwise severe hypotension may occur. β-blockade *alone* may precipitate a hypertensive crisis, and must never be given prior to adequate α-blockade. Labetalol is predominantly a β-blocker and should not be used alone. Long-acting α-blockers prevent escape episodes.

- Adequate fluid replacement with CVP monitoring.
- Acute hypertensive crises should be controlled with **phentolamine** (2–5mg iv bolus, repeated as necessary) – see p126.
- Preparation for surgery:-
  - Initiate oral α-blockade: **phenoxybenzamine** 10mg daily increasing gradually to 40mg tds. Monitor bp closely. Tumour β-stimulation may produce excessive vasodilatation and hypotension requiring inotropic support.
  - When the blood pressure is controlled with phenoxybenzamine, add propranolol 10–20mg tds.
  - Invasive monitoring pulmonary artery (Swan-Gantz) catheter and arterial line is mandatory.
- Hypotension commonly occurs intra-operatively when the tumour is removed, and this should be managed with blood, plasma expanders, and inotropes as required. Inotropes should only be used when the patient is appropriately fluid replete. Expansion of intravascular volume 12 hours before surgery significantly reduces the frequency and severity of post operative hypotension. Angiotensin II should be available as an alternative inotrope for cases of resistant hypotension.

Autosomal dominant conditions with a high risk of developing phaeochromocytoma include:

- ***Von-Recklinghausen disease*** [neurofibromata, café au lait spots, Lisch nodules (iris hamartomas) and axillary freckling].
- ***Von-Hippel Lindau disease*** (cerebellar haemangioblastomas, retinal haemangiomas, and other neoplasms including hypernephroma).
- ***Multiple endocrine neoplasia types 2a*** (hyperparathyroidism and medullary thyroid carcinoma) ***and 2b*** (medullary thyroid carcinoma, bowel ganglioneuromatosis, and hypertrophied corneal nerves).

Polyuria

Definition: > 3 litre urine per day

Presentation

- Confusion (hyponatraemia or dehydration)
- Coma
- Proteinuria on screening
- Depression or other psychiatric manifestations
- Renal stones

Causes

- Excessive fluid intake (e.g. psychogenia polydipsia)
- Endocrine dysfunction (DM, diabetes insipidus, hypercalcaemia)
- Hypokalaemia
- Intrinsic renal disease (polycystic kidneys, analgesic nephropathy, medullary cystic disease, amyloidosis) or renal recovery from ATN. Post obstructive, e.g. after catheterization of patient in chronic retention. Post renal artery angioplasty.
- Drugs (frusemide, alcohol, lithium, amphotericin B, vinblastine, demeclocycline, cisplatinum).

History

- Duration and severity (nocturia, frequency, water consumption at night)
- FH of diabetes mellitus, polycystic kidneys, renal calculi
- Drug history (diuretics, analgesics, lithium, etc., see above)
- Renal calculi (hypercalcaemia)
- Weakness (low potassium), depression (hypercalcaemia)
- Pschiatric history
- Endocrine history (menses, sexual function, lactation, pubic hair) for pituitary lesions.
- Other significant pathology (e.g. causes of amyloid)

Investigations

- U&Es (renal disease, hypokalaemia)
- Glucose
- Calcium, phosphate and alkaline phosphatase
- Plasma and urine osmolality [a U:P osmolality of < 1.0 indicates diabetes insipidus, intrinsic renal disease (including hypokalaemia), or hysterical drinking]
- AXR (nephrocalcinosis)
- Lithium levels if appropriate
- Dipstick protein and quantitation if indicated

Management

- Assess fluid status (JVP, bp, postural drop, weight charts, CVP).
- Strict fluid balance and daily weights.
- Insert central line to monitor the CVP.
- Measure urinary sodium and potassium (random samples will give an indication of the loss of sodium or potassium initially, and if losses are great, accurate timed samples of < 6 hours are possible).
- Replace fluid losses as appropriate to maintain a normal homeostasis, using combinations of saline and dextrose.
- Monitor potassium, calcium, phosphate, and magnesium daily, or twice daily if necessary.
- If lithium toxicity is present see p652.
- Avoid excessive fluids. Once the patient is optimally hydrated avoid replacing fluids with large volumes to allow physiological homeostasis to occur.
- If diabetes insipidus suspected, arrange water deprivation test (see table opposite).

Water deprivation test

- Stop all drugs the day before the test; no smoking or caffeine.
- Supervise the patient carefully to prevent surreptitious drinking.
- Empty the bladder after a light breakfast. No further fluids po.
- Weigh the patient at time 0, 4, 5, 6, 7, 8 hours into the test. (Stop the test if >3% of body weight is lost).
- Measure serum osmolality at 30min, 4h and hourly till the end of the test. (Check that the plasma osmolality rises to > 290mosmol/kg to confirm an adequate stimulus for ADH release).
- Collect urine hourly and measure the volume and osmolality. (The volume should decrease and osmolality rise. Stop test if urine osmolality > 800mosmol/kg as DI is excluded).
- If polyuria continues, give desmopressin 20μg intranasally at 8h.
- Allow fluids po (water) after 8h. Continue to measure urine osmolality, hourly, for a further 4 hours.

Interpretation

- *Normal response:* Urine osmolality rises to > 800 mosmol/kg with small rise after desmopressin.
- *Cranial DI:* Urine osmolality remains low (< 400mosmol/kg) and increases by > 50% after desmopressin.
- *Nephrogenic DI:* Urine osmolality remains low (< 400mosmol/kg) and only rises a little (< 45%) with desmopressin.
- *Psychogenic polydipsia:* Urine osmolality rises (> 400mosmol/kg) but is typically less than the normal response.

Malignant hyperthermia

Malignant hyperthermia is a drug- or stress-induced catabolic syndrome characterized by excessive muscular contractions, a sudden rise in body temperature, and cardiovascular collapse. The incidence is ~ 1:15000, with a 30% mortality. The cause is unknown, but may involve abnormal calcium homeostasis in skeletal muscle cells. The condition seems to be inherited in an autosomal dominant manner with variable penetrance.

Drugs precipitating malignant hyperthermia	
• Halothane	• Ketamine
• Succinylcholine	• Phencyclidine
• Methoxyflurane and enflurane	• Cyclopropane

Halothane and succinycholine account for 80% of cases

Drugs considered safe in malignant hyperthermia	
• Barbiturates	• Tubocurare
• Nitrous oxide	• Pancuronium
• Diazepam	• Opiates

Diagnosis

- Malignant hyperthermia most commonly presents in the early 20s. The early signs are muscular rigidity, sinus tachycardia and SVTs, increased carbon dioxide production, and hypertension.
- Hyperthermia occurs late, and may be rapidly followed by hypotension, acidosis, and hyperkalaemia, which gives rise to ventricular tachycardia.
- The condition almost always occurs peri-operatively.
- The differential diagnoses includes phaeochromocytoma, thyrotoxic crisis, narcotic-induced hyperthermia in patients taking MAOIs, and drug-induced hyperthermia (caused by cocaine, phencyclidine, amphetamine, LSD, tricyclics, or aspirin).
- Plasma CPK is high.

Management

The aim is to decrease thermogenesis, and promote heat loss.

- ***Dantrolene:*** 1–2.5mg/kg intravenously every 5–10 minutes to a maximum dose of 10mg/kg. The dantrolene should then be continued at a dose of 1–2mg/kg (iv or orally every 6 hours for 2 days).
- Stop any anaesthetic agent.
- External cooling by submersion is helpful. All administered fluids should be chilled.
- Procainamide should be given to all patients to prevent ventricular dysrhythmias (↑ uptake of calcium and may reduce hyperthermia).
- Hypotension should be treated with saline/colloids ± isoproterenol. Dopaminergic and α-adrenergic agonists reduce heat dissipation and should be avoided.
- Some authorities advocate prophylactic anticonvulsants as seizures are common.

Neuroleptic malignant syndrome

The neuroleptic malignant syndrome results from an imbalance of dopaminergic neurotransmitters following neuroleptic drug use. The incidence is ~ 0.5% in patients taking neurolpetic drugs. This syndrome is clinically distinct from malignant hyperthermia (p476); it is not an allergic reaction. The mean age of onset is 40 years. Mortality is ~ 10%.

Drugs associated with neuroleptic malignant syndrome	

• Haloperidol
• Phenothiazines
• Loxapine
• Thioxanthenes
	• Dopamine-depleting drugs
	  – metoclopramide
	  – tetrabenazine
	  – withdrawal of levadopa or
	    amantadine

Clinical features
- Muscular rigidity with dysphagia, and dysarthria early on (96%).
- Extra-pyramidal signs (pseudoparkinsonism), tremor (90%).
- Catatonia – muteness (95%).
- Increased serum CPK/AST (97%).
- Pyrexia (rarely > 40°C) follows onset of rigidity.

The syndrome can occur within hours of initiating drug therapy, but typically takes ~ 1 week. It can also occur following a dosage increase of a well-established drug.

Complications
- Rhabdomyolysis (p294)
- Renal (15%) and hepatic failure
- Fitting is rare
- Cardiovascular collpase
- Disseminated intravascular coagulation
- Respiratory failure

Differential diagnoses
- Malignant hyperthermia (p476)
- Heat stroke (p746)
- Other causes of catatonia
- Thyrotoxic crisis (p462)
- Phaeochromocytoma (p470)
- Drug-induced hyperthermia (caused by cocaine, phencyclidine, amphetamine, LSD, tricyclics, and aspirin)

Management
- Withdrawal of causative agent.
- Dantrolene (1–2mg/kg every 6 hours up to a maximum 300mg/day).
- Paralysis and ventilation (curare, pancuronium).
- Bromocriptine, amantadine, levodopa (increase dopaminergic tone and reduce rigidity, thermogenesis, and extra-pyramidal symptoms).

9 Gastroenterological emergencies

Acute upper gastrointestinal bleeding

Assessment

Presentation

- Haematemesis (bright red, dark clots, coffee grounds)
- Melaena (black, sticky, smelly). This may arise from anywhere proximal to and including the caecum. Blood is cathartic and takes 4–6h to be passed. With massive bleeding (e.g. variceal) there may be dark clots in the stool. Other causes of dark stool include iron therapy, bismuth (present in De-Nol®), liquorice, or excessive consumption of Guinness.
- Weakness/sweating + palpitations
- Postural dizziness and fainting
- Collapse or shock

Causes

Common
- Peptic ulcer (~ 60% of cases, DU > GU)
- Mallory-Weiss tear
- Oesophagitis
- Gastric or oesophageal malignancy
- Varices (oesophageal or fundal)
- Gastritis/gastric erosions

Rare
- Vascular malformations
- Meckel's diverticulum (rare if > 25 years old)
- Small bowel tumours (melaena)
- Crohn's disease
- Coagulation disorders

Assessment of severity – (poor prognostic signs on presentation)
- Age > 60 years
- Shock (bp < 100mmHg systolic in patients < 60 years or < 120mmHg in patients > 60 years. Remember, young patients can tolerate blood volume loss remarkably well – look for both postural drop in bp and/or rise in pulse rate) see p206.
- Inappropriate bradycardia or HR > 120 per min.
- Chronic liver disease
- Other chronic disease (e.g. cardiac, respiratory, renal)
- Bleeding diathesis
- Decreased conciousness level

Management

Liaise with specialists early (On-call endoscopy team and surgeons). Most patients will have stopped bleeding by the time they are seen; however, all upper GI bleeds should be taken seriously as they may re-bleed in hospital, and the mortality following a re-bleed is high.

Priorities are:-

1 Stabilize the patient; protect the airway, restore the circulating volume
2 Identify the source of the bleeding
3 Definitive treatment of the cause to stop the bleeding.

Acute upper gastrointestinal bleeding

Initial management

- ***Protect the airway:*** (position the patient on side)
- ***iv access:*** Use 1 or 2 large bore (14G-16G) cannulae into peripheral vein for initial fluid rescuscitation. If peripheral access is difficult, access via jugular, subclavian, or femoral vein may be necessary. CVP monitoring (see p768) allows early identification of re-bleeding and is essential in older patients or with massive haemorrhage. A fall of 5cm H_2O over 2h is suggestive of re-bleed.
- Take blood for ***Hb and PCV*** (does not fall till the plasma volume has been restored, but if low at presentation suggests massive blood loss or acute on chronic bleeding). ***WCC*** may be elevated but usually < 15000/mm³-look for concomitant sepsis. ***Platelet count*** (if low suggests hypersplenism and chronic liver disease). ***U&Es*** ↑ urea out of proportion to the creatinine indicates protein absorption by the gut. ***Blood glucose*** (may be low in patients with chronic liver disease). ***PT, PTT, and LFTs*** (if liver disease suspected), ***group and X-match*** 4–8 units. Monitor ***arterial blood gases*** in severely ill patients.
- ***Restore the circulating volume***
  - If there are no signs of haemodynamic compromise use a slow infusion of N saline (0.9%) to keep the iv line patent and for maintenance fluids. In patients with excess body sodium (e.g. those with ascites and peripheral oedema) use 5% dextrose infusions.
  - Tachycardia, hypotension, or a postural fall in bp suggests a low intravascular volume. Give 500ml-1 litre colloid over 1 hour (e.g. 4.5% albumin or Haemaccel®) and continue until blood is available. Stable bp takes precedence over body sodium balance.
  - Use compatible blood when it is ready (give 1 unit/h): if the rate of bleeding is slow, packed cells are preferred. If there is massive haemorrhage, ask for 'O'-negative blood which may be given without cross-matching. Save serum for retrospecetive cross-match.
- ***Monitor urine output*** and catheterise the patient if there are signs of haemodynamic compromise. Aim for > 30ml/h. Prompt rescuscitation should restore urine output (see p298 – oliguria).
- ***Watch for the usual signs of overload*** (raised JVP, pulmonary oedema, peripheral oedema). Too rapid transfusion may precipitate pulmonary oedema even before the total lost volume has been replaced.
- Consider passing an ***NG-tube*** This may help confirm 'coffee-grounds' or blood in the stomach and is useful in diagnosing re-bleeding. Saline lavage is of no proven benefit and is not routine. However, the NG-tube is uncomfortable for the patient, may cause further bleeding, gastro-oesopheal reflux, and pulmonary aspiration.
- Keep the patient ***nil by mouth*** for the endoscopy.

Acute upper gastrointestinal bleeding

Determine the source

- **History:** Ask specifically about dyspepsia, alcohol, drug history (e.g. NSAIDs, anti-coagulants), risk factors for liver disease, normal vomit prior to haematemesis (Mallory-Weiss tear, variceal bleed), previous GI bleeds, ulcers, or surgery.

- **Physical examination:** Look for stigmata of chronic liver disease (including hepatomegaly and splenomegaly), scars of previous surgery, telangiectasia (Osler-Weber-Rendu syndrome), abdominal bruit, bruises. Rectal examination is essential.

- **Upper GI endoscopy** should ideally be done within 12 hours of the bleed. It may be difficult to precisely locate the site of bleeding due to clots in the stomach, but it is easy to exclude possible areas of bleeding which may help decide further management. Remember, upper GI bleeding in cirrhotics has a non-variceal origin in ~ 30% of cases.

- **Selective arteriography** of the coeliac axis, superior mesenteric or inferior mesenteric artery is of value when the bleeding site cannot be identified, usually after 2 or more negative endoscopies and bleeding is brisk (0.5–1ml/min). **Barium studies** have been surpassed by endoscopy for diagnostic purposes but are used to diagnose small bowel causes of melena (e.g. Crohn's or tumour).

- **Meckel's scan** may be useful in younger patients (< 25 years) to identify a Meckel's diverticulum.

Stop the bleeding: general measures

- Correct any coagulopathy
  - Platelet count below $50,000/mm^3$ should be treated with platelet support (6–12 units of platelets).
  - If the patient is on anti-coagulants, one must assess the need for anti-coagulation before reversal. If the patient may require re-anti-coagulation (e.g. prosthetic mitral valve), correct with fresh frozen plasma and/or a very low dose of vitamin K (0.5–1mg, iv). Otherwise give fresh frozen plasma (2–4 units) and iv vitamin K (5–10mg).
  - Cryoprecipitate may be required if the fibrinogen levels are low.

- **Serum calcium** may fall after several units of citrate-containing blood transfusion. Give 10ml (4.5mEq) of calcium gluconate for every 3–4 units transfused. Supplement **magnesium** and **phosphate** as necessary (low in alcoholics).

- **Ulcer healing agents** There is no evidence that iv H_2-antagonists or omeprazole decrease the rate of re-bleeding acutely. They assist in healing of peptic ulcers and prevent gastric erosions in the acutely ill, but may predispose to pneumonia in the ventilated patient.

- Give ranitidine 50mg iv (in 20ml N saline) q8h.

- Alternatively, sucralfate 1–2g q6h po or via NG-tube.

Peptic ulcer disease

Bleeding peptic ulcers form the mainstay of upper GI bleeding, accounting for 60% of all cases, and one third of these have been taking a NSAID. Patients may give a history of epigastric discomfort relieved by food, but often there is no prior history.

- **Endoscopy** allows the bleeding site to be visualized. Identification of the bleeding vessel or adherent clot has prognostic significance- > 80% of these patients will re-bleed, cf. < 5% without these stigmata.
  - The bleeding point may be treated endoscopically by electro-coagulation, injection sclerotherapy (1 in 10,000 adrenaline or alcohol injected into the base), heat probe, or laser photo-coagulation, depending on the local facilities.
  - Keep the patient NBM for 6–8 hours post endoscopy in case a repeat endoscopy/surgery is deemed necessary.
- Indications for surgery see table below
- Medical management
  - Treat with H_2–antagonists for 4–8 weeks,
  - Repeat endoscopy at 6–8 weeks to check the lesion has healed.
  - A biopsy should be taken at the original endoscopy for the urease test for *Helicobacter pylori*. If positive add an *H. pylori* eradication regimen (take the advice of the local gastroenterologists).
  - Resistant ulcers warrant treatment with omeprazole 20mg od for 4–6 weeks (+ *H. pylori* eradication if necessary).
- Prognosis Overall mortality is < 10%. Mortality is reduced by early surgery in high risk patients.

Erosive gastritis/oesophagitis

These generally present as relatively minor bleeds, though not always. Represents ~ 20% of upper GI bleeds and are associated with prior use of asprin or other NSAIDs in previously fit patients, or 'stress' in the critically ill patient.

- **Management:** At endoscopy there is commonly a generalized ooze of blood from the inflamed mucosa. Initial management is as before.
- Give H_2–antagonists or sucralfate 1–2g q6h po or via NG-tube.
- Omeprazole is better than H_2–antagonists in healing oesophagitis and oesophageal ulcers. (Give 20mg po od.)
- Correct any clotting disorder.
- If the lesions are too diffuse and the bleeding continues, partial gastric resection may be performed.
- Prognosis ~ 6% of patients with haemorrhagic gastritis require surgery. Overall mortality is < 10%.

Indications for surgery
• Exanguinating haemorrhage (too fast to replace)
• Profuse bleeding   – > 6 units blood in initial rescuscitation
– continued bleeding at > 1 unit per 8 hours
– persistent hypotension
• Re-bleed in hospital
• Lesions which are at high risk of re-bleeding
• Patients with poor prognostic features (p480)
• Special situations, e.g. patients with a rare blood group or patients refusing blood transfusion, should be explored earlier

Peptic ulcer disease
Erosive gastritis/oesophagitis 487

Variceal haemorrhage: Medical management

Oesophageal and gastric varices develop with portal hypertension of whatever cause. Bleeding from them is typically vigorous and difficult to control and often occurs in the setting of abnormal clotting, thrombocytopenia, encephalopathy, and ascites.

- **Diagnosis** History and physical examination may raise the suspicion of a variceal source of bleeding but ~ 30% of patients with cirrhosis have a non-variceal source of haemorrhage. The most reliable method is **upper GI endoscopy** which should be performed as soon as is feasible. Bleeding may occur from either gastric or oesophageal varices, or, rarely, portal hypertensive gastropathy.

Medical management

- Initial rescuscitation is as described earlier (p482).

- Transfuse with blood, fresh frozen plasma, and platelets, as necessary according to haematological parameters to try to stop the bleeding. Give vitamin K 10mg iv daily (for two days). Avoid overtransfusion as this increases portal pressure and the risk of re-bleeding.

- Give a bolus dose of metoclopramide 20mg iv or domperidone 10mg iv. This transiently increases the lower oesophageal pressure and decreases azygous blood flow.

- **Vasopressin** is effective in controlling variceal bleeding by causing splanchnic vasoconstriction. Side-effects include colic and intestinal hurry, profound peripheral vasoconstriction which may produce significant hypertension, skin, coronary and splanchnic ischaemia. **Nitrates** are used to reduce the peripheral effects of vasopressin and also augment the fall in portal pressure. **Octreotide** is a synthetic analogue of somatostatin. It does not have the cardiac side-effects of the other agents and nitrates are not required. Its efficacy is currently under investigation. A typical regimen is shown in the table opposite.

- **Endoscopic injection** of sclerosant into the varices or para-variceal can control the bleeding acutely. Side-effects include retrosternal pain and fever immediately post injection, mucosal ulceration and late oesophageal strictures. Gastric varices are more difficult to inject.

- **Band ligation** of the varices is sometimes used but is technically more difficult in the setting of acute haemorrhage.

- **Balloon tamponade** A Sengstaken-Blakemore tube may be inserted (p824). Inflation of the gastric balloon only, usually suffices. This should not be left in place for more than 12 hours as ischaemic ulceration may occur, a risk increased by the co-administration of vasopressin. The Linton tube has a larger gastric balloon and is more effective.

- **Liver failure regimen** (p522) Give lactulose 15ml q8h po or per-NG-tube to prevent encephalopathy and supplement with thiamine and multivitamins. Use magnesium or phosphate enemas.

Drugs to control variceal haemorrhage	
Vasopressin	• Add 120 units to 250ml 5% dextrose • Infuse 50ml (24 units) over 15 minutes then 50ml/h (0.4U/min) for 12 hours.
Nitrates	• Nitroglycerin 50mg in 50ml 5% dextrose infused at 2–20ml/h keeping systolic bp > 90mmHg. • Isosorbide dinitrate 25mg in 50ml, infused at 2–10ml/h. Keep systolic bp > 90mmHg. • Transdermal patch (10–20mg).
Octreotide	• 100µg iv bolus followed by a continuous infusion at 25–50µg/h (500µg in 50ml; 2.5–5ml/h).

Note: Nitrates are only used in conjunction with vasopressin. They are never used as monotherapy.

Variceal haemorrhage: Further management

Radiological management

- **Transvenous intrahepatic portosystemic shunting (TIPS)** is available in specialized units. Using a femoral or jugular approach, the hepatic veins are cannulated and an expandable stent is placed between the hepatic veins (low pressure) and the portal venous system (high pressure). The portal pressure should be decompressed to below 12mmHg to prevent further bleeding.

Surgical management

- **Emergency portocaval or mesocaval shunting** is effective in controlling the bleed (> 95%) but has a high mortality (~ 40%) and does not influence long-term survival.
- **Oesophageal transection** with a staple-gun has a low operative mortality (~ 10–20%) but re-bleeds occur in up to 80% of survivors within one year.
- **Selective decompression** (e.g. Warren shunt) is technically difficult and has a high operative mortality.

Prognosis

Overall mortality is 30%. This is highest in those with severe liver disease (Child's Grade C, see table opposite).
Success rates for cessation of acute bleeding varices:-

- Injection sclerotherapy or banding   ~ 90%
- Balloon tamponade   ~ 80%
- Vasopressin + nitrates   ~ 65%

Long-term management

- **Injection sclerotherapy** with 0.5–1ml sclerosant para-variceal or 1–5ml intravariceal at weekly intervals until the varices are obliterated; then 3–6 monthly.
- **Band ligation** involves a similar regimen to injection therapy but achieves variceal obliteration more rapidly (39 days vs 72 days).
- **Propranolol** (80mg tds: aim for a 30–40% reduction in resting heart rate) reduces the rate of re-bleeding from varices and portal hypertensive gastropathy. It has not been shown to decrease mortality.
- **TIPS or shunt procedures** provide a more definite cure and bleeding tends to recur only when the shunt blocks, but there is an increased incidence of chronic hepatic encephalopathy.

Mallory-Weiss tear

This a tear in the mucosa at the gastro-oesophageal junction following severe retching and is particularly common following large bouts of alcohol. The vomit is normal initially and becomes bright red.

Management

- Most stop bleeding spontaneously.
- Tamponade with a Sengstaken-Blakemore tube may be used.
- Surgical oversewing of bleeding point or selective arteriography and embolization of the feeding artery may be necessary.

Child-Pugh Score			
Clinical or biochemical measurement	**Points scored**		
	1	**2**	**3**
Encephalopathy grade	None	1–2	3–4
Ascites	Absent	Mild	Moderate-severe
Bilirubin	<35 μmol/l	36–60 μmol/l	>60 μmol/l
Albumin	>35 g/l	28–35 g/l	<28 g/l
Prothrombin time (secs prolonged)	1–4 s	4–6 s	> 6 s

The Child-Pugh scoring system is a very effective way to get an index of severity of liver disease in patients with cirrhosis. It is not directly applicable to primary biliary cirrhosis of sclerosing cholangitis.

Child-Pugh A   Score ≤ 6
Child-Pugh B   Score 7–9
Child-Pugh C   Score ≥ 10

Acute gastroenteritis: Assessment

Food-poisoning is an acute attack of abdominal pain, diarrhoea ± vomiting 1–40 hours after ingesting contaminated foodstuffs and lasting 1–7 days. With the exception of an acute attack of inflammatory bowel disease and mesenteric ischaemia (see acute colitis, p498) the majority of acute onset diarrhoea has an infective aetiology.

Differential diagnosis of acute diarrhoea

Common
- Gastroenteritis (bacterial, viral, protozoal)
- *Clostridium difficile* diarrhoea (pseudomembranous colitis)
- Inflammatory bowel disease
- Food intolerance/allergy (e.g. lactase deficiency)
- Drugs (see table p496)
- Constipation with overflow

Less common
- Coeliac disease
- Tumour (benign or malignant)
- Carcinoid syndrome
- Bacterial overgrowth
- Pancreatic insufficiency
- Bile salt enteropathy
- Hyperthyroidism
- Autonomic neuropathy

Presenting features Ask specifically about:
- Recent eating habits esp. restaurants and food prepared by caterers. Anyone else (family/friends) with similar symptoms?
- Time interval between eating any suspicious substance and onset of symptoms. Early onset of vomiting or diarrhoea (6–12h) suggests ingestion of preformed toxin (e.g. *Staph* exotoxin). Enterotoxin producing organisms may take 1–3 days to produce symptoms.
- Recent travel? (Enterotoxigenic *E. coli*, *Salmonella*, *Giardia*, or amoeba). Recent medication? Any antibiotics (*Cl. difficile*)?
- PMH, e.g. gastric surgery or immunosuppression (drugs or HIV).
- Anal intercourse increases the risk of amoebiasis, giardiasis, shigellosis, rectal syphilis, rectal gonorrhoea, *Chlamydia trachomatis*, HSV of rectum and perianal area. Diarrhoea in HIV positive patients is discussed on p273.
- The gross appearance of the diarrhoea may help: frankly bloody stool (*Campylobacter* or *Shigella*), watery, 'rice-water stool' (classically typhoid fever, occasionally inflammatory bowel disease or secretory diarrhoea due to cholera, enterotoxigenic *E. coli*, or pancreatic tumours).
- Abdominal pain may be present usually cramp-like, or tenesmus.
- Fever: common with the severe bacterial diarrhoeas and acute exacerbations of Crohn's or UC.

Investigations
- FBC   ↑ WBC; ↑ haematocrit (dehydration)
- U&Es   ↑ urea (dehydration); ↓ K$^+$
- Blood cultures   Systemic infection may occur.
- Stool cultures   Fresh samples, mandatory for wet mount microscopy for ova, cysts and parasites, culture, and antibiotic sensitivities. WBC in stool implies intestinal inflammation (mucosal invasion, toxin, inflammatory bowel disease, ischaemic colitis)
- *Clostridium difficile* toxin   Specifically request this for all patients who have recently taken antibiotics.
- Sigmoidoscopy and rectal biopsy   Useful for bloody diarrhoea and to rule out inflammatory bowel disease or melanosis coli (laxative abuse).

Gastroenterological emergencies

General approach to treating acute diarrhoea

Severity of symptoms	Management
• Mild (1–3 stools/day)	Oral fluids only
• Moderate (3–5 stools/day)	Oral fluids, loperamide (Imodium®)
• Severe (> 6 stools/day, fever)	Fluids (± ivi), antimicrobial agent

Viral gastroenteritis

In addition to diarrhoea, URTI-like symptoms, abdominal cramps headache, and fever may occur. The causative agent is usually not found but many viruses implicated (e.g. echovirus, Norwalk virus, and adenoviruses). Self-limiting illness (3–5 days). *Management:* Oral fluids and restricting solid foods and dairy product intake usually suffice.

Bacterial gastroenteritis

Salmonella sp. may produce acute gastroenteritis (e.g. *S. enteritidis*, ~ 70–80% of cases), enteric fever (*S. typhi* and *S. typhimurium*, see p246), or asymptomatic carriage. Acute gastroenteritis often occurs in epidemics, and is derived from poultry, eggs or egg products, and occasionally pets (terrapins). *Symptoms:* Gastroenteritis occurs 8–48h after ingestion with headache, vomiting (more prominent than either *Shigella* or *Campylobacter*), fever, and diarrhoeas lasting 2–4 days (rarely bloody with mucus). Reactive arthritis is occasionally seen in HLA-B27 positive individuals. (Enteric fever – see p246). Bacteraemia is seen occasionally (esp. *S. dublin* and *S. choleraesuis*). *Management:* Usually self-limiting after 2–5 days, and treatment should only be supportive. Antibiotics prolong carriage of the illness, and make clinical relapse more likely.

Clostridium perfringens (type A) spores are heat resistant and may germinate during reheating or slow cooking of meats. Enterotoxin is released when sporulation occurs in intestine. Accounts for 15–25% of cases of bacterial food-poisoning. Incubation 8–22h. *Symptoms* diarrhoea, abdominal pain, nausea (rare to get vomiting). No fever. Lasts 12–24h. *Management:* Supportive.

Campylobacter infections are common (5–10% of patients with acute diarrhoea). The incubation period is 3–7 days, symptoms last for 1–2 weeks. Presentation often follows eating contaminated poultry. *Symptoms:* Flu-like illness followed by headache, myalgia, abdominal pain (continuous then colicky), diarrhoea, rectal bleeding occasionally. Rarely complicated by reactive arthritis (1–2%), Guillain-Barré syndrome, or Reiter's syndrome. *Management:* The disease is usually self-limiting within 5 days. Treatment comprises either erythromycin or tetracycline. Anti-diarrhoeals are contraindicated.

Staph. aureus (2–5% of cases of bacterial food-poisoning) can multiply at room temperature in foods rich in carbohydrates and salt (dairy products, cold meats, mayonnaise). A heat-stable exotoxin produces nausea vomiting, and diarrhoea 1–6 hours after ingestion of contaminated foods Fever is uncommon. Treatment is supportive.

Bacillus cereus infection is usually associated with slow-cooking food and re-heated rice (fast-food takeaways). It produces an emetic toxin tha results in vomiting in 1–5 hours or infection, may result in diarrhoea 8–1 hours later. Treatment is supportive.

Vibrio parahaemolyticus produces epigastric pain (cf. those above) diarrhoea, vomiting and fever 12–18h after ingestion of raw seafoo (shellfish). May last up to 5 days. *Vibrio cholerae* is uncommon in th Western nations. It produces a profuse secretory diarrhoea requirin vigorous rehydration and salt replacement. The disease is usually sel limiting (5–7days) but tetracyclines may be used.

Yersinia enterocolitica: Incubation period 4–10 days after contact wit infected animals, water or ice-cream. *Symptoms:* Diarrhoea (80% abdominal pain (80%), fever (40%), bloody stool in 10%, mesenter adenitis, lymphadenopathy, reactive arthritis. Diagnosed by serolog rather than culture. *Management:* Supportive.

Gastroenterological emergencies

Pseudomembranous colitis

This is produced by a necrolytic toxin produced by *Clostridium difficile*. Infection typically follows antibiotic therapy; most commonly with clindamycin, ampicillin, cephalosporins, or aminoglycosides, though almost all antibiotics have been implicated. Diarrhoea may occur during or up to 4 weeks following cessation of treatment.

Symptoms: Diarrhoea is usually profuse, watery, and without blood (may be bloody in ~ 5%). It is commonly associated with abdominal cramps and tenderness, fever, and an elevated white cell count.

Diagnosis is based on detection of *Clostridium difficile* toxin in stool. Culture of the organism itself is unhelpful; ~ 5% of healthy adults carry the organism. Sigmoidoscopy is not diagnostic, but may show mucosal inflammation together with multiple yellow plaques.

Management: Patients should be isolated and barrier nursed. Rehydrate and correct electrolyte abnormalities. Mild disease responds to oral metronidazole (500mg tds). *Oral* vancomycin 250mg qds for 7–14 days is an alternative. Severe disease requires iv therapy. Complications include toxic megacolon and colonic perforation.

Giardiasis

Giardia lamblia is transmitted by the faeco-oral route. Risk factors include recent travel, immunosuppression, homosexuality, and achlorhydria. *Symptoms:* More chronic diarrhoeal illness with epigastric discomfort due to duodenal infestation. Malaise, bloating, flatulance, and occasionally malabsorption occur. Diagnosis is by stool microscopy for cysts or trophozoites or duodenal aspiration. If negative, consider blind therapeutic trial. *Management:* Metronidazole is the treatment of choice – 2g daily for 3 days or 400mg tds for 5 days orally. Alternatively include tinidazole (2g single dose) or mepacrine hydrochloride 100mg tds for 5–7 days. Lactose-intolerance post infection may persist for up to 6 weeks.

Travellers' diarrhoea

Travel through developing countries is commonly associated with self-limiting acute diarrhoeal illness transmitted through food and water. The most frequent pathogen is enterotoxigenic *E. coli*. The illness lasts 3–5 days with nausea, watery diarrhoea, and abdominal cramps. Oral rehydration is usually sufficient; anti-motility agents (e.g. loperamide) may be used with caution. Antibiotic treatment (co-trimoxazole) may help patients with more protracted illness. Bismuth (*Pepto-Bismol®*) is reported to reduce the severity of symptoms, and prophylaxis with doxycycline reduces the incidence: avoiding ingestion of contaminated foodstuffs remains the most effective measure.

HIV and diarrhoea, see p273

Common drugs that may cause acute diarrhoea		
Laxatives	Colchicine	Propranolol
Antacid (Mg^{2+}, Ca^{2+})	Quinidine	Aspirin
Lactulose	Digitalis	NSAIDs
Diuretics	Theophyllines	Cytotoxic therapy
Antibiotics	Cholinergic agents	Captopril

There are many drugs other than those listed above that can cause diarrhoea.

Gastroenterological emergencies

Bloody diarrhoea

Causes

- Acute infectious colitis
  - Bacillary dysentery (*Shigella* spp.)
  - Salmonellosis (p494)
  - Campylobacter (p494)
  - Pseudomembranous colitis (p496)
- Inflammatory bowel disease (IBD – ulcerative colitis or Crohn's)

Presenting features

- Ask about duration of symptoms and recent eating habits. Anyone else with similar symptoms? Recent travel? (Enterotoxigenic *E. coli*, *Salmonella*, *Giardia*, or amoeba). Recent medication? Any antibiotics (*Cl. difficile*)?
- The gross appearance of the stool may help. Inflammatory bowel disease may result in rectal bleeding (fresh red blood) in patients with disease largely confined to the rectum and sigmoid colon. Diffuse disease tends to be associated with diarrhoea. Infectious colitis results in frankly bloody stool (*Campylobacter* or *Shigella*).
- Abdominal pain may be present, usually cramp-like or tenesmus
- Vomiting is uncommon in acute inflammatory bowel disease.
- Systemic features such as general malaise and lethargy, dehydration electrolyte imbalance, or fever are seen with the severe bacterial diarrhoeas and acute exacerbations of Crohn's or UC. Skin, joints, and eyes may be involved in either IBD, or follow acute infection.
- Previous altered bowel habit, weight loss, smoking history, vascular disease (mesenteric infarction), mesenteric angina may be relevant.

Examination Look for:

- Fever, signs of dehydration (tachycardia, postural hypotension), abdominal distension. Abdominal tenderness or rebound over affected colon (IBD) may indicate colonic dilatation or perforation. An abdominal mass may indicate tumour or inflammatory mass.
- Mouth ulcers and perianal disease are common in active IBD.
- Erythema nodosum and pyoderma gangrenosum occur in inflammatory bowel disease; *Yersinia* may produce erythema nodosum. Rose spots indicate typhoid fever.
- Joint involvement – often an asymmetrical, non-deforming synovitis, involving large joints of the lower limbs – may occur in active IBD, but also in infectious colitis (e.g *Campylobacter*, *Yersinia*). Spondylitis does not reflect disease activity.
- Uveitis is associated with both IBD and acute infectious colitis.

Investigations

The priority is to exclude any infectious cause for the bloody diarrhoea and to monitor for complications.

Blood tests	FBC, U&Es, LFTs and albumin, CRP, ESR, coagulation studies
Microbiology	Stool culture and microscopy, blood cultures, *Clostridium difficile* toxin
Sigmoidoscopy ± biopsy	May help to distinguish between acute infectious colitis and inflammatory bowel disease
Imaging	Plain AXR may help monitor colonic dilatation. Contrast studies are contraindicated acutely. Nuclear imaging studies (e.g. WBC-scans) are used in IBD to demarcate extent of disease (p502)

Bloody diarrhoea

Bacterial dysentery

This is due to infection with shigella *(S. dysenteriae, S. flexneri, S. boydii, S. sonnei)* or some shigella-like *E. coli* (0157:H7). Transmitted by the faeco-oral route, and clusters of cases are often found.

Symptoms

- It causes mild diarrhoea to a severe systemic illness between 1 and 7 days following exposure.
- Fever (usually resolves in 3–4 days).
- Abdominal cramps with tenesmus.
- Watery diarrhoea ± nausea and vomiting (resolves by day 7). Bloody diarrhoea occurs later (after 24–72 hours) due to invasion of the mucosa.
- Diagnosed by stool culture. *E. coli* infections may be complicated by haemolytic uraemic syndrome (p562).

Management

- Patients may require iv fluid replacement.
- Antibiotics should be reserved for the most severe cases. Ampicillin (250mg po qds × 5–10 days) is usually effective, but in resistant cases co-trimoxazole or ciprofloxacin may be used.
- Anti-motility agents such as loperamide and codeine are contraindicated as they prolong carriage and worsen symptoms.
- May be complicated by haemolytic uraemic syndrome.

Amoebic dysentery

Entamoeba histolytica can produce intermittent diarrhoea or a more severe illness that resembles inflammatory bowel disease. There is an increased risk in homosexuals, and those with recent travel to third world countries. It is transmitted by the faeco-oral route.

Symptoms

- Diarrhoea or loose stool (± blood), abdominal discomfort, mild fever. In severe cases, liver abscess.
- Fulminant attacks present abruptly with high fever, cramping abdominal pain, and profuse bloody diarrhoea.
- Marked abdominal tenderness is present.
- Diagnosis is made by identifying amoebic cysts on stool microscopy.

Treatment

- Aimed at replacement of fluid, electrolyte and blood loss, and eradication of the organism.
- In acute-invasive intestinal amoebiasis, oral metronidazole 800mg tds for 5–10 days is the treatment of choice. Tinidazole (2g daily for 2– days) is also effective. This should be followed with oral diloxanid furoate 500mg tds for 10 days to destroy gut cysts.
- Metronidazole (or tinidazole) and diloxanide furoate are also effectiv for liver abscesses, and USS-guided aspiration may help improv penetration of the drugs and shorten illness.
- Diloxanide furoate is the treatment of choice for asymptomat patients with *E. histolytica* cysts in the stool, as metronidazole an tinidazole are relatively ineffective.

Gastroenterological emergencies

Inflammatory bowel disease (IBD) 1.

Presentation

Diarrhoea is dependent on disease activity and extent. Nocturnal diarrhoea and urgency are common symptoms of severe (IBD). Mucus and frank pus, or blood, is often mixed in with the stool. *Abdominal pain* is not a prominent feature, though lower abdominal cramping pain relieved by defecation is common. Severe abdominal pain suggests a severe attack with acute dilatation or perforation, or ischaemic colitis.

Examination

Look for *fever*, signs of dehydration (tachycardia, postural hypotension), abdominal distension. *Abdominal tenderness* or rebound over affected colon may indicate colonic dilatation or perforation. This may be masked if the patient is on steroids. An abdominal mass may indicate tumour or inflammatory mass. *Systemic features:* examine carefully for mouth ulcers and perianal disease; erythema nodosum and pyoderma gangrenosum; uveitis; joint involvement – (often an asymmetrical, non-deforming synovitis, involving large joints) – spondylitis does not correlate with disease activity.

Investigations

- **Blood tests:** Anaemia may be present if the colitis is acute and florid severe and iron-deficiency picture may be observed. ↑ WCC (neutrophilia) and ↑ platelets reflect disease activity.

  ↓ K^+ may follow severe diarrhoea. There may also be an element of pre-renal dehydration. Albumin – in severe colitis this often falls to 20–30g/l.

  ESR and CRP – reflect disease activity, though are often not elevated in distal (rectal) disease. They are useful to monitor therapy.

- **Stool culture and microscopy:** Treatment should be delayed, except in the most severe cases, until results of the above are available.

- **Supine AXR ± erect CXR:** To look for wall thickening (moderate-severe) and mucosal oedema, with loss of haustration and colonic dilatation (more severe cases). Colonic diameter > 6cm indicates toxic dilatation, with risk of perforation. The extent of the disease can be indirectly assessed; distal colitis is often associated with proximal faecal loading.

  In the acute stages of a severe attack abdominal films should be performed daily, or twice daily if there is borderline toxic dilatation. Free air under the diaphragm on an erect CXR indicates perforation.

- **White cell scan:** [111]Indium-labelled WBC accumulate in areas of active inflammation, and are a useful adjunct to plain AXR to assess the extent of active disease. Crohn's typically shows patchy uptake and involvement of the small bowel, while UC is commonly limited to colon.

- **Sigmoidoscopy ± colonoscopy:** Bowel preparation is unnecessary and may cause reddening of the mucosa. Flexible sigmoidoscopy has a lower risk of bacteraemia and is easier than rigid sigmoidoscopy. Non-specific findings such as hyperaemia and contact or spontaneous bleeding are common. Ulceration suggests acute disease; pseudo-polyps and atrophy of the bowel mucosa indicates chronic UC. Rectal biopsy from the posterior wall below 10cm should be taken from all patients (less risk of perforation).

Markers of a severe attack

- > 6 bloody stools/day
- Systemically unwell – pyrexia and tachycardia (HR > 100)
- Hb < 10g/dl
- Albumin < 30g/l
- Toxic dilatation (transverse colon > 6cm)
- Diffuse abdominal tenderness

Inflammatory bowel disease (IBD) 2.

Differential diagnosis of inflammatory bowel disease	
Infection	**Miscellaneous**
Bacteria: *Shigella, Salmonella, E. coli, Camplyobacter, Cl. difficile*, TB,*Gonococcus, Chlamydia, Yersinia*	Ischaemic colitis
	Lymphoma
	Trauma
Parasites: amoebiasis, schistosomiasis	Radiation colitis

Management

- Rehydrate patient with iv fluids and correct any electrolyte imbalance (hypokalaemia in particular). Inform and discuss the patient with surgical colleagues, especially if moderate-severe.
- The differentioal diagnosis is wide (see above). Exclude infectious colitis (normal stool microscopy and culture) and systemic infections as far as possible.
- Avoid anti-motility opiate drugs (such as loperamide and codeine) and anti-spasmodics as they cause proximal constipation and may precipitate paralytic ileus and megacolon.
- ***Corticosteroids:*** Acute attacks of UC may respond to rectal steroids (e.g. *Predfoam®* or *Predsol®* enema, 20mg 1–2 times daily) especially if disease is confined to the rectum. However, severe attacks require intravenous steroids (hydrocortisone 100mg qds iv) until remission is achieved.
- ***Aminosalicylates:*** Sulphasalazine or the newer agents (mesalazine and olsalazine) should be started in addition to steroids – they help induce, and maintain, remission after steroids are tailed off. They are of doubtful value in Crohn's disease of the small bowel.
- ***Other immunosuppressants:*** Some authorities advocate azathioprine 2mg/kg daily for patients resistant to steroids (unlicensed indication), or iv cyclosporin (5mg/kg over 24h in 2 divided doses – monitor levels).
- ***Antibiotics:*** There is little evidence that broad spectrum antibiotics are useful. Metronidazole may be of benefit in Crohn's disease. Other antibiotics should only be used if specifically indicated and should be considered for patients developing toxic megacolon.
- ***Nutrition:*** There is no evidence for keeping the patient 'nil by mouth'. However, a low residue or elemental diet, and early institution of TPN may be of benefit, especially if the patient is likely to come to surgery. When the patient is recovering, stool bulking agents (e.g. methyl-cellulose) may be used to adjust stool consistency.

Indications for surgery

- Failure of symptoms to resolve after 5 days is an indication for proctocolectomy (7–10 days in some centres).
- Colonic perforation, uncontrollable bleeding, toxic megacolon, and fulminating disease requires *urgent* proctocolectomy; ~ 30% of all patients with UC will require a colectomy at some stage.
- Toxic dilatation prior to treatment is not an indication for surgery: failure of the colonic diameter to decrease after 24 hours is. The development of dilatation *during* treatment is an indication for surgery.
- Surgery in Crohn's disease is not 'curative' and is only indicated for perforation, obstruction, abscess formation, and fistulae (entero-cutaneous or enterovesical). Recurrence rate after surgery is high.

Jaundice: Assessment

Jaundice requires urgent investigation and diagnosis. It may herald the onset of a severe hepatitis and acute liver (± renal) failure (see p518). It may indicate an obstructive jaundice which can be complicated by cholangitis, and septicaemia (p514). Exclude these complications first: further investigations may be done later.

506

History

- Non-specific symptoms (as regards aetiology) include anorexia, pruritus, malaise, lethargy, drowsiness, confusion, or coma. Dark urine and pale stools may be features of both post hepatic and hepatic jaundice.
- Colicky RUQ pain, previous biliary colic, or known gall-stones suggests biliary colic (see p512). Fever, rigors, abdominal pain, and fluctuating jaundice should raise the suspicion of cholangitis (p514). Painless jaundice and weight loss suggest pancreatic malignancy.
- Take a detailed drug history including homeopathic or proprietary preparations. Ask specifically about use of paracetamol and alcohol.
- Risk factors for infectious hepatitis – blood transfusion, iv drugs, homosexual, travel, ethnic origin, ingestion of shellfish, etc.

Examination

- Note the degree of jaundice (mild, moderate, or severe) and look for stigmata of chronic liver disease (spider naevi or telangiectasiae, palmar erythema, Dupuytrens' contractures, etc). Lymphadenopathy may reflect malignancy or cirrhotic liver disease. Hepatic encephalopathy results in falling conscious level, and liver flap.
- Note the bp and the diastolic carefully: it falls with liver failure p518). Oliguria or shock may occur with acute liver failure (see p518). Examine for pleural effusions (may occur with ascites).
- Examine the abdomen for ascites, hepatomegaly, splenomegaly (portal hypertension or intravascular haemolysis), or masses. If there is hepatomegaly, is it hard?

Urgent investigations for jaundice (on the day of admission)

U&Es, LFTs	Exclude renal failure (hepatorenal syndrome, p296).
Glucose	DM is common in haemochromatosis or pancreatic carcinoma; hypoglycaemia in acute liver failure.
PT	↑ in severe liver injury or DIC.
FBC	↓ platelets (chronic liver disease with hypersplenism, malaria or alcoholism etc); ↑ WBC (sepsis, alcoholic hepatitis ± sepsis).
Urinalysis & septic screen	Absence of bilirubin in the urine in a jaundiced patient (acholuric) indicates haemolysis or a conjugation defect (Gilbert's). Culture urine, blood, and ascitic fluid.
CXR	Tumour or metastases, effusion assoc. with ascites.
USS scan ± CT scan	If patient is unwell or septic, exclude biliary obstruction which may require urgent decompression (p514). Note spleen size and any masses in the liver.
Paracetamol	If overdose is suspected or possible.

Non-urgent investigations for jaundice

UViral serology	(anti-HAIgM, HBsAg and anti-HBc, anti-HCV,cMV serology, EBV capsig antigen IgM)
Immunology	ANA, Anti-SM, AMA and Igs (CAH, PBC).
Ferritin, iron, transferrin	↑ Ferritin is seen in any acute illness, but may indicate haemochromatosis. (↑ in alcoholic liver disease also.)

Causes of jaundice

- Viral hepatitis
- Alcoholic hepatitis ± cirrhosis
- Drug-induced hepatitis (including paracetamol)
- Advanced cirrhosis (alcoholic, chronic viral hepatitis, haemochromatosis, Wilson's, cryptogenic cirrhosis, etc.)
- Haemolytic anaemias
- Gilbert's syndrome
- Extrahepatic biliary obstruction (stones or tumour)
- Intrahepatic cholestasis, post hepatitic, (primary biliary cirrhosis, primary sclerosing cholangitis, sepsis, drugs)
- Autoimmune hepatitis
- Ischaemic hepatitis
- Sepsis

Viral hepatitis

Detailed management protocols are beyond the scope of this book, and the outlines below are a guide only.

- Characterized by prodromal 'flu-like' illness and very high transaminase (up to ~ 5000U/l) with less rise in ALP.
- If there is **no** coagulopathy, encephalopathy, or renal failure, send the patient home, and await virology results. Advise the patient to avoid alcohol. See the patient again within a week. Instruct the patient to return if increasingly unwell, or drowsy. Arrange repeat LFTs and clotting after 1–2 days, and **see** the results. Repeat after 24h if LFTs worse.
- For anti-HAV IgM positive patients no specific treatment is required but *all* household and school contacts should receive normal human immunoglobulin (0.02ml/kg IM) if not already immune to HAV.
- For HBsAg positive patients, vaccinate family. Follow up for at least 6 months to ensure virus is cleared (HBsAg -ve, HBeAb +ve). Prophylactic specific hepatitis B immunoglobulin ('HBIG' 500 units im) has been shown to be protective if given within 10 days of exposure to HBV; however, only use for persons with clear exposure to HBsAg-contaminated material (needle-stick or sexual contacts who are HbsAb negative).
- For anti-HCV positive patients, try and determine source. Follow-up for years. Check LFTs and HCV RNA to exclude continued viral replication; refer to a liver centre if necessary.

Alcoholic hepatitis

- Acute hepatitis may be asymptomatic or present with nausea, vomiting, and anorexia, rarely RUQ pain. Fever may reflect severe liver damage but infection needs to be excluded.
- Investigations: ↑ transaminases (usually < 400U/l); bilirubin may be up to 800μM; albumin is often reduced; prolonged PT (> 7–10 seconds) carries a worse prognosis; ↑ WBC with left shift may occur (even without infection), anaemia and ↓ platelets suggest cirrhosis with hypersplenism; renal failure may occur in severe alcoholic hepatitis.
- Admit most patients to hospital, unless mild (bilirubin < 50mM, normal PT). Give thiamine, folic acid and multivitamins. Monitor and correct K^+, mg^{2+}, PO_4^{3-}, and glucose. Start a high calorie diet.
- Delirium tremens or severe agitation may be managed with chlormethiazole iv or po (p397). Treat seizures in the standard way (p370).
- Calculate the discriminant function for alcoholic hepatitis:-

$$\frac{Bilirubin}{17} + (Prolongation\ of\ PT \times 4.6)\ (40\%\ mortality\ if > 32)$$

[E.g. bilirubin = 340 μM, PT = 17s, (control 12s), would score (340 ÷ 17) + (17 – 12) × 4.6 = 43]

- A value > 32, or the presence of encephalopathy, should be treated with prednisolone 40mg/day for 4 weeks. The only practical contraindication is untreated sepsis. If there is doubt, then broad spectrum antibiotics should be given for 24–48 hours prior to steroids.

Drug-induced hepatitis

Most cases of drug-induced jaundice should be monitored three times per week or admitted for observation, since many are serious and may not resolve. Withdraw suspected drug and observe. Look for rash and eosinophilia and exclude other causes (see table p511) (For paracetamol overdose see p662.) Drugs causing jaundice are listed in the table opposite. Drugs causing a rise in transaminases, but rarely causing jaundice, are not listed. All drug-induced causes of jaundice should be reported to the CSM (yellow pages at the back of the BNF).

Autoimmune hepatitis

This is characterized by elevated transaminases, up to several thousand, usually < 2000U/l, anti-smooth muscle antibody positive, ANA positive, raised IgG (polyclonal). Confirm with liver biopsy. Treatment is with steroids ± azathioprine as a steroid-sparing agent once viral hepatitis has been excluded (i.e. HBsAg negative). If there is failure to respond in a young patient (< 30 years), consider Wilson's disease.

Acholuric jaundice

This is characterized by the absence of bilirubin in the urine. This may be caused by haemolytic anaemia (previous history, excess urinary urobilinogen, splenomegaly, reticulocytosis, etc.) or a congenital disorder of conjugation (Gilbert's syndrome, 1–2% of population). Fasting (< 400 calories) for 48–72 hours (or iv nicotinic acid 50mg) will increase serum unconjugated bilirubin in patients with Gilbert's. These usually cause mild icterus (bilirubin rarely > 80μM).

Sepsis

Any severe infections may cause jaundice (incl. pneumonia). Most severe with intra-abdominal sepsis. LFTs may be cholestatic, or characterized by a predominant rise of the bilirubin only. Exclude other causes and treat infection with antibiotics ± surgical drainage.

Ischaemic hepatitis

Presentation: Usually occurs in any individual with significant hypotension or hepatic arterial occlusion. In its mildest form it manifests as mildly deranged LFTs (hepatitic picture, ↑ PT) in a patient with CCF and in its most severe form may present as acute liver failure. Look for hypoxia, hypotension (may have normalized by the time of assessment), signs of arteriopathy (abdominal bruits from hepatic arterial occlusion) and signs of right ventricular failure. May cause confusion ± encephalopathy. Exclude other causes of liver failure (p520).

Management: Most will respond to correction of the underlying aetiology. Correct hypotension (see p210) and give oxygen to correct hypoxia. If hepatic artery or coeliac axis are occluded prognosis is poor, and depends on the extent of hepatic necrosis. Usually age and extent of disease preclude salvage surgery. Discuss with specialist centre. If signs of severe (acute) liver failure present see p522 for guidance. Most patients are not fit enough for liver transplantation.

Obstructive jaundice (see biliary obstruction, p514)

Common drugs that cause jaindice		
Hepatitic	**Cholestatic**	**Mixed**
Paracetamol	Chlorpromazine	Co-amoxiclav
Rifampicin	Flucloxacillin	Sulphonamides
Allopurinol	Azathioprine	Sulphasalazine
Ethanol	Captopril	Carbamazepine
Halothane	Cyclosporin	Dapsone
Methyldopa	Penicillamine	Ranitidine
Hydralazine	Erythromycin	Amitriptyline
Isoniazid	Anabolic steroids	Nitrofurantoin
Phenytoin	Oral contraceptive	

Gall-stone disease

Gall-stone disease affects 10–20% of the population. The stones may be predominantly cholesterol (account for > 80% of all gall-stones; pure cholesterol stones are usually solitary), pigment stones (< 25% cholesterol; multiple, irregular, friable), or mixed (faceted, calcium containing). The majority are asymptomatic and diagnosed incidentally.

Complications of gall-stones

- Biliary colic
- Cholecystitis ± empyema and gangrene of gall-bladder
- Acute pancreatitis (p528)
- GB fistula, gall-stone ileus
- Obstructive jaundice
- Cholangitis ± septicaemia or liver abscesses (p514)
- Perforation and peritonitis

Biliary colic

Presentation: Abdominal pain (RUQ) radiating to epigastrium, back, or shoulders, associated with nausea and vomiting. Attacks commonly follow a heavy meal and pass spontaneously. Differential diagnoses includes acute MI, leaking aortic aneurysm, peptic ulcer, intestinal obstruction or ischaemia, pancreatitis, renal colic, and pneumonia.

Investigations: USS to detect the stone and gall-bladder distention. Urine microscopy, CXR, ECG will help exclude other conditions.

Management
- Pain relief (pethidine 50–100mg im q4h + prochlorperazine 12.5mg im q8h); avoid morphine.
- Cholecystectomy in the longer term. Stone dissolution therapy (e.g. ursodeoxycholic acid) may be an alternative for selected patients.

Acute cholecystitis

Presentation: Sudden onset severe RUQ pain and symptoms similar to biliary colic with fever and persisting symptoms. Persistent vomiting suggests a bile duct stone. Physical signs include fever, tachycardia, sweating, RUQ tenderness, and peritonism, especially in inspiration (Murphy's sign) ± palpable gall-bladder. Jaundice (~ 33%) suggests obstruction of CBD. Differential diagnosis is as above. *Acalculous cholecystitis* is seen in elderly or patients with co-existing disease or trauma, in the ITU, and patients on TPN. Mortality is high (up to 50%) if not diagnosed early.

Investigations
- Blood tests — ↑ WCC is usual. LFTs show ↑ bilirubin, and cholestatic liver function tests; ± ↑ amylase.
- USS — Should demonstrate gall-stones or biliary sludge ± thickening of gall-bladder wall .
- AXR — Gall-stones visble in ~ 10% of patients. Local peritonitis may produce a 'sentinal loop'.
- HIDA scan — Using ^{99}Tc-label is usually diagnostic.

Management
- NBM and iv fluids; insert an NG-tube if there is severe vomiting.
- Antibiotics should cover enteric organisms and enterococcus (e.g cefuroxime 750mg iv q8h + metronidazole 500mg iv q8h).
- Cholecystectomy is the treatment of choice. Liaise with surgeons fo optimal timing of surgery.
- Complications include perforation, gall-stone ileus, or fistula.

Biliary obstruction

Biliary obstruction or apparent biliary obstruction will be associated with either a dilated or undilated biliary system and the patient may be either

septic or aseptic. Biliary dilatation in patients with mechanical biliary obstruction may not always be apparent on USS.

Presentation
- Jaundice (painful or painless) ± fluctuation
- RUQ pain ± tenderness
- Fever (indicates infection or cholecystitis)
- Itching
- Dark urine ± pale stools (not very useful in practice)
- Septic shock

Investigations
- Blood tests ↑ WCC indicates sepsis. U&Es may indicate renal failure or pre-renal uraemia. LFTs show ↑ bilirubin, ↑↑ ALP and ↑↑ γ-GT; ↑ amylase with concomitant pancreatitis; transient ↑ ALT,AST with passage of a stone and persistent in cholangitis (usually ≤ 400U/l;) higher suggests hepatitis. AST may be >1000u/l. Blood cultures, and CRP mandatory.
- USS This is mandatory, and should be performed within 12 hours if possible, to demonstrate the presence of dilated ducts ± gall-stones. Post cholecystectomy slight dilatation (~ 0.8cm) of CBD is normal.
- AXR Aerobilia may indicate a gas-forming organism or recent instrumentation. There may be localized ileus.
- ERCP Shows stones in CBD and allows examination of GI tract and ampulla to exclude other pathology. Give broad spectrum antibiotics if intervention is planned.

Poor prognostic features (depends on the cause)
- Elderly (> 65 yrs)
- Shock
- Renal failure
- Cholangitis with cirrhosis, liver abscess, or high malignant stricture
- Cholangitis following transhepatic percutaneous cholangiography
- Acute pancreatitis

Indications for specialist referral
For patients with PBC, PSC, or cholestatic drug reactions
- Bilirubin > 100 μM
- Coagulopathy (uncorrected by vitamin K)
- Hypoalbuminaemia
- Ascites

Management (see algorithm on facing page)
- Analgesia (pethidine 50–100mg imq4h), NBM, iv fluids.
- Antibiotics (e.g. cefotaxime or ciprofloxacin+amoxycillin) if septic.
- Emergency decompression of the biliary system by:
  - i ERCP
  - ii Percutaneous drainage
  - iii Surgical decompression
- Follow up with LFTs, CRP, and temperature.
- Repeat ERCP when well to exclude missed stones or further anatomic abnormality.
- Repeat USS or CT liver scan to look for hepatic abscesses.

Causes of biliary obstruction	
Mechanical obstruction	***Non-mechanical obstruction***
• Gall-stones	• Primary sclerosing cholangitis
• Malignancy (pancreatic	(PSC)
carcinoma, nodes, secondary	• Primary biliary cirrhosis (PBC)
deposits, cholangiocarcinoma)	• Cholestatic drug reaction
• Post operative stricture	
• Parasitic infection (e.g.	
onchocerciasis)	
• Cavernous transformation of portal vein	

Management algorithm for biliary obstruction

Obstructive jaundice
ALP > 4 × normal
γ-GT > 10 x normal
Ultrasound liver
?? bile duct dilation

Dilated ducts
(see table above)

Undilated ducts
(May be mechanical obstruction
but with apparently normal ducts)

• Antibiotics if septic
• Urgent ERCP or
• Percutaneous cholangiography
• Discuss with surgeons (PRIOR
to decompression)

• Antibiotics if septic
(makes PSC more likely)
• Autoantibodies (AMA, pANCA)
• When stable, consider:-
  • ERCP
  • Liver biopsy

NB In cirrhosis there may be no duct dilatation with biliary obstruction.

Ascites

Presentation

The patient may present with symptoms due to the fluid (abdominal distension, weight gain, abdominal pain), the underlying cause (jaundice, haematemesis, fever, or night sweats), or complication of the ascites (dyspnoea, anorexia, reflux oesophagitis, herniae, pleural effusions, scrotal or leg oedema, peritonitis). Ask specifically about alcohol, risk factors for chronic liver disease, GI bleeding (portal hypertension), previous pancreatitis, risk factors and contacts for TB, cardiac history, exercise tolerance, and menstrual history (?ovarian malignancy).

Differential diagnoses

- Ovarian cyst
- Pregnancy
- Obesity (simple or metabolic)
- Abdominal mass

Investigations

- Blood tests — U&Es, glc, FBC, PT, LFTs blood cultures. Amylase.
- Ascitic tap (see p820) — An ascitic tap should be carried out in ALL patients unless a diagnosis of malignant ascites is certain. Inoculate blood culture bottles and send fluid in sterile pot for microscopy. Use of EDTA tubes and coulter counters is probably unreliable at the low, but pathological, WBC counts encountered.
- Imaging — Plain AXR shows a glass-ground pattern with loss of psoas shadow. USS can detect as little as 30ml. Note the size and texture of the liver and spleen, check patency of hepatic veins. CT scan may be required.
- Urine — Urine sodium (cirrhotic ascites), 24h protein.

Management

Admit all patients with symptomatic ascites. Treat the underlying cause.

Cirrhotic ascites: Do NOT start diuretics if there is renal impairment. *Salt restrict* to 40 mmol/day. *Paracentese* if tense or moderate ascites: drain ALL ascites as quickly as possible (maximum 25 litres in 5 hours !), and then give 200ml 20% albumin. Start *spironolactone* 200mg/day increasing to 400mg/day after 2 weeks if urine sodium < 40mmol/l. Water restrict (< 1l/day) if serum Na^+ < 135mM. If there is renal impairment (creatinine > 140mM), give an extra *colloid challenge* (400ml 20% albumin) in association with paracentesis. There is NO hurry to commence diuretics, which should be started after the patient has settled from paracentesis. Much harm can result from diuresing patients who are effectively hypovolaemic.

Malignant ascites: Treatment is palliative, and may include total paracentesis to make the patient more comfortable. Specialist advice should be sought for future management of the malignancy.

Pancreatic ascites: Usually associated with a pancreatic pseudocyst and should be managed in consultation with surgical colleagues.

Spontaneous bacterial peritonitis occurs in up to 25% of patients admitted with cirrhotic ascites, and is frequently asymptomatic. It rarely, if ever, occurs in non-cirrhotic ascites. The risk is increased with low ascitic protein. > 90% will yield +ve ascitic cultures if inoculated into blood culture bottles; < 40% will yield +ve cultures if sent to lab. in sterile pot. Diagnosis: ascitic WCC > 250PMN/mm³. If culture +ve but ascitic WBC low repeat tap for microscopy and treat if WBC > 250PMN/mm³. Treat with broad spectrum antibiotic for enteric organisms and Gram +ve cocci (e.g. cefotaxime). Suspect tuberculous ascites if there is a predominant lymphocytosis.

Causes of ascites

- Cirrhosis and portal hypertension
- Malignant ascites
- Congestive cardiac failure
- Pancreatic ascites
- Hepatic venous obstruction
- Nephrotic syndrome
- Hypothyroidism
- Infection (e.g. TB ascites)
- It does **not** occur with portal vein thrombosis, congenital hepatic fibrosis, or other causes of non-cirrhotic portal hypertension

Acute liver failure: Assessment

Acute liver failure (fulminant hepatic failure) is defined as a potentially reversible severe liver injury, with an onset of hepatic encephalopathy within 8 weeks of the appearance of the first symptoms and in the absence of pre-existing liver disease. A more recent classification is:-

Hyper-acute liver failure: Encephalopathy within 7 days of jaundice

Acute liver failure: Encephalopathy within 8–28 days of jaundice.

Sub-acute liver failure: Encephalopathy 29–84 days of jaundice.

Presentation

- The history may point to a cause (see table p520). Ask specfically about recent viral illnesses, paracetamol, alcohol, and drug history. Signs of chronic liver disease are typically not present (unless 'acute-on-chronic'). Splenomegaly does not occur. If present consider an acute presentation of Wilson's disease, autoimmune chronic active hepatitis, or lymphoma. Frequently, the presenting feature is a complication of liver failure. Patients with paracetamol overdose may present with severe abdominal pain and retching, and often have subconjunctival haematoma.

- *Encephalopathy:* Present in all cases (by definition) and conventionally divided into 4 grades (see table below). Cerebral oedema is heralded by spikes of hypertension, dysconjugate eye movements; papilloedema is rare. Unless treated this progresses to posturing (back, arms, and legs rigid, hands in flexion, opisthonus), and brainstem coning. (see also p525)

Grades of hepatic encephalopathy	
Grade 1	Drowsy but coherent; mood change
Grade 2	Drowsy, confused at times, inappropriate behaviour
Grade 3	Very drowsy and stuparose but rousable; alternatively restless, screaming
Grade 4	Comatose, barely rousable

- *Metabolic disturbances:* Hypoglycaemia and hyponatraemia are common. Other abnormalities include hypokalaemia, respiratory alkalosis, and severe hypophosphataemia. Lactic acidosis carries a poor prognosis.

- *Cardiovascular abnormalities:* Spikes of systolic hypertension reflect cerebral oedema. The diastolic bp falls as disease progresses with a vasodilated hyperdynamic circulation ($\downarrow$ SVR, $\uparrow$ cardiac output).

- *Respiratory failure:* Hypoxia is relatively common and may be worsened by localized infection, aspiration, or atelectasis. Non-cardiogenic pulmonary oedema is seen in ~ 10%.

- *Renal failure:* Usually indicates a poor prognosis and may be due to hepatorenal syndrome (see p296) or ATN (paracetamol).

- *Bleeding problems:* The PT is prolonged and reflects the progression of the disease. Low-grade DIC may occur with bleeding from the GI tract from gastritis or elsewhere. Subconjunctival haematoma is common in paracetamol-induced liver failure.

- *Infections:* Bacterial and fungal infections (septicaemia, pneumonia, peritonitis, UTIs) are more frequent due to impaired neutrophil function.

Acute liver failure: Investigations

Investigations

- **Blood tests** (daily)

  U&Es, glucose (and 2 hourly BM stix), FBC, PT, LFTs (albumin is usually normal on admission unless 'acute-on chronic'), phosphate, arterial blood gases.

  Blood group and cross-match on admission.

- **Blood tests** (for diagnosis)

  Viral serology (HAV IgM, HBsAg, HBcore Ab IgM, delta in HBsAg +ve, EBV,CMV, EBV, HSV), drug screen (esp. paracetamol), plasma caeruloplasmin (if < 50 yrs ± 24h urine copper).

- **Bacteriology**

  Blood cultures, urine and sputum MC&S daily (incl. fungal cultures). Throat and vaginal swabs.

- **USS (liver)**

  To assess hepatic veins, portal vein patency, size (if possible), spleen size, nodes (lymphoma).

- **ECG / CXR**

  Repeat CXR daily (infection/ARDS).

- **EEG**

  May be helpful in the assessment of hepatic encephalopathy though not widely used.

- **Liver biopsy**

  Rarely necessary but will exclude underlying malignant infiltration or cirrhosis where the diagnosis is in doubt. The transjugular approach is preferred as it carries lower risk of haemorrhage (p826).

Causes of acute liver failure in the UK	
Drug-induced hepatitis (58%) (see p511)	Paracetamol od (p662). Less commonly halothane, isoniazid, sulphonamides, NSAIDs, phenytoin, valproate, penicillins, MAOIs, sulphasalazine, disulphiram, ketoconazole,
Viral hepatitis (36%) (see p508)	Hepatitis A, B, delta co-infection in HBsAg +ve carrier, NANB (*not* HCV in UK), E; less commonly CMV, EBV, and HSV.
Toxins	*Amanita phalloides* (these fungi are found in the UK), herbal remedies, CCl_4
Malignancy	Lymphoma, malignant infiltration
Vascular	Budd-Chiari syndrome, veno-occlusive disease, ischaemic injury (shock and hypotension).
Miscellaneous	Wilson's (not strictly acute, since many are cirrhotic, but in all clinical respects similar), autoimmune hepatitis, malignant hyperthermia (incl. ecstasy), fatty liver of pregnancy, PET / HELLP syndrome, Reye's syndrome.

Acute liver failure: Management

The mainstay of treatment is support until the acute insult resolves. If a patient has criteria approaching those for liver transplantation (see table opposite) on or during their admission they should be referred to a centre where liver transplantation is available. (These are listed on p854).

*It is **vital** to discuss all cases of severe liver injury with one of the regional centres* even though patients may not fulfil the criteria above, since it generally takes up to 48h to obtain an emergency graft, and delay in referral can result in failure to procure an adequate graft. All of these centres are also experienced in managing this serious illness.

None of the known causes of acute liver failure respond well to medical therapy in terms of enhanced recovery. Steroids may be of benefit in patients with lymphoma or autoimmune hepatitis, but by the time most patients present it is usually too late. All patients should be admitted to a high dependency or intensive care unit.

- *Paracetamol overdose:* Give N-acetyl cysteine (see p664) unless already given. The benefit of N-acetyl cysteine may be evident up to 48 hours and possibly longer.
- *General measures:* Nurse supine (at 10° head-up tilt). Keep in a peaceful environment. Insert an arterial line and CVP line for monitoring and if possible a pulmonary artery catheter (Swann-Gantz) to optimize the haemodynamic status.
- *Coagulopathy:* The PT is the best indicator of liver function. Avoid giving FFP unless there is bleeding or unless undergoing surgical procedures or line insertion. Factor concentrates may precipitate DIC. The PT may rise and fall precipitously and should be measured twice daily if deteriorating. Give vitamin K daily. Give platelet support if thrombocytopenic and bleeding.
- *Cerebral oedema:* ICP monitoring is used in some centres. If signs of cerebral oedema are present then give mannitol (100mls of 20% mannitol); if in renal failure, watch for fluid overload. Hyperventilation decreases ICP at the expense of cerebral blood flow and should be avoided. Prostacyclin and N-acetyl cysteine have been reported to decrease ICP. Hypertension is almost always secondary to raised ICP and should be treated with mannitol as above; antihypertensive drugs may precipitate brainstem coning. There is no evidence that giving lactulose or neomycin affects prognosis or prevents Grade 3–4 encephalopathy. Flumazenil is reported to improve encephalopathy but does affect outcome. Seizures should be treated in the usual way (p370).
- *Haemodynamic support:* Correct hypovolaemia with colloid or blood but avoid fluid overload. Persistent hypotension may respond to noradrenaline or vasopressin infusion, though these have not been shown to improve overall survival.
- *Metabolic changes:* Monitor *glucose* (BM stix) 2 hourly, and give 10% or 50% glucose to keep glc > 3.5mM. Monitor serum *phosphate* (often very low), replace with iv (9–18mmol/24 hours) or oral (effervescent Phosphate-Sandoz® 2 tabs tds) if less than 0.6mM. *Nutrition*: preferably enteral but avoid NG feeds if ileus is present.
- *Renal failure* (p296): Monitor renal function (renal failure occurs in ~ 70% cases). Treat by haemodiafiltration rather than haemodialysis.
- *Respiratory support:* Monitor oxygen saturations continuously and give oxygen by mask if $S_aO_2 < 90\%$. Ventilate when Grade 3 or 4 coma (avoid ET tube ties which compress the IJ veins).
- *Infection:* Start prophylactic antibiotics and antifungals (e.g. cefotaxime and fluconazole).
- *Wilson's disease:* Consider penicillamine and iv vitamin E.

Indications for liver transplantation

Paracetamol induced liver failure

- pH < 7.3 (after volume expansion) *OR*
- *ALL* of the following
  - PT > 100s
  - Creatinine > 300μM
  - Grade 3–4 encephalopathy

Non-paracetamol induced liver failure

Any 3 of the following

- PT > 50s
- Jaundice to encephalopathy > 7 days
- Aged < 10yrs or > 40 yrs
- Bilirubin > 300 μM
- Unfavourable aetiology *(i.e. non-paracetamol, not Hep A, not Hep B)*

Decompensated chronic liver disease

Patients with chronic liver disease from cirrhosis may present with acute decompensation due to a variety of causes (see table below).

Clinical features
- Ask specifically for a history of previous hepatitis, jaundice, alcohol intake, previous drug history. Weight loss may point to a malignancy. Pruritus, pigmentation, and xanthelasma in a young woman may be due to primary biliary cirrhosis.
- Examine for evidence of long-standing liver dysfunction: leuconychia, palmar erythema, clubbing, spider naevi, gynaecomastia, and small testes. Splenomegaly and distended abdominal veins signify portal hypertension.
- Examine specifically for features of decompensation: encephalopathy (confusion, 'liver flap'), ascites, oedema, jaundice, or fever.

Causes of acute decompensation of chronic liver disease	

• Intercurrent infection
  – spontaneous bacterial peritonitis
  – pneumonia
  – skin infections
• Acute GI haemorrhage
• Additional hepatotoxic insult
  – alcoholic binge
  – acute viral hepatitis
  – hepatotoxic drugs (see p571)
	• Drugs
	  – sedatives/narcotics
	  – diuretics
	• Metabolic derrangement
	  – hypoglycaemia
	  – electrolyte disturbance
	• Major surgery
	• Constipation
	• Progression of disease

Investigations

Unless the cause for the decompensation and the diagnosis for the pre-existing liver disease is known, the patient warrants full investigation (see p520).

Management

As for patients with acute liver failure, the mainstay of treatment is supportive. The decision on how aggressively you manage the patient (i.e admission to ICU, invasive monitoring, etc.) depends on the previous diagnosis, on a reversible element to the acute insult, and whether the patient is a candidate for liver transplantation. They have less capacity to regenerate their hepatocytes and prognosis of patients requiring mechanical ventilation and haemodynamic support is very poor without transplant.

- *Sepsis:* Start 'blind' treatment if there is a fever or increased WCC (e.g. cefotaxime): be guided by culture results. Bacterial peritonitis, see p516.
- Management of *coagulopathy*, *cardiovascular* and *respiratory support*, *metabolic disturbances*, and *renal failure* is discussed on p522. *Ascites* – see p516.
- *Upper GI haemorrhage* – see p480.

Hepatic encephalopathy

Hepatic encephalopathy is a neuropsychiatric disturbance of cognitive function in a patient with acute or chronic liver disease (see p518). It is said that patients with cirrhosis do NOT develop cerebral oedema, although we have seen extensor posturing in alcoholic cirrhotics following variceal haemorrhage.

Clinically it can be assessed by the presence of altered conscious level, asterixis (liver flap), abnormal EEG, impaired psychometric tests and an elevated arterial ammonia concentration. Patients may present with Parkinsonian features. However in patients with chronic liver disease, it may be sub-clinical with subtle changes in awareness, or attention span. It is graded as shown on p518.

Treatment The aim of treatment is to improve morbidity.
- Exclude other causes of confusion (see p394).
- Dietary restriction is controversial, and may be harmful in malnourished patients. Ensure adequate calorie intake.
- Give lactulose: This semi-synthetic disaccharide is poorly absorbed. It is digested in the large bowel and undergoes fermentation. This alters faecal pH and nitrogen-utilization by bowel flora.
- Lactitol has a similar action to lactulose but has less side effects
- Phosphate enemas help to purge the large bowel. Most useful in the context of an acute food load (e.g. GI bleeding).

Liver abscesses

Presentation

- Commonly present with fever and night sweats, weight loss, or right upper quadrant or intercostal pain.
- The underlying cause (e.g. appendicitis) may be silent or barely noticed. Ask about recent abdominal pain, altered bowel habit, diarrhoea, biliary colic, blood p.r, or inflammatory bowel disease
- The travel history, occupation (farming is a risk factor for amoebiasis), or contact with infected persons (TB) may help.
- Examine for jaundice, hepatomegaly, pleural effusions (commonly right-sided), intercostal tenderness (characteristic of amoebic abscesses), abdominal masses (tumour or inflammatory mass), and lymphadenopathy. Perform a rectal examination for pelvic tumour.
- Severe infection may be associated with septic shock (p216).

Causes

- Pyogenic organisms (appendicitis, diverticulitis, carcinoma, biliary)
- Amoebic abscess (*Entamoeba histolytica*)
- Hydatid cyst (*Echinococcus granulosus*)
- Tuberculous (very rare)

Investigations

- U&Es (renal impairment with sepsis).
- LFTs (non-specific, tend to be cholestatic; may be normal with amoebic abscess).
- Prothrombin time may be prolonged with multiple abscesses.
- FBC (leucocytosis, eosinophilia, non-specific anaemia).
- Blood cultures, CRP, ESR.
- Amoebic and hydatid serology.
- Stool may contain amoebic cysts or vegetative forms.
- CXR (looking for effusion, or pulmonary TB).
- USS of liver, biliary tree, and abdomen (iliac fossae in particular) ± CT scan with contrast, looking for masses. Both pyogenic and amoebic abscesses tend to be thick-walled; hydatid cysts are thin-walled and there may be daughter cysts. Solid tumours are echodense but may have necrotic hypodense centres.
- Gallium scan (or indium-111 labelled WBC scan) will show up pyogenic foci in the liver and elsewhere (e.g. terminal ileitis); amoebic abscesses do not take up the label.
- Aspirate any large abscesses and send for Gram stain, and culture. If there is a suspicion of hydatid disease aspiration is contraindicated.

Management

- Aspirate any large abscesses under USS. It is pointless to try and drain multiple abscesses. If there is a continuing intra-abdominal source it is virtually impossible to eradicate liver abscesses without removing or dealing with that source (e.g. appendix or biliary infection).
- *Pyogenic abscess:* Percutaneous aspiration of any large abscesses. Broad spectrum antibiotics (e.g. cefotaxime and metronidazole).
- *Amoebic abscess:* (see p500). Treat with metronidazole (or tinidazole) and diloxanide furoate. USS-guided aspiration may help improve penetration if the drugs and shorten illness. Secondary bacterial infection occurs in up to 20%.
- *Hydatid disease:* Open surgical drainage is the treatment of choice. Albendazole may help reduce the risk of recurrence post surgery or used in inoperable cases.
- Give anti-tuberculous therapy for tuberculous abscesses

Acute pancreatitis: Assessment

Acute pancreatitis is occasionally managed by physicians, particularly if it presents in an unusual way (e.g. chest pain).

Presentation

- Abdominal pain: Epigastric or generalized, of rapid onset, but may occur anywhere (including chest); dull, constant, and boring. Radiation to the back or between the scapulae, often relieved by leaning forward. (Differential diagnosis is leaking aortic aneurysm.)
- Nausea, vomiting, and dehydration ± jaundice.
- Peritonitis with epigastric tenderness, localized rebound tenderness or generalized abdominal rigidity. An abdominal mass may indicate a pancreatic pseudocyst or abscess. Bowel sounds usually absent.
- Tachycardia and hypotension; shock/collapse and respiratory failure in severe cases (especially in the elderly).
- Very rarely signs of bleeding in the pancreatic bed, Grey-Turner's sign (ecchymosis in the flanks) or Cullen's sign (peri-umbilical bruising), tender red skin nodules (due to sub-cutaneous fat necrosis).
- Hypocalcaemic tetany.

Investigations

• Amylase	Elevated, but not specific (see table opposite), especially if only up to 4 × upper limit of normal. A persistently raised amylase (several days-weeks) may indicate the development of a pseudocyst.
• FBC	Raised haematocrit and leukocytosis.
• U&Es	Urea may be raised with hypovolaemia.
• Glucose	May be raised.
• LFT's	AST and bilirubin often elevated especially in gall-stone pancreatitis. Disproportionately elevated γ-GT may indicate an alcohol aetiology.
• Calcium	Hypocalcaemia (unless precipitant was ↑ Ca^{2+})
• ABGs	Mandatory. Hypoxia ± metabolic acidosis.
• AXR	Generalized ileus or sentinel loops (dilated gas filled loops in the region of the pancreas). Look for evidence of pancreatic calcification or biliary stone.
• CXR	May show a pleural effusion, elevated diaphragm, or pulmonary infiltrates.
• USS	May confirm diagnosis and detect gall-stones ± biliary obstruction, pseudocysts, and abscesses.
• CT abdomen	Dynamic contrast-enhanced is reliable at detection of pancreatic necrosis and grading severity
• Misc.	Pancreatic lipase, trypsin activated peptides, or pancreatic amylase are more specific than amylase. CRP is often elevated and may be used to monitor progression of the attack

Assessment of severity

The severity of disease has NO correlation with the elevation of serum amylase. Several prognostic indices have been published, but it takes 48 hours to fully appreciate disease severity. See table opposite.

The mortality from acute pancreatitis is approximately 10%, and rises to 40% in those developing a pancreatic abscess. The mortality is highest in those with a first episode of pancreatitis. Around 15% of patients presenting with acute pancreatitis have recurrent disease.

Causes of abdominal pain and elevated serum amylase

- Acute pancreatitis
- Stomach or small bowel perforation
- Perforated peptic ulcer
- Mesenteric infarction
- Acute liver failure
- Acute cholecystitis or cholangitis
- Renal failure (modest elevation)
- Diabetic ketoacidosis

Markers of severity in acute pancreatitis*

At presentation
- Age > 55 years
- WBC > 16 x 10^9/litre
- Glucose > 10mM (non-diabetic)
- LDH > 350IU
- AST > 250 iu/litre

During the first 48 hours
- Haematocrit fall > 10%
- Urea rise > 10mM
- Serum Ca^{2+} < 2.0mmol/litre
- Base excess > 4mEq/litre
- P_aO_2 < 8kPa
- Serum albumin < 32g/litre
- Estimated fluid sequestration > 6 litres

Mortality: 0–2 criteria = 2%; 3–4 = 15%; 5–6 = 40%; > 7 = 100%.

* Data compiled from Imrie CW *et al* (1978) *Br. J. Surg.* **65**:337 and Ranson JH *et al* (1974) *Surg. Gynaecol. Obstet.* **139**:69.

Acute pancreatitis: Management

The principles of management are:
• Liaise with surgeons.
• Supportive measures – the majority will subside in 3–10 days.
• Careful observation for the development of complications.
• Identify the cause (see table opposite).

Supportive treatment
• Establish iv access. If there is shock, markers of moderate-severe pancreatitis, elderly patient, hypoxia not readily correcting with oxygen, or other co-existent disease, insert a CVP line to help control fluid input/output.
• Patients are usually severely volume depleted: give prompt fluid replacement with colloid (e.g. Haemaccel®) or 0.9% saline. Monitor urine output and insert a urinary catheter if required.
• Oxygen should be given if there is hypoxia on air (use continuous pulse oximetry in severe cases and 6 hourly for the first 48 hours for the rest, to monitor for respiratory failure).
• Keep nil by mouth ± nasogastric suction. If the course of the illness is protracted consider early use of TPN.
• Monitor blood glucose regularly and treat with insulin if high.
• Narcotic analgesia: *pethidine* causes less spasm of the sphincter of Oddi and is preferred to morphine.
• Antibiotics: are not indicated unless there is evidence of sepsis (see below). Give cefuroxime and metronidazole.
• Octreotide (somatostatin analogue): This suppresses pancreatic enzyme secretion and so makes theoretical sense but is of unproven benefit (see p489 for one regimen for iv infusion).
• Peritoneal lavage. There is no proven benefit from removing toxic materials from peritoneal exudate.
• H_2-antagonists have not been shown to affect mortality.

Complications (seen in ~ 20%)

Local	Systemic
• Abscess	• Electrolyte imbalance
• Pseudocyst ± infection	• $\downarrow Ca^{2+}$, $\downarrow Mg^{2+}$
• Biliary obstruction	• Acute renal failure
• Ascites, pleural effusion	• Shock
• Fistula	• Respiratory failure
• Splenic, portal, or mesenteric vein obstruction	• Sepsis

Septic complications
Sepsis is the most common cause of death. This should be suspected when there is a persistent fever, leucocytosis, pain/tenderness, or an overall clinical deterioration. These signs are an indication for multiple blood cultures and an abdominal CT. Pancreatic pseudocysts are more common in alcoholic pancreatitis (15% v 3% in gall-stone AP), but infection is more common in gall-stone pancreatitis,

Biliary pancreatitis: Urgent ERCP within 72h of presentation reduces complications and mortality in patients with severe gall-stone pancreatitis. The benefit has not been demonstrated in mild cases.

Indications for surgery
• Infected pancreatic necrosis
• Pancreatic abscess
Radiologically guided percutaneous drainage is now preferred to surgery for pancreatic pseudocysts.

Gastroenterological emergencies

Acute pancreatitis

Causes of acute pancreatitis

Common (80%)
- Gall-stones (including biliary microlithiasis or sludge) (60%)
- Alcohol (20%)

Rare (10%)
- Iatrogenic (ERCP or any form of abdominal surgery)
- Trauma (even seemingly minimal trauma, as pancreas is in a very vulnerable position e.g. 'seat-belt sign' or bicycle handle-bar injury)
- Infections

  Viral – mumps, rubella, coxsackie B, EBV, CMV, Hep A and B)

  Bacterial – mycoplasma

  Others – ascaris, flukes (*Clonorchis sinensis*) .
- Systemic vasculitis (SLE, polyarteritis nodosa, etc.)
- Drugs (e.g. thiazides, frusemide, NSAIDs, sulphonamides, azathioprine, tetracyclines, and valproate; possibly steroids)
- Hypertriglyceridaemia (serum amylase falsely low)
- Hypercalcaemia or iv calcium infusions
- Hypothermia
- Pancreatic carcinoma (3% present with acute pancreatitis)
- Misc.: Anatomical abnormalities (pancreas divisum, duodenal or peri-ampullary diverticulae); scorpion bites, cystic fibrosis

Unknown (10%)

---

10 Haematological emergencies

Blood transfusion reactions: Assessment

Presentation	Causes	Timing
Shock (major haemolysis) Lumbar pain, headache Chest pain, SOB Rigors, pyrexia Urticaria, flushing Hypotension Oliguria Haemoglobinuria Jaundice DIC	**Red call antibodies** ABO incompatibility Other antibodies	**Immediate** (mins/hours)
Shock (septic) Rigors, pyrexia Hypotension Oliguria DIC	**Bacterial contamination**	**Immediate** (min/hours)
Fever Isolated pyrexia Rigors Pulmonary infiltrate (rare)	**White cell antibodies** Bacterial pyrogens	**Early** (30–90 min)
Allergic reactions Urticaria Pyrexia Rigors Facial oedema Dyspnoea	**Donor plasma proteins**	**Early** (mins/hours)
Circulatory overload Breathlessness Cough Pulmonary/peripheral oedema	**Rapid transfusion**	**Early** (hours)
Delayed haemolysis Pyrexia Anaemia Jaundice	**Minor red cell antibodies**	**Late** (7–10 days)
Delayed thrombocytopenia Purpura Mucosal bleeding	**Platelet antibody** (commonly anti-Pl^{A1})	**Late** (2–10 days)
Infection	**Hep. B,C, non A/B/C CMV, EBV, HIV Toxoplasmosis Malaria, syphilis**	**Late** (days/months)

Blood transfusion reactions

Blood transfusion reactions: Management

The main problem encountered in practice is differentiating a (common) rise in temperature during a blood transfusion from (the rare but potentially lethal) major transfusion reactions. The common patterns of reactions are outlined on p534.

Pointers to a severe reaction include:
- Symptoms – does the patient *feel* unwell?
- Pattern of temperature – a *rapid* rise in temperature to > 38°C is common in minor reactions.
- Hypotension or tachycardia.

Management
- Stop the transfusion
- *Give*   Hydrocortisone 100mg iv
  Chlorpheniramine 10mg iv
  Adrenaline 1:1000 1ml im if severe reaction
  If severe shock give adrenaline 100µg slowly iv, repeating as necessary, stopping once the patient responds
- *Treat shock* iv colloids, crystalloid, inotropes (see p212)
  Antibiotics – if bacterial contamination is possible
  Monitor fluid balance
  Watch for hyperkalaemia/haemoglobinuric ARF
- *Take blood* FBC, U&Es
  Repeat cross-match and Coomb's test
  Full coagulation screen
  Blood cultures
- *Urine*   Bilirubin, free Hb, methaemoglobinuria
  (repeat at 6h and 24h)
- *Return donor blood* for repeat cross-match and culture
- *Examine urine for haemoglobinuria* (dipstick)

Non-haemolytic transfusion reaction

• Isolated pyrexia	Slow transfusion
• Allergic symptoms	Stop transfusion Give hydrocortisone 100mg iv and chlorpheniramine 10mg iv
• Anaphylaxis (see p212)	Stop transfusion and give oxygen Adrenaline 1:1000, 1ml im; if severe give 100µg (1ml of 1:10,000) slow iv injection) Hydrocortisone 100mg iv Chlorpheniramine 10mg iv IV colloid to restore circulatory volume
• Circulatory overload (see p74)	Oxygen, frusemide iv (40–120mg) Nitrate infusion (0–10mg/h)
• Delayed haemolysis	Repeat cross-match, and Coomb's test Transfuse with fresh cross-matched blood
• Thrombocytopenia	Immune mediated – Treat with Pl^{A1} negative transfusions, high dose iv IgG, steroids and plasmapheresis. [↓ platelets seen if > 5 units transfused due to dilution]

Sickle cell crisis: Presentation

A small percentage of sufferers with sickle cell disease have recurrent crises, and repeated hospital admissions. There is an unwarranted tendency to attribute this to a low pain threshold, or to 'dependence' on opiates, rather than to severity of disease. Analgesia should never be denied to patients. This group of patients has the *highest* rate of serious complications and mortality as a result of their severe disease.

Painful (vaso-occlusive) crisis
- This is the most common presentation in adults and children.
- Severe/excruciating pain is felt at one or more sites, especially long bones (small bones in children), back, ribs, sternum.
- There may be associated pyrexia (usually < 38.5°C), tenderness, local warmth and swelling, or there may be no objective features.
- Haemolysis may be increased (increased bilirubin, fall in Hb), but is not a good correlate.
- *There are no reliable clinical markers for severity of crisis.*

Chest crisis
- The commonest cause of mortality.
- Vaso-occlusion of pulmonary microvasculature results in reduced perfusion and local infarction.
- May be heralded by rib/sternal pain.
- Often precipitated by a chest infection.
- Symptoms (which may be minor initially) include pleuritic chest pain, breathlessness.
- Signs are minimal; usually reduced air entry at lung bases.
- CXR shows uni/bilateral consolidation, usually basal.
- P_aO_2 is often markedly reduced.

Cerebral infarction
- Usually in children < 5 yrs, rare in adults.
- Presents as acute stroke.
- High risk of recurrence.

Splenic/hepatic sequestration
- Usually in children < 5 yrs.
- RBCs trapped in spleen and/or liver.
- Causes severe anaemia; circulatory collapse.

Aplastic crisis
- Usually in children, young adults.
- Mainly caused by parvovirus infection
- Exacerbated by folate deficiency.
- Sudden fall in Hb, reduced reticulocyte count.

Haemolytic crisis
- Often accompanies painful crises.
- Fall in Hb; *increased* reticulocyte count.

Cholecystitis/cholangitis/biliary colic
- Pigment stones common due to haemolytic anaemia.
- Can be misinterpreted as vaso-occlusive crisis.

Priapism
- Prolonged, painful erections due to local vaso-occlusion.
- May result in permanent impotence.
- This is a urological emergency. On-call urologists should be informed on the patient's arrival in casualty.

Sickle cell crisis: Management

General measures

Control pain

- Oral analgesia (e.g. dihydrocodeine) may be sufficient for minor crises.
- Usually parenteral opiates are necessary, often in high doses,
  - e.g. pethidine 100–150mg im every 2 hours.
    diamorphine 20–25mg sc every 2 hours.
- Failure to control pain using these regimes usually indicates the need for a continuous opiate infusion, or a patient-controlled analgesia (PCA) pump.
- Supplementary analgesics, such as diclofenac 50mg tds po, and dothiepin 75–150mg nocte po, may have a small additional benefit.

Ensure hydration

- iv crystalloids are preferred, but venous access is often a problem.
- Aim for an input of 3–4l/day.

Give oxygen

- Surprisingly not of proven benefit (except in chest crises), but often provides symptomatic relief.
- In a severe chest crisis, CPAP/full ventilation may become necessary. Transfer to ITU early.

Give folic acid

- Give 5mg po od (continue long-term in all patients).

Give antibiotics

- If an infective precipitant, or component, of the crisis is suspected, start 'blind' antibiotics (e.g. cefuroxime 750mg iv tds) after infection screen.

Investigations

- FBC — Hb (?fall from steady state).
  WCC – often artefactually raised, due to the presence of nucleated RBCs.
- Reticulocytes — Raised in haemolysis, reduced in aplastic crisis.
- HbS% — Can guide transfusion requirements.
- Blood cultures — If pyrexial.
- Stool cultures — If diarrhoea + bone pain ?salmonella osteomyelitis.
- CXR — Regardless of symptoms.
- Pulse oximetry — +/- Arterial blood gases if hypoxic.
- Bone XR — ?osteomyelitis (persisting pain, pyrexia, or bacteraemia). ?avascular necrosis (chronic hip / shoulder pain).
- Viral serology — If aplastic crisis (?parvovirus).
- X-match — If transfusion/exchange indicated (see below).

Exchange transfusion

This is performed by venesection of 1–2 units, with fluid replacement, (N saline 1 litre over 2–4 hours) followed by transfusion of cross-matched blood. If a larger exchange is required, or fluid balance is precarious, the exchange can be performed on a cell separator. Aim for Hb between 7–9g/l in either case; *a higher Hb can increase blood viscosity and pre cipitate further sickling*. In severe crises, red cell exchange should be repeated until the HbS% is < 40%.

Sickle cell crisis

Indications for urgent exchange transfusion

- Chest crisis
- Cerebral infarction
- Severe, persisting painful crisis
- Priapism

Bleeding disorders: General approach

Presentation

- Normal haemostasis requires the interaction of platelets, fibrin from the clotting cascade, and the microvasculature. An abnormality of any of these components may present as easy bruising, purpura, or spontaneous or excessive bleeding.
- Muscle haematomas or haemarthroses suggest clotting factor deficiencies (e.g. haemophilia), whereas purpura or bruising suggests abnormalities of platelet function.
- Mucosal haemorrhage (acute GI bleed) may occur without any haemostatic abnormalities, e.g. due to peptic ulcer disease.
- If a coagulation or platelet abnormality is uncovered on 'routine' testing, examine the patient for occult bleeding (e.g. iron-deficient anaemia, fundal haemorrhages).

Causes

These can be divided into:
1. Coagulation abnormalities
2. Platelet abnormalities (too few or dysfunctional)
3. Microvascular abnormalities

Investigations

All patients should have:-
- Coagulation screen (PT, APTT, TT)
- FBC and film
- U&Es
- LFTs
- X-match

Where appropriate consider:-
- Bleeding time
- Platelet function tests
- Bone marrow aspirate and trephine
- Autoantibody screen
- Anti-platelet antibodies
- Specific coagulation factor levels
- Acquired factor inhibitors

Management

General measures

- Avoid non-steroidal medications, especially aspirin
- Never give intramuscular injections
- Avoid arterial punctures
- Enlist expert help with invasive procedures. Use internal jugular rather than subclavian route for central line insertion.
- Avoid automated blood pressure measurement devices as they may provoke bleeding into the upper arm.
- Examine skin, oral mucosa, and fundi daily for evidence of fresh bleeding. Remove any IUD.
- Restore circulatory volume with iv colloid if there is haemodynamic compromise. Give blood as soon as available but remember that blood transfusions can exacerbate existing platelet or clotting factor deficiencies (dilutional effect).

Specific therapy

- Look for any local cause for the bleeding (e.g. oesophageal varicies, vascular damage causing epistaxis, chest infection causing haemoptysis) that may be amenable to treatment.
- Stop any drug that may be exacerbating bleeding (see table opposite).
- Correct coagulation abnormalities if appropriate (p546).
- Correct platelet abnormalities if appropriate (p550).

Drugs that may cause bleeding disorders

Coagulation abnormalities
- Heparin
- Warfarin
- Asparaginase ($\downarrow$ vitamin K-dependent factors)
- Heparin analogues (argatroban, hirudin)

Thrombocytopenia

Immune
- Heparin
- Quinine
- Penicillin
- H_2-receptor antagonists
- Thiazide diuretics

Non-immune
- Cytotoxic chemotherapy
- Chloramphenicol
- Primaquine
- Alcohol

Abnormal platelet function
- Aspirin, NSAIDs
- Ticlopidine
- Antibiotics (e.g. piperacillin, cefotaxime)
- Dextran
- Alcohol

Abnormal microvasculature
- Corticosteroids

Bleeding disorders: Abnormal coagulation

Common causes
- Anti-coagulants
- Liver disease
- Vit. K deficiency
  - obstructive jaundice
  - small bowel disease
- DIC

Rarer causes
- Massive transfusion
- Haemophilia A, B
- von Willebrand's disease
- Acquired Factor VIII inhibitors
- Amyloid (acquired Factor X deficiency)
- α_2-plasmin inhibitor deficiency

544

Diagnosis

Defect	Interpretation	Consider
↑ PT	Extrinsic pathway defect	Warfarin, liver disease, vitamin K deficiency
↑ APTT	Intrinsic pathway defect	Heparin, haemophilia, von Willebrand's disease, lupus anti-coagulant (anti-phospholipid syndrome). Bleeding time will be abnormal in vW's disease
↑ PT and APTT	Multiple defects (usually acquired)	Liver disease, DIC, warfarin
↑ TT	Abnormal fibrin production	Heparin effect, fibrinogen defect, excess FDPs (which interfere with reaction)
↑ PT, APTT, TT	Multiple (acquired) defects	Deficient or abnormal fibrinogen or heparin. Reptilase time* will be normal if due to heparin
↓ Fibrinogen	Excess consumption of clotting factors and fibrinogen	Consumptive coagulopathy (but not necessarily full DIC), severe liver disease
↑ FDPs	↑ Fibrin(ogen) degradation	The exact interpretation depends on the lab. test used. Some do not distinguish between fibrin and FDPs. Some are more specific to fibrin degradation (e.g. D-dimers) and thus suggest widespread clot formation and breakdown (i.e. DIC)
↑ Bleeding time	Abnormal platelet function	vW's disease (↑ APTT), congenital or acquired platelet dysfunction (see table p543). Consider platelet aggregation studies

The lupus anticoagulant usually confers a pro-thrombotic rather than a bleeding tendency. *Reptilase is a snake venom not inhibited by heparin. It converts fibrinogen to fibrin.

Haematological emergencies

Bleeding due to abnormal coagulation:
Management

Options are:

- **Fresh frozen plasma**: Indicated for rapid treatment of prolonged PT or APTT of whatever cause. Give approximately 2 units for every 5 seconds the PT is prolonged above normal; recheck PT after every 4 units. Watch for signs of fluid overload and give iv frusemide if necessary.

- **Vitamin K**: 10mg iv slowly (daily for 3 days) if deficiency is suspected (e.g. warfarin or obstructive jaundice). If bleeding is not severe, and complete reversal of anti-coagulation is contraindicated (e.g. in patients with prosthetic valves) give 1mg vitamin K iv once only and give FFP to control bleeding acutely.

- **Protamine sulphate** (1mg iv neutralizes 100 iu heparin) is rarely used in practice. Stopping a heparin infusion will normalize an APTT in 2–4h.

- **Cryoprecipitate** should be used only if the fibrinogen is below 200g/l.

- **Factor concentrates** can be used in the treatment of isolated factor deficiencies, e.g. haemophilia. Concentrates of Factors II, VII, IX, and X are also available in some centres for specific reversal of warfarin effects.

- **Anti-fibrinolytics** are used occasionally for the treatment of life-threatening bleeds following thrombolytic therapy or prostatectomy, and in certain conditions associated with hyperplasminaemia (e.g. acute promyelocytic leukaemia, certain malignancies). Give *aprotonin* 50–100ml (0.5–1MU) slow iv followed by 20ml (200kU) every hour until bleeding stops; alternatively, *tranexamic acid* 0.5–1g slow iv injection tds.

- **Miscellaneous**. DDAVP (see p558) and oestrogens are occasionally used for haemophilia and renal failure.

Circulating inhibitors of coagulation

Autoantibodies (IgG or IgM and occasionally IgA) which inhibit clotting factors are seen with:-

- Autoimmune diseases (e.g. SLE, rheumatoid arthritis)
- In response to therapy with factor concentrates (e.g. haemophilia)
- Drug induced (e.g. isoniazid, chlorpromazine, streptomycin)
- Post partum

Clotting tests most commonly show a prolonged APTT which is not corrected by 1:1 mixture with normal plasma.

Dysproteinaemias (e.g. myeloma or macroglobulinaemia) interfere with fibrin polymerization, impaired platelet function, and may be associated with factor deficiencies.

Management: Strategies include:

- Removal of immunoglobulin (e.g. plasmapheresis)
- Infusion of large amounts of factor
- Bypassing the factor inhibitor (e.g. with prothrombin complex concentrates, Factor VIIa or porcine factors)
- High dose iv immunoglobulin
- Cytotoxic chemotherapy

Haematological emergencies

Bleeding disorders: Abnormal platelets

Causes

Thrombocytopenia	

Increased platelet consumption
Immune
• Idiopathic (ITP)
• Drug-induced
• SLE
• HIV – related
• Massive transfusion
Non-immune
• Hypersplenism
• DIC, TTP
	Reduced platelet production
	• Myelosuppressants
	  drugs, alcohol
	  viral infections
	• Marrow infiltration / failure
	• B_{12} or folate deficiency
	• Wiscott-Aldrich syndrome
	  (eczema, immunodeficiency, and
	  thrombocytopenia)

Abnormal platelet function

• Drugs (e.g. aspirin)
• Uraemia
• Liver disease
• Myeloproliferative disorders
• Myelodysplasia
• Dysproteinaemia (e.g. myeloma)
• Inherited disorders
  Glanzman's disease (GP Ia deficiency)
  Bernard-Soulier disease (GP IIb/IIIa deficiency)
  Chediak-Higashi syndrome (abn. platelet granules)

Investigations

- Peripheral blood film — Evidence of haemolysis (DIC? TTP?), blasts; pancytopenia (marrow failure or infiltration? hypersplenism?).
- Coagulation screen — ?DIC
- Bone marrow aspirate — Increased megakaryocytes generally indicates ↑ peripheral consumption; decreased or abnormal megakaryocytes suggest a marrow problem.
- Autoantibody screen — Associated autoimmune diseases
- Anti-platelet antibodies
- Platelet function tests — For bleeding in the presence of adequate platelet numbers on the blood film.

- Low platelets ($< 20 \times 10^9$/l) may cause spontaneous bleeding and require platelet transfusion ± treatment for the underlying cause.
- Moderately low counts ($20–140 \times 10^9$/l) will rarely cause spontaneous bleeding, unless there is an associated clotting abnormality (e.g. DIC) or a primary marrow defect, with production of defective platelets (e.g. myelodysplasia). Transfuse only if there is continued bleeding or in preparation for major surgery.
- High counts ($500–1000 \times 10^9$/l) may also indicate a primary production problem, with abnormal platelets (e.g. myeloproliferative disorders). (Note: A moderately raised platelet count is a normal response to bleeding and is also seen in chronic inflammation.)

Bleeding due to abnormal platelets:

Management

This depends on the platelet count and severity of bleeding.

- If a *non-immune cause* is suspected and thrombocytopenia is profound ($< 20 \times 10^9/l$), transfuse 1–2 pools of platelets (5–6 units per pool).
- In *immune-mediated thrombocytopenia*, platelet transfusions are usually ineffective as sole therapy. Other measures include:
  - Prednisolone (60mg po od)
  - Immunoglobulin (0.25–1g/kg iv infusion): this usually works quicker than steroids, and can be combined with platelet transfusion if bleeding is severe. Start the infusion very slowly, as anaphylactic reactions (fever, urticaria, bronchospasm, and hypotension) are not uncommon. Treat as on p212.

Platelet transfusion

- These are available as pooled single-donor or random-donor platelet concentrates (PCs). 1 PC will raise the platelet count by $5–8 \times 10^9/l$, depending on the size of the patient and presence of anti-platelet antibodies. Pools of 5–6 units (PCs) are usually given.
- The platelet increment and survival should be monitored by FBC taken 30–60 minutes post transfusion and at 18–24h.
- Poor increments acutely may be due to the development of platelet alloantibodies; the patient should be switched to single donor platelets from a matched donor.
- Low counts at 18–24 hours may reflect co-existent conditions that reduce platelet survival (e.g. DIC, splenomegaly, sepsis).

Bleeding disorders: Over anti-coagulation

Warfarin

- Warfarin overdose (accidental or deliberate self-harm) results in a prolonged PT (and thus INR).
- Risk factors for significant bleeding include poor control, local lesion (e.g. peptic ulcer, angiodysplasia of the colon), high level of anti-coagulation (INR > 2.5), co-existent haematological abnormality (e.g. thrombocytopenia, myelodysplasia, etc.).

Management

- Moderate warfarin overdose (INR 6–9) without overt bleeding does not usually require specific treatment and may be managed as an out-patient provided the patient can attend for daily INR. Withhold warfarin until the INR falls to the therapeutic range. Try to identify the cause (incorrect tablets, alcohol binge, etc.).
- Asymptomatic patients with INR > 9 should be admitted to hospital overnight as the risk of severe haemorrhage is high. Withhold warfarin and give 2 units FFP iv and 0.5–1mg vitamin K iv slowly. Check INR in 18–24 hours and if < 7 treat as above.
- Bleeding in patients on warfarin requires urgent correction of clotting. If anti-coagulation needs to be continued (e.g. prosthetic heart valve) give FFP 2–4 units iv (p546) and vitamin K 2–4mg iv (this dose does not usually interfere with re-anti-coagulation, whereas higher doses make subsequent anti-coagulation difficult). Identify and treat the local lesion from which the patient is bleeding.

Heparin

- Risk factors for bleeding include increasing age, recent surgery or trauma, renal or liver failure, malignancy, bolus iv dosing rather than continuous infusion, APTT ratio > 3, co-existent haematological abnormality. Bleeding may occur even with the APTT within the therapeutic range.

Management

- Stop heparin: the APTT usually normalizes in 3–4 hours.
- Protamine sulphate (1mg iv neutralizes 100U heparin) may be used; halve the dose if heparin has been turned off 1 hour previously.

Low molecular weight heparins are thought to have fewer bleeding complications . However, their plasma half-life is longer and they are less easily reversed with protamine. Treatment of overdose is as above, but with repeated protamine if the APTT remains prolonged.

Heparin-associated thrombocytopenia (see p564)

Bleeding with fibrinolytic therapy

Risk factors for bleeding with fibrinolytic therapy are given on p20. Severe haemorrhage should be managed with:

- Supportive measures (colloid and blood transfusion to support circulatory volume).
- *Cryoprecipitate* transfusion as a source of fibrinogen.
- *Aprotonin* 50–100ml (0.5–1MU) slow iv followed by 20ml (200kU) every hour until bleeding stops. (Alternatively, give tranexamic acid 0.5–1g slow iv injection tds.)

Haematological emergencies

Bleeding in liver disease

The liver is involved in the synthesis of Factors II, VII, IX, and X (the vitamin K-dependent factors) as well as the clearance of 'activated' coagulation factors, fibrin molecules, and tissue plasminogen activator. The abnormalities most commonly found are:

Obstructive jaundice: Prolonged PT (vitamin K deficiency)

Acute liver failure: Prolonged PT and later prolonged APTT and TT (DIC).

Cirrhosis: Prolonged PT, APTT, and TT; low fibrinogen and/or dysfibrinogenaemia; raised FDPs, decreased clearance of tPA; low platelets (hypersplenism, DIC ± marrow dysfunction).

Management

Treatment is required for active GI bleeding or as prophylaxis for surgery or liver biopsy.

- Give *vitamin K* 10mg iv slowly (single dose).
- *FFP transfusion* is more effective.
- *Factor IX concentrate* contains Factors II, IX, and X and may be used in life-threatening bleeding. Discuss with your haematologist – this may paradoxically result in thrombosis as synthesis of the anti-coagulant proteins (antithrombin III, protein C and S) are reduced in liver failure.

Bleeding in uraemia

Uraemia results in both platelet dysfunction (impaired aggregation, adhesion, and activation) and endothelial dysfunction.

Management

- The treatment of choice is haemodialysis.
- Other measures that have been shown to be effective include
  – cyroprecipitate infusion,
  – desmopressin (DDAVP) (p558),
  – conjugated oestrogens,
  – blood transfusion or erythropoietin to raise the haematocrit to > 0.25.

Massive transfusion/cardiopulmonary bypass

- Transfusion results in dilutional thrombocytopenia and coagulopathy since transfused blood has lost functioning platelets and certain coagulation factors (e.g. V and VIII). This is particularly marked when packed red cells and colloids are used for volume expansion. With cardiopulmonary bypass, the extracorporeal circuit further damages the native platelets and depletes coagulation factors.
- Abnormalities include ↑ PT, ↑ APTT, ↑ bleeding time, ↑ FDPs, hypofibrinogenaemia, reduced Factor V and VIII levels.
- Post transfusion thrombocytopenia is a distinct disorder seen 8–10 days following transfusion and is due to a platelet-specific antibody (see p536).

Management

- *Prevent by* giving 1 unit FFP and 2 units platelets for every 5 units of stored blood.
- *Treatment* should be discussed with the haematology team and involves FFP, platelet and cryoprecipitate transfusion, and occasionally purified factor concentrates.

Haematological emergencies

Haemophilia and related disorders

Assessment

Haemophilia A X-linked recessive deficiency of Factor VIII ($\uparrow$ APTT; $\downarrow$ Factor VIII activity)

Haemophilia B X-linked recessive deficiency of Factor IX ($\uparrow$ APTT; $\downarrow$ Factor IX activity)

Clinical presentation depends upon the degree of factor deficiency.

- Patients with $< 2\%$ activity have a serious bleeding diathesis. Most are on home therapy.
- Patients with 2–5% activity are moderately affected; they bleed rarely but should be treated as severe haemophiliacs when they do.
- Patients with 5–40% factor activity rarely bleed spontaneously.

von Willebrand's disease

- Autosomal dominant (Types I, IIa and IIb) or recessive (Type III) with varying expression.
- Reduced levels of vW factor, which normally promotes platelet adhesion and protects Factor VIII from destruction (hence $\downarrow$ Factor VIII activity; $\uparrow$ bleeding time; $\uparrow$ or normal APTT).
- Less severe than the haemophilias, with haemarthroses and muscle bleeds being rare. Mucous membrane bleeding (esp. epistaxis) and post traumatic bleeding are the main problems.

Acute presentations

- *Acute haemarthroses* often occur at sites of previous bleeding, particularly if this has led to degenerative joint disease. Ankles, knees, hips, elbows are the most common sites. Symptoms include local tenderness, warmth and swelling, and may take days or weeks to resolve.
- *Intramuscular bleeds* can cause a compartment-type syndrome, leading to ischaemic necrosis and contracture. *Iliopsoas bleed* causes entrapment of femoral nerve and produces the triad of groin pain, hip flexion, and sensory loss over femoral nerve distribution. The pain may radiate to the abdomen, and mimic appendicitis.
- *Intracranial bleeding* is infrequent, but is still a common cause of mortality. It often follows minor head injury. Prognosis of intracerebral haemorrhage is generally poor. Extradural and subdural haemorrhage have a better prognosis.
- *Bleeding post trauma:* Classically there may be an initial period of haemostasis; bleeding then becomes persistent or intermittent over days/weeks.
- *Haematuria/ureteric clot colic* is rare in haemophilia. Usually there is no detectable underlying abnormality of renal tracts.
- *Problems relating to co-existent HIV or hepatitis B/C infection* are now the commonest cause of mortality, due to infected Factor VIII administered during the 1980s.

Investigations

Generally, acute investigations are not necessary for simple joint and muscle bleeds in a known haemophiliac. Consider:

- USS – for muscle haematomas (e.g. iliopsoas bleed).
- CT scan- history of head trauma; headache; abnormal neurology.
- Factor VIII levels- if bleed is severe and treatment is necessary.
- Factor VIII inhibitor titre – if refractory bleeds/history of inhibitor development.

Haemophilia and related disorders

Management
Most patients contact their haematologist directly unless they bleed when away from home. Be guided by your local haematologist.

General measures
- *Rest* of the affected part and ice packs may be of benefit.
- *Analgesia:* Avoid NSAIDs and intramuscular injections. Oral analgesia (e.g. dihydrocodeine) for minor bleeds; iv injections or infusions of high-dose opiates may be necessary. *NO im injections.*

Moderate or severe haemophiliac
- Treat with iv Factor VIII concentrate (minor bleeds – DDAVP).

Mild haemophiliac
- Factor VIII deficiency only: Mild or moderate bleeds should be treated with DDAVP. Severe bleeds or those not responding to DDAVP – treat with iv Factor VIII concentrate.
- Factor IX deficiency only – treat with Factor IX.

von Willebrand's disease
- *Mild and moderate bleeds*
  Type I and IIa – treat with DDAVP + tranexamic acid
  Type IIb – NOT DDAVP as this may result thrombocytopenia. Use Factor VIII concentrate.
- *Severe bleeds* – treat with Factor VIII concentrate and if bleeding continues, give cryoprecipitate and platelet transfusions.

N.B. *All CNS and perispinal bleeds are regarded as severe.*

Factor VIII replacement (see table opposite)
- Minor bleeds may respond to a single, slow, iv bolus of Factor VIII
- Major bleeds should be managed by 12 hourly treatment (8 hourly in severe bleeding) with frequent monitoring of Factor VIII levels, pre- and post treatment.
- Patients with *Factor VIII inhibitors* present a particular problem. This can sometimes be circumvented by the use of alternative forms of Factor VIII (human or porcine, depending on the type of inhibitor), or by the use of other products (e.g. FEIBA: Factor VIII inhibitor bypassing activity).

Factor IX replacement (see table opposite)
- Plasma half-life is longer than Factor VIII, and once daily administration is sufficient (twice daily in severe bleeds).
- Never give > 3 doses (each a maximum of 50U/kg) of Factor IX in 36 hours as it is highly thrombogenic.

DDAVP
- *Indications:* Mild – moderate haemophilia A, especially in children, von Willebrand's disease Type 1 and some Type II.
- *Dosage:* 0.4µg/kg in 100ml N saline iv over 20 mins; may be repeated 8–12 hours later. Peak haemostatic effect in 60–90 minutes.
- Monitor pulse and bp every 5 minutes: side-effects include flushing, hypotension, tachycardia, headache, nausea, rare reports of MI (caution in patients > 40 years or with cardiac history)

Tranexamic acid
- Give with DDAVP in vW or mild haemophilia A. Most useful in mucosal bleeds. Avoid in renal tract bleeding (may cause clots).
- *Dosage:* 1g po qds (adults). Mouthwash 4.8% every 10 minutes for oral bleeding.

Cryoprecipitate
- Give for severe bleeding in von Willebrand's disease not responding to DDAVP and tranexamic acid.
- *Dosage:* 10 – 20 units (bags) for 70 kg adult

Haemophilia and related disorders

A rough guide to Factor VIII and IX replacement			
	Desired Factor level	*Approx. amount of Factor VII required for 70kg patient*	
Mild/early bleeds	10–20%	500 units	(2 bottles)
Moderate bleeds	30–50%	1000 units	(4–6 bottles)
Severe bleeds	50–100%	1500–2000U	(> 8 bottles)

Factor VIII dose $= \dfrac{\text{Desired rise} \times \text{Body Wt}}{2}$

Factor IX dose $= \text{Desired rise} \times \text{Body Wt}$

Combined thrombotic and haemorrhagic disorders

A group of disorders in which the pathways of haemostasis become dysregulated, leading to microthrombus formation, platelet consumption, and, to a variable extent, clotting factor consumption. The exact pathogenesis varies, but in each case microthrombi cause organ damage, and thrombocytopenia results in bleeding. This co-existence of thrombosis and bleeding makes management very difficult.

Disseminated intravascular coagulation

An inappropriate activation of the coagulation pathways leading to:-

• Depletion of clotting factors, causing *prolongation of PT and APTT*
• Widespread thrombin activation, causing *prolongation of TT and reduced levels of fibrinogen*
• Formation of microthrombi, leading to *end-organ damage*
• Destruction of red cells in fibrin mesh, causing *microangiopathic haemolysis*
• Consumption of platelets leading to *thrombocytopenia* and increasing the bleeding tendency
• Activation of thrombolysis *(raised FDPs)* and further bleeding

The 'full house' of abnormalities does not need to be present initially, as the process is a progressive one.

Management

• *Treat the underlying cause* (60% have underlying sepsis).
• Supportive measures such as correction of shock, acidosis, and hypoxia may lead to an improvement in the coagulopathy.
• Transfuse blood to correct anaemia – massive transfusion may exacerbate coagulopathy by dilution of coagulation factors and platelets.

Specific therapy

• *Heparin:* This may be indicated when the coagulopathy results mainly in thromboses (e.g. in deep veins, peripheral gangrene). Give 15,000–24,000 units/24h iv infusion; aim for APTT ratio 1.5–2. Oral anticoagulants are generally ineffective.
• *Clotting factors:* Continued haemorrhage in spite of treatment of the underlying cause may respond to FFP (to correct abnormal PT / APTT), platelet (to correct thrombocytopenia) and cryoprecipitate (if fibrinogen level < 200g/l) transfusions. Purified antithrombin III has been used with some success in small trials.
• *Anti-fibrinolytics:* These may be used when there is marked fibrinolysis (↑ FDPs and ↓ fibrinogen) and haemorrhage. Give aprotinin 500,000 units (50ml) iv over 15–20 min followed by 200,000 units (20ml) iv every 4 hours. Heparin (15–24,000 units/24h) should be given simultaneously to try to prevent widespread thrombosis.

Prognosis

Overall mortality is > 50%. Obstetric complications have the best prognosis if managed expediently. There is little evidence that measures to prevent thrombosis (heparin, antithrombin III) or prevent thrombolysis improve the general prognosis.

Combined thrombotic and haemorrhagic disorders
Disseminated intravascular coagulation

Causes of DIC

Common
- Gram -ve septicaemia
- *Staph. aureus* sepsis
- Meningococcal septicaemia
- Malaria (esp. *falciparum*)
- Disseminated malignancy
  - mucinous adenocarcinomas
  - prostatic carcinoma
- Liver failure

Rarer
- Incompatible blood transfusion
- Severe trauma/burns
- Acute promyelocytic leukaemia
- Obstetric emergencies
  - abruptio placentae
  - amniotic fluid embolism
  - retained dead foetus
  - severe pre-eclampsia
- Anaphylaxis (e.g. snake bites)
- Hypoxia
- Haemangioma

Thrombotic thrombocytopenic purpura (TTP) and haemolytic-uraemic syndrome (HUS)

The primary event appears to be endothelial damage, causing micro-thrombus formation, end-organ damage (esp. brain, kidneys), and platelet consumption. The clinical picture tends to vary with age, renal abnormalities being more common in children; neurological problems in adults, but with considerable overlap.

Presentation

- Fever
- Anaemia (haemolytic picture: associated with jaundice, and haemo-globinuria)
- Thrombocytopenia with purpura and bleeding
- CNS-(confusion, headache, aphasia, visual disturbance, fits, coma, paralysis, psychoses – often fluctuating)
- Renal involvement (oliguria, anuria, haematuria) often mild initially
- The spleen is often slightly enlarged
- The presentation is usually acute, but there may be a history of neuropsychiatric disturbance going back over months or years
- HUS is often preceded by gastroenteritis or URTI

Investigations

- **FBC** — Anaemia with thrombocytopenia. Moderate leukocytosis with left shift.
- **Blood film** — Fragmented RBCs, polychromasia, thrombocytopenia, neutrophilia. Often not time for reticulocytosis.
- **Clotting** — *Mild or no abnormalities* initially; may deteriorate.
- **U&Es** — In adults, creatinine slow to rise over a few days; rapid deterioration more common in children.
- **LFTs** — ↑ Bili. (unconjugated) ↑ LDH (from haemolysis).
- **Haptoglobins** Decreased.
- **Urinalysis** — Proteinuria frequent; haematuria, haemoglobinuria.
- **Stool** — Culture – especially for *E. coli* strains.

Associations of TTP and HUS	
Recognized	*Controversial*
- Normal pregnancy	- SLE

- Drugs (OCP, cyclosporin, FK506, chemotherapeutic agents, metronidazole, penicillin, penicillamine, sulphonamides)	- HIV infection
	  – symptomatic or
	  – asymptomatic

- Gastroenteritis
  – esp. with E. coli
    (type 0157:H7 in children)
	- Coxsackie B infection
	- *Mycoplasma*
	- Malignancies
	- Bee stings
	- Radiotherapy

Thrombotic thrombocytopenic purpura (TTP) and haemolytic-uraemic syndrome (HUS)

Management

- Refer to specialist unit (renal and/or haematology).
- Give FFP while arranging urgent plasma exchange.
- Plasma exchange – aggressive regimen (65–140ml/kg/d) with FFP results in improvement (and possibly cure) of TTP in many patients. Tail off only after remission obtained.
- Steroids – used with plasma exchange at high doses (200mg/day) may be effective in mild cases without CNS involvement.
- Dialysis (haemodialysis or peritoneal dialysis) is used for acute renal failure (usually children).
- Broad spectrum antibiotics – unproven benefit, but seem sensible given infectious aetiology in some patients.
- Blood transfusion – to correct anaemia.
- Avoid platelet transfusion – exacerbates thrombosis.
- Other agents of unproven benefit include anti-coagulant therapy (heparin), thrombolytic therapy, anti-platelet agents (aspirin, dipyridamole, prostacyclin), vincristine, and gammaglobulin.

Prognosis

- Children/predominant HUS picture – 5–30% mortality. Renal impairment and hypertension is common in survivors.
- Adults / predominant TTP picture – 20–50% mortality.

Heparin-associated thrombocytopenia

- An idiosyncratic reaction seen in 1–2 %.
- It may be transient in the first week, often resolving spontaneously with continued therapy, without significant haemorrhage.
- Late-onset thrombocytopenia is seen 2–4 weeks after starting therapy and is caused by an IgG autoantibody that results in platelet activation, haemorrhage, and, in ~ 40%, thromboembolic events.
- Consider the diagnosis if the problem demanding heparinization does not resolve or worsens while the patient is on heparin (e.g. propagation of DVT) or a new thrombotic event takes place in a heparinized patient.
- Coagulation tests initially reflect heparin effects, but may become more abnormal with increasing clotting factor consumption.

Management

- Stop heparin immediately. Do not wait to see what happens to the platelet count
- Consider heparin alternatives. Both low molecular weight heparin and heparin substitutes can have a cross-over effect, and perpetuate the problem. Switch to warfarin as soon as possible.
- Do not give platelets to treat thrombocytopenia, as this can lead to further platelet activation and thrombosis.

Haematological emergencies

Acute leukaemias: Presentation

Types of acute leukaemia

Acute lymphoblastic leukaemia (ALL)

- B-, T-, null (undifferentiated), and common forms
- Mainly children and young adults

Acute myeloid leukaemia (AML)

- Classified into types M1–M7 ('FAB types')
- Mainly adults, including elderly

Both AML and ALL can develop by transformation of chronic myeloid leukaemia, or secondary to an underlying myelodysplastic syndrome , as well as occurring *de novo*. Rarer associations include paroxysmal nocturnal haemoglobinuria, Fanconi's anaemia, Down's syndrome.

Poor prognostic factors

- Increasing age.
- High white cell count at presentation.
- Severe sepsis.
- Single or multiple organ failure.
- Underlying myelodysplastic syndrome.
- Philadelphia chromosome positive acute leukaemia.
- Depends upon sub-classification of leukaemia on basis of morphology, chromosomal abnormalities, and cell surface markers.

Presentation

Red cell problems

- *Anaemia* – caused by suppression of erythropoiesis by leukaemia cells; also by bleeding due to low platelets or deranged clotting. The MCV is usually normal or high, unless blood loss is predominant. The reticulocyte count is often inappropriately low, reflecting myelosuppression.

White cell problems

- *High blast count* – may cause 'leukostasis' (crudely, sludging of white cells in small vessels), causing respiratory impairment, myocardial ischaemia/infarction, renal impairment, acute confusion, stroke, fits, migraine.
- *Leukaemia-related phenomena*–pyexia, malaise, muscle and joint pains
- *Neutropenia* – secondary to marrow infiltration by leukaemic cells.

Platelet problems

- *Thrombocytopenia* due to myelosuppression by leukaemic infiltrate. Existing platelets may have sub-normal function. Risk of bleeding increases if platelets are $< 15 \times 10^9/l$, or $< 20 \times 10^9/l$ if there is concomitant sepsis or coagulation abnormality.

Coagulation problems

- Range from a *prolongation of PT* to *DIC*, and may be due to sepsis, or effects of the leukaemia itself, especially acute promyelocytic leukaemia

Priorities

1. Stabilize the patient
2. Treat immediate problems, e.g.bleeding, sepsis
3. Confirm diagnosis
4. Define treatment strategy

Acute leukaemias: Management

Stabilize the patient

- *Airway:* Stridor may be secondary to mediastinal obstruction in certain cases of leukaemia – mainly T-ALL. If present, call anaesthetist immediately and arrange transfer to ITU
- *Breathing:* Breathlessness may be due to infection (including atypical organisms), leukostasis (high WCC), severe anaemia, cardiac failure (leukostasis; severe sepsis), pulmonary haemorrhage (rarely due to thrombocytopenia, alone – ?concurrent infection).

  Give oxygen. Where possible, use pulse oximeter to monitor oxygen saturation, avoiding arterial puncture with thrombocytopenia.
- *Circulation:* Shock is usually secondary to sepsis, but consider the possibility of blood loss if low platelets/clotting abnormalities, or cardiac failure from leukostasis.
  - Restore circulatory volume
  - Give broad spectrum antibiotics immediately (after blood cultures) if sepsis suspected (see febrile neutropenia).
- ***Refer to a haematologist.***

Treat immediate problems

- *Infection*: Until the blood film has been reviewed by a haematologist, assume the patient is neutropenic, and treat all infections aggressively. See section on febrile neutropenia (p580).
- *Severe bleeding*
- Transfuse cross-matched blood.
- If platelets $< 50 \times 10^9$/l, give 1 adult pool platelets (5–6 units).
- If platelets $< 20 \times 10^9$/l, give 2 adult pools.
- If prothrombin time prolonged, give 2 units FFP for every 5 seconds above normal PT (approximate guide).
- If fibrinogen < 200g/l, consider cryoprecipitate in addition.
- *Minor bleeding/bleeding risk*
  - Transfuse 1 adult pool platelets if platelets $< 15 \times 10^9$l, or if platelets $< 20 \times 10^9$/l and there is a clotting abnormality or pyrexia (sepsis can precipitate bleeding).
- *Anaemia:-*
  - Transfuse CMV-screened blood if symptomatic UNLESS
    – Platelets $< 15 \times 10^9$/l (give platelets first, as transfusion will lower platelet count further)
    – WCC $> 100 \times 10^9$/l

Transfusion in the presence of a high WCC is dangerous, and can precipitate the complications of leucostasis.

- *High WCC* Discuss with haematologists. May require urgent leuko-pheresis, preferably in an ITU setting.

Confirmation of diagnosis

Take a full history, looking for possible aetiological factors. Length of illness (was there a preceding chronic condition, e.g. myelodysplasia?). PMH (?Down's syndrome, radiation/chemotherapy exposure). Occupation (?exposure to irradiation; benzenes; other mutagens). Family history (rare familial syndromes, e.g.Fanconi's anaemia).

Examine the patient, looking for accessory clues to diagnosis (?lymphadenopathy, hepatosplenomegaly, gum hyperplasia) and identifying potential sites for infection (dental caries, skin lesions, etc.)

Final confirmation then rests upon a bone marrow aspirate, with samples being sent for morphology, chromosome analysis, and cell surface markers.

Acute leukaemias: Treatment

The treatment of acute leukaemia depends upon the type of leukaemia, and involves several courses of chemotherapy, taking months or even years to complete. The prognosis has improved in recent years and depends upon the exact diagnosis; mortality in the first few months is still, however, 20–40%. The impact of the diagnosis on – often young – patients and their families is devastating, and extensive time is needed in discussion.

Before embarking on chemotherapy, the following must be considered.

Sperm/oocyte banking

Almost all forms of chemotherapy carry a high incidence of subsequent infertility. When desired by the patient, every attempt must be made to provide for banking of sperm or, if possible, oocyte collection prior to starting chemotherapy. Unfortunately, in practice, the presence of leukaemia itself often makes sperm non-viable, and the need to start treatment precludes repeated collections.

Discussion about side-effects

Patients need to be warned about hair loss, sterility, emesis (less of a problem with current anti-emetics, but varies with individual), infections, bleeding, mucositis, etc. Patient-orientated literature is available on acute leukaemia and chemotherapy, and may be helpful.

Other considerations

- Lumbar puncture (?CNS involvement). Indicated in:-
  - Acute lymphoblastic leukaemia
  - AML if high WCC at presentation
  - Any neurological symptoms / signs
- HLA typing of patient/siblings may be considered, with a view to possible bone marrow transplant in the future. This is usually left to a later stage, once the patient has achieved clinical remission.
- CMV status should be determined, and CMV negative products administered to all CMV negative patients throughout their treatment.

Prior to commencement of chemotherapy

- Commence allopurinol 24h in advance.
- Prescribe regular antiseptic mouthwashes, to be used 4–5 × /day in conjunction with anti-thrush prophylaxis (nystatin suspension and/or amphotericin lozenges).
- Ensure adequate hydration. Give iv fluids if fluid input < 3l/d.
- Give an anti-emetic one hour before chemotherapy, and at regular intervals during treatment with chemotherapy. Appropriate regimes include:
  - ondansetron 4–8mg iv/po bd
  - metoclopramide 10–20mg iv po plus dexamethasone 2–4mg iv po 4–8 hourly.

Complications of bone marrow transplantation (BMT) 1.

- *Always contact and refer the patient back to their BMT centre*

The morbidity and mortality following BMT (especially allogeneic BMT) is high, particularly within the first 100 days. The patients are very reliant on close medical and nursing surveillance to ensure that they do not perish from preventable/treatable causes. The following is a guide to some of the problems encountered; most units have well defined policies on management and you should be advised by the local guidelines.

Skin rash

Causes: drug reaction, GVHD (acute or chronic), infection (?HSV)

Fever (see p580 – the neutropenic patient)

Causes: infection (bacterial, viral, fungal, protozoal), GVHD, drug reaction.

GI complications

1 *Nausea and vomiting*

Causes: chemotherapy, radiotherapy, the memory of previous chemotherapy, reaction to antibiotics, GVH disease of upper GI tract.

Management

- Correct dehydration and electrolyte abnormalities (iv fluids)
- Appropriate regimes include:-
  - Lorazepam (2mg po q8h) with dexamethasone (4–8mg po/iv q8h) and metoclopramide (10–20mg q6–8h)
  - Alternatively ondansetron 4–8mg po/iv q8–12h.

2 *Mucositis*

Presentation: oral pain, retrosternal or epigastric discomfort, nausea, vomiting, GI bleeding.

Causes: chemotherapy (busulphan, methotrexate), radiotherapy, infection (HSV, candida, CMV), GVHD.

Management

- Endoscopy ± biopsy.
- Adequate analgesia: local measures (paracetamol gargles, throat lozenges, H$_2$–antagonists); opiate analgesia is frequently required, e.g. diamorphine infusion.
- Search for an infectious cause (mouthwash and swabs for HSV and *Candida*).
- Start parenteral nutrition if required.

3 *Diarrhoea*

Causes: chemo/radiotherapy related, antibiotic related, pseudo-membranous colitis (*C. difficile*), acute GVHD, other GI infections (bacterial, CMV enteritis, fungal).

Management

- Rehydrate, NG suction, plain abdominal X-ray, endoscopy.
- Examine stool – *C. difficile* toxin or culture; green, watery diarrhoea ± strands of epithelial cells in GVHD; culture for other pathogens.
- Blood cultures.
- Specific treatment – for *C. difficile* (metronidazole po/iv; po vancomycin), for CMV enteritis (see p588), for GVHD (immuno-suppression). Start broad spectrum iv antibiotics if febrile (p582).

Complications of BMT

Early complications of BMT	

• Skin rash
• GI complications
  – Nausea and vomiting
  – Mucositis
  – Diarrhoea
• Abnormal LFTs (p574)
• Haemorrhagic cystitis (p576)
	• Interstitial shadowing on CXR (p574)
	• Cardiovascular complications
	  – Cardiac failure (p574)
	  – Hypertension (p576)
	  – Endocarditis (p576)
	• Deteriorating renal function (p576)
	• CNS complications (p576)

Complications of BMT   2.

Abnormal liver function tests

Causes: drug-induced hepatitis (methotrexate, cyclosporin), infection (viral, fungal, bacterial), GVHD (veno-occlusive disease), acalculous cholecystitis, biliary obstruction. Some may progress to severe jaundice, hepatorenal syndrome, ascites, acute abdominal pain, mental confusion.

Management

- Supportive measures: monitor fluid balance, coagulation tests, renal function; adjust drug doses accordingly.
- For progressive liver failure, try to avoid loop diuretics in severe hepatic dysfunction – consider dopamine (2–5µg/kg/min) and spironolactone (200–400mg/24h); consider salt-poor albumin if hypo-albuminaemic; paracentesis for ascites (p516); etc.
- Search for an infectious aetiology.
- Liver ultrasound with Doppler of the hepatic and portal veins (reversed hepatic-portal flow seen in veno-occlusive disease).
- Consider liver biopsy (transjugular if possible).
- *Specific treatment:* Intravenous heparin, prostacyclin and rt-PA have been tried for veno-occlusive disease with limited success; broad spectrum antibiotics ± anti-viral and anti-fungal agents for suspected infections; immunosuppression for GVHD ± ursodeoxycholic acid; liver transplantation may be required.

Interstitial shadowing on CXR

These may be diffuse or localized and associated with varying degrees of fever, breathlessness, and hypoxia.

Causes

- Pulmonary oedema [fluid overload, cardiac failure due to chemo/ radiotherapy, non-cardiac (ARDS) – related to sepsis or drug toxicity];
- Infection [bacterial, viral (esp. CMV), fungal, *Pneumocystis*];
- Thromboembolic;
- GVHD;
- Pulmonary haemorrhage;
- Idiopathic.

Management

- Supportive treatment: oxygen, diuretics (if pulmonary oedema) and ventilatory support depending on degree of ventilatory failure (pXX).
- Exclude an infectious cause – neutropenic patients may have only minor changes on CXR with bacterial infections until the neutrophil count rises: blood and sputum culture, bronchoscopy ± broncho-alveolar lavage, lung biopsy may be necessary for diagnosis.

Cardiac failure

- Cardiac toxicity may be secondary to high-dose cyclophosphamide, total body irradiation, and/or anthracycline exposure.
- Transient ST and T wave abnormalities and LV dysfunction on ECHO are seen in up to 30% following conditioning prior to BMT.
- Overt cardiac failure may be seen with repeated high-dose steroid therapy that is required for episodes of GVHD.

Management: Standard therapy with diuretics and ACE inhibitors is usually sufficient. Cardiac transplantation may be the only option.

Complications of BMT 3.

Hypertension

Very common in the early days post BMT and most commonly due to cyclosporin therapy ± renal impairment.
Treatment: calcium antagonists (e.g. Nifedipine SR. 10–20mg po bd) are most effective.

Endocarditis

Both bacterial (related to pre-existing cardiac lesion ± intravenous lines) and non-bacterial thrombotic (marantic) endocarditis (NBTE) are recognized in up to 7% of patients post BMT.
Diagnosis is difficult and depends on clinical suspicion, multiple embolic events, persistent bacteraemia, ECHO (bacterial vegetations are usually easily visible, cf. NBTE vegetations).
Management: see p90.

Deteriorating renal function

Causes
- Drug therapy [cyclosporin A, amphotericin, aminoglycosides. vancomycin, methotrexate (high-dose), mitomycin C, nitrosoureas, cisplatinum, acyclovir, allopurinol]
- Pre-renal (dehydration, shock, bleeding)
- Renal (hepatorenal syndrome, sepsis, anaemia, radiotherapy)
- Tumour lysis syndrome (see p592)
- *Haemolytic uraemic syndrome* (see p592): this may be related to cyclosporin therapy (mild symptoms usually and responds to cessation of the drug), CMV infection, GVHD, chemo/radiotherapy.

Haemorrhagic cystitis

- Frequency, dysuria, and haematuria occurring days to weeks after conditioning therapy; commonly related to cyclophosphamide (caused by acreolin, a metabolite), but also seen with anthracyclines, cytosine arabinoside, etoposide, adenovirus, and BK virus infection.
- Prevent with Mesna (see data sheet for dose).

Management: supportive therapy with blood and platelet transfusion is usually sufficient; surgical intervention may be necessary.

CNS complications

Symptoms may include seizures, drowsiness/confusion, focal neurological signs, stroke.
Causes
- Metabolic ($\downarrow Mg^{2+}$, $\downarrow Ca^{2+}$, hypoxia, liver failure, renal failure)
- Infection [bacterial, viral (e.g. HSV), fungal (esp. *Aspergillus*), *Toxoplasma*]
- Drug toxicity (cyclosporin, imipenem, ciprofloxacin, high-dose acyclovir, opiates, cytosine arabinoside, busulphan cisplatinum, intrathecal methotrexate)
- Intracranial haemorrhage
- Cerebral infarction (embolic)
- Relapse of disease

Investigate with CT scan, LP (after correcting clotting and platelets), blood cultures, serology, Mg^{2+} and Ca^{2+} levels, ECHO.
Management: prophylactic phenytoin (300mg daily) for patients receiving high-dose busulphan conditioning; specific therapy for underlying cause.

Acute graft-versus-host disease (GVHD)

- An immunological reaction of T cells against RECIPIENT antigens and rarely manifest until engraftment takes place – i.e. day 14–21 following transplantation.
- Usually confined to allogeneic / matched-unrelated-donor transplants.
- Can occur at any time up to 6 months post transplant. Thereafter, the manifestations are somewhat different, and it is termed *chronic GVHD*.
- There is a (poorly understood) temporal and pathological correlation between acute GVHD and CMV infection. Always consider both when one is suspected.

Manifestations

- Erythema, soreness, and desquamation of palms and soles.
- Skin rash (widespread or localized, maculopapular, non-pruritic).
- Mucositis in mouth and GI tract. Profuse, green, watery 'mincemeat' diarrhoea.
- Deranged liver function – may be isolated hyperbilirubinaemia or rising ALP only.

Management

- Mild GVHD is considered acceptable, and even preferable to complete absence of GVHD, as the causative donor T cells may also have a 'graft-versus-leukaemia' effect. However, involvement at more than one site or deterioration in the patient's condition often necessitates intervention (discuss with senior haematologist).
- Treatment may involve simply increasing cyclosporin if levels are low, but usually requires daily high-dose methylprednisolone (e.g. 1g iv daily for 3 days, reducing to 500mg-250mg-125mg-stop over next 4 days).

Cyclosporin-related toxicity

Cyclosporin is used as an immunosuppressant in all allogeneic and MUD bone marrow transplants. Frequent measurement of trough cyclosporin levels acts as a rough guide to the possibility of toxic effects, but the therapeutic and toxic ranges overlap.

Side-effects such as hypertension, $\uparrow K^+$, and deterioration in renal function are common, but in an acute situation, neurotoxicity can present as a medical emergency.

Presentation

- Acute confusion, tremor, cerebral irritation, seizures, renal impairment, hypertension.
- Cyclosporin levels are raised by ciprofloxacin, erythromycin, grapefruit juice, NSAIDs, allopurinol, amiodarone – see BNF.

Management

- Control fits with iv diazepam (p370).
- Stop cyclosporin (usually needs to be reintroduced cautiously at a later stage).
- Take blood for random cyclosporin level, U&Es, and serum Mg^{2+} ($\downarrow Mg^{2+}$ can predispose to cyclosporin toxicity).
- Exclude other causes, e.g. CNS infection, other drugs, intracerebral bleed.

Haematological emergencies

The febrile neutropenic patient: Diagnosis

- Neutropenia (in this context) may be defined as a total neutrophil count of $< 1 \times 10^9$/l, regardless of total WCC. This usually coincides with the period of maximal mucositis post BMT.
- Significant infections are usually associated with a fever; and a 'spike' to $\geq 38°$C is regarded as warranting action. Severely ill patients may not be able to mount a fever.
- The site of infection is not usually obvious; potential sites include chest, Hickman or other central line (or inflammation around exit site of line), mouth, perianal area / perineum, urine, or skin.

Organisms

Common

Gram-positive (60%)
Coagulase -ve staphylococci
  S. epidermis
Streptococci
  viridans streptococci
Gram-negative (30%)
Escherichia coli
Klebsiella spp.
Pseudomonas aeruginosa

Other (10%)
Staph. aureus
Corynebacterium JK
  Acinetobacter sp.
  Mixed infections
  Anaerobes
Fungal infections
  Candida sp.
  Aspergillus fumigatus
Viral infections (VZV, CMV)
  Pneumocystis carinii

- A microbiological diagnosis is reached only in ~ 40%.
- Coagulase -ve staphylococci: Hickman or other iv lines.
- Viridans streptococci : mucositis ± previous exposure to quinolones.
- Fungal infections: occur after prolonged and profound neutropenia, previous antibiotic therapy, underlying lung disease (pulmonary aspergillosis).

Basic microbiological investigations

- ***Blood cultures*** taken from Hickman line and by venepuncture. This allows line infections to be differentiated from bacteraemias.
- ***Culture of urine and faeces*** including stool for *C. difficile*.
- ***Cultures from other suspected sites*** – e.g. line exit sites, sputum, skin lesions, throat.
- ***Viral serology*** – less useful, as a rising titre is often necessary to diagnose infection. Viral antigen/particle detection (e.g. CMV DEAFF test), where possible, may be more helpful in an acute situation.
- ***Line tips*** – rush to laboratory. Do not allow to dry out on ward bench or store overnight in fridge.

Important points

- ***Antibiotic therapy should never be delayed to await further assessment of clinical progress, or lab. results.***
- Neutropenic patients may not show a localized response to infection. The most common presentation is that of a fever of unknown origin.
- A pyrexia lasting > 48h, despite iv antibiotics, usually requires some alteration to the antimicrobial regime.
- ***Platelet requirements increase with sepsis.*** Neutropenic patients are commonly also thrombocytopenic, and platelet counts should be kept above 20×10^9/l.
- Thrombocytopenia also demands care with invasive procedures. Central lines and urinary catheters should be inserted with platelet cover, and ***arterial puncture is best avoided*** (use pulse oximetry).

The febrile neutropenic patient

Immediate management

Given the above caveats, the stabilization of a septic neutropenic patient is the same as the management of any other septic patient.

- Oxygen, iv colloid, crystalloid, and inotropes should be administered as is appropriate to the patient's clinical condition.
- CVP readings may be taken from existing central lines to assess the patient's hydration status, but – with Hickman lines in particular – the readings are frequently not accurate, and should be interpreted in the context of the clinical assessment.

Antimicrobial regime

When in doubt, take microbiological advice; use hospital policy. Regimes for empirical therapy are based on broad spectrum, bactericidal antibiotics. Monotherapy is hardly ever appropriate, even when an organism has been isolated: the patient may well have more than one infection.

A typical policy is shown below.

Empirical antibiotic therapy for febrile neutropenia		
1st Line :	**Ceftazidime** +	**Vancomycin**
	2g iv q8h	1g iv q12h (guided by levels)
2nd Line :	**Piperacillin** +	**Gentamicin**
	4g iv q8h	120mg loading dose
		80mg iv q8h (guided by levels)
3rd Line :	**Imipenem / cilastatin**	
	500mg iv q8h	

Notes

1 Doses of **vancomycin** and **gentamicin** will need to be adjusted according to serum levels.

2 Add **metronidazole** 500mg iv q8h to 1st or 2nd line regimens if fever persists and anaerobic infection possible (mucositis).

3 Add **amphotericin B** 200µg/kg/day iv increasing stepwise to 1mg/kg/day for 4 weeks for proven (or possible) fungal infection.

4 The **change from 1st to 2nd line therapy** should be considered under the following circumstances:
- Persistent pyrexia > 48h (or less if the patient's condition markedly deteriorates).
- A new spike of temperature once the fever has settled on 1st line antibiotics (suggesting emergence of another, resistant organism).
- Rising CRP in the face of apparently appropriate antibiotics.

5 Choice of **3rd line antibiotics** is often more arbitrary, and combinations should again be discussed with the microbiologists. Duration of neutropenia is an important factor, as fungal infections become more likely the longer the period of neutropenia.

The febrile neutropenic patient

Particular situations

• **Infections of the mouth, perianal area, or elsewhere in the GI tract:** consider adding **metronidazole**.

• **Suspected line infections:** ensure good Gram-positive cover (**vancomycin** or **teicoplanin**)

• **Diarrhoea after prolonged antibiotic therapy:** suspect *Clostridium difficile*; consider empirical oral **vancomycin** or **metronidazole** while awaiting stool culture results.

• Orophryngeal mucositis due to **reactivation of herpes simplex virus** is common. It is effectively treated with **acyclovir**; the main complication is bacterial super infection.

• **Pyrexias associated with a normal CRP** virtually exclude bacterial or fungal infection as a cause of the fever.

• **Deteriorating renal function:** avoid nephrotoxic agents, particularly in combination (e.g. vancomycin, amphotericin, gentamicin)

• **Systemic candidiasis** may be manifest only as fever unresponsive to antibiotics: blood cultures are rarely positive; signs of local invasion, (e.g. endophthalmitis) are seen in a minority. Have a high index of suspicion and treat aggressively with amphotericin or fluconazole.

• **Invasive aspergillosis** presents as fever, abnormal CXR and dyspnoea, or sinusitis (invasive disease of sinuses). There is extensive local tissue destruction with cavitating lung lesions or bone destruction of sinuses. Treat aggressively with iv amphotericin.

• **Granulocyte transfusions**, in small studies, have been shown to be beneficial in neutropenic patients. This has largely been superseded by recombinant colony stimulating factor (CSF) either **GM-CSF** (granulocyte-macrophage CSF) or **GCSF** (granulocyte CSF) – take advise from your haematologists (see p720).

When selecting an antimicrobial regime, it is worthwhile reviewing all recent microbiology results, including skin swabs (axilla, groin, perineal).

Causes of failure to respond to empirical antibiotics
1 Wrong microbiological diagnosis
Consider infection with fungi, viruses, protozoa, mycobacteria
2 Line-associated fever
3 Graft versus host disease
(also possible with liver transplantation)
4 Drug fever
5 Inadequate antibiotic doses
6 Underlying disease (e.g. relapse)

The febrile neutropenic patient

Infections in the transplant patient

Infectious diseases are a major cause of mortality and morbidity following both solid organ and bone marrow transplantation, related to the immunosuppression [and in the case of bone marrow transplantation (BMT), the innate immuno-incompetence in the neutropenic and early engraftment phases].

Different pathogens are typically implicated in infections depending on the degree of immunocompetence of the patient.

• The neutropenic patient (see p580).

• The non-neutropenic transplant patient
Cell-mediated immunity may be impaired for several months after bone marrow (and solid organ) transplantation. This predisposes to viral (CMV, HSV, adenovirus) and protozoal (*Pneumocystis carinii*, toxoplasmosis) infections.

• **Cytomegalovirus infections (see p588)**

• **Suspected *Pneumocystis* pneumonia**: Treat with *high-dose septrin*; (0.96–1.44g q12h iv); consider urgent bronchoscopy/broncho-alveolar lavage (p260).

• **Toxoplasmosis:** Usually due to reactivation of latent infection. Presents as intracranial space occupying lesion, meningoencephalitis, or diffuse encephalopathy. Seizures and focal neurological signs are common. Treatment is with *pyrimethamine* and *sulphonamides* (p268).

• **Other viral infections**

• **HSV** commonly produces localized infection and dissemination is rare but recognized to produce encephalitis and pneumonia – treat with *high-dose acyclovir* iv.

• **VZV** (varicella) reactivation is frequently seen and most infections are mild; encephalitis and pneumonitis are usually fatal – treat with high dose acyclovir (10mg/kg iv q8h).

• **Adenovirus** infection produces an interstitial pneumonitis similar to CMV and may disseminate.

Infections in the transplant patient

CMV infections in transplant patients

- Also see p269.
- May be acquired from the reactivation of previous CMV infection in recipient, due to immunosuppression.

- May be acquired from the bone marrow from a CMV positive donor or CMV positive blood products. (**All BMT recipients should receive CMV negative blood products if they are CMV IgG negative prior to BMT.** CMV IgG positive recipients can receive unscreened blood products.)
- Do not usually occur until day 21 following BMT.
- Occur more commonly in allogeneic and unrelated donor transplants, due to the greater immunosuppression.

Presentation of acute CMV infections

- Fever of unknown origin.
- Antigenaemia (detected by routine weekly CMV antigen testing – blood and urine – currently only in certain centres; becoming more widely available).
- Graft failure/myelosuppression (anaemia, thrombocytopenia, leukopenia).
- Interstitial pneumonitis: deteriorating oxygen saturation, with widespread bilateral interstitial opacities on CXR.
- Enteritis (oesophagitis, gastritis, colitis): pyrexia, diarrhoea.
- Hepatitis.

Immediate management

- Ensure adequate respiration; consult anaesthetists and consider CPAP or ventilation early if oxygen requirements are increasing, or the patient is becoming exhausted.
- Inform haematologist responsible for patient's care.
- Take blood for CMV antigen, culture, and antibody testing.
- Send urine sample for CMV antigen.
- If CMV is strongly suspected, commence ganciclovir treatment immediately. Otherwise, consider:
  - (a) bronchoscopy/ bronchoalveolar lavage if pulmonary infiltrate (send washings for CMV antigen)
  - (b) upper GI endoscopy and biopsy

Treatment

- **Ganciclovir** should be commenced at 2.5mg/kg iv tds and continued for three weeks, reducing the dose after the first week to 2.5mg/kg bd (modify in renal impairment).
- Studies suggest that where organ damage is present (i.e. rather than antigenaemia only), **combined ganciclovir and intravenous immunoglobulin** is more effective than ganciclovir alone.
- Side-effects of ganciclovir include nephrotoxicity, and myelosuppression/graft failure – which may be difficult to distinguish from the effects of CMV itself. If side-effects become a serious problem, consider changing to **foscarnet**.

Hyperviscosity syndrome

Causes

Increased cellularity	Raised plasma proteins
Polycythaemia ($1°$ or $2°$) – Haematocrit > 50–60%	Waldenstrom's macroglobulinaemia – IgM paraprotein, level > 30 g/l
Leukocytosis (acute leukaemias) – WCC > 50–100 $\times 10^9$/l	Myeloma usually IgA subtype – paraprotein level > 80 g/l

Presentation

Most patients develop symptoms when serum viscosity reaches 5–6 centipoises (normal < 1.8).

General features
- Muscle weakness
- Lethargy, headache
- Mental confusion, proceeding to coma
- Visual disturbance
- Congestive cardiac failure
- Fundoscopy   – engorgement and sludging in the veins
  - – haemorrhage, exudates
  - – papilloedema

Specific features
The predominant symptoms vary with the underlying cause.

- *Raised paraprotein*
  - Bleeding/purpura: platelet dysfunction and factor deficiency
  - Neuropathies
  - Renal impairment
  - Cardiac conduction abnormalities
- *Leukostasis*
  - Myocardial ischaemia / infarction
  - Pulmonary infiltrates
- *Polycythaemia*
  - Peripheral ischaemia
  - Transient ischaemic attacks / strokes
  - Myocardial infarction

Management

Arrange urgent intervention (same day) depending on cause.

- Polycythaemia   – venesect 1–2 units
  - – replace with N saline
- Leukaemia   – leucapheresis
- High paraprotein   – plasmapheresis

Tumour lysis syndrome

A syndrome of metabolic abnormalities and renal impairment that can occur within hours or days of commencing chemotherapy, due to rapid lysis of tumour cells. It is most likely to occur with bulky, highly chemosensitive disease (e.g. lymphomas; high blast-count leukaemias; germ-cell tumours).

Features
- Hyperuricaemia ± urate nephropathy and oliguric renal failure.
- Hyperkalaemia (especially with progressive renal impairment).
- Hyperphosphataemia.
- Hypocalcaemia and hypomagnesaemia (due to rising phosphate).
- Cardiac arrhythmias (secondary to ↑ K^+, ↓ Ca^{2+}, and ↓ Mg^{2+}).
- Weakness, twitching, tetany (hypocalcaemia).
- Severe metabolic acidosis (renal failure).

Management
- Emergency treatment of hyperkalemia (see p282).
- Exclude bilateral ureteric obstruction by ultrasound.
- Alkalinize the urine (p668).
- Arrange urgent haemodialysis if the patient is oliguric.
- Monitor U&Es, PO_4^{3-}, Ca^{2+} and urate at least twice daily for the first few days of treatment.
- Strict fluid balance measurements, with urinary catheter if necessary.

Prevention
- Start **allopurinol** 300mg od 48h prior to chemotherapy
- **Hyperhydrate** (iv fluids, 3–5 litres / 24h) prior to chemotherapy. Urine alkalinization helps promote urate excretion.
- **Leucopherese** if high peripheral blast count
- Continue iv fluids during therapy, giving frusemide to maintain diuresis and prevent volume overload.

Tumour lysis syndrome

Hypercalcaemia of malignancy (See p452)

Urgent intervention required if $Ca^{2+} > 3$ mmol/l

[N.B. True Ca^{2+} = measured $Ca^{2+} + (40 - albumin) \times 0.02$]

Causes
- Bony metastases – probable local cytokine effect
- Myeloma – secretion of an osteoclast-activating factor
- Secretion of PTH-related peptide (non-small cell lung cancer)

Presentation
- Nausea, vomiting, drowsiness, confusion, nocturia, polyuria, bone and abdominal pains, constipation

Management
- Hydration: 3–4l over 24h, continuing for 4–5 days.
- Frusemide to maintain diuresis; has an additional Ca^{2+}-lowering effect.
- Following overnight hydration recheck Ca^{2+}, albumin.
- If symptoms persist, and/or Ca^{2+} remains > 3mmol/l, give pamidronate disodium iv: a typical dosing regimen is

    $Ca^{2+} < 3$mmol/l   30mg over 4h

    Ca^{2+} 3–4mmol/l   60mg over 8h

    $Ca^{2+} > 4$mmol/l   90mg over 24h

- For myeloma, consider prednisolone 30–60mg po daily.

Superior vena cava obstruction

Presentation
- Awareness of fullness of head and tightness of collar
- Symptoms exacerbated by bending down
- Syncope
- Breathlessness
- Facial suffusion and oedema
- Engorgement of veins (with downwards flow) in neck, arms, and upper thorax

Causes
- Usually bronchogenic carcinoma (+/– secondary thrombosis of SVC)
- Other tumours, including lymphoma, more rarely

Management
- FBC and film
- U&Es, Ca^{2+}, albumin
- CXR
- Doppler USS of neck veins if diagnosis uncertain
- Consider iv heparin infusion, providing platelet count and clotting function are normal
- Arrange urgent radiotherapy (within 24h)

11 Rheumatological emergencies

Acute monoarthritis: Presentation

An acute monoarthritis should always be treated as sepic arthritis until proved otherwise. Failure to treat sepitic arthritis is a medical disaster. 50% of cartilage proteoglycan is lost within 48 hours; bone loss is evident within 7 days; mortality of *Staph. aureus* arthritis is 10%.

Presentation

- Hot, swollen red joint
- Joint line tenderness
- Restricted range of movement
- Systemic features of fever and malaise

Assessment

Look for any risk factors for infection

- Diabetes mellitus.
- Immunodeficiency state (monoarthritis is rare in AIDS).
- Underlying structural joint disease (e.g. rheumatoid arthritis or other deforming arthropathy, prosthesis).
- Sexual impropriety, intravenous drug abuse (predisposes to sacro-ileitis and acromioclavicular joint infection).

Ask for risk factors for gout

- Alcohol
- High purine diet (protein, e.g. meat)
- Drugs (e.g. thiazides, frusemide, ethambutol)
- High cell turnover states (e.g. lymphoma, polycythaemia, psoriasis)

Examine for evidence for multi-system disease

- Rash
- Ocular involvement
- Orogenital ulceration
- Gastrointestinal symptoms
- Renal involvement
- Pulmonary manifestations

Conditions that mimic monoarthritis

- Bone pain or fracture close to a joint
- Tendinitis (especially at the wrist)
- Bursitis (commonly olecranon or pre-patellar bursae; no joint line tenderness)
- Neuropathic pain
- Soft tissue pain

Differential diagnosis of a monoarthritis

Traumatic
- Traumatic synovitis
- Haemarthroses
  - Fracture
  - Haemophilia
  - Ruptured anterior cruciate ligament

Non-traumatic

Infective
- *Neisseria gonococcus*
- *Staphylococcus aureus*
- *Staphylococcus albus*
- Streptococcal
- Gram-negative rods

Crystals
- Uric acid (gout)
- Calcium pyrophosphate (pseudo-gout)
- Hydroxyapatite [usually a monoarthritis (shoulder) in elderly pts]

Monoarticular presentation of
- Rheumatoid arthritis
- Seronegative arthritis (e.g. Reiter's, psoriasis)
- SLE

Miscellaneous
- Pigmented villonodular synovitis
- Secondary deposits
- Osteosarcoma

Acute monoarthritis: Investigations

1 *Synovial fluid analysis*
Aspirate the joint to dryness (see p840) and send fluid for :-

- WBC — Fluid may be placed in EDTA tube
- Microbiology — Fluid into sterile container and a sample into blood culture bottles
- Polarized microscopy — For crystals – fluid into sterile container

2 *Take blood for:*
- Blood cultures
- FBC — WBC high in infection and crystal arthritis
- CRP / ESR — Elevated with an inflammatory arthritis
  Elevated ESR and normal CRP suggest SLE
- U&Es, LFTs — May be impaired with sepsis
- Glucose — ?Diabetes mellitus
- Uric acid — ?Gout
- Clotting — Bleeding diathesis causing haemarthrosis
- Immunology — RF, ANA, anti-dsDNA, complement levels (?RA or SLE)

3 *X-ray the joint*
But <u>not</u> helpful in the early diagnosis of a septic arthritis as the appearance may be unchanged for up to 2 weeks in infection. Chondrocalcinosis suggests pseudo-gout.

4 *Sepsis screen*
Cervical, rectal and throat swabs. Aspirate any cutaneous pustules for Gram stain in patients with suspected gonococcal infection.

Indications for synovial fluid aspiration in casualty
• Suspected septic arthritis • Suspected crystal arthritis • Suspected haemarthrosis • Relief of symptoms by removal of effusion in degenerative arthritis.

Contraindications to joint aspiration
• Overlying sepsis • Bleeding diathesis

Septic arthritis

The commonest pathogen in the UK is *N. gonorrhoeae*. World-wide the causes include *Staph. aureus* (70%), *Streptococci* (20%), *H. influenzae* (in children).

Management

- Admit and inform orthopaedic team.
- Aspirate the joint to dryness. Liaise with the orthopaedic team and consider early arthroscopy to facilitate effective joint washout, especially if inflammatory markers are slow to fall.
- Strict rest for the joint (bed rest) and no weight bearing on infected joints.
- Analgesics (NSAIDs) – consider adding H_2–antagonist if history of dyspepsia
- **Antibiotics**
  - Initially intravenous for 2 weeks, then oral for a further 4 weeks.
  - Emperically start with **flucloxacillin** 1g q6h and **benzyl penicillin** 1.2g q4h. For penicillin allergy **use vancomycin and clindamycin**. In young children use cefotaxime to cover *H. influenzae*.
  - (N.B. Aminoglycosides are not effective in the acid pH of an infected joint; erythromycin penetrates the synovial fluid poorly.)
  - Review antibiotics when microbiology available.
  - For gonococcal arthritis, treat with iv **benzyl penicillin** 1.2g q4h for 7 days and then p.o. **amoxycillin** 500mg tds for 10 days. Remember to trace and treat contacts. (Liaise with G.U. Medicine team.)

Crystal arthropathy

Management

- May usually be managed as an out-patient.
- Bed rest.
- Analgesics. **NSAIDs**, e.g. diclofenac SR 75mg bd. (Use cautiously in the elderly, or patients with peptic ulceration, or patients with cardiac failure, renal, or liver disease).
- **Colchicine** is a good alternative if NSAIDs are contraindicated. Give 1mg initially followed by 500µg every 6 hours for the first 48 hours, maintenance dose 500µg bd.
- Give one dose of corticosteroid (**prednisolone** EC 30mg po) to help reduce the inflammation acutely and reduce symptoms. Do NOT give steroids if there is any possibility of septic arthritis.
- Rheumatology consultation if symptoms fail to settle – intra-articular corticosteroid may be given.
- Both allopurinol and probenecid are contraindicated during acute gout since both may prolong symptoms. They may be started for prophylaxis when the acute attack has settled if the patient has had more than three attacks of acute gout in one year, if tophi are present, or serum uric acid levels are high. Initiation of these drugs should be accompanied by either a NSAID or colchicine for the first two weeks.

Polyarthritis

Presentation

- Pain
- Stiffness (esp. early morning)
- Loss of function
- Joint inflammation

Differential diagnoses

Rheumatoid arthritis
Seronegative arthritis

- Psoriatic arthropathy
- Reactive arthritis
- Ankylosing spondylitis
- Enteropathic arthritis
- Systemic lupus erythematosus

Crystal arthropathy

- Chondrocalcinosis
- Gout

Infections

- Viral
- Bacterial

Miscellaneous

- Sarcoid: Associated with erythema nodosum (20%), and a transient RA like polyarthritis or acute monoarthritis.
- Behçet's syndrome: Polyarthritis (± *erythema nodosum*) with painful orogenital ulceration and iritis.
- Familial Mediterranean Fever: Occurs in middle eastern individuals with recurrent attacks of fever, arthritis (usually monoarticular), abdominal, or chest pain (pleurisy).
- Transient polyarthritis may be associated with SLE, bacterial endocarditis (p86), para-infectious, Reiter's, reactive arthritis, and Henoch-Schönlein purpura.

Investigations

- Aspirate a large affected joint and analyse synovial fluid (see p840)
- Blood cultures if appropriate
- FBC with differential count
- CRP and or ESR
- Biochemical profile (U&Es, LFTs, urate) and glucose
- Rheumatoid factor, ANA, anti-dsDNA (RA and SLE)
- Complement levels
- Viral serology
- X-rays (may show chondrocalcinosis, typically knees and wrists, or early changes of rheumatoid arthritis with periarticular osteoporosis).

Management

General measures

- Bed rest – rest for the affected joints.
- NSAIDs – e.g. indomethacin 50mg tds adjusting dose according to symptoms and response. (Caution in elderly patients, patients with dyspepsia, asthmatics and patients on anti-coagulants.)
- Consider specific treatment of underlying condition (see above).
- Consider the need for physiotherapy and exercise regimens to reduce long-term disability.

Antibody	Association
Rheumatoid factor	Rheumatoid arthritis
ANA	Many autoimmune disorders
Anti-dsDNA	SLE
ENA	Mixed connective tissue disease (MCTD)
	SLE
RO (SSA)	Primary Sjogrens' syndrome, SLE
LA	Primary Sjogrens' syndrome
Anti-sm	SLE, chronic active hepatitis
Centromere	CREST, PACK syndrome
Nucleolus	Systemic sclerosis
SCL-70	Systemic sclerosis
Jo-1	Polymyositis
Cardiolipin	SLE, anti-phospholipid syndrome

Rheumatoid arthritis

Clinical features
- Typically young women (F:M 3:1)
- Symmetrical polyarthritis involving the small joints of the hands and feet.
- May present as a relapsing or persistent monoarthritis.
- All synovial joints are involved – signs most common in hands, feet, knees but remember synovial joints of spine (and atlantoaxial joint or ligaments) and larynx (aryetenoid joints).
- Extra-articular manifestations – vasculitis, sub-cutaneous nodules, lymphadenopathy, peripheral neuropathy, anaemia (normochromic normocytic, Fe-deficiency, drug-induced aplasia, haemolytic), ocular involvement, pleurisy, pericarditis, pulmonary fibrosis.

Management
- General measures as before (p602).
- Early steroids reduce long-term joint destruction.
- Symptomatic treatment with NSAIDs.
- Long-term immunosuppressive therapy with penicillamine, gold, azathioprine, methotrexate, hydroxychloroquine, and sulphasalazine are all used.

Psoriatic arthropathy

Clinical features
- May present as an asymmetrical large or small joint oligoarthritis, symmetrical polyarthritis, or clinical picture similar to RA or AS. Joint destruction may be extensive (arthritis mutilans).
- Look for rash (scalp, behind ears, umbilicus, natal cleft), nail changes (pitting, onycholysis, ridging).

Management
- Treatment is as for rheumatoid arthritis with NSAIDs as the mainstay.
- Avoid chloroquine as this precipitates psoriasis.

Reactive arthritis

Clinical features
- Typically young, sexually active individual with orogenital ulcers (painless), conjunctivitis (which may progress to iritis), rash (soles – keratoderma blenorrhagica).
- May occur following non-specific urethritis or infection with *Shigella*, *Salmonella*, *Yersinia*, or *Campylobacter*.

Treatment
- NSAIDs are the main therapy.
- See p606 for Reiter's syndrome

Rheumatological emergencies

Reiter's syndrome

Clinical features

- Comprises a triad of seronegative arthritis, non-specific urethritis, and conjunctivitis
- Skin lesions are psoriasiform (keratoderma blennorrhagicum) with brown macules progressing to pustules on the soles and palms.
- The arthritis begins ~ 2 weeks after infection and the lower limb joints are most commonly affected (asymmetrical) and resolves over months; occasionally the skin lesions and arthritis progresses to typical psoriatic arthropathy.
- It may be associated with a sterile urethral discharge and mild dysuria. Erosive lesions may affect the penis (circinate balanitis) or mouth.
- Rarely progresses to give aortic incompetence, heart block, pericarditis.

Treatment

- NSAIDs, and sometimes steroids, are the mainstay of therapy.

Ankylosing spondylitis

Clinical features

- Enquire about axial skeleton involvement (lower lumbar back pain with early morning stiffness).
- Peripheral joint involvement (~ 40%), uveitis (p326), anaemia of chronic disease, and progressive immobility may be found.

Management

- NSAIDs for pain.
- Exercise to try to prevent progressive immobility.
- Sulphasalazine may be tried for joint disease.
- Refer to a rheumatologist for long-term management.

Enteropathic arthritis

- Large joint arthritis often coincides with active inflammatory bowel disease.
- Arthritis may predate the onset of intestinal symptoms. Commonly there are other extraintestinal manifestations (e.g. erythema nodosum and iritis).
- Treatment of colitis improves arthritic symptoms.

Infections

- **Viral** – Rubella, parvovirus B19 (common, often presents with a generalized rash), and HIV seroconversion illness may present with polyarthritis.
- **Bacterial** – *Gonococcus* (rash, tenosynovitis, sexually active), *Staphylococcus* (immunosuppressed with septicaemia and seeding to several joints), infective endocarditis – (vasculitic lesions, heart murmur).
- **Treatment** – see p600.

Rheumatological emergencies

Vasculitis

The term vasculitis denotes an inflammatory reaction with destructive change of blood vessel walls. The vasculitides are classified into *primary* and *secondary* types.

Classification

Primary systemic vasculitis (simplistic classification)

	Granulomatous	Non-granulomatous
Large vessel	Giant cell arteritis	Takayasu's arteritis
Medium vessel	Churg-Strauss synd.	Polyarteritis nodosa
Small vessel	Wegener's arteritis	Microscopic polyarteritis
		Henoch-Schonlein purpura
		Hypersensitivity vasculitis

Causes of secondary vasculitis

- Infective endocarditis
- Malignancy
- Rheumatoid arthritis
- Systemic lupus erythematosus
- Cryoglobulinaemia (strongly associated with hepatitis C)
- Drug reaction
  Organ involvement varies with the type of vasculitis but commonly includes skin, joints, kidneys, lung, and nervous system.

Presentation

- Arthralgia or arthritis, myalgia
- PUO (pyrexia of unknown origin)
- Generalized systemic illness, e.g. weight loss, malaise
- Rashes – splinter haemorrhages, nail fold infarcts, purpura, livedo, nodules
- Renal disease – haematuria, proteinuria, hypertension, renal failure.
- Lung disease – haemoptysis, cough, breathlessness, pulmonary infiltrates.
- Neurological disease – mononeuritis multiplex, sensorimotor polyneuropathy, confusion, fits, hemiplegia, or other acute cerebral syndrome.

Causes of lung haemorrhage and renal failure	Causes of renal failure only (no lung haemorrhage)
• Goodpasture's syndrome	• Anti-GBM disease
• Wegener's granulomatosis	• Small vessel vasculitis
• Microscopic polyarteritis	• Secondary vasculitis
• Systemic lupus erythematosus	• Medium vessel vasculitis (rare)
• Leptospirosis (rarely)	

Anti-neutrophil cytoplasmic antibody (ANCA)

c-ANCA (anti-neutrophil α-proteinase 3)
- Wegener's granulomatosis (very sensitive and specific)
- Microscopic polyarteritis

p-ANCA (anti-myeloperoxidase or elastase)
- Any secondary vasculitis
- Microscopic polyarteritis
- Churg-Strauss syndrome
- Ulcerative colitis (also c-ANCA)
- Sclerosing cholangitis

If positive, test for anti-myeloperoxidase antibody:
- if negative ignore the p-ANCA as a false positive
- if positive investigate for vasculitis

Systemic lupus erythematosus (SLE)

Assessment

This is a chronic autoimmune disorder characterized by the production of a wide range of autoantibodies against both intracellular and cell surface antigens, though most often with anti-nuclear antibodies (ANA). It commonly affects young women (1:3000 in the UK) and is ten times commoner in West Indian blacks.

Patients with SLE may present to the A&E Dept. in one of two ways:
1 Known diagnosis of lupus having become acutely unwell. Clinically one has to determine whether their symptoms reflect disease activity, an underlying infection which may precipitate a flare up of the disease, or an unrelated condition.
2 As a presenting diagnosis – the attending physician should be alert to the varied presentations of lupus.

Clinical features

Constitutional (90%)	Fever; malaise; weight loss
Musculoskeletal (90%)	Arthralgia; myalgia; myositis
Deforming arthropathy	(Jaccoud's) 2% to ligament and capsular laxity; aseptic necrosis 2% to steroid therapy
Cutaneous (80–90%)	Butterfly rash; photosensitive rash; discoid lupus; Raynaud's phenomenon; purpura; scarring alopecia; livedo reticularis; urticaria
Haematological (75%)	Thrombocytopenia Anaemia (normochromic normocytic, Coomb's positive in 15%) Leukopenia and lymphopenia
Neuropsychiatric (55%)	Depression; psychosis; fits; hemiplegia; cranial nerve lesions; ataxia; chorea; aseptic meningitis/encephalitis
Renal (50%)	Glomerulonephritis; nephritis or nephrotic syndrome; proteinuria; hypertension
CVS or RS (40%)	Pleurisy; pericarditis; pleural or pericardial effusion; Libman-Sacks endocarditis; shrinking lung syndrome
Aphthous ulcers (40%)	

Urgent investigations

• FBC	Anaemia, ↓ WCC and ↓ plts (see above)
• U&Es, creatinine	Renal failure
• ESR	Elevated with disease activity
• CRP	Typically normal. ↑ suggests infection.
• APTT	Prolonged if there is an 'anti-cardiolipin' antibody (IgG or IgM)
• Blood cultures	Infection-induced flare-ups
• Urine	Dipstick for proteinuria or haematuria. Microscopy for casts. Culture for infection
• CXR	Infection or pleurisy
• ABG	Hypoxia with infection.

Systemic lupus erythematosus (SLE)

Management
Other investigations

612

- Immunology   ANA, DNA, ENA, ACA, complement levels.
- LFTs   Usually normal.
- Viral serology   e.g. DEAFF tests (for cytomegalovirus).
- Urine   24h collection for creatinine clearance and protein excretion.

Points to note
- Immunology:
  - > 80% of patients are ANA +ve (anti-dsDNA is almost pathognomonic of SLE)
  - Anti dsDNA antibody titre may correlate with disease activity
  - Low complement levels correlate with disease activity (and renal involvement)
  - 40% are rheumatoid factor positive
- Pneumococcal and meningococcal infections are more common in patients with SLE as a consequence of either hereditary or acquired deficiencies of the components of the complement pathway.
- Immnosuppressive therapy renders patients susceptible to the usual range of opportunistic infections, including pneumocystis, cytomegalovirus, and mycobacteria.
- Chest and urine are the commonest sources of infection.
- Patients with disease activity classically have an elevated ESR but a relatively normal CRP.
  An elevated CRP should alert you to look for an underlying infection.

Management
- **Prednisolone** 30–60mg od.
- Additional **immunosuppressive therapy** such as pulsed methyl prednisolone, azathioprine, or cyclophosphamide should be given on consultation with a rheumatologist.
- **Antibiotics** if infection is suspected (e.g. cefotaxime) which will treat most chest or urinary tract infections. If the source is known then antimicrobial therapy can be more rationally prescribed.
- **Hydroxychloroquine** (200mg/day) may be added if there is cutaneous or joint involvement.

Systemic lupus erythematosus

Wegener's granulomatosis and microscopic polyarteritis 1.

- Both of these small vessel vasculitides may present to casualty with acute renal failure (rapidly progressive glomerulonephritis).
- Wegener's granulomatosis classically involves the upper and lower respiratory tracts and the kidneys.

Clinical features

- Systemic features — Fever, malaise, weight loss.
- Upper respiratory — Nasal discharge, nose bleeds, sinusitis, collapse of the nasal bridge, deafness (all suggest a diagnosis of Wegener's granulomatosis).
- Lower respiratory — Dyspnoea, haemoptysis, cavitating lung lesions.
- Kidneys — Nephritis with deranged renal function, haematuria, proteinuria, and active urinary sediment.
- Musculoskeletal — Myalgia, arthralgia.
- Neurological — Both peripheral and central.
- Ask about smoking — Strongly associated with lung haemorrhage.

Urgent investigations

- FBC — Anaemia

  Neutrophil leukocytosis

  Thrombocytosis
- Renal function — Impaired renal function or acute renal failure
- LFTs — Low albumin (nephrotic syndrome). Elevated AST, ALT and ALP with hepatitis
- CK and AST — Elevated due to myositis
- PT and APTT — Prolonged with widespread vasculitis and DIC
- ESR and CRP — Elevated
- Blood cultures — Sepsis
- ABG — Hypoxia (haemorrhage or infection) Metabolic acidosis (renal failure)
- Urine — Dipstick for blood or protein

  Microscopy and culture

  24h collection for creatinine clearance and protein excretion
- Sputum — Culture (infection often precipitates lung haemorrhage)
- Calcium/phosphate — Low corrected calcium and high phosphate suggest chronicity
- CXR — Shadowing seen in lung haemorrhage or infection; cavitating lesions typically occur in Wegener's granulomatosis
- USS of the kidneys — If in renal failure to exclude obstruction

Wegener's granulomatosis and microscopic polyarteritis 2.

Immunology

- c-ANCA — Positive (see opposite).
- ANA, anti-dsDNA — To exclude SLE.
- RF — To exclude rheumatoid arthritis.
- Complement levels
- Anti-GBM antibody — A positive test suggests primary anti-GBM disease such as Goodpasture's syndrome, in which there is rapid progressive glomerulonephritis and lung haemorrhage.
- Cryoglobulins — To exclude as a secondary cause of vasculitis.
- Hepatitis serology — Hepatitis B and C.

Miscellaneous investigations

- ECG — Baseline ± changes of hyperkalaemia if ARF is present.
- Lung function tests — Measurement of KCO (increased with lung haemorrhage).
- ECHO — To rule out unsuspected indolent infective endocarditis (secondary cause of vasculitis).
- X-ray sinuses — Commonly involved in Wegener's.
- Renal biopsy — Histological diagnosis (light/ immuno-fluorescence / EM – see p836).

Management

Involve specialists early – rheumatology and renal.

Emergency management

- Patients commonly die from hypoxia (pulmonary haemorrhage, pulmonary oedema), arrhythmias, (secondary to electrolyte abnormalities), and concomitant infection.
- Ensure adequate **oxygenation** and consider ventilation if necessary.
- Assess **fluid balance** and monitor urine output carefully.
- Consider **invasive haemodynamic monitoring** (CVP, arterial line, Swan-Ganz catheter).
- Patients with nephritis may be volume overloaded with **pulmonary oedema**. Treat with intravenous frusemide (80–120mg; high doses may be required), GTN infusion, venesection, or haemodialysis or haemofiltration.
- **Correct electrolyte abnormalities:** Hyperkalaemia (see p282)
- Consider urgent haemodialysis or haemofiltration in patients with ARF or hyperkalaemia (consult renal physicians).
- Treat precipitating infections empirically with **cefotaxime** until a pathogen is identified.
- Treat underlying vasculitis
- High-dose prednisolone (60mg/day)
- Cyclophosphamide (only after renal or rheumatological opinion)
- Plasmapheresis (Renal Units)

Wegener's granulomatosis and microscopic polyarteritis

Points to note

- The ANCA test provides a rapid screening test and shows high sensitivity for patients with small vessel vasculitis.

- Patients with Wegener's granulomatosis are classically c-ANCA positive (cytoplasmic pattern of immunofluorescent, antibody against neutrophil α-proteinase 3), whilst patients with microscopic polyarteritis may be either p-ANCA (perinuclear pattern of immunofluorescence, antibody against myeloperoxidase) or c-ANCA positive. A negative ANCA does not however preclude the diagnosis of a small vessel vasculitis.

- Underlying infection, especially infective endocarditis and chronic meningococcaemia, should always enter the differential diagnosis of a patient with small vessel vasculitis.

- An infectious episode such as an upper respiratory tract infection often will precipitate the presentation of a small vessel vasculitis.

Cryoglobulinaemia

Cryoglobulins are immunoglobulins that precipitate at low temperatures and dissolve on rewarming. They precipitate in the superficial capillaries or outside vessels in the coldest part of the skin to produce microinfarcts or purpura. Cryoglobulinaemia occurs in several conditions.

- Essential cryoglobulinaemia implies the absence of an identifiable cause.
- Renal disease is associated with all three types, and is thought to involve immune-complex pathways.

Type 1. Monoclonal

- Associated with myelo- or lymphoproliferative disease.
- Heavy proteinuria, haematuria, and renal failure may occur (membranoproliferative glomerulonephritis).
- Serum C4 and C1q are low.

Type 2. Mixed

- Monoclonal immunoglobulin (usually IgM) directed against polyclonal IgG.
- Associated with immune complex vasculitis and 50% have evidence of renal disease.

Type 3. Mixed polyclonal

- Associated with SLE, hepatitis B and C, and systemic infections (post streptococcal nephritis, leprosy, and syphilis).
- Renal involvement is also seen.

Clinical features

- Renal involvement (haematuria, proteinuria, renal failure)
- Raynaud's phenomenon
- Purpura (esp. legs)
- Arthralgia and fever
- Confusion and weakness (2% to hyperviscosity)
- Hepatosplenomegaly (probably a manifestation of underlying aetiology).

Management

- There is no specific treatment.
- Plasmapheresis and immunosuppressive therapy may be tried.

Giant cell arteritis (temporal arteritis)

- The commonest type of primary large-vessel vasculitis in clinical practice, with an incidence of 1:10,000. This is typically a disorder of the elderly (mean age 70 yr, with a female to male ratio of 2:1).
- The diagnosis is made clinically (see below) and is supported by an elevated acute phase response (ESR, CRP, and thrombocytosis), and temporal artery histology.
- The classical pathological description is of a segmental granulomatous pan-arteritis, but in the early stage changes may be confined to thickening of the internal elastic lamina associated with a mononuclear cell infiltrate.

Clinical features

- Headache   90%
- Temporal artery tenderness   85%
- Scalp tenderness   75%
- Jaw claudication   70%
- Thickened/ nodular temporal artery   35%
- Pulseless temporal artery   40%
- Visual symptoms (incl. blindness)   40%
- Polymyalgic symptoms   40%
- Systemic features   40%
- CVA or myocardial infarction   rare

Investigations

- FBC   Normochromic anaemia, thrombocytosis
- Biochemistry Elevated alkaline phosphatase
- ESR   ESR > 50mm in the first hour, 95% of cases
- CRP   Elevated
- Chest X-ray   Exclude underlying bronchial carcinoma
- Urinalysis   Exclude haematuria and proteinuria
- Temporal artery biopsy

Management

- Patients with suspected giant cell arteritis should be started on **high-dose prednisolone immediately,** since delay may result in blindness. For most patients 40mg od is sufficient but higher dosages, 60–80mg may be used if the patient has visual symptoms.
- All patients should have a temporal artery biopsy performed within 48 hours of commencing steroids to try to confirm the diagnosis. A normal biopsy does not exclude the diagnosis because of the 'skip' nature of the disease.
- **Polymyalgia rheumatica** – see p622

Giant cell arteritis

Polymyalgia rheumatica (PMR)

Polymyalgia rheumatica is a clinical syndrome characterized by an acute phase response (high ESR or high CRP) which predominantly affects the elderly Caucasian population, median age of onset 70 years, females > males, annual incidence approximately 1:2500.

Clinical features

- Proximal muscle stiffness and pain without weakness or wasting.
- Systemic symptoms of malaise, fever, and weight loss.

Causes of proximal upper and lower girdle stiffness or pains	
• Cervical spondylosis ± adhesive capsulitis	No acute phase response, CPK (N)
• Lumbar spondylosis	
• Osteomalacia	
• Fibromyalgia	
• Hypothyroidism	No acute phase response, ↑ CPK
• Polymyositis/dermatomyositis	↑ acute phase response, ↑ CPK
• Inflammatory arthritis	↑ acute phase response

Investigations

- FBC   (Normochromic normocytic anaemia)
- U&Es, LFTs   (Elevated alkaline phosphatase is common (50%))
- CPK   Normal (if high consider polymyositis or hypothyroidism)
- ESR   High (> 40mm/h initially)
- CRP   High
- RF   PMR may be the presenting feature of rheumatoid arthritis
- CXR   PMR symptoms may be the presenting feature of a neoplasm

Treatment

- **Steroids** – Prednisolone 20mg po od initially reducing to 5–10mg od over 2–3 months and very slow reduction thereafter. Some patients may require treatment for years.
- Monitor response with symptoms and ESR.

Points to note

- Polymyalgia rheumatica and giant cell arteritis form part of a clinical spectrum of disease and up to 40% of patients with biopsy-proven giant cell arteritis have polymyalgic symptoms.
- Polymyalgic symptoms may be the presenting feature of an underlying neoplasm or connective tissue disease.
- Polymyalgic symptoms should respond dramatically to prednisolone. Failure to respond should alert the clinician to the possibility of an underlying neoplasm or connective tissue disease.

Polymyalgia rheumatica

Back pain: Assessment

Approximately 5% of all medical consultations in the UK are for back or neck pain. In the majority of patients no definite anatomical diagnosis is made (non-specific back pain) but it is important not to miss the sinister causes of back pain.

Causes of back pain	
Mechanical back pain	***Inflammatory back pain***
• Spondylolisthesis	• Rheumatoid arthritis
• Spondylosis	• Seronegative spondyloarthritides
• Intervertebral disc prolapse	– Psoriatic
• Spinal stenosis (claudication type pain)	– Ankylosing spondylitis
	– Reiter's
• Apophyseal joint disease (exacerbated by lumbar extension, cervical, or thoracic rotation)	– Enteropathic
	– Behçet's
	Referred pain
	• Aortic aneurysm
• Non-specific back pain	• Pyelonephritis, renal calculus
• Trauma	• Pancreatitis

Causes of 'sinister' back pain	
• Infection – discitis	• Myeloma
– epidural abscess	• Osteoporotic crush fracture
• Malignancy	• Paget's disease

History

Is pain likely to be mechanical, inflammatory, or sinister in origin?

- Mechanical back pain is exacerbated by prolonged sitting or standing, is relieved by movement and precipitated by trauma.
- Inflammatory back pain is characterized by prolonged early morning stiffness and is relieved by exercise.
- Sinister back pain (e.g. malignancy and infection) often leads to pain at night, constant pain, local bony tenderness, and may be accompanied by other systemic symptoms.
- Are there any sensory or motor symptoms? Ask specifically for any change in bowel or bladder function.

Examination

- General – look for evidence of malignancy.
- Spine (palpation for tenderness, muscle spasm, cervical spine flexion, extension, rotation and lateral flexion, thoracic spine rotation, lumbar spine flexion, extension, side flexion, compression of sacroiliac joints).
- Neurological examination looking specifically for absent ankle jerk (slipped disc) or long-tract signs in the legs. S1 nerve root signs and symptoms can be produced by a lesion in the region of the upper lumbar cord (central disc prolapse compressing the S1 nerve root).
- Always do a rectal examination and test perineal sensation.

Back pain: Management

Investigations

Patients with back pain occurring at night and patients with neurological signs warrant investigation.

- X-rays of spine ± CXR (?malignancy)
- FBC and ESR (elevated with sinister causes of pain)
- Biochemical profile (calcium, alkaline phosphatase, and phosphate)
- Immunoglobulins and protein electrophoresis (?myeloma)
- Acid phosphatase
- Prostate specific antigen (PSA)
- Bence-Jones protein and urine protein electrophoresis

Further imaging

- CT scan
- MRI scan (superior to CT for imaging the spinal cord and roots)
- Technetium bone scan ('hot-spots' identify neoplastic or inflammatory lesions)
- Myelography
- Radiculography (to look for cord or root compression)

Management

General measures

- Analgesics
- Bed rest
- Physiotherapy
- Appropriate referral to a specialist

Prolapsed intervertebral disc

Acute postero-lateral herniation of a lumbar disc, usually L4–L5 or L5–S1, is a common cause of acute incapacitating lower back pain. There is often a clear precipitating event (e.g. lifting) and pain may radiate in the distribution of the L5 or S1 nerve root.

Patients should be examined carefully for:

- Paraspinal muscle spasm is often prominent.
- Straight leg raising is typically reduced on the affected side.
- Look for nerve root signs and test sacral and perineal sensation. Always do a rectal examination.
- L5 lesion leads to weakness of extensor hallus longus, ankle dorsiflexion and ankle eversion, and altered sensation is perceived in the L5 dermatome.
- S1 lesion leads to weakness of ankle plantar flexion, ankle eversion and a diminished or lost ankle jerk, and altered sensation is perceived in the S1 dermatome.

Treatment

- If the X-rays reveal a fracture, refer the patient to the orthopaedic team; severe pain from inflammatory arthritides should be referred to the rheumatologists.
- Majority of patients respond to conservative management.
- Bed rest until the acute pain subsides followed by mobilization and physiotherapy (Patients may often be managed at home with instructions to return to the GP or doctor for review in 2–3 weeks.)
- Non-steroidal anti-inflammatory agents.
- Physiotherapy.

Neurosurgical emergencies presenting as back pain

An acute disc prolapse at the L2/3 level may cause bilateral multiple root lesions and may affect bladder and bowel function (cauda equina syndrome).

This requires immediate investigation.

1 **Acute cauda equina compression** (p404)
2 **Acute cord compression** (p404)

C$_1$-esterase inhibitor deficiency (Angioneurotic oedema)

This condition may be inherited or acquired, occurring approximately in 1:50,000 in the UK.

Hereditary

- Autosomal dominant inheritance.
- Usually presents in the second decade.
- Characterized by low serum concentrations of complement components C2, C4 and C$_1$–inhibitor, but normal C1 and C3 levels.

Acquired

- Paraneoplastic syndrome – autoantibody against C$_1$-esterase inhibitor
- Characterized by low serum concentrations of complement components C1, C2, C4, and C$_2$–inhibitor levels.

Clinical features

- Laryngeal oedema (48% of attacks) – may be life-threatening.
- Sub-cutaneous oedema (91% of attacks) – affecting face, buttocks, genitals, and limbs. Usually non-itchy.
- Abdominal symptoms – pain, vomiting, and diarrhoea.

Precipitating factors include:-

- Stress
- Infection
- Pre-menstrual
- Oestrogen-containing contraceptive pill
- Angiotensin converting enzyme inhibitors

Management

Acute severe attack

- C$_1$-esterase inhibitor plasma concentrate – an intravenous infusion of 1000 to 1500 units – usually effective in 30–60 minutes.
- Fresh frozen plasma 2–4 units may be given if C$_1$-esterase inhibitor plasma concentrate is not available.

Laryngeal oedema

- If a patient is admitted with laryngeal oedema 60% oxygen should be given immediately, blood gases should be checked and a senior anaesthetist or ENT surgeon called as intubation or tracheostomy may be required (p202).
- Intramuscular adrenaline 0.5–1ml 1: 1000 (see p212).
- Hydrocortisone 200mg iv.
- Chlorpheniramine 10mg iv may be administered initially prior to the infusion of C$_1$-esterase inhibitor.

Prophylaxis

Those with greater than 1 attack per month

- Tranexamic acid (1–1.5g 2–4 times daily) – effective in 28%.
- Attenuated androgens – e.g. danazol (unlicensed indication).

C_1-esterase inhibitor deficiency
(Angioneurotic oedema) **629**

12 Drug overdoses

Overdoses: General approach

- The history may be unreliable. Question any witnesses or family about where a patient was found and any possible access to drugs.

- 65% of drugs involved belong to the patient, a relative, or friend.
- 30% of self-poisonings involve multiple drugs.
- 50% of patients will have taken alcohol as well.
- Examination may reveal clues as to the likely poison (e.g. pin-point pupils with opiates) and signs of solvent or ethanol abuse and iv drug use should be noted.

Management

Priorities are:

1 Resuscitate the patient
2 Prevent absorption of the drug if possible
3 Give specific antidote if available

- Supportive care is crucial to the survival of the unconscious, intoxicated patient. Monitor their airway (place in the recovery position) and ventilation, bp, body temperature, acid-base and electrolytes, and treat seizures or dysrhythmias.
- Take account of any active medical problems that the patient may have, e.g. iv drug-users may have concurrent septicaemia, hepatitis, SBE, corpumonale from pulmonary granuloma or HIV-related disease.
- Prevention of gut absorption is common to the treatment of most ingested poisons. Measures include:
  - **Ipecac-induced emesis** (30ml in adults repeated after 20 minutes if ineffective) may be used for alert co-operative patients. It is contraindicated in patients with impaired consciousnessness or who have ingested petroleum distillates or corrosives.
  - **Gastric lavage** is equally effective in most circumstances. Protect the airway with endotracheal intubation if consciousness level is impaired.
  - **Activated charcoal** will absorb many drugs if given within 1h of ingestion, although its effectiveness falls off rapidly thereafter. This decline may be reduced if gastric emptying is delayed pharmacologically (e.g. opiates or anticholinergics), by the formation of tablet bezoars (e.g. salicylates), or ingestion of sustained-release preparations (e.g. theophyllines).
  - Repeated administration of activated charcoal may also accelerate whole-body clearance of some drugs by interrupting enterohepatic cycling, e.g. phenobarbitone, phenytoin, carbamazepine, and quinine. Charcoal is rather unpleasant to drink repeatedly and will be more reliably taken if given down a nasogastric tube.

Always seek advice from the local Poisons Unit (listed inside the front cover of the BNF and on p854).

Drug	Action	Antidote / Therapy
Antidepressants	Activated charcoal	Diazepam for convulsions, Cardiac monitoring
Aspirin	Gastric lavage or ipecac if < 12h post overdose	Alkaline diuresis. Haemodialysis
Benzodiazepines	Protect airway	Flumazenil if severe
Beta-blockers	Check bp, HR, and breathing	Atropine (3mg) Glucagon 7mg im Consider pacing
Calcium antagonists	Calcium gluconate	Anticholinergics
Carbon monoxide	Give 100% oxygen	Treat cerebral oedema with mannitol Consider hyperbaric oxygen
Cyanide	Give 100% oxygen	Dicobalt edetate Sodium thiosulphate Sodium nitrite
Digoxin	Check K$^+$ and ECG	Digibind® (digoxin binding antibody)
Ethylene glycol	Gastric emptying	Infuse ethanol 4–Methyl pyrazole
Heavy metals	Gastric emptying	Dimercaprol Penicillamine Sodium calcium edetate
Iron tablets	Gastric emptying	Desferrioxamine
Lithium	Gastric emptying	Diuresis / dialysis
Mefenamic acid	Convulsions may occur Treat with diazepam	None
Methanol	Monitor U&Es, Glc	Infuse ethanol Phenytoin for seizures Dialysis if severe
Organophosphorus insectides	Gastric emptying, Remove clothes, and decontaminate	Atropine Pralidoxime
Opiates	Ensure breathing is adequate	Naloxone
Paracetamol	Gastric emptying if within 4 hours	N-Acetyl cysteine (or methionine)
Paraquat	Gastric emptying	Fuller's Earth (or bentonite or activated charcoal) Intravenous vitamin E may be of benefit
Theophylline	Check plasma potassium urgently	Repeat does of activated charcoal

Amphetamines

This agent (and its cogener methamphetamine) is widely abused for its effects on CNS arousal. A number of its methylenedioxy derivatives (e.g. **'Ecstasy'** or MDMA) are also available on an illicit basis and have additional hallucinogenic actions (LSD-like).

Presentation

Sympathomimetic effects

- Mydriasis
- Hypertension
- Tachycardia
- Skin pallor

Central effects

- Hyperexcitability
- Agitation
- Talkativeness
- Paranoia (esp. with chronic use)

Complications

- Intracranial (and subarachnoid) haemorrhage: Although attriubted to its hypertensive effect this can occur after a single dose.
- Vasospasm may be seen on angiography ('string-of-beads' sign).
- **Ecstasy** is associated with a heat-stroke-like syndrome (p746).

Poor prognostic features

- Hyperpyrexia ($> 42°C$)
- Rhabdomyolysis
- Disseminated intravascular coagulation
- Acute renal failure
- Acute liver failure

Management

- Sedate agitated patients with a benzodiazepine (e.g. 5–10mg diazepam iv or 1–2mg lorazepam im). Frankly psychotic patients may require haloperidol (5–10mg im).
- Monitor core temperature at least hourly initially.
- Seizures should be controlled with diazepam (5–10mg iv stat.). New focal signs should prompt urgent CT scanning looking for evidence of intracranial bleeding.
- Hypertension should be controlled with labetalol, a combined α- and β-blocker: give 50mg stat iv followed by an infusion of 1–2mg/minute which should be stopped when the bp is controlled. (Selective β-blockers such as propranolol may actually worsen the hypertension.) In the absence of labetalol, phentolamine may be substituted (2–5mg iv bolus prn see p126).
- Hyperpyrexia requires prompt cooling with tepid sponging or even chilled iv fluids as necessary to keep the rectal temperature $< 38.5°C$. Chlorpromazine (25–50mg im) will decrease the core temperature but may cause sedation and hypotension. Dantrolene is reported to decrease hyperpyrexia.
- Acidification of the urine can substantially increase drug elimination but can exacerbate electrolyte and pH disturbances. There is no evidence that it influences the outcome and should not be routinely used. Contact your local poison's unit for advice (p854).

Ecstasy

Ecstasy, "E" and "XTC" are street names for MDMA (methylenedioxy-metamphetamine). It produces a positive mood state with feelings of increased sensuality and euphoria. Side-effects with chronic use include anorexia, palpitations, jaw stiffness, grinding of teeth, sweating, and insomnia. Most deaths from Ecstasy result from disturbance of thermo-regulation resulting in hyperthermia. MDMA also causes life-threatening cardiac dysrhythmias, abnormal liver function tests, acute liver failure, and has been associated with cerebral infarction and haemorrhage.

The hyperthermic syndrome occurs within hours of ingestion, and often follow intense physical activity. Features include core temperature $> 40°C$, severe metabolic acidosis, muscle rigidity, DIC, and rhabdomyolysis.

Management: Consider other causes of hyperthermia (p476). Patients should be treated with dantrolene 1mg/kg up to a maximum of 5mg/kg. Dantrolene inhibits release of calcium from the SR in cells. Rhabdomyolysis should be treated in the usual way (p294).

Benzodiazepines

Deliberate overdose with this group of compounds is very common. Unless combined with other sedatives (e.g. alcohol or tricyclics) effects of overdosing are generally mild.

Presentation

- Drowsiness
- Slurred speech
- Nystagmus
- Hypotension (mild)

- Ataxia
- Coma
- Respiratory depression
- Cardiorespiratory arrest (with iv administration)

The elderly are generally more susceptible to cardiorespiratory depression with benzodiazepine overdose.

Management

- If patients present within a few hours of ingestion, empty the stomach with ipecachuanha or gastric lavage. Ensure the patient can protect their airway. No further intervention is usually required for mild to moderate overdoses.

- Severe overdose may require use of the benzodiazepine antagonist, flumazenil, e.g. comatose patients, particularly where the diagnosis is uncertain and, patients with significant cardiorespiratory depression. **Flumazenil** is given as an iv bolus of 0.2mg followed by further bolus dose of 0.1mg every 2–3 mins until the patient is rousable. Most benzodiazepines have a substantially longer duration of action than flumazenil and an ivi of 0.1–0.4mg/h will be needed to prevent early resedation.

- Avoid giving excess flumazenil to completely reverse the effect of a benzodiazepine. In chronic benzodiazepine abusers this can cause marked agitation and may precipitate seizures in patients who have taken an overdose of a combination of benzodiazepines and proconvulsants (e.g. dextropropoxyphene, theophyllines, and tricyclics).

Beta-blockers

These agents competitively antagonize the effects of endogenous catecholamines. They cause profound effects on atrioventricular conduction and myocardial contractility, and their effects are predictable based on their known pharmacology.

Presentation

- Sinus bradycardia
- Hypotension
- Cardiac failure
- Cardiac arrest (asystole or VF)
- Bronchospasm (rare in non-asthmatics)

- Drowsiness
- Hallucinations
- Fits (esp. with propranolol)
- Coma
- Hypoglycaemia (rare)

Prognostic features

- Subjects with pre-existing impaired myocardial contractility are less likely to tolerate even moderate overdoses of beta-blockers.
- The ECG may provide some indication as to the dose ingested: mild overdose is suggested by first-degree heart block; widening of the QRS and prolongation of the QT interval (particularly after sotalol) are associated with moderate to severe overdose.

Management

- Establish iv access.
- Check a 12–lead ECG and then monitor ECG continuously.
- Record bp regularly (at least every 15 minutes).
- *Gastric lavage* should be attempted if seen within 4h of ingestion. Give atropine (0.6–1.2mg iv) BEFORE lavage to prevent vagal-induced cardiovascular collapse.
- *Hypotension*: Treat with an iv glucagon (50–150µg/kg followed by an infusion of 1–5mg/h). This peptide is able to exert an inotropic effect independent of beta-receptor activation by raising myocardial cAMP levels.
- *Bradycardia*: May respond to atropine alone (0.6–1.2mg iv 6–8 hourly). Isoprenaline infusions (5–50µg/min) may be tried but are often ineffective. If the bradycardia persists and the patient is in cardiogenic shock a transvenous pacing wire should be inserted (see p782).
- *Convulsions*: Treat in the standard way (p370). Give diazepam 5–10mg iv initially.
- *Bronchospasm*: Treat initially with high-dose nebulized salbutamol (5–10mg). Nebulized ipratropium bromide (250–500µg) may be tried but it is unlikely to offer additional bronchodilatation in a fully atropinized subject. If nebulized bronchodilators are ineffective, an aminophylline infusion should be used (e.g. 0.5mg/kg/min, see p167 for regime).
- *Monitor blood glucose* regularly (hourly BM stix). If hypoglycaemia develops give 25mls of 50% dextrose followed by an ivi infusion of 10% dextrose adjusting the rate as necessary.

Carbon monoxide (see smoke inhalation p760)

The commonest sources are smoke inhalation, poorly maintained domestic gas appliances, and deliberate inhalation of car exhaust fumes. It causes intense tissue hypoxia by two mechanisms. Firstly, it interrupts electron transport in mitochondria. Secondly, it reduces oxygen delivery both by competing with O_2 for binding to Hb (its affinity for Hb is 220–fold that of O_2) and altering the shape of the HbO_2 dissociation curve (making it less sigmoidal).

Presentation

Patients present with signs of hypoxia without cyanosis. Skin and mucosal surfaces may appear 'cherry-red' (most obvious post mortem). Levels of COHb below 30% cause only headache and dizziness. 50–60% produces syncope, tachypnoea, tachycardia, and fits. Levels over 60%, cause increasing risk of cardiorespiratory failure and death.

Complications

These are the predictable result of local hypoxia. Sites at particular risk are: CNS, affecting cerebral, cerebellar or mid-brain function, e.g. Parkinsonism and akinetic-mutism; the myocardium, with ischaemia and infarction; skeletal muscle, causing rhabdomyolysis and myoglobinuria; skin involvement ranges from erythyema to severe blistering.

Prognostic features

Anaemia, increased metabolic rate (e.g. children), and underlying ischaemic heart disease all increase susceptibility to CO. Neurological recovery depends on the duration of hypoxic coma; complete recovery has been reported in young subjects (under 50) after up to 21h versus 11h in older ones.

Management

- An arterial blood gas should be taken. Although pO_2 may be normal and COHb measurements are often not readily available, any evidence of metabolic acidosis indicates severe poisoning.

  N.B. Monitoring O_2 saturation with a pulse oximeter is unhelpful since it will not distinguish HbO_2 and COHb (hence the apparent oxygen saturation will be falsely high).

- Apply a tight fitting face mask and give 100% O_2. Check a 12–lead ECG and continuously monitor rythm. Take blood for FBC, U&E, CPK, and cardiac enzymes.

- If the patient is comatose they should be intubated and ventilated with a 100% F_iO_2 (this reduces the half-life of COHb to 80 mins, cf. 320 mins on room air). This should also be considered in patients who are severely acidotic or show evidence of myocardial ischaemia.

- Fits should be controlled with iv diazepam (5–10mg). The metabolic acidosis does not generally require correction with iv $NaHCO_3$.

- Hyperbaric oxygen will shorten the washout of COHb further (half-life of 25 mins at 2 atmospheres), but access and transfer times to a hyperbaric chamber makes this an impractical option. Ventilatory stimulation by adding CO_2 (4–7%) to the inspired O_2 also reduces washout times (to < 15 mins) but worsens the metabolic acidosis.

Ensure medical follow-up since the neuropsychiatric sequelae may take many weeks to evolve.

Cocaine

Intoxication during its therapeutic use as a topical analgesic is extremely rare. It is rapidly absorbed, when applied intranasally ('snorting') or smoked (free-basing 'crack'). Occasionally it presents in drug smugglers as massive overdosing when the swallowed packets of illicit cocaine rupture. Its subjective and sympathomimetic actions are often indistinguishable from amphetamine.

Presentation

- Hypertension
- Tachycardia
- Skin pallor
- Ventricular arrhythmias
- Paranoid delusions (with chronic use)

- Seizures (common), may occur in epileptics even at low doses
- CNS depression (with high doses) esp. the medullary centres
- Cardiorespiratory failure

Complications

- Vasoconstrictor effects on the coronary circulation can cause myocardial ischaemia and infarction even in subjects with angiographically normal vessels.
- In the cerebral circulation the hypertension may precipitate stroke.
- Psychotic reactions (similar to amphetamine psychosis) may occur.

Prognostic features

- The lethal dose of cocaine is approximately 1200mg (regular users often tolerate doses considerably in excess of this).
- Cocaine can cause seizures in epileptics in 'recreational' doses, but, for non-epileptics presentation in status epilepticus, generally implies massive overdose and carries a poor prognosis.
- Rhabdomyolysis, hyperpyrexia, renal failure, severe liver dysfunction, and DIC have been reported and carry a high mortality.
- Patients with deficiency of serum pseudocholinesterase appear to be at particular risk of life-threatening cocaine toxicity.

Management

- Establish iv access, taking blood for U&Es and CPK.
- Ensure the airway is clear and if the patient is comatose intubate and mechanically ventilate early.
- Monitor ECG continuously for arrhythmias.
  Ventricular arrythmias may be treated with labetalol (50mg iv bolus and ivi of 1–2mg/min), provided the patient is conscious. Lignocaine should be used with caution as it may precipitate seizures. Give 100mg stat. then an ivi of 1–4mg/min. Phenytoin may be tried if labetalol is ineffective (250mg given as a slow bolus over 5min) particularly in the presence of seizures.
- Monitor core temperature for evidence of *hyperpyrexia*. If necessary, start cooling measures (see p746), e.g. tepid sponging, or chilled iv fluids, as necessary to keep the temperature below 38.5°C. Chlorpromazine 25–50mg im may be useful but sedation and hypotension may occur.
- *Hypertension* should be controlled with labetalol (50mg stat. iv followed by an ivi of 1–2mg/minute which should be stopped when the bp is controlled). Pure β-blockers, such as propranolol, may actually worsen the hypertension. In the absence of labetalol, phentolamine may be substituted (2–5mg iv bolus prn).
- *Seizures* should be controlled with diazepam (10–30mg iv stat. and if necessary an ivi of up to 200mg/24h). Presentation with new focal seizures after cocaine ingestion usually implies ischaemic or haemorrhage stroke: arrange an urgent brain CT scan.

Cyanide

Poisoning is most commonly seen in victims of smoke inhalation (HCN is a combustion product of polyurethane foams). Cyanide derivatives are, however, widely employed in industrial processes and fertilizers. Children may also ingest amygdalin, a cyanogenic glycoside, contained in kernels of almonds and cherries. Cyanide acts by irreversibly blocking mitochondrial electron transport.

Presentation

HCN gas can lead to cardiorespiratory arrest and death within a few minutes. Onset of effects after ingestion or skin contamination are generally much slower (up to several hours). Early signs are dizziness, chest tightness, dyspnoea, confusion, and paralysis. Cardiovascular collapse, apnoea, and seizures follow. Cyanosis is not a feature. The classical smell of bitter almonds is unhelpful (it is genetically determined and 50% of observers cannot detect it).

Pulmonary oedema and lactic acidosis are common in severe poisoning.

Prognostic features

- Ingestion of a few hundred mg of a cyanide salt is usually fatal in adults. Absorption is delayed by a full stomach and high gastric pH (e.g. antacids).
- Patients surviving to reach hospital after inhalation of HCN are unlikely to have suffered significant poisoning.
- Acidosis indicates severe poisoning.

Management

- Do NOT attempt mouth-to-mouth resuscitation. Give 100% O_2 by tight fitting face mask or ventilate via ET tube if necessary.
- Establish iv access.
- Check arterial blood gases. Acidosis indicates severe poisoning.
- Providing there are no signs of cyanide toxicity, ingested cyanide should be removed by gastric lavage. Skin contamination requires thorough washing of the affected area with soap and water.
- If signs of cyanide toxicity are present, give 300mg of dicobalt edetate (*Kelocyanor*®) iv over 1 min. If there is no response in 1 min repeat upto a max. of 900mg. Alternatively, give sodium nitrite (10ml of a 3% solution) and sodium thiosulphate (25ml of 50% solution).

Digoxin

Deliberate overdosing with digoxin is unusual. Significant toxicity is, however, a common adverse drug reaction in patients taking digoxin therapeutically (up to 25% of patients in some series). It is particularly common when renal impairment occurs (digoxin is almost totally cleared by the kidneys), and is exacerbated by hypokalaemia.

646

Presentation
- Nausea, vomiting, confusion, and diarrhoea.
- Visual disturbance (blurring, flashes, disturbed colour vision).
- Cardiac dysrhythmias (tachyarrhythmias or bradyarrhythmias).

Complications
- Hyperkalaemia
- Cardiac dysrhythmias. The initial effect is usually a marked sinus bradycardia which is vagally mediated. This is followed by atrial tachyarrhythmias (with/without heart block), accelerated junctional rhythms, ventricular ectopy, and finally VT or VF.

Prognostic features
- Digoxin level > 15ng/ml represents a severe overdose.
- A serum K^+ of > 5mmol/l indicates severe toxicity.
- Susceptibility to digoxin toxicity is increased by:-
  - Renal impairment
  - Electrolyte disturbance (hypokalaemia or hypomagnesaemia)
  - Hypothyroidism

Management
- Take blood for a digoxin level and U&Es.
- Baseline 12-lead ECG and continuous ECG monitoring.
- *Ipecachuanha or gastric lavage* should be attempted if seen within 4 hours of ingestion of an overdose, followed by activated charcoal (100g stat.). Patients presenting > 4h should be given cholestyramine orally (4g qds).
- Sinus bradyarrhythmias and AV block usually respond to atropine (0.6mg iv repeated to a total of 2.4mg). Asymptomatic ventricular ectopics do not require specific treatment.
- *Ventricular tachyarrhythmias* should be treated with phenytoin (250mg over 5 minutes). If this is not effective, give amiodarone (600mg over 1h) or lignocaine (100mg iv loading dose followed by an ivi of 1–4mg/min) may be effective.
- Patients with haemodynamic instability, resistant ventricular tachyarrhythmias, or high serum K^+ require specific treatment with *digoxin-binding antibody fragments* (Fab, *Digibind*®). Dose is: (No. of vials) = $1.67 \times$ amount ingested (mg). If latter unknown give 20 vials (infused over 30 mins). Patients intoxicated during chronic therapy: dose (No. of vials) = digoxin level (ng/ml) $\times$ wt (kg) $\times$ 0.01. Fab therapy will terminate ventricular tachyarrhythmias in 20–40 minutes.
  The potassium and free serum digoxin levels should be monitored for 24h after Fab therapy. A substantial hypokalaemia can develop and, not infrequently, there is a rebound in digoxin levels which may require administration of additional Fab. In patients with renal impairment this rebound is delayed and monitoring should be extended to 72h.
- Patients with severe renal failure who require *Digibind*® therapy are obviously unable to clear the Fab-digoxin complexes. Plasmaphoresis is indicated to clear the bound digoxin.
- If *Digibind*® is not available, insert a transvenous pacing wire and try to control arrhythmias with a combination of overdrive pacing, DC shock, and drugs (see p40–72).

Ethylene glycol

Ingestion may be deliberate but usually it is taken accidentally as an ethanol 'substitute'; it is present in 'anti-freeze'. Ethylene glycol (EG) toxicity is due to accumulation of toxic metabolites (aldehydes, glycollate, oxalates, and lactate). This metabolic route may be blocked by competitive antagonism with ethanol.

Presentation
- Impaired conciousness ('inebriation' without alcohol on the breath)
- Seizures and focal neurological signs (e.g. ophthalmoplegias) are seen in the first 24 hours.
- Loin pain, haematuria, and ATN occurs over the next 48 hours.

Prognostic features
- As little as 30ml of ethylene glycol can be fatal in adults.
- It is often taken with ethanol, which is actually protective through blocking the metabolism of glycol to toxic metabolites.
- Renal failure can be averted if specific treatment is instituted early.
- Plasma levels of EG > 500mg/l (8mmol/l) indicate severe overdose
- The degree of acidosis is the best indicator of likely outcome.

Complications
- Oliguric renal failure (crystal nephropathy)
- Non-cardiogenic pulmonary oedema
- Cerebral oedema
- Cardiovascular collapse
- Myocarditis

Management
- Perform *gastric lavage* if presenting within a few hours of ingestion. This will also enable confirmation that EG has been taken; commercial 'anti-freeze' often contains fluorescein which is easily detected with a UV light source (also detectable in urine).
- Establish iv access and take blood for U&Es, glucose, biochemical profile incl. Ca^{2+}, plasma osmolality, and ethanol and EG levels.
- Check arterial blood gases to assess degree of acidaemia
- Microscope a fresh urine sample looking for the needle-shaped crystals of calcium oxalate monohydrate which are pathognomonic.
- The half-life of EG is short (3h). To prevent significant metabolism an *ethanol infusion* should be started as soon as possible (detailed under 'methanol' poisoning, p656). The infusion should be continued until plasma EG is undetectable. Infusion of ethanol will cause intoxication.
- *4–methylpyrazole* (10–20mg/kg/d orally) has also been used as an inhibitor of alcohol dehydrogenase and has the advantage that, unlike ethanol, it does not cause CNS depression. It is not widely available.
- The metabolic acidosis should be treated with $NaHCO_3$

$$\left[\begin{array}{c}\text{Volume of 8.4\%}\\\text{bicarbonate (mls)}\end{array}\right] = 0.15 \times \left[\begin{array}{c}\text{Base deficit}\\\text{(BE on ABG printout)}\end{array}\right] \times \left[\begin{array}{c}\text{Body weight}\\\text{(kg)}\end{array}\right]$$

8.4% $NaHCO_3$ must be given only through a central line and slowly (over 20–40 minutes). Isosmolar bicarbonate (1.26% $NaHCO_3$) may be given through a peripheral line (multiply the volume by 6.7): e.g. for a 70kg man with a base deficit of -7, give 73ml 8.4% bicarbonate (490mls of 1.26%). Recheck ABGs and administer further amount according to the above formula

Indications for dialysis: Severe acidosis (declining vital signs or a EG level > 500mg/l) or oliguria requires haemodialysis or peritoneal dialysis (the former is 2–3 fold more effective). Normal renal function is generally restored in 7–10 days although permanent impairment has been reported.

Iron

Accidental ingestion is almost exclusively a problem in children. In overdose, iron binding mechanisms are rapidly saturated leading to high concentrations of free iron. The latter catalyses the widespread generation of free radicals which is the basis of the toxic manifestations of iron overdose.

Presentation

- Iron is extremely irritant and causes prominent abdominal pain, vomiting and diarrhoea, haematemesis and rectal bleeding.
- Usually the initial GI symptoms subside before secondary signs develop 12–24h after ingestion. Hepatic failure, jaundice, fits, and coma are common.
- Very large overdose can cause early cardiovascular collapse and coma.
- In children, 1–2g of iron may prove fatal. Patients alive 72h after ingestion usually make a full recovery
- Late sequelae of gastric fibrosis and pyloric obstruction have been reported occasionally.

Management

- The stomach should be emptied either by *lavage or ipecacuanha*. The lavage fluid should contain 1% $NaHCO_3$. 50–100ml of a solution of 5–10g desferrioxamine in 50–100ml water should be instilled and left in the stomach to prevent further absorption.
- A *plain AXR* may be useful to assess the number of tablets ingested.
- Establish iv access. Take blood for U&Es, LFTs, FBC, serum iron, and TIBC (total iron binding capacity).
- *Parenteral chelation therapy* is indicated if the serum iron level is $> 90\mu M$ or exceeds the TIBC.
  - Desferrioxamine should be given im (2g for adults and 1g for children) every 6–12h (N.B. 100mg of desferrioxamine binds 8.5mg of elemental iron).
  - If the patient is hypotensive give desferrioxamine iv at a rate of 15mg/kg/h (recommended max daily dose is 80mg/kg; although if the patient tolerates it, and it is indicated by the serum iron, higher doses may be given). The ivi is continued until the serum iron falls below the TIBC.
- *Dialysis:* Haemodialysis is indicated for very high serum iron levels that respond poorly to chelation therapy or if the urine output is not maintained during chelation therapy, since the iron-chelate is only excreted in the urine.
- *Exchange transfusion* has also been used successfully for very severe intoxication.

Lithium

Lithium has a low therapeutic index and toxicity can and does occur much more frequently than deliberate self-administration. Toxicity is commonly precipitated by adminstration of diuretics or intercurrent dehydration, e.g. following vomiting or a febrile illness.

Presentation

- Thirst, polyuria, diarrhoea, vomiting, and coarse tremor are common.
- In severe toxicity the effects on the CNS generally predominate, with impairment of conciousness, fine tremor, hypertonia, seizures, and focal neurological signs.
- Cardiac arrythmia and hypotension are seen in very severe poisoning.

Prognostic features

Features of toxicity are usually associated with Li^+ levels of > 1.5 mmol/l. However, Li^+ enters cells relatively slowly so that the levels taken shortly after a large overdose may be very high with the patient showing few if any signs of toxicity. Levels > 4 mmol/l will probably require haemo- or peritoneal dialysis.

Management

- Patients presenting within 6–8h of ingestion should be given ipecachuanha or undergo gastric lavage. If slow-release preparations are involved cathartics (e.g.$MgSO_4$) may decrease absorption. Activated charcoal is NOT useful.
- Check serum Li^+ level (ensure the tube used does not contain lithium-heparin anti-coagulant).
- Check U&Es: If hypernatraemia is present check serum osmolality.
- Any diuretic or other drug likely to alter renal handling of Li^+ (e.g. NSAIDs) should be stopped.
- Correct any fluid or electrolyte deficits. Forced diuresis using iv 0.9% saline, e.g. 3–4 litres/24h should be started if there are any signs of severe toxicity or levels > 3mmol/l. (Watch for fluid overload). The serum Na^+ and osmolality must be monitored daily since both are likely to rise.
- If levels are > 4mmol/l or oliguria precludes diuresis then the patient should be haemodialysed. Although Li^+ can be effectively cleared from the extracellular compartment with dialysis, movement out of cells is much slower. Dialysis should be continued until Li^+ is not detected in the serum or dialysate. Levels should be measured daily for the next week in case Li^+ rebounds due to slow release from intracellular stores.

LSD (lysergic acid diethylamide)

LSD is the prototypical psychedelic drug. Although its abuse was a feature of the 1960s and early 1970s, it has reappeared in the last few years in increasing amounts. It is no longer manufactured for medicinal use but illicit sources are surprisingly pure, i.e. free of adulterants. The preferred route is ingestion, although it is occasionally injected and has been reported to be active if snorted.

654

Presentation

A typical dose of around 100μg causes:-

- Pupillary dilatation
- Sweating
- An acute anxiety state
- Tachycardia
- Depersonalization, visual illusions, and distortion of time

Large doses can cause convulsions, focal neurological deficit (due to vasospasm), and coma.

Complications

- Acute psychosis with visual hallucination, paranoia, or features of mania is well described.
- Very large overdoses have been associated with a mild bleeding disorder due to blockade of 5–HT-induced platelet aggregation.
- Rhabdomyolysis has been reported in the past but appears to have reflected the physical restraints used, i.e. 'straight-jackets'.
- Death from even large overdoses is unusual and usually reflects suicide or accidental trauma while under the psychedelic effects of LSD.

Management

- Absorption is likely to be complete by the time symptoms are manifest. Lavage may actually worsen the behavioural disturbance.
- Most patients will need a quiet side room and verbal reassurance only ('talking down'). The visual illusions fade in 4–8h.
- Very agitated patients can be sedated with im lorazepam (1–2mg) and/or im haloperidol 5–10mg.
- Seizures respond to diazepam iv (5–10mg bolus).
- The development of focal neurological signs should prompt a CT scan and probably cerebral angiography. Occasionally, intense vasospasm is seen involving even the intracranial carotids.
- Comatose patients require full supportive care (p306) but generally recover fully in 24h. Aspiration appears to be a definite risk and protection of the airway is particularly important.
- There are no specific antidotes or methods for enhanced drug elimination.

Methanol

Poisoning usually follows ingestion of contaminated alcohol beverages or 'methylated spirits'. Intoxication in industrial settings follows absorption across the skin or lung. Alcohol dehydrogenase metabolizes it to form-aldehyde which is oxidized to the toxic formic acid.

Presentation
- Signifcant ingestion causes nausea, vomiting, and abdominal pain.
- Its effects on the CNS resemble those of ethanol although in low doses it does not have an euphoric effect.
- Visual symptoms present with falling visual acuity, photophobia, and the sensation of 'being in a snow storm'.

Complications
- Up to 65% of patients have a raised amylase but this does not necessarily represent pancreatitis (usually salivary-gland amylase type). If pancreatitis is suspected clinically, measure serum lipase (haemorrhagic pancreatitis has been reported at post mortem).
- Seizures are seen in severe intoxication. CT scanning usually shows cerebral oedema or even necrosis in the basal ganglia (a Parkinsonian-like state is sometimes seen with recovery).
- Patients with visual syptoms may develop irreversible visual impairment even with aggressive intervention.
- Rhabdomyolysis and acute renal failure.
- Hypoglycaemia.

Prognostic features
- 10ml of methanol can cause blindness and 30ml can be fatal.
- Peak plasma methanol is useful although in practice the 'peak' is often unclear; > 0.2g/litre (6.25mmol/l) indicates significant ingestion and 0.5g/l (15.6mmol/l) is severe.
- Arterial pH seems to correlate best with formate levels and pH < 7.2 is a severe intoxication.

Management
- Ipecachuanha or gastric lavage is useful only if presenting within 2 hours of ingestion. Activated charcoal is not indicated.
- Take blood for U&E, CPK, glucose, amylase, and ethanol/methanol levels; ABG (acidosis), urine (myoglobin, p294).
- **Seizures** are probably best treated with phenytoin (250mg iv over 5 mins) since this will have less of a CNS depressant effect than diazepam. Exclude hypoglycaemias, a cause of seizures.
- **Ethanol infusion:** This should be given to:
  - All patients, pending methanol levels
  - Those patients with methanol levels > 0.2g/l (6.25mmol/l)
  - Acidotic patients
  - Anyone needing haemodialysis
- Give iv as a 10% solution in 5% dextrose or N saline (i.e. take 50ml from a 500ml bag and replace with 50ml ethanol). A loading dose of 10ml/kg should be given followed by an ivi of 0.15ml/kg/h for non-drinkers (regular drinkers-0.3ml/kg/h). Titrate to a plasma ethanol level of 1–1.5g/litre (21.7–32.6mmol/l). The ethanol ivi should be continued for at least 48h as ethanol and severe methanol overdose prolong the half-life of methanol to > 30h.
- Metabolic acidosis should be corrected with iv NaHCO₃.
- Hypoglycaemia is treated with 25ml of 50% glucose iv stat. followed by an ivi of 10% glucose adjusted as necessary.
- **Haemodialysis** is reserved for those patients with renal failure, ANY visual impairment or a plasma methanol level of > 0.5g/l (15.6 mmol/l). The ethanol infusion rate should be doubled during dialysis (or ethanol may be added directly to the dialysis fluid).

Ethanol: Acute intoxication

Patients may present either with acute intoxication (often on a background of chronic misuse), withdrawal syndromes, nutritional deficiency syndromes, or chronic toxicity (liver, CNS, peripheral neuromyopathy, etc).

Presentation

Ethanol initially results in disinhibition and euphoria, and with increasing serum levels, this progresses to incoordination, ataxia, stupor, and coma. Chronic alcoholics tend to require higher blood ethanol levels than 'social' drinkers for intoxication. Try to obtain a history from friends or relatives. Examine the patient for signs of chronic liver disease, trauma, or signs of infection.

Complications

- Acute gastritis causes N&V, abdominal pain, and GI haemorrhage.
- Respiratory depression and arrest, inhalation of vomit (with ARDS-Mendelson's syndrome), and hypothermia may accompany the profound sedation.
- Hypoglycaemia is common and should be excluded.
- Alcoholic ketoacidosis or lactic acidosis.
- Accidental injury, particularly head injury (subdural).
- Rhabdomyolysis and acute renal failure.
- Infection (septicaemia, meningitis).

Management

- Mild to moderate intoxication usually requires no specific treatment: the need for admission for re-hydration and observation depends on the individual patient. Admit all patients with stupor or coma.
- Check the airway is clear of vomitus and the patient is able to protect it. Nurse in the recovery position.
- Ipecachuanha, gastric lavage, or charcoal are not indicated.
- Take blood for U&E, CPK, glucose, anylase, and ethanol (and methanol) levels, ABG (acidosis), lactate, ammonia. Analyse, urine (myoglobin, p294). Consider the possibility of other drug overdose.
- Monitor closely for respiratory depression, hypoxia, cardiac arrhythmias, and hypotension and withdrawal syndromes (see p396).
- Check BM stix. In comatose patients, there is a good argument for giving 25–50ml of 50% dextrose immediately for presumed hypoglycaemia because this will usually not cause any harm. Follow with an ivi of 10% glucose if necessary.
- The only concern is that glucose may precipitate Wernicke's encephalopathy in malnourished individuals. Some clinicians therefore favour giving a bolus of thiamine 1–2mg/kg iv beforehand.
- Rehydrate with intravenous fluids (avoid excessive use of saline in patients with signs of chronic liver disease); monitor urine output.
- Naloxone reduces the effects of alcohol toxicity but its use is not standard at present.
- Rarely, haemodialysis is used if intoxiciation is very severe or in the presence of acidosis.
- Watch for complications (see above) any treat as necessary.
- After recovery from the acute episode arrange for a psychiatric or medical assessment and follow-up and referral to an alcohol rehabilitation programme if appropriate.

Alcohol withdrawal and delirium tremens (DTs) see p396

Isopropanol

As a cause of poisoning with alcohols this is second after ethanol. It has twice the potency of ethanol on the CNS (its major metabolite, acetone, compounds this) and isopropanol-induced coma can last > 24h. Effects are seen within 30–60mins of ingestion and large overdoses cause coma and hypotension as the major effect. Haemodialysis is indicated if the hypotension fails to respons to iv fluids, vital signs decline, or blood levels are > 4g/l (66.7mmol/l). Monitor for hypoglycaemia and myoglobinuria.

Opiates

Overdosing with opiates usually occurs in regular drug-users, where the most commonly abused agent is diamorphine (heroin). It may be taken intravenously, smoked, or snorted. A number of other opiates have been similarly abused. Opiates such as dextropropoxyphene and dihydrocodeine (present in combination formulations with paracetamol) are often taken with alcohol by non-addicts with suicidal intent.

Presentation

Pin-point pupils, severe respiratory depression ± cyanosis, and coma are typical. The depressive effects are exacerbated by alcohol. bp may be low but is often surprisingly well maintained, and with pentazocine overdose actually increases. Although some opiates, e.g. dextropropoxyphene and pethidine, increase muscle tone and cause fits in overdose, in general opiates cause marked hypotonia.

Prognostic features
- Non-cardiogenic pulmonary oedema carries a poor prognosis (it is not naloxone reversible).
- Patients with underlying ischaemic heart disease seem more susceptible to haemodynamic disturbance after naloxone is given to reverse opiate intoxication (see below).
- Renal impairment reduces the elimination of many opiates and prolongs their duration of action.

Management
- Ensure a patent airway and monitor respiratory rate, depth of respiration, and continuous pulse oximetry. Give oxygen by mask.
- Establish iv access and take blood for U&Es and CPK. If opiate and paracetamol combinations have been ingested measure a paracetamol level (see p662).
- Monitor the ECG continuously for arrhythmias.
- Any patient who is comatose or has respiratory signs requires a CXR (signs of infection, septic emboli, interstitial shadowing, p154).
- The specific antidote is ***naloxone*** (a pure opiate antagonist) which should be given iv in boluses of 0.4mg at 2–3 minute intervals until the patient is rousable and any evidence of respiratory depression corrected. Doses of up to 2mg (and above) may be required but if no response is seen at this level then the diagnosis of opiate overdose should be revised.
- The duration of action of naloxone is shorter than many opiates hence an infusion should be started to avoid resedation (starting with 0.2mg/h and increasing as necessary). In the case of overdose with long-acting opiates such as methadone, infusion of naloxone may be necessary for 48–72h.
- Avoid giving sufficient naloxone to completely reverse the effect of opiates in an opiate-dependent subject. This is likely to precipitate an acute withdrawal reaction. If this occurs and hypertension is marked then iv labetalol is probably the most suitable agent (50mg stat. followed by an ivi of 1–2mg/min until the bp is controlled).
N.B. Marked hypertension, acute pulmonary oedema and VT/VF have been observed in non-addicts given naloxone to reverse the effects of high therapeutic doses of opiates for pain.
- Convulsions which are opiate-induced (usually pethidine or dextropropoxyphene) will respond to iv naloxone. Additional anti-convulsant therapy is generally not required.
- Pulmonary oedema present on admission requires ventilation with pressure support (p802). It does not respond to naloxone.
- Rhabdomyolysis and acute renal failure, see p294.

Complications
- All opiates can cause non-cardiogenic pulmonary oedema although it is most frequently seen with iv heroin.
- Rhabdomyolysis is common in opiate-induced coma and should be looked for in all cases.
- The substances used to dilute ('cut') illicit opiates may also carry significant toxicity when injected (e.g. talc and quinine).
- iv drug-users may develop right-sided endocarditis and septic pulmonary emboli (several localized infiltrates on CXR).
- Ingestion of paracetamol, containing preparations (e.g. co-dydramol) may develop renal or hepatic failure.

Important points

1 Dextropropoxyphene in combination with alcohol can cause marked CNS depression. Respiratory arrest can evolve rapidly within < 30 mins of ingestion. Give naloxone even if the patient is only mildly drowsy. It also causes an acute cardiotoxicity with arrythmias due to a membrane-stabilizing effect (naloxone ineffective).
2 The respiratory depressant effects of buprenorphine are not fully reversed by naloxone. Doxapram has been used in milder cases of buprenorphine overdose as a respiratory depressant (1–4mg/min), although severe cases may require mechanical ventilation.

Paracetamol: Assessment

The toxicity of this analgesic stems from its saturable metabolism. In therapeutic doses, only a minor fraction is oxidized to the reactive/toxic species (NABQI, N-acetyl-benzoquinoneimine) which is detoxified by conjugation with glutathione. In overdose, an increased fraction is metabolized to these metabolites, whose detoxification rapidly depletes hepatic glutathione stores.

Presentation

- Apart from mild nausea, vomiting, and anorexia, patients presenting within 24h of ingestion are generally asymptomatic.
- Hepatic necrosis becomes apparent in 24–36h with right subchondral pain/tenderness, jaundice (and acute liver failure), vomiting.
- Confusion and encephalopathy develop over 36–72h.
- Oliguria and renal failure.
- Lactic acidosis may be seen early (i.e. within 12 hours) and late.

Complications

- Acute liver failure (see p518) with hypoglycaemia, cerebral oedema, and GI bleeding.
- Severe metabolic (lactic) acidosis.
- Pancreatitis (alone or with liver failure).
- Some 10% of patients develop acute renal failure from acute tubular necrosis which may be seen in the absence of liver failure.
- Very rarely patients with G6PD deficiency develop methaemoglobinaemia and haemolysis.

Investigations

- **Paracetamol**   Measure levels at least 4h post ingestion and plot on the graph in the figure on p665.
- **U&Es**   Renal failure generally occurs on day 3.
- **Glucose**   May fall with progressive liver failure. Give iv dextrose (25–50ml of 50% dextrose) if necessary.
- **FBC**   In patients with severe overdoses and liver failure, thrombocytopenia is common and may be severe.
- **LFTs**   Transaminases rise early (up to 20,000 U/l).
- **PT**   This may be normal despite high transaminases. The PT is the best indicator of the severity of liver failure.
- **ABGs**   To assess degree of acidosis.

Prognostic features

Fatal overdose may occur with $< 10g$ but usually involves $> 30g$. The cause of death is usually acute liver failure. Chronic alcoholics or patients on phenobarbitone or phenytoin are more susceptible to developing hepatotoxicity and nephrotoxicity.

- Refer to a liver unit all patients with acidosis (pH < 7.32) and coagulopathy (INR > 1.5). Refer early.
- If renal failure occurs in isolation (no coagulopathy but transaminase levels high), then refer to a renal unit.
- **Indications for liver transplantation**
  - Late acidosis (> 36 hours post-overdose) with arterial pH < 7.3
  - Prothrombin time (PT) $> 100s$.
  - Serum creatinine $> 300\mu M$
  - Grade 3 encephalopathy (confused, distressed, barely rousable)

Paracetamol: Management

- Patients presenting within 4h of ingestion should undergo *gastric lavage* or be given *ipecachuanha*.
- Measure paracetamol levels at least 4h post ingestion and plot on the graph in the figure opposite.
- All patients on or above the **'Normal' treatment line** (and presenting up to 24h after ingestion) should be given *N-acetylcysteine* (see table below). If allergic to N-acetyl cysteine or if presenting WITHIN 10–12 hours, with oral *methionine* (see table below) may be used.
- Patients on enzyme-inducing drugs (e.g. phenytoin, carbamazepine, rifampicin, phenobarbitone) or with a history of high alcohol intake may develop toxicity at lower plasma levels and should be treated if the level is above the **'High-Risk' treatment line** (figure opposite).
- If the initial levels indicate no treatment is necessary, repeat the paracetamol levels 4 hours later. Occasionally there may be delayed absorption and treatment is inappropriately witheld.
- Give N-acetyl cysteine to all severe overdoses (> 10g) who present at 24–72h with symptoms or derranged investigations (LFTs, PT).
- *Monitor* U&Es, FBC, PT, LFTs, glucose, and arterial blood gases daily. Monitor glucose with BM stix at least 6 hourly.
- *Give vitamin K* iv 10mg (in case body stores are deficient) but *avoid giving FFP* unless there is active bleeding. The PT is the best indicator of the severity of liver failure; FFP may only make management decisions (e.g. liver transplantation) more difficult. All patients who are encephalopathic or have a rapidly rising PT must be referred to a liver unit.
- Management of *acute liver failure* is discussed on p522.

Specific treatment for paracetamol poisoning

• N-acetyl cysteine infusion

150mg/kg in 200ml 5% dextrose over 15min, followed by 50mg/kg in 500ml 5% dextrose over 4h, and finally 100mg/kg in 1 litre 5% dextrose over 16h.
[Up to 10% of patients have a rash, bronchospasm, or hypotension during the infusion. Stop the ivi and give chlorpheniramine (10mg iv); restart the ivi when symptoms settle].

• Oral methionine

This may be given orally once vomiting has occurred if the patient presents within 10–12 hours of ingestion of the overdose. Give 2.5g stat. and 3 further doses of 2.5g every 4 hours

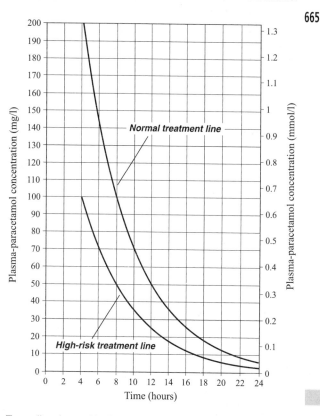

Treat all patients with plasma paracetamol concentrations above the normal treatment line with iv acetylcystein. Patients on enzyme inducing drugs (eg carbamazepine, phenobarbitone, phenytoin, rifampicin, and alcohol) or those who are malnourished (eg anorexia, alcoholism, or HIV-positive) should be treated if their plasma-paracetamol concentrations are above the high-risk treatment line. (British National Formulary Number **33** (March 1997) p21; BMA, London and the Royal Pharm. Soc., Wallingford, with permission).

Paraquat

This bipyridilium herbicide (*Gram:noxone*® is a 20% solution, cf. *Weedol*® 2.5%) is notoriously toxic in overdose. Children may drink it inadvertently and horticulturists have occasionally been poisoned through skin splashing. Death is usually due to delayed pulmonary fibrosis and respiratory failure. The mechanism is thought to be due to the generation of cytotoxic oxygen radicals.

Presentation

- Nausea and vomiting are seen within a few hours of ingestion.
- Mouth and oesophageal ulceration are common.
- Oliguric renal failure develops with doses of $> 2g$ within 12 hours of ingestion.
- Very high doses (e.g. 50–100ml 20% solution, i.e. $> 10g$) may cause acute dyspnoea with an ARDS-like picture and rapid evolution of multi-organ failure.
- Insidious pulmonary fibrosis develops in the second week after exposure (often as the oliguria is resolving). This is not reversible and occasional survivors invariably have a severe handicap.
- Liver failure and myocarditis are also reported and thought to reflect the same free radical-mediated cell damage.

Prognostic features

- The dose ingested is a good predictor of outcome: death has been reported after only 10–15ml of the 20% solution (3g) of paraquat and is universal after 50ml (10g).
- Plasma levels of paraquat e.g. $> 2mg/l$ at 4 hours or $0.1mg/l$ at 24 hours are associated with a poor prognosis.
- A low WBC on admission carries a poor prognosis.

Management

- Patients presenting within 6h of ingestion should *receive gastric lavage* with the instillation of a 30% solution of *Fuller's Earth* (250ml) repeated 4 hourly. If the latter is not available then activated charcoal should be given (50–100g).
- Blood should be taken for FBC, U&E, LFT, and paraquat levels.
- Perform a baseline CXR and arterial blood gases.
- Monitor urine output (catheterize if necessary).
- iv fluids (but not a forced diuresis) are indicated when oesophageal ulceration is severe enough to produce dysphagia.
- The use of *haemoperfusion* or *haemofiltration* should be reserved for subjects whose outcome is borderline. It is only in these cases that the very small amounts of paraquat removed by either process (perhaps a few tens of mg) could conceivably affect outcome. Haemodialysis may of course be needed independently of drug elimination if renal failure develops.
- Attempts have been made to prevent or slow the process of pulmonary fibrosis, and include radiotherpay to the lungs and immunosuppression with dexamethasone $\pm$ cyclophosphamide. Neither has proved to be effective and cannot be recommended. A single report exists of acute lung transplantation to salvage a patient with terminal fibrosis but the patient subsequently died of a late paraquat-induced myopathy.

Salicylates

Aspirin is probably the commonest drug to be ingested deliberately in overdose. Occasionally, poisoning follows the topical application of salicylic acid in keratolytics or ingestion of methyl salicylate ('oil of wintergreen'). Its primary toxic effect is to uncouple oxidative phosphorylation.

Presentation

- The typical features of moderate salicylate toxicity are sweating, vomiting, epigastric pain, tinnitus, and blurring of vision.
- In adults, there is also an early increase in respiratory rate causing an alkalosis that precedes the later development of a metabolic acidosis (children do not develop the early respiratory alkalosis).
- In severe overdose, the acidosis reduces the ionization of salicylic acid which enhances tissue penetration. In the CNS, this presents as agitation, tremor and fits, coma, and respiratory depression.

Complications

- Disturbance of electrolytes (hypokalaemia and either hyper- or hyponatraemia) and blood glucose ($\uparrow$ or $\downarrow$) are common.
- Pulmonary oedema (non-cardiogenic, ARDS).
- Acute renal failure.
- Abnormal clotting due to hypoprothrombinaemia is very rare.
- Significant GI bleeds are surprisingly infrequent.

Prognostic features

- Therapeutic levels of salicylate are generally < 300mg/l (2.2 mmol/l). Levels of 500–750mg/l represents moderate overdose and > 750mg/l (5.4 mmol/l) is severe.
- Severe metabolic acidosis is associated with a poor outcome.

Management

- Gastric lavage should be attempted where possible up to 12h after ingestion (or longer if there is evidence of continued absorption, since tablets may adhere to form large masses in the stomach).
- Take blood for U&Es, PT, and salicylate (& paracetamol) level on admission (ideally repeat 4h later to assess continued absorption).
- Check arterial blood gases to assess degree of acidosis.
- Monitor blood glucose regularly (lab. and/or BM stix every 2 hours)
- Mild or moderate salicylate overdose requires only oral or iv rehydration with particular attention to K^+ supplements.
- Marked signs/symptoms of salicylism or levels > 750mg/l need specific elimination therapy (below, in order of use).
  - Activated charcoal should be given orally (50g 4 hourly).
  - Forced alkaline diuresis is no more effective than simple alkalinization of the urine, e.g. 1 litre 1.26% $NaHCO_3$ over 2h and repeat as necessary to keep the urinary pH > 7.5).
  - Haemodialysis is indicated for: levels > 1000mg/l (7.25 mmol/l); persistent or progressive acidosis; deteriorating level of conciousness.
- Pulmonary oedema may indicate either fluid overload or increased vascular permeability. Admit to ITU and insert a pulmonary artery catheter for measuring wedge pressures (p774). Non-cardiogenic pulmonary oedema will require mechanical ventilation (p188).

Theophylline

Intoxication can be deliberate or iatrogenic due to the low therapeutic index of theophylline.

Presentation

- The features of acute ingestion reflect the local irritant GI effects of theophylline, i.e. nausea, vomiting, abdominal cramps, and diarrhoea. GI bleeding is also well recognized.
- Features of systemic toxicity include cardiac arrythmias, hypotension, and seizures.

Complications

- Acid-base disturbance: An initial respiratory alkalosis which gives way to a secondary metabolic acidosis.
- Marked hypokalaemia is common.
- Theophylline-induced fits carry a high mortality (up to 30%) and usually reflect serum theophylline levels of > 50mg/l (0.28 mmol/l).

Management

- Gastric lavage should be attempted if seen within 1–2h of ingestion. Activated charcoal should also be given both to prevent further absorption and enhance systemic clearance (50–100g stat. then 50g 4–hourly), although this may not be practical in the presence of severe nausea and vomiting.
- Take blood for U&E and theophylline level.
- *Hypokalaemia* should be corrected aggressively with iv supplements (40–60mmol/h may be needed).
- Record a 12–lead ECG and then monitor ECG continuously for arrhythmias.
- Verapamil (10mg iv, p51) and propranolol (2–5mg iv, p51) are useful for treating supraventricular and ventricular *tachyarrhythmias*, respectively. Lignocaine appears to have little effect on ventricluar ectopy.
- *GI bleeding* should be managed in the usual way (p482). Avoid cimetidine which substantially inhibits theophylline metabolism (ranitidine is safe, e.g. 50mg iv tds).
- *Seizures* should be controlled with diazepam (10mg iv prn).
- *Haemoperfusion* (charcoal or resin) should be considered in severe overdoses, particularly those with recurrent seizure activity or intractable vomiting. The latter represents direct stimulation of the area postrema and generally responds poorly to anti-emetics, e.g. metoclopramide and prochlorperazine.

Tricyclic antidepressants

First-generation agents (e.g. amitriptyline, imipramine, and desipramine) are the most likley to cause lethal intoxication. The newer second-generation tri- (e.g. lofepramine) and tetracyclics are generally much safer in overdose. There are, however, exceptions, e.g. the tetracyclic maprotiline is probably as cardiotoxic and induces even greater seizure activity; the second-generation tricyclic amoxapine, although less cardiotoxic, induces seizures and, in 10% of cases, acute renal failure.

Presentation

- Anticholinergic features are prominent early on with dry mouth, blurred vision, sinus tachycardia, urinary retention, myoclonic jerking, agitation, and even hallucinations.
- Cardiac arrhythmias from a quinidine-like (type Ia) effect on the heart, profound hypotension, convulsions, and coma follow.

Complications

- Severe intoxication causes deep coma with respiratory depression, hypoxia, and a metabolic acidosis.
- Neurological signs include a temporary loss of oculocephalic and oculovestibular reflexes, long tract signs, and internuclear ophthalmoplegia.
- Hypothermia, skin blistering (cf. barbiturates), and rhabdomyolysis are also reported.

Prognostic features

- Death may follow ingestion of as little as 1000mg of a tricyclic.
- Prolongation of the QRS > 100ms suggests significant intoxication with a high risk of convulsion; a QRS > 160ms is generally seen before ventricular arrythmias develop. Patients with ischaemic heart disease (especially post MI) and conduction defects are particularly at risk.

Management

- Patients with CNS depression should be monitored closely preferably on an ITU or high-dependency area.
- Gastric lavage should be attempted if seen within 12h of ingestion. Activated charcoal should be given orally (50–100g, single dose).
- Record a 12-lead ECG and monitor continuously for up to 48h.
- Respiratory failure may evolve rapidly necessitating intubation and ventilation.
- Severe hypotension requires inotropic support (see p210).
- Acidosis should be corrected with iv $NaHCO_3$ (see p716).
- Control seizures with diazepam (5–10mg iv bolus prn).
- Sinus tachycardias and arrhythmias that do not compromise cardiac output do not need treatment. If output is failing then correct any acidosis or hypoxia before considering anti-arrhythmics.
- Most class I arrhythmic agents are ineffective or worsen the conduction disturbance. Phenytoin (250mg iv over 5min) or amiodarone (300mg ivi over 30 min) are probably the most useful.
- If all measures fail then an induced alkalosis (by hyperventilation or 50–100mmol $NaHCO_3$ over 15min, i.e. 50–100ml 8.4% $NaHCO_3$) may help by increasing binding of the tricyclic to plasma proteins.
- Tricyclic coma may last 24–48h. In many patients recovery is marked by profound agitation and florid visual and auditory hallucination (a 'central anticholinergic syndrome'). Sedation may be necessary (e.g. po diazepam or chlormethiazole).

13 Pharmacotherapy

Anti-arrhythmics

Anti-arrhythmics are often classified using the Vaughan-Williams scheme (below), although this is not comprehensive, leaving the cardiac glycosides and adenosine unclassified. Group I is subdivided into A, B, or C depending on the effect on action potential duration (QT interval on the ECG): it is respectively lengthened, shortened, or unchanged. IA and IC agents act on both the atria and ventricles and slow conduction in the ventricles.

Class I	Class II	Class III	Class IV
A Quinidine	β-blockers	Bretylium	Verapamil
Disopyramide	Bretylium	Amiodarone	
Procainamide		Sotalol	
B Lignocaine		Disopyramide	
C Flecainide			
Propafenone			

Lignocaine

Pharmacology

Its effect on the cardiac action potential is due to slowing of depolarization, and thus the generation of nerve impulses by sodium channel blockade. The duration of the action potential and the effective refractory period are both reduced in the presence of lignocaine.

Uses

The prevention and treatment of ventricular arrythmias, and as a local anaesthetic agent.

Dosing

A loading intravenous dose of 1mg/kg is given iv over 2mins followed 5 minutes later by half this dose. (*N.B.* 10ml of 1% lignocaine contains 100mg of drug). The effect is maintained with an ivi infusion of 1–4mg/min to produce levels in the range of 1–5mg/l.

Pharmacokinetics

There is high first pass metabolism (70%). The V_d is ~ 100litres. Approximately 65% is plasma protein bound and has a half-life of 1.6h.

Side-effects

- Toxic effects on the CNS are restlessness, tremor, nystagmus, convulsions and eventually medullary depression/coma.
- Because of its extensive metabolism in the liver, the toxicity of lignocaine is increased in patients with either impaired hepatocellular function or reduced portal blood flow (e.g. CCF).
- Allergic reactions are rare

Drug interactions

Drugs such as cimetidine and propranolol also substantially inhibit the hepatic metabolism of lignocaine. Reduce the rate of infusion by 50%.

Contraindications

- Hypersensitivity to local anaesthetics.
- Congestive cardiac failure

Adenosine

Pharmacology

A purine nucleoside that activates adenosine receptors (A1 and A2) non-selectively. Stimulation of A2 receptors causes vasodilatation in vascular smooth muscle, and A1 receptor stimulation in the heart has a negative inotropic effect with a negative chronotropic effect on the SA node and reduces conduction through the AV node. The half-life of adenosine is < 2 seconds *in vivo*, making it an ideal agent for stopping tachyarrhythmias.

Uses

- Treatment of paroxysmal SVT in which the AV node forms part of the re-entrant circuit (AVRT and AVNRT): over 90% of these are terminated by adenosine, and although 30% recur they can usually be terminated by a further dose of adenosine. 10% of patients with atrial flutter or fibrillation will cardiovert following adenosine therapy.
- Diagnosis of tachycardias: The ventricular rate in atrial arrythmias may be slowed by adenosine to reveal the underlying dysrhythmia, e.g. AF. Broad complex tachycardias are either ventricular in origin (and unresponsive) or atrial in origin with abberant conduction (and respond to adenosine).
- It is occasionally used during thallium-201 imaging.

Dosing

It is given by rapid iv bolus with a starting dose of 3mg. Further boluses of 6 or 12mg can be given at 1–2min intervals. It cannot be given orally.

Pharmacokinetics

There is a highly efficient system for the uptake, conversion, metabolism, and recycling of adenosine resulting in a plasma half-life < 2s.

Side-effects

Angina-like chest pain, flushing, breathlessness, and hypotension are well recognized. Asthmatics may also suffer bronchospasm. However, the rapid metabolism of adenosine means that these effects are rarely significant. Trasnsient arrhythmias may occur, e.g. AF, atrial flutter, bradycardia, and VEs.

Drug interactions

- Dipyridamole markedly potentiates the effect of adenosine by blocking cellular uptake. Use a starting dose of 0.5mg iv in these patients.
- Methylxanthines (theophylline and caffeine) are non-selective adenosine receptor antagonists. Patients with therapeutic levels of these drugs may need > 12mg of adenosine for an effect.

Contraindications

- 2nd or 3rd degree heart block
- Sick sinus syndrome
- Asthma. A few patients with asthma may worsen when given adenosine.

Amiodarone

Pharmacology

This class III agent prolongs the action potential in both the atrium and ventricle. There is a corresponding increase in refractoriness. Used acutely its major effect seems to be depression of the AV node which reflects, in part, a non-competitive adrenergic blockade.

Uses

- Atrial fibrillation, flutter or tachycardia. Effective in 75% of patients.
- It is the treatment of choice for paroxysmal AF or re-entry AV tachycardias complicating Wolf-Parkinson-White syndrome (effective in 50–75%).
- Useful in non-sustained paroxysmal VT in patients with impaired ventricular function or HOCM.

Dosing

Because of its very prolonged elimination (mean half-life of > 50d) oral loading is necessary, e.g. 200mg tds for 1 week, 200mg bd for a further 1 week and a final maintenance dose of 200mg od. iv administration is needed for life-threatening arrythmias, preferably via a central line. Up to 2g/d may be given intravenously, and if required up to 5mg/kg can be given over 20 mins. Higher doses cause hypotension from the polysorbate vehicle; N.B. amidarone for iv use must be made up in 5% dextrose.

Pharmacokinetics

Amiodarone is slowly absorbed from the GI tract, and peak levels are found at 5 hours. It has poor bioavailability (~ 50%), has a $t_{1/2}$ of 50 days, and a V_d of 62l/kg.

Side-effects

- Almost all patients on long-term amiodarone develop corneal deposits which do not impair visual acuity.
- Skin photosensitization to UV-A is also common (and often the reason for the drugs withdrawal).
- Significant derangement of thyroid function (hypo- or hyper-thyroidism) occurs in 2% of patients.
- Other problems include slate-coloured skin pigmentation, alopecia, tremor, nightmares (25%), neuropathy, abnormal liver function tests (20%), hepatitis, and pulmonary alveolitis (5% with high doses).

Drug interactions

- Amiodarone substantially reduces the clearance of both digoxin and warfarin. Digoxin levels and the INR should be closely monitored and maintenance doses reduced as necessary.
- Amiodarone has an additive effect with β-blockers, calcium antagonists, and class I anti-arrhythmic agents (disopyramide, quinidine, mexilitene, propafenone).

Contraindications (relative)

- Thyroid disease
- Pregnancy

Bretylium

Pharmacology

This quaternary ammonium compound has both direct and indirect electrophysiological effects. The latter are due to its action on catecholamine release from adrenergic nerves; at the high concentrations achieved by iv bolus administration it releases catecholamines, while the lower subsequent circulating levels actually block impulse-induced release. The direct effect on ventricular and purkinje tissue is a reduction in action potential duration.

Uses

The treatment of resistant ventricular tachyarrhythmias that have not responded to conventional treatment (either class I drugs or cardioversion). There are no controlled trials on its use.

Dosing

At cardiac arrests it can be used as an iv bolus of 5mg/kg (for VF use 10mg/kg). This can be repeated at 15–30 min intervals up to a total dose of 30mg/kg. In less urgent settings, an ivi is used of 5–10mg/kg in 50ml of 0.9% saline or 5% dextrose over 10 min. This can be repeated 6–8 hourly or a maintenance infusion started of 1–2mg/min. The doses used for ivi can be given im and undiluted, but no more than 5ml can be given at one site. It is not recommended that it is given iv/im for > 3–5 days.

Pharmacokinetics

It is poorly absorbed when given orally. Intramuscular bretylium is rapidly absorbed with effect in 15 minutes. There is no protein binding, it has a $t_{1/2}$ of 10 hours, and a V_d of 5l/kg.

Side-effects

- Pulse and blood pressure usually rise within the first 15 min of iv administration
- Hypotension is the major side-effect due to adrenergic neuronal blockade. This can be severe enough to require iv fluids or vasopressor support
- Facial flushing and transient diplopia

Drug interactions

- It should **not** be used for digitalis-induced arrythmias.
- If catecholamine infusions (dopamine, adrenaline, or noradrenaline) are used they should be started at low doses due to the marked potentiation possible with bretylium.
- Tricyclic antidepressants block uptake of bretylium into adrenergic nerve terminals. Tricyclic drugs therefore reduce the hypotensive effects of bretylium, and antagonize its anti-arrhythmic potency.

Contraindications

- Primary treatment of cardiac arrhythmias
- Digoxin induced arrhythmias
- Arrhythmia prophylaxis post MI

Digoxin

Pharmacology

The therapeutic effects of cardiac glycosides are attributable to blockade of the Na,K-ATPase. In atrial fibrillation it slows the ventricular rate largely by reducing the sympathetic drive and a vagotonic action. It has no direct effect on the SA node or conduction in the AV node.

Uses

- Control the ventricular rate in chronic atrial fibrillation or flutter. However, the rate is often not controlled during exercise.
- It is often ineffective in paroxysmal AF.
- It occasionally restores an SVT to sinus rhythm (not 1st line therapy).
- Its use as an inotrope for patients in sinus rhythm and CCF is still debated.
- Recent evidence suggests it may be useful in those with ECHO-proven systolic dysfunction as a fourth-line agent (after diuretic, ACEI, and vasodilator).

Dosing

Oral dosing requires a loading dose of 12–20µg/kg (in severe renal failure use 12µg/kg) given as 3 divided doses 6–8h apart. The maintenance dose should reflect renal function and plasma levels. Intravenous loading is possible (the loading dose given in 50–100ml of 0.9% saline or 5% dextrose). The onset of action by this route is 15 min, versus 30–60 min after oral dosing. im injection should not be used.

Pharmacokinetics

Digoxin is well absorbed orally, but absorption may be delayed by food. Bioavailability following im injection is 80%. It is 20% protein bound, it has a $t_{1/2}$ of 36 hours, and a V_d of 6l/kg. It is excreted unchanged by the kidney.

Side-effects

- Cardaiac arrhythmias (any type but SVT is most common)
- Anorexia, nausea, and vomiting. Diarrhoea rarely
- Confusion, dizziness, agitation, psychosis
- Gynaecomastia
- For overdosage see p646

Drug interactions

- Potassium lowering drugs such as diuretics
- Spironolactone and triamterene increase plasma digoxin by 25%
- Amiodarone, quinidine, and verapamil reduce digoxin clearance with corresponding rises in digoxin levels.
- The absorption of digoxin is reduced if its administration is combined with either antacids or anion exchange resins (e.g. colestipol).

Contraindications

- Hypertrophic cardiomyopathy.
- Arrhythmias due to accessory pathways.
- Electrolyte disturbances ($\downarrow K^+$, $\downarrow Mg^{2+}$, and $\uparrow Ca^{2+}$) increase the sensitivity of the myocardium and should be corrected where possible.
- Hypothyroidism also sensitizes the myocardium to digoxin.
- Even in therapeutic usage digoxin toxicity is common (see section on drug overdoses for the signs and management of digoxin toxicity).
- The risk of arrhythmia is also increased in patients with cor pulmonale, acute myocarditis, and some dilated cardiomyopathies.

Disopyramide

Pharmacology

Disopyramide is a Ia anti-arrhythmic with negative inotropic and prominent atropine-like side effects (approx. 10% of the potency of atropine). Its N-desacetyl metabolite has less effect as a Ia agent but has increased atropine-like properties.

Uses

- It is used primarily in the treatment of atrial tachyarrhythmias including AF, SVT, and Wolff-Parkinson-White.
- It is sometimes effective at cardioverting patients with AF when used with digoxin.
- Ventricular tachycardia and arrhythmias of acute myocardial infarction
- In HOCM patients at risk of VT, its negative inotropic effect (reducing outflow gradients) may be an advantage. Generally, however, its anticholinergic and negative inotropic effects limit its overall usefulness.
- Control of digoxin-induced arrhythmias

Dosing

Oral dosing is started with a 300mg loading dose followed by 100–150mg 6 hourly (or bd if a sustained release preparation is available). The dosing interval should be increased in renal failure (creatinine clearance 30–40ml/min 8 hourly, 15–30ml/min 12 hourly and < 15ml/ml once daily). It can be given as a slow iv bolus (2mg/kg to a maximum of 150mg) over at least 5 minutes. Stop the injection if the arrythmia terminates.

Pharmacokinetics

The drug is completely and rapidly absorbed with a peak plasma concentration at 2 hours. 50% is eliminated by the kidneys and 10% by bile, the rest being metabolized. The $t_{1/2}$ is ~ 8 hours, and is prolonged in renal impairment. The V_d is 0.7 l/kg. 25–80% of drug is protein bound.

Side-effects

- Negative inotropic effects causing cardiac failure
- Hypoglycaemia (< 1%)
- QT prolongation and torsade de pointes. Disopyramide should be stopped in patients developing significant QT prolongation (> 25%) without therapeutic benefit due to the risk of VT/VF.
- Overdose is associated with apnoea, loss of consciousness, and cardiac arrhythmias. Treatment is with lavage, inotropes.

Drug interactions

- Phenytoin (lowers disopyramide levels)
- Other negative inotropes may exacerbate effect
- Tricyclic antidepressants, amiodarone, and sotalol which prolong the QT interval should not be co-administered.

Contraindications

- Left ventricular dysfunction
- 2nd or 3rd degree heart block
- Hypotension or shock
- Concurrent administration of other class Ia agents
- Digoxin toxicity
- Use with caution in patients who will not tolerate its atropinic side-effects, i.e. glaucoma, urinary obstruction, and myasthenia gravis

Flecainide

Pharmacology

Flecainide is a local anaesthetic related to procainamide (approx. 10–fold more potent). It is a class IC agent which reduces conduction throughout the heart by depression of sodium channels, but is most marked within the His-purkinje conduction system. The PR interval and QRS interval are both increased. It has minimal depressant effect on the sinus node, and does not affect normal sinus rhythm. Although it does have a negative inotropic action, this is less than that observed with disopyramide.

Uses

Largely used for control of ventricular tachyarrhythmias. However, in the light of the CAST study Ic agents are not generally regarded as first-line drugs. It has been employed for paroxysmal SVT and AF, especially where they complicate Wolff-Parkinson-White.

Dosing

- Oral administration is started at 50mg bd for supra- and 100mg bd for ventricular arrythmias. Dosing is increased at 3–5 day intervals to a maximum of 400mg/d if required. In renal failure the starting dose should not exceed 100mg/d and future adjustments should ideally be made on the basis of plasma levels (therapeutic range 200–1000ng/ml).
- Flecainide can be given as a slow iv bolus of 2mg/kg over 10 min although an injection over 30 min is safer (especially if there is heart failure). The ECG should be monitored continuously and the injection stopped if the arrhythmia is controlled. A maintenance ivi can be given of 0.1–0.25mg/kg/h but no more than 600mg should be infused in 24h. For renal failure patients, i.e. creatinine clearance < 30ml/min, these doses should be halved.

Pharmacokinetics

The drug is rapidly absorbed from the GI tract. There is no significant first pass metabolism. The bioavailability is ~ 90%. The $t_{1/2}$ is 14h in normal subjects, 20h in cardiac patients, and 26h in severe renal failure. The V_d is 10l/kg, and 40% is protein bound. 86% of the drug is excreted in urine unchanged; renal clearance is decreased by alkalinization of urine.

Side-effects

- Cardiac failure
- Ventricular proarrhythmic effects
- Pre-syncope blurred vision, nausea, headache, anxiety, metallic taste

Drug interactions

- Amiodarone increases plasma levels of flecainide
- Drugs with negative inotropic potential (e.g. disopyramide, verapamil β-blockers) may execerbate the decrease in ventricular performance

Contraindications

- Patients in cardiogenic shock should not be given flecainide, and in those with an ejection fraction < 30% it should be used with extreme caution.
- Flecainide may worsen the degree of block (even sinus arrest o complete AV block) in patients with significant conduction defects.
- Most deaths during long-term treatment are, however, probably the result of its proarrhythmic effect
- Flecainide may dramatically increase the pacing threshold in patient with pacemakers or implantable defibrillators.

Inotropes

General points

- Ensure all patients given inotropes have an adequate intravascular volume (CVP or Swan-Ganz catheter).
- The aim of inotropic support is to maximize tissue oxygenation (e.g. as assessed by plasma lactate and mixed venous oxygenation) and not cardiac output.
- The inotropes in widespread clinical use are catecholamines or their derivatives. Their haemodynamic effects are complex and reflect the relative importance of a and b adrenergic effects for each agent. They are summarized in the table below:

	HR	SVR	MAP	CO	CP
Isoprenaline	+++	−	+/−	+	±
Adrenaline	+	+	+	++	++
Dopamine					
(low dose)	+	−	±	+	+
(high dose)	++	++	++	++	±
Dobutamine	++		−/+	++	++
Noradrenaline	−	++	++	−/+	−/+

Abbreviations: HR, heart rate; SVR, systemic vascular resistance; MAP, mean arterial pressure; CO, cardiac output; CP, coronary perfusion; +, increase; −, decrease; ±, no change.

Isoprenaline

Pharmacology

Isoprenaline is a synthetic β-adrenoceptor agonist (β_1 & β_2) with no activity on a-receptors. It is a bronchodilator, acts as a cardiac stimulant in heart block by stimulating the sino-atrial node, increasing conduction velocity and shortening the refractory period of the AV node. It has a positive inotropic effect. It also acts on skeletal muscle and blood vessels. It has a plasma half life of 5 minutes.

Drug interactions

- Tricyclic antidepressants enhance the effects
- Beta-blockers anatgonise the effects
- Sympathomimetic amines may produce an additive effect
- Anaesthetic gases sesnsitize the myocardium an may trigger arrhythmias
- Digoxin - increased risk of tachyarrhythmias

Preparation of inotrope infusions for a typical 70kg patient				
Inotrope	Formulation	Volume to add to 500ml 5% Dextrose	Starting infusion rate	Maintenance dose
Adrenaline	1:1000 soln	2ml (2mg)	15ml/h (1µg/min)	15–180ml/h (1–12µg/min)
Dopamine	40mg/ml	20ml (800mg)	6ml/h (2.25µg/kg/min)	"Renal" dose 2.5–13ml/h (1–5µg/kg/min) "Cardiac" dose 13–26 ml/h (5–10 µg/kg/min)
Dobutamine	12.5mg/ml	40ml (500mg)	10 ml/h (2.5µg/kg/min)	10–60ml/h (2.5–15µg/kg/min)
Noradrenaline	2mg/ml	2ml (4mg)	15ml/hr (2µg/min)	7.5–90ml/h (1–12µg/min)
Isoprenaline	1mg/ml	5ml (5mg)	3ml/h (0.5µg/min)	3–60ml/h (0.5–10µg/min)

Adrenaline

Pharmacology

- Adrenaline is a β_2 selective agonist (10–fold over β_1) but makes little distinction between α_1 and α_2 receptors.
- It has generally little effect on MAP except in the presence of a non-selective β-blocker, when the loss of β_2-mediated vasodilatation converts adrenaline into an extremely potent pressor agent (α_1 selective blockers do not produce this effect).

Uses

- Anaphylactic shock angioedema and acute allergic reactions
- The use of adrenaline as an inotrope is largely restricted to septic shock were it may have advantages over dobutamine (see p688). It causes, however, a marked reduction in renal blood flow (up to 40%) and should only be used with a renal dose of dopamine.
- Cardiac arrest
- Open angle glaucoma
- Adjunctive with local anaestheic agents

Doses

- 0.2–1mg im for acute alleric reactions and anaphylaxis, respectively
- 1mg (10ml of 1:10,000, or 1ml of 1:1000) for cardiac arrest
- In shock infuse doses of 1–10μg/min.

Pharmacokinetics

It is extensively metabolized with 50% protein binding and a $t_{1/2}$ of 3 minutes, being metabolized by the liver and neuronal tissue.

Side-effects

- Cardiac arrhythmias
- Cerebral haemorrhage (overdose)
- Pulmonary oedema (overdose)
- Local ischaemic necrosis
- Anxiety, dyspnoea, palpitations, tremors, weakness, cold extremities

Drug interactions

- Tricylclic antidepressants
- Anaesthetic agents
- β-blockers
- Quinidine and dogoxin (cardiac dysrthmias more common)
- α-antagonists block the α-effects

Contraindications

- Hyperthyroidism
- Hypertension
- Ischaemic heart disease
- Closed angle glaucoma

Dopamine

Pharmacology

Dopamine acts on different receptors. At low doses D_1 and D_2 receptors are activated. D_1 receptors are found in vascular smooth muscle, and cause vasodilatation in the renal, mesenteric, cerebral, and coronary vascular beds. D_2 receptors are found on post ganglionic sympathetic nerve endings, and autonomic ganglia. At the next dose, β_1 receptors are activated with a postive chronotropic and inotropic effect, and at higher doses α_1 and α_2 receptors are also activated, which inhibit renal vasodilatation.

Uses

To increase renal blood flow in patients with impaired renal perfusion, usually in the setting of multi-organ failure. There is little evidence that dopamine affects clinical outcome.

Dosing

Dopamine at low infusion rates (0.5–2µg/kg/min) selectively vasodilates the renal (and mesenteric) vascular beds, increasing renal blood flow and GFR. At higher rates (2–5µg/kg/min) there is activation of β_1 and α receptors, and subsequent decrease of renal blood flow.

Pharmacokinetics

Dopamine is rapidly distributed by active uptake into sympathetic nerves. The $t_{1/2}$ is 9 minutes with a V_d of 0.9 l/kg, but steady state is achieved within 10 minutes (i.e. more rapidly than predicted). It is metabolized by the liver.

Side-effects

- Cardiac arrhythmias rarely
- Hypertension if dosing too high
- Extravasation may cause skin necrosis. The antidote is infiltration of phentolamine in the ishaemic area
- Nausea, vomiting, headache, palpitations, and mydriasis
- Increased catabolism

Drug interactions

- Monoamine oxidase inhibitors
- α-blockers may exacerbate vasodilatation
- β-blockers may exacerbate hypertension
- Ergot alkaloids exacerbate peripheral vasoconstriction

Contraindications

- Phaeochromocytoma
- Tachyarrhythmias (untreated)

Dobutamine

Pharmacology

Dobutamine is an isoprenaline derivative acting on β_1, β_2, and α_1 receptors. It is used as a racemate with the d-isomer showing β_1 ($+\beta_2$) selectivity and the l-isomer α_1 selectivity. The β_2 effects (vasodilation of mesenteric and skeletal muscle bed) and α_1 effects (vasoconstriction) tend to cancel each other out, so that it has little effect on bp unless high doses are used. It is less arrythmogenic than dopamine.

Uses

- Inotropic support for cardiac failure
- Inotropic support for septic shock and liver failure is controversial since it may cause vasodilatation.
- Pharmacological cardiac stress testing

Dosing

It is administered intravenously at a dose of 2.5–10 μg/kg/minute (rarely up to 40 μg/kg/min). The onset of action is within 2 minutes, with a peak effect at 10 minutes. In congestive cardiac failure it may increase PCWP, through an unknown mechanism.

Pharmacokinetics

The drug is extensively metabolized by the liver. It has a $t_{1/2}$ of 2.5 minutes, and V_d of 0.2l/kg.

Side-effects

- Cardiac arrhthmias
- Myocardial ischaemia may occur if cardiac output increases
- Hypotension may be minimized by cocomitant use with dopamine at a dose to cause vasoconstriction. May occur in patients with sepsis or liver disease.
- Allergies are very rare
- Tissue necrosis at site of administration

Drug interactions

- α-antagonists may execerbate vasodilatation causing hypotension

Contraindications

- Low cardiac filling pressures
- Cardiac arrhythmias
- Cardiac tamponade
- Valvular heart disease (AS, MS, HOCM)
- Known hypersensitivity

Noradrenaline

Pharmacology

Noradrenaline has similar α_1 effects to adrenaline but it is slightly less
potent on most β_1 receptors, and has very little β_2 activity. This lack of β_2-mediated vasodilatation makes it a much more potent pressor agent than
adrenaline. It is sometimes employed in acute hypotension, but it has
relatively little effect on cardiac output and the intense vasoconstriction
actually worsens tissue ischaemia (especially in kidney, skin, liver, and
skeletal muscle).

If a noradrenaline infusion is used it should be never be stopped abruptly
because of the risk of a sudden collapse of the bp.

Drug interactions

- Tricylic antidepressants (which block re-uptake into catecholamine
  nerve terminals) cause a 2–4-fold increase in sensitivity to adrenaline
  or noradrenaline infusions. MAO inhibitors (e.g. tranylcypromine and
  pargyline) markedly potentiate the effects of dopamine infusions which
  should be started at one-tenth the usual infusion rate, i.e. $0.2\mu g/kg/min$.
- Dobutamine is <u>not</u> a substrate for MAO.

Milrinone

Milrinone is a potent inhibitor of phosphodiesterase (type III) and causes
a concentration dependent increase in cellular cAMP. It acts as a positive
inotrope and vasodilator, with little chronotropic activity. Its cardiac
actions probably involve effects on calcium channels or fast entry sodium
channels. The positive inotropic effects are enhanced by β-agonists. It has
a $t_{\frac{1}{2}}$ of ~ 1h. It is used in the short term treatment of severe heart failure
unresponsive to other therapy and acute heart failure following cardiac
surgery.

Doses (for 70kg patient)
- Add 10mg to 40ml 5% dextrose (50ml final volume)
- Loading dose 17.5 ml ($50\mu g/kg$) over 10 minutes
- Maintenance dose 6-15ml/hr (0.3–0.8 $\mu g/kg/min$): max 24mg/kg/day

Side-effects
- Hypotension and/or cardiovascular collapse in hypovolaemic patients

Enoximone

Enoximone is a potent inhibitor of phosphodiesterase (type IV) and
causes a concentration dependent increase in cellular cAMP. It acts as a
positive inotrope and vasodilator, with little chronotropic activity; these
effects are not associated with increased myocardial oxygen consumption.
It is over 20 times more potent than theophylline, and has a $t_{\frac{1}{2}}$ of ~ 1.5
hours,. It is metabolised to an active metabolite which has 10% of
potency and a half life of 15 hours. It is used in the treatment of congestive
cardiac failure, and can be given either orally or intravenously.

Doses (for 70kg patient)
- Add 50mg to 40ml normal saline (50ml final volume)
- Loading dose 63ml ($90\mu g/kg/min$) over 10 minutes
- Infusion of 20-80ml/hr (5-$20\mu g/kg/min$): max. 24mg/kg/day

Side-effects
- Hypotension and/or cardiovascular collapse in hypovolaemic patients

Nitroprusside

Pharmacology

Sodium nitroprusside is a potent rapid-acting vasodilator, acting via a nitric oxide-dependent pathway by increasing cGMP within smooth muscle cells. It is light sensitive.

Uses

- Hypertensive emergencies
- Hypotensive anaesthesia
- Dissecting aortic aneurysm
- Acute cardiac failure (rarely)
- Acute VSD and acute mitral regurgitation

Dosing

It is administered intravenously with continuous arterial monitoring of the blood pressure, and the dose titrated to achieve the desired effect. The starting dose should be low (e.g. $0.1\mu g/kg/min$) and increased slowly up to between 2–$6\mu g/kg/min$ (average $3\mu g/kg/min$, or $200\mu g/minute$ total).

Pharmacokinetics

The $t_{1/2}$ is unknown, but it takes between 30–60 seconds to achieve a fall in blood pressure. Its metabolic byproducts include cyanide and thiocyanate.

Side-effects

- Hypotension (if excess administered)
- Nausea, sweating, headache, twitching
- Overdose can be associated with cyanide accumulation (see p64)

Drug interactions

None reported, but since cysteine can react with nitroprusside to form cyanide, it seems wise to avoid co-administration with N-acetyl cysteine.

Contraindications

- Coarctation of the aorta
- Arteriovenous shunt (relative)
- B_{12} deficiency (cyanide and thiocyanate interfere with cyanacobalamin)
- Severe liver disease or Leber's optic atrophy

Interferons

Pharmacology

These lymphocyte-derived proteins have complex and potent effects on the immune system. There are 3 types in clinical use, namely α, β and γ-interferon. They are given by injection (e.g. thrice weekly).

Uses

α-interferon
- Hepatitis B (50% long-term response)
- Hepatitis C (50% respond, 20% long-term)
- Hairy cell leukaemia
- AIDs-related Karposi's sarcoma
- Condylomata acuminata
- Renal cell carcinoma
- Chronic myeloid leukaemia
- Certain lymphomas

β-interferon
- Multiple sclerosis

γ-interferon
- Adjunct to antibiotics to reduce risk of infection in chronic granulomatous disease

Dosing

Refer to specialist centres.

Side-effects
- Nausea
- Influenza-like symptoms (relieved by paracetamol)
- Lethargy
- Depression
- Hypersensitivity
- Myelosuppression

Drug interactions
- Metabolism of warfarin and phenytoin impaired
- Decreased activity of certain cytochrome p450 enzymes affecting metabolism of cimetidine, theophylline, diazepam, and propranolol.

Contraindications
- Pregnancy

Disodium pamidronate

Pharmacology

Biphosphonates were designed to inhibit calcium phosphate precipitation. Pamidronate is an amino-substituted biphosphonate, and inhibits calcification and bone resorption *in vivo*, by acting on osteoclasts. Treatment with pamidronate inhibits bone resorption within 2 days of administration, causing a reduction of plasma and urinary calcium and alkaline phosphatase if increased (e.g. Paget's). This is accompanied by a reduction of bone pain. In cancer-associated hypercalcaemia-bone resorption remains supressed for up to 6 weeks. 30% of patients exhibit an acute phase response on commencing treatment.

Uses

- Cancer-associated hypercalcaemia
- Accelerated bone resorption in other conditions
- Paget's disease
- ?Osteoporosis in post menopausal women

Dosing

- Intravenous infusions of 15–60mg are given over 2–8h at < 15mg/hour.
- Rapid infusions are nephrotoxic.
- iv infusion of 30mg once/week for Paget's disease (max. 180mg).

Pharmacokinetics

Poor oral absorption. Low protein binding and elimination is predominantly by the kidneys (> 50%). The $t_{1/2}$ is 30 min with a V_d of 0.5l/kg.

Side-effects

- Pyrexia and acute phase response in 30%
- Hypocalcaemia (usually asymptomatic)
- Hypophosphataemia

Drug interactions

- None known

Contraindications

- Known hypersensitivity

Chlormethiazole

Pharmacology

Chlormethiazole has sedative, tranquilizing, and anticonvulsant properties, mediated by an indirect action on GABA receptors. It also inhibits alcohol dehydrogenase.

Uses

- Control of alcohol withdrawal/delirium tremens (iv/oral) – see p396
- Management of restlessness/insomnia in the elderly (oral)
- Hypertension in pregnancy (pre-eclampsia)
- Status epilepticus

Dosing

Avoidance of overdosage is important. For oral use, doses ranging from 1 capsule 3 times/day (restlessness) to 3 capsules 4 times daily are given. For intravenous use (solution of 0.8%), doses ranging from an acute bolus of 40–100ml over 10 minutes followed by an infusion of 0.5–4ml/minute depending on response.

Pharmacokinetics

Rapidly and well absorbed with a peak concentration within 1 hour. There is extensive presystemic metabolism by the liver (75%). 65% is protein bound, with a $t_{1/2}$ of 5–8h, and a V_d of ~ 10 litres/kg.

Side-effects

- Respiratory arrest
- Dependency
- Tingling sensation of nose and sneezing
- Thrombophlebitis

Drug interactions

- Cimetidine reduces clearance of chlormethiazole

Contraindications

- Poor respiratory function
- Pregnancy
- Lactation

Heparin

Pharmacology

Heparin inhibits coagulation by augmentation of antithrombin III's inhibition of activated factors XIIa, XIa, IXa, Xa, and thrombin. It also impairs platelet function *in vivo*.

Uses

- Prophylaxis of deep vein thrombosis
- Treatment of DVT and pulmonary emboli
- Myocardial infarction and unstable angina
- Prevention of thrombosis in dialysis, haemofiltration, bypass surgery
- Consumptive coagulopathies
- Maintenance of patency of iv lines
- Taking blood gases

Dosing

Dosing depends on close monitoring of the partila thromboplastin time (APTT)

- DVT prophylaxis, 5000U bd or tds sc
- Treatment 5000U bolus, then 30,000–60,000U/day iv
  It can be given sub-cutaneously depending on form used,
  5000U bolus then 1000U/h to an APTT ratio of 1.5–2.0 for mi
- iv patency 50U tds through line

Pharmacokinetics

It is well absorbed following sub-cutaneous injection. Peak levels occur at 5 hours, and the effect lasts 12 hours. The $t_{1/2}$ is 20–60 minutes and has a V_d of 0.05l/kg.

Side-effects

- Bleeding (see p552)
- Osteoporosis
- Skin necrosis
- Hypoaldosteronism
- Excessive heparin in ABG samples mimics metabolic acidosis

Drug interactions

- Aminoglycosides interact with heparin in cannulae
- Anti-platelet drugs
- Zinc salts inhibit heparin

Contraindications

- Current bleeding or recent trauma/surgery
- Cerebral haemorrhage
- Cerebral infarction (controversial risk of secondary haemorrhage)
- Heparin-induced thrombocytopenia
- Proliferative retinopathy (relative contraindication)
- Hypersensitivity

Warfarin

Pharmacology

Warfarin is an antagonist of vitamin K and inhibits γ-carboxylation of the glutamyl residue of coagulation factors II, VII, IX, and X. The onset of action is delayed until existing clotting factors are catabolized. It is said to have a prothrombotic effect on initiation, and therfore it is advised that all patients are heparinized prior to commencing treatment. It also has an immunomodulatory effect on T-cell responses.

Uses

- Deep vein thrombosis/pulmonary embolism
- Atrial fibrillation or valvular disease
- Transient ischaemic attacks
- Reconstructive arterial surgery
- Budd-Chiari syndrome

Dosing

Oral dosing is adjusted to the size and age of the patient on initiation, and monitored by measurement of the prothrombin ratio (INR) which should be maintained at ~ 2–3 times normal. In a young adult, commence with 10mg on day 1, 10mg on day 2 and measure the prothrombin time. In the elderly or those with cardiac failure, commence with 10mg on day 1, and 5mg on day 2, then measure the INR. Seek advice for further dosing increments if needed.

Pharmacokinetics

Warfarin is completely absorbed with minimal presystemic metabolism. It has a $t_{1/2}$ of 36 hours, and a V_d of 0.15l/kg. It is eliminated by hepatic metabolism.

Side-effects

- Bleeding (see p552)
- Other rare side-effects include alopecia, hypersenitivity, and skin necrosis

Drug interactions

There are many drug interactions of warfarin, and the reader is referred to the BNF. The most important ones to note are:

- Alcohol enhances the effects of warfarin
- Anti-epileptics (may reduce warfarin effect, phenytoin variable)
- Cimetidine potentiates warfarin
- Co-trimoxazole and metronidazole increase warfarin effect
- Cholestyramine reduces warfarin absorption

Contraindications

- Active haemorrhage
- Severe liver or renal disease (relative)
- Hypersensitivity

Phenytoin

Pharmacology

Phenytoin protects against seizures by limiting the spread of seizure discharges, rather than preventing initiation. It inhibits voltage-dependent sodium channels.

Uses

- Prevention of epilepsy (intermittent and status)
- Prophylaxis against supraventricular dysrhythmias
- Prophylaxis against certain varieties of migraine
- Tic douloureux
- Myotonia

Dosing

Oral phenytoin is administered once or twice daily at a dose to obtain a therapeutic range of 10–20mg/l for epilepsy. The average dose in adults is 5mg/kg/day (300–400mg/day). In view of the zero-order kinetics, the dose should only be increased by 50mg/day if the blood levels are within the therapeutic range but epileptic seizures persist. For parenteral administration the drug is irritant to veins and should be given at < 50mg/minute. It is relatively insoluble.

Pharmacokinetics

Phenytoin follows zero-order kinetics. In other words, there is a limit on the dose such that a given individual will have an exponential rise in plasma concentrations once the maximum therapeutic dose is exceeded. The half-life is approximately 20 hours with a V_d of 0.6l/kg.

Side-effects

- Nystagmus, blurred vision and ataxia (cerebellar), and dyskinesias
- Nausea, vomiting, drowsiness, and stupor
- Gum hypertrophy, pseudolymphoma, hypocalcaemia, and hyperglycaemia

Drug interactions

- Steroids and warfarin
- Other interactions should be viewed in the BNF

Contraindications

- Acute intermittent porphyria
- Hypersensitivity

Amphotericin B

Pharmacology

Amphotericin B is a polyene antibiotic used as an anti-fungal agent. It acts by binding to ergosterol in the fungal cell membrane, increasing its permeability, and disrupting potassium channels within the fungal cell. At low concentrations it stimulates macrophages, and lymphocyte responses. It is active against a wide range of fungi and moulds including *Candida, Aspergillus, Cryptococcus, Histoplasma, Blastomyces, Coccidoides, Trichophyton, Microsporum*, and *Epidermiophyton*.

Uses

- Candidiasis of mouth and GI tract
- Systemic fungal or mould infections, esp. candidaemia and aspergillosis
- Prophylaxis in immunocompromised, subjects prone to vaginal candidosis, and following major surgery.
- Denture stomatitis
- Cutaneous and mucocutaneous candidosis
- Leishmaniasis

Dosing

Oral amphotericin is not absorbed. It is available as a tablet lozenge or suspension. It is also available as a pessary. See BNF. For parenteral administration amphotericin is usually given as a complex with sodium desoxycholate. Give a test dose of 1mg over 2 hours in 250ml 5% dextrose. Follow with 5mg over 4 hours, then 10mg over 6 hours. The daily dose is 0.6–1mg/kg up to a maximum of 50mg/day.

If there is a reaction (bronchospasm, N&V, fever and hypotension) then consider other agents. If amphotericin is essential, give hydrocortisone cover ± chlorpheniramine, and give the test dose over a longer period of time, and gradually increase the dose depending on tolerance.

Pharmacokinetics

Only 10% remains in the blood, and is mostly protein bound (95%), esp. to lipoproteins, the rest binding to membranes. It has a half-life of 24–48h and a V_d of 4l/kg. It is not dialysable.

Side-effects

- Anaphylaxis
- Nephrotoxicity causing renal failure, renal tubular acidosis, loss of potassium, impaired renal concentration. Renal toxicity may be irreversible (esp. with total doses > 4g). Virtually all patients receiving amphotericin for more than 2 weeks have some nephrotoxicity, when the dose should be reduced.
- Fevers, chills, nausea, and vomiting. Often respond to hydrocortisone, antihistamines, and paracetamol.

Drug interactions

- It precipitates in solution if mixed with slats including other antibiotics.
- Ketoconazole and miconazole may have antagonistic anti-fungal effects.

Liposomal amphotericin

There is good evidence to demonstrate reduced nephrotoxicity of this formulation. It has excellent efficacy against leishmaniasis, but controlled trials comparing its efficacy (and thus bioavailability) in the prohylaxis and treatment of severe fungal infections are not currently published.

Vasopressin

Pharmacology

Vasopressin is native anti-diuretic hormone (ADH). It binds to V_1 and V_2 receptors, which are responsible for the pressor and anti-diuretic effects, respectively. At low concentrations it has an anti-diuretic effect, and at high concentrations a pressor effect. It preferentially decreases splanchnic blood flow and lowers portal pressure.

Uses
- Bleeding oesophageal or gastric varices
- Diabetes insipidus (cranial) treatment and diagnosis
- Hepatorenal syndrome (used as a pressor agent)

Dosing
Bleeding varices: 24U over 15 minutes followed by 0.4U/min. Do not continue infusion beyond 24 hours. Prevent chest pain (coronary vasospasm) by co-administration of iv GTN.
Diabetes insipidus: either by sub-cutaneous or im routes at a dose of 0.5–10U. Its effects last 2–8 hours.

Pharmacokinetics
The plasma half-life is 7 min, and there is no binding to plasma proteins.

Side-effects
- The vasoconstrictor properties may cause angina in acute MI.

Contraindications
- Known ischaemic heart disease or uncontrolled hypertension
- Renal disease (except hepatorenal syndrome)
- Polydipsia

Octreotide

Pharmacology

Octreotide is a long-acting octapeptide analogue of somatostatin which inhibits the secretion of peptides from the gastro-enteropancreatic system and of growth hormone from the pituitary. It binds to somatostatin receptors, but unlike somatostatin has no rebound hypersecretion following cessation of its action.

Uses
- Control of symptoms in endocrine tumours (e.g. carcinoid tumours, VIPomas, glucagonomas)
- Acromegaly: either prior to pituitary surgery or until effects of radio-therapy become fully apparent. Occasionally required as long-term therapy in patients not adequately controlled on other therapy.
- Bleeding oesophageal or gastric varices.

Dosing
- For endocrine tumours, 50µg 1–2 times daily sub-cutaneously increasing to max. 200µg tds depending on tolerance and response.
- For bleeding varicies, 100µg iv bolus followed by a continuous infusion at 25–50µg/h (500µg in 50ml; 2.5–5ml/h), see p489.

Pharmacockinetics
- It has half-life of approximately 90 minutes and a V_d of 0.3l/kg.

Side-effects
- GI: nausea, abdominal pain, flatulence, diarrhoea, steatorrhoea
- Biliary and gall-bladder stones with long-term treatment (abrupt withdrawal may precipitate biliary colic)

Drug interactions
- Reduces insulin and oral hypoglycaemic requirements in DM.
- Reduces absorption of cyclosporin.

Sodium bicarbonate

Pharmacology

Sodium bicarbonate is an important buffering mechanism *in vivo*. Its
effects are short lived. The administration of sodium bicarbonate results
in both a sodium load and generation of carbon dioxide. It causes
intracellular acidosis, and is negatively inotropic, and for these reasons
should be used cautiously. It may also produce a left shift in the oxygen
dissociation curve, and decrease effective oxygen delivery. Mild acidosis
also causes cerebral vasodilatation, and thus correction could
compromise cerebral blood flow in those with cerebral oedema.

Uses

• Severe metabolic acidaemia (use in DKA is controversial)
• Severe hyperkalaemia
• Its use is best avoided in cardiac resuscitation, since adequate
  ventilataion and chest compression usually suffice.

Dosing

It is available as either an 8.4% solution (hypertonic, contains 1mmole
HCO_3^-/ml) or a 1.26 % solution (isotonic). It is usually administered as
intermittent boluses of 50–100ml, and the effect on arterial pH and
haemodynamics monitored. According to the UK Resuscitation Council
Guidelines, the approximate dose of 8.4% solution required can be
calculated as follows:-

$$\text{Dose in ml (mmoles)} = \frac{\text{Base excess} \times \text{Weight (kg)}}{3}$$

Thus a patient of 60kg with a base excess of -20, would require 400ml. of
8.4% bicarbonate to normalize the pH. This contains the equivalent of
400mmole of sodium. Our personal view is that this is too much, and one
should try to correct the arterial pH to 7.0–7.1 by giving 50–100ml sodium
bicarbonate followed by repeat arterial blood gases, and repeating the
bicarbonate as necessary. This should buy enough time for more effective
and safer measures to be employed to try to correct the underlying cause
for the acidosis.

Side-effects

• Tissue extravasation causes severe necrosis. Give via a central line
  where possible.
• It precipitates in the line when given with calcium chloride, and can
  cause microemboli.

Drug interactions

• Precipitates with calcium salts

Contraindications

• Arterial pH > 7.2

Doxapram

Pharmacology

Doxapram hydrochloride is a respiratory stimulant acting by selectively stimulating chemoreceptors. At high doses it is an analeptic agent.

Uses

In practice doxapram is used to stimulate respiration in patients who for various reasons are not generally considered candidates for ventilatory support, but in whom some support is generally felt warranted. There are many who feel that it has no place in clinical practice, but it is the editors' view that occasionally there are patients with severe chronic airways obstruction whom the ITU would not wish to give the option of ventilatory support, but in whom buying an extra 24 hours of self ventilation is adequate for respiratory recovery. It is easy to argue in retrospect that a particular patient should have been ventilated, but there are situations in which there is disagreement about such a course and the physician is left to either force the issue or try alternatives such as doxapram.

- Ventilatory support for chronic and acute respiratory failure.
- Respiratory depression following anaesthesia (rare)

Dosing

It is provided as a solution of 20mg/ml (check with local formulary) and given iv at a dose of 1–4mg/minute, depending on response (see p182).

Pharmacokinetics

The half-life is 3–4 hours, and it has a V_d of 1.5l/kg.

Side-effects

- Hypertension
- Exacerbation of apparent dyspnoea
- Agitation, confusion, sweating, and cough
- Headaches and dizziness
- Nausea and vomiting, and problems with micturition

Drug interactions

- Incompatible with alkaline solutions of aminophylline, frusemide, or thiopentone.
- Concurrent use with theophylline may enhance agitation

Contraindications

- Heart disease
- Epilepsy
- Cerebral oedema
- CVA
- Asthma
- Hypertension (relative contraindication)
- Hyperthyroidism or phaechromocytoma

Granulocyte macrophage colony stimulating factor (GMCSF)

Pharmacology

GMCSF is a recombinant haemopoietic growth factor, which is being increasingly used in patients with life-threatening neutropenia. Natural GMCSF is produced by T lymphocytes, monocytes, macrophages, endothelial cells, and fibroblasts. It binds to specific receptors on myeloids cells. It enhances survival of cells committed to the granulocytic and macrophage lineages, and stimulates proliferation of these cells. It also enhances the immune function of these cell types. *In vivo* it increases the neutrophil, monocyte, and eosinophil count.

Uses

- Reduction of severity of neutropenia (and so reduction of risk of infection) following chemotherapy or bone marrow transplantation.
- Stimulation of myeloid recovery in bone marrow failure or following bone marrow transplantation.
- Treatment of neutropenia following other drug therapy (e.g. after gancyclovir therapy for patients with CMV retinitis).
- Stimulation of circulating colony forming unit granulocyte macrophages (CFU-GM) for use in autologous BM transplantation.

Dosing

- Consult haematologists

Pharmacokinetics

Little known at present

Side-effects

Side-effects are common.
- Pericardial effusion and pericarditis
- Fluid retention
- Peritonitis with collection of ascites
- GI disturbances, fever, bone pain, myalgia, and arthralgia
- Dyspnoea may follow first dose
- Serum enzyme rises

Drug interactions

- None known

Contraindications

- Myeloid malignancies
- Ineffective in congenital neutropenia

14 Dermatological emergencies

Cutaneous drug reactions: Presentation

- *Maculopapular erythema* with variable pruritus and scaling. Resolves once the drug is stopped. 46% of cutaneous drug reactions.
- *Urticaria/angioedema:* Accounts for ~ 25% of drug reactions. Sudden onset of ind ividual pruritic erythematous lesions which resolve within 24 hours. Angioedema may involve mucous membranes and can be associated with life-threatening anaphylaxis (see p212). Aspirin, morphine, codeine act directly in mast cells to liberate histamine in sensitive individulas. Penicillin (and aspirin) can cause an IgE mediated or IgG complement-fixing allergic reaction. Urticarial eruptions associated with serum sickness may be persistent and can be associated with systemic symptoms.
- *Fixed drug eruption:* Characterized by a few well-demarcated painful erythematous lesions often involving the face, hands, forearms, and genitalia. Local hyperpigmentation persists after recovery. Rechallenge is associated with recurrent lesions in the same location. Drugs implicated include sulphonamides, tetracyclines, barbiturates, salicylates, dapsone. Represents 10% of cutaneous drug reactions.
- *Photosensitive drug eruptions:* Cutaneous reaction limited to exposed sites with characteristic sparing of certain areas. May be due to either a photoallergic (immune-mediated, e.g. chlorpromazine, sulphanilamide, amiodarone) or phototoxic (non-immune, e.g. tetracyclines, sulphonamides, griseofulvin, naproxen, high-dose frusemide) reaction. Some drugs may induce photosensitive disorders such as porphyria cutanea tarda or photo-onycholysis.
- *Erythema multiforme/Stevens-Johnson syndrome:* Associated with 10% of drug reactions. Sudden onset of erythematous lesions affecting the skin and mucous membranes. Acral sites are preferentially involved and ind ividual lesions may have necrotic or targetoid appearances. Associated with fever, malaise', and sore throat due to mucous membrane involvement (Stevens-Johnson syndrome) and rarely confluent epidermal necrolysis as seen in toxic epidermal necrolysis (see p738). Drugs implicated include salicylates, sulphonamides, penicillin, sulphonylureas, and barbiturates. Stop the drug; give steroids in severe cases.
- *Exfoliative dermatitis:* Presents as erythroderma. 4% of drug reactions. Causative drugs include barbiturates, salicylates, penicillin, sulphonamides, and sylphonylureas.
- *Toxic epidermal necrolysis:* There are two types: in adults it is an immunological disease provoked by drug hypersensitivity, but in babies it is due to the direct necrolytic effect of a *Staphylococcal* toxin. It may be caused by penicillins, sulphonamides and other antibiotics, blood products, NSAIDs, and anti-convulsants.

Cutaneous drug reactions: Management

Points to note

- Usually develop within 1–2 weeks following initiation of therapy but occasionally reactions present later (due to cumulative toxicity).
- Development of extensive angioedema is associated with a risk of anaphylaxis and shock characterized by hypotension, bronchospasm, oropharyngeal irritation associated with angioedema, flushing or urticaria, and acral oedema.
- Patients who present with either erythema multiforme or Stevens-Johnson syndrome may develop confluent areas of epidermal necrolysis as seen in toxic epidermal necrolysis (p738).
- Peripheral blood eosinophilia is rare.
- Intravenous routes of drug administration are more likely to be associated with anaphylaxis.
- Cutaneous drug reactions are common in treatment of HIV disease.

Management

- Severe angioedema and anaphylaxis require immediate treatment (see p212).
- Seek specialist advice for severe Stevens-Johnson syndrome or toxic epidermal necrolysis.
- Stop any responsible drugs and prescribe an alternative if necessary. Hospitalized patients receiving numerous drugs should be assessed carefully and all non-essential therapy discontinued.
- Prescribe oral non-sedating or sedating antihistamines with simple emollients and medium potency topical steroids. Short courses of systemic steroids may be required in erythema multiforme or Steven's Johnson syndrome.
- Pyrexia may occur with cutaneous drug reactions but underlying infection should always be excluded.
- There should be clinical improvement within a few days: persistent reactions should prompt a search for other causes.
- Although rechallenge with a suspected drug can provide a definitive diagnosis, reactions may be more severe and can lead to fatal anaphylaxis or severe toxic epidermal necrolysis.
- Specific RAST can be used to measure serum IgE antibody production in patients with penicillin allergy. However, a positive RAST for penicillin is only seen with the major antigenic determinants and a negative reaction does not exclude penicillin allergy.
- Skin biopsies can be useful for specific forms of cutaneous drug reactions such as fixed drug eruption and erythema multiforme.

Erythroderma

Presentation

- Erythroderma may be acute or chronic. Acute erythroderma is more likely to present as an emergency.
- There is generalized erythema associated with exfoliation.
- Scaling can be fine (pityriasiform) or coarse (psoriasiform).
- Patients may be febrile or hypothermic because of loss of temperature control mechanisms.
- Chronic erythroderma may be associated with nail dystrophy, diffuse hair loss, and ectropion. Palmo-plantar hyperkeratoses and peripheral lymphadenopathy may be prominent.

Causes

Common causes: Eczema, psoriasis, drug reactions
Rare causes: Cutaneous T-cell lymphoma, pityriasis rubra pilaris, toxic shock syndrome, Kawasaki disease, sarcoidosis.

Investigations

- Monitor FBC U&Es, albumin, calcium, and LFTs regularly.
- Blood cultures and skin swabs should be performed and sustained pyrexia, hypotension or clinical deterioration should prompt a search for underlying sepsis.

Management

General measures

- Nurse in a warm room with regular monitoring of core temperature and fluid balance. Patients should be nursed on *Lyofoam*® if necessary.
- **Encourage** oral fluids and high calorific food and protein supplements. Nasogastric feeding may be required. Avoid intravenous cannulae because they can act as a potential source of infection.
- Monitor fluid balance closely: daily weights and clinical examination (as allowed by the exfoliation).

Specific therapy

- The skin should be treated at least four times daily with emollients such as 50% white soft paraffin/50% liquid paraffin.
- A daily bath should be supplemented with emollients such as oilatum or balneum.
- Oral sedating antihistamines such as hydroxyzine (10–100mg in divided doses) may be used and the dose adjusted according to severity and weight.
- Application of mild or potent topical steroids may be appropriate but liaise with specialist at early opportunity.
- In eczema, systemic treatment with prednisolone, azathioprine, or cyclosporin may be appropriate, and in psoriasis, acitretin, methotrexate, or cyclosporin may be required. Liaise with specialist prior to embarking on this approach.

Complications

- Infection
- Hypoalbuminaemia
- High output cardiac failure.

Erythroderma

Urticaria: Assessment

Presentation

- Urticaria presents as erythematous pruritic evanescent areas of oedema involving the superficial dermis which may be small weals or larger plaques. Lesions present suddenly and will resolve within 24 hours, although new lesions may develop repeatedly.

- In severe urticaria systemic symptoms may predominate with the development of anaphylaxis characterized by histamine shock and collapse (see p212). Features include hypotension, bronchospasm, angioedema, and diffuse urticaria.

- Presence of extensive urticarial lesions does not imply anaphylaxis in the absence of systemic features. Drug sensitivities and reactions to radiocontrast media are more likely to produce anaphylaxis.

Causes

- Bee/wasp stings, drug reactions (penicillin common, aspirin and non-steroidal anti-inflammatory drugs), radiocontrast media, blood products, food sensitivity such as nuts and shellfish.

- Physical causes of urticaria such as dermographism, pressure, vibration, cold, aquagenic, solar, and cholinergic (heat/exercise).

- Contact urticaria

- Hereditary angioedema associated with a genetic deficiency of the enzyme C_1-esterase inhibitor (see p628).

- Malignancy and autoimmune disorders such as lupus associated with a functional defiency of C_1-esterase inhibitor.

- Chronic idiopathic urticaria possibly due to autoantibodies produced against the low affinity IgE receptor.

Diagnostic points

- A family history may suggest hereditary angioedema.

- In patients with chronic urticaria, ask specifically about possible physical causes (e.g. induced by cold, exercise, water, pressure, heat and rarely light and vibration. Dermographism is the most common form of physical urticaria; briskly stroking the skin with a firm object produces linear weals).

- Contact urticaria usually occurs within minutes after direct contact with various agents such as plants, aeroallergens, foods such as cheese, eggs and fish, and, in healthcare workers, after contact with latex. Contact sensitivity to latex products is also associated with a high incidence of anaphylaxis.

- If individual urticarial lesions persist for more than 24 hours a diagnosis of urticarial vasculitis is likely. Such lesions are tender and painful rather than pruritic and may appear bruised. Unlike other forms of urticaria this diagnosis should be established by histology.

- Patch tests are not indicated in urticaria. Prick tests will indicate if individuals are atopic but, rarely, may also be useful in establishing a specific cause of contact urticaria (should only be carried out under medical supervision because of a risk of anaphylaxis). Total serum IgE levels may be elevated in atopic individuals. Specific IgE RAST may be used to identify potential sensitivities but can produce false negative/positive results.

Urticaria: **Management**

- Anaphylactic reactions require immediate treatment (see p212).
  - Secure the airway and give oxygen.
  - Give intramuscular adrenaline 0.5–1mg (0.5–1ml of 1 in 1000 adrenaline injection) and repeat every 10 minutes according to bp and pulse. iv adrenaline may be required if the patient is severely ill with poor circulation (see p212).
  - Start iv fluids if hypotensive.
  - Give iv hydrocortisone 100–300mg and chlorpheniramine 10–20mg. Continue H_1-antagonist (e.g. chlorpheniramine 4mg q4–6h) for at least 24–48h; longer if urticaria and pruritis persist.
  - If the patient continues to deteriorate, start iv aminophylline infusion (see p167). Patients on beta-blockers may not respond to adrenaline injection and require iv salbutamol infusion.
- Hereditary angioedema may present with extensive urticaria and angioedema associated with systemic features including anaphylaxis. Management is discussed on p628.
- Severe acute urticaria with or without angioedema is usually not life-threatening unless associated with systemic features of anaphylaxis.
  - Give oral antihistamines such as hydroxyzine 25mg or chlorpheniramine 4mg.
  - A single dose of prednisolone 50mg orally may be prescribed but should not be continued indefinitely without specialist advice.
  - When the patient's condition has stabilized, they can be discharged on regular maintenance treatment with an oral non-sedating antihistamine such as cetirizine 10–20mg daily, loratadine 10–20mg daily or terfenadine 120mg daily. (Sedative antihistamines such as hydroxyzine or chlorpheniramine are usually not required for maintenance treatment of chronic urticaria.)
- Patients with no specific identifiable cause of acute urticaria and all patients with chronic or physical forms of urticaria should be referred for specialist advice.
- Patients with contact sensitivity to latex should use alternatives such as *allergard*® gloves (Johnson and Johnson), vinyl gloves, or non-sterile copolymer gloves. Such individuals should be warned to avoid the use of condoms.

Autoimmune bullous disease

Presentation
- Intact, pruritic, fluid filled blisters.
- Very itchy urticated erythematous plaques (pre-bullous eruption).
- Cutaneous and/or mucosal erosions.

Causes
Common: Bullous pemphigoid, pemphigus vulgaris
Rare: Pemphigoid gestationes (second/third trimester), dermatitis herpetiformis, pemphigus foliaecus, epidermolysis bullosa acquisita, bullous lupus, linear IgA disease, paraneoplastic pemphigus.

Poor prognostic features
- Pemphigus (higher mortality than other autoimmune bullous disease)
- Age > 60 years
- Extensive involvement

Diagnosis
- Biopsy of a fresh blister for histology and a small fragment of perilesional skin should be sent for direct immunofluorescence studies (transported in Michel's medium: contact the Histopathology lab.).
- Serum should also be sent for indirect immunofluorescence studies.

Management (Liaise with specialist at an early opportunity)

General measures
- Intact blisters should be aspirated. Examine for new blisters daily.
- Patients should be bathed daily with emollients and, if necessary, chlorhexidine bath additive in order to prevent secondary bacterial infection. Use diluted potassium permanganate soaks for eroded and weeping areas with non-adherent dressings such as *Lyofoam®*. Nurse the patient on a *Clinitron®* bed.
- Give oral sedating antihistamines (e.g. hydroxyzine) for pruritis, titrating dose to age and severity.
- Potent topical steroids (*Dermovate-NN®* cream) should be applied to individual lesions twice daily.
- Prescribe prophylactic sc heparin for immobile elderly patients.
- Monitor fluid balance carefully. FBC, U&Es, and LFTs regularly.

Specific systemic therapy (liaise with specialists)
- Pemphigus requires high dose immunosuppressive therapy (prednisolone 80–100mg daily) but mild disease may be controlled with a less intensive regime.
- Subepidermal bullous disease such as pemphigoid can occasionally be controlled with dapsone or high-dose minocycline, but extensive disease will require immunosuppressive therapy. Prednisolone 30–60mg daily is usually required and the dosage gradually reduced according to response.
- Steroid sparing agents such as azathioprine 50–100mg daily should also be considered for extensive disease.
- Alternatives for resistant disease include pulsed methylprednisolone, intramuscular gold, cyclophosphamide, and cyclosporin.
- Mucosal disease requires regular use of *Diflamm®* and tetracycline mouth washes with *Corlan®* lozenges (hydrocortisone 2.5mg) for painful erosions.
- Refer severe conjunctival disease to an ophthalmologist early.
- If condition deteriorates consider secondary bacterial or viral infection of cutaneous or mucosal sites.

Autoimmune bullous disease

Teaching points

Pemphigus is characterized by *intraepidermal* separation and acantholysis of ind ividual keratinocytes. In pemphigus vulgaris the split is suprabasal while in pemphigus foliaecus the separation is much higher in the epidermis. Penicillamine, captopril, rifampicin and other drugs can, rarely, induce a pemphigus-like syndrome which is indistinguishable from pemphigus vulgaris. This accounts for < 10% of all cases of pemphigus.

Bullous pemphigoid is characterized by a *subepidermal* split and an inflammatory infiltrate containing eosinophils. Specialist advice is required. Exclude other causes of bullous disease such as porphyrias, drugs (NSAIDs, barbiturates, frusemide), diabetes mellitus, and bullous amyloid. Also consider bullous insect bite reaction and bullous impetigo in the differential diagnosis, particularly for localized blisters. Tense blisters on the palms and soles may be due to endogenous eczema (pompholyx) or fungal infection (tinea).

Eczema herpeticum

Presentation

- Patients with atopic endogenous eczema are predisposed to secondary herpes simplex infection. This may occur as a primary infection following an episode of herpes labialis or after contact with an affected individual.

- Patients present with a sudden deterioration of their eczema characterized by widespread vesiculo-pustular lesions which are tender and gradually become necrotic. Resolution of the condition produces extensive crusting and exudation.

- Patients are usually pyrexial and toxic with a tachycardia. Cardio-respiratory collapse is unusual.

Management

- The condition can progress rapidly and, therefore, localized disease should be treated aggressively. Patients should be admitted and early specialist advice is required.

- Refer patients with ocular disease to an ophthalmologist urgently.

- Extensive mucosal disease may make oral nutrition difficult and patients may require intravenous fluids.

- Perform bacterial swabs daily: secondary bacterial infection is common and if present requires treatment with systemic antibotics.

- Topical therapy
  - Do not use topical steroids.
  - Use simple emollients such as aqueous cream and *Lyofoam*® dressings.
  - Chlorexidine (topical antiseptic) and diluted potassium permanganate (1/10,000) as a soak once or twice daily for brief periods to areas of excessive exudation.

- Give oral non-sedating antihistamines.

- Start high dose intravenous acyclovir at the earliest opportunity (maximum 2mg/kg/h). If intravenous therapy is not possible, give valacyclovir 1000mg tds for seven days.

- Patients with severe atopic eczema should be advised about prompt treatment of herpes labialis and to avoid contact with herpes simplex.

Herpes zoster see p238.

Eczema herpeticum

Generalized pustular psoriasis

Presentation

- Rapid onset of superficial pustules, usually in a patient with typical plaque psoriasis. Pustules may be confluent or pin-point and may be studded around the periphery of typical psoriatic plaques.
- Irritant topical therapies (e.g. potent topical steroids, vitamin D analogues, coaltar and dithranol preparations) may precipitate generalized pustular psoriasis in patients with 'unstable' psoriasis (hot tender erythematous psoriatic plaques).
- Rarely, patients develop generalized pustular psoriasis without a previous history, and similar presentations can occur in pregnancy.
- Pyrexia is often accompanied by systemic symptoms such as malaise, anorexia, and arthralgia. Cutaneous infection with *Staphylococcus aureus* is common and may result in septicaemia.
- Differential diagnosis includes bullous impetigo, toxic epidermal necrolysis, staphylococcal scalded skin syndrome, autoimmune bullous disorders, and, in particular, subcorneal pustular dermatosis, pustular vasculitis, particularly due to herpes simplex infection or drugs, eczema herpeticum.

Natural history

- Repeated acute episodes of generalized pustulation associated with pyrexia and systemic symptoms which resolve within 5–7 days to produce extensive superficial crusting and resolution of fever. Episodes recur every 7 to 10 days.
- Patients with localized palmo-plantar pustular psoriasis have a mild chronic disease which is not associated with systemic abnormalities.
- Patients with generalized disease may develop ARDS and shock due to release of cytokines or the presence of septicaemia.
- Elderly patients with generalized pustular psoriasis (Von Zumbusch) have a worse prognosis.

Management

- Liaise with specialists at an early opportunity.
- Admit all patients with pustular psoriasis and enforce bed rest.
- *Investigations*
  - Monitor FBC, U&Es, and LFTs regularly. A neutrophil leukocytosis is invariable. Abnormal LFTs and ↓ Ca^{2+} may occur.
  - Primary bacterial or viral infection should be excluded by appropriate bacterial and viral swabs. Blood cultures should be performed when patients are pyrexial.
  - Obtain a CXR and pulse oximetry on all patients. Perform ABGs in hypoxic patients or those with an abnormal CXR.
- *Topical therapy*
  - The early phase of pustulation can be associated with extensive crusting and exudation. Treat with topical diluted potassium permanganate (1/10,000) soaks.
  - Patients with extensive disease should have their skin dressed with *Lyofoam*® and may require nursing on a *Clinitron*® bed.
  - Bathe daily with emollients and antiseptic washes.
  - Avoid topical steroids, vitamin D analogues, coaltar, and dithranol (may cause severe irritation and exacerbation of the disease).
- *Systemic therapy*
  - Give regular oral sedative antihistamines (e.g. hydroxyzine).
  - Bacterial infection should be treated with appropriate antibiotics.
  - Severe generalized pustular psoriasis may require systemic treatment with retinoids, methotrexate, or cyclosporin: seek specialist advice.

Generalized pustular psoriasis

Toxic epidermal necrolysis (TEN)   1.

Presentation

Acute onset of morbilliform or confluent erythema associated with widespread blistering (necrolysis) and skin tenderness.

Diagnostic points

- Necrolysis is used to describe confluent blistering of the skin associated with epidermal separation, rather like a large burn. It should be distinguished from discrete, intact blisters which are characteristic of autoimmune bullous diseases.

- There may be clinical overlap between toxic epidermal necrolysis and erythema multiforme as seen in the Steven's Johnson syndrome. Mucocutaneous involvement is common and both oral and conjunctival erosions may be present.

- TEN should be distinguished from the **staphylococcal scalded skin syndrome (SSS).** This usually occurs in children or immuno-suppressed adults and is associated with the production of staphylococcal toxins. A skin biopsy is diagnostic: in TEN there is full thickness epidermal necrosis, subepidermal separation, and a sparse or absent dermal infiltrate, while in SSS there is suprabasal epidermal separation with an intact basement membrane.

Causes

- Idiopathic
- Drug induced [sulphonamides and occasionally other antibiotics, anticonvulsants (not described with sodium valproate), NSAIDs].

Adverse prognostic factors

- Age greater than 60 years (25% overall mortality).
- Area of cutaneous involvement greater than 50%.
- Blood urea greater than 17mmol/l.
- Neutropenia (neutrophil count $< 1 \times 10^9$/l).
- Idiopathic aetiology.

Management

The priorities are:
1 Try to identify the cause and treat.
2 Supportive care – fluid balance and nutrition.
3 Prevent complications
   - Eye care
   - Screening and treatment of sepsis

Toxic epidermal necrolysis

Toxic epidermal necrolysis (TEN)   2.

1 Identify the cause

- A specific drug is unlikely to be responsible if treatment was started after the onset of erythema, necrolysis, or mucous membrane involvement.
- A drug aetiology should be considered if TEN develops 7 to 21 days after the first administration of a drug, or within 48 hours if the drug has caused an eruption in the past.
- If patients are on several different drugs, stop all that may be a potential cause.

2 General supportive care

- Patients should be nursed on an air fluid or *Clinitron*® bed in a side room. A single designated nurse should attend the patient continuously and the room should be kept warm in order to prevent hypothermia.
- Core temperature should be continuously monitored via a rectal probe and a space blanket may be required if the patient becomes hypothermic because of cutaneous vasodilatation. However, patients frequently also develop hyperthermia which may necessitate temporary cooling of the room with fans.
- *Lyofoam*® dressings should be used between the patient and bedding in order to ease mobility and skin dressings. Emollients should be applied every two to four hours for all areas.
- Oral mucosal surfaces should be cleaned every 4 to 6 hours and sprayed with clorhexidine and *Diflamm*®. Mucosal involvement may produce oral erosions or constrictions affecting the oral aperture or pharynx.
- Mucous membrane involvement usually antedates skin necrolysis for several days before presentation. Gastrointestinal involvement may be characterized by bleeding and/or a protein-losing enteropathy. The net result is a profound negative fluid and nitrogen balance.
- Monitor fluid balance closely, preferably by daily weights.
- If possible, fluids should be administered orally or via a nasogastric route. Avoid iv lines to reduce the risk of sepsis. 5–7 litres are usually required during the first 24 hours. A protein and energy rich nasogastric feed should be administered (1–1.5 litres per day). Colloids or FFP may be required.
- Daily FBC, U&Es, LFTs, glucose (hyperglycaemia may cause an osmotic diuresis aggravating dehydration), amylase ($\downarrow$), and phosphate (may fall).
- Chest X-rays should be performed regularly. Pulmonary oedema and adult respiratory distress syndrome are frequent complications. Arterial blood gases should be assessed if there is a deterioration of respiratory function and have a low threshold for admission to ITU and mechanical ventilation.
- Prophylactic anti-coagulation should be used (sub-cutaneous calcium heparin 5000 units tds).
- Patients are frequently terrified and in considerable pain. Adequate analgesia and tranquillizers should be administered.
- Post inflammatory pigmentary changes are common and will gradually resolve.

Toxic epidermal necrolysis

3 Prevent complications: Infection

- Central venous lines should be avoided if possible. iv lines should be discontinued as soon as possible in order to reduce infection risk.

- Several cutaneous and mucuous membrane sites should be swabbed daily. Culture sputum and urine daily. Intravenous and in-dwelling catheters should be changed frequently and tips sent for culture. Perform blood cultures daily if febrile. Remember that pyrexia is a feature of TEN and does not always indicate infection.

- Prophylactic antibiotics are only indicated if the risk of sepsis is extremely high such as severe neutropenia or a heavy single strain bacterial colonization of the skin.

- Antibiotics should be started if there is positive blood, urine, or sputum culture, or indirect evidence of sepsis such as hypothermia, hypotension, fever, decreasing level of consciouness, reduced urinary output, or failure of gastric emptying.

- Weeping, crusted, and exudative areas of the skin should be treated by local application of potassium permanganate soaks (1:10,000).

- Necrotic epidermis should be carefully removed because it forms a focus for infection. Affected skin that has not become necrotic should not be removed. Topical flamazine should be avoided as this can cause neutropenia when applied to large surface areas.

4 Prevent complications: Ocular involvement

- Corneal scarring and blindness are the commonest sequelae of TEN.

- The cornea should be examined daily by an ophthalmologist and antibiotic or antiseptic eyedrops should be applied every 1–2 hours.

- Synechiae form usually in the second week. These can be separated using a blunt instrument several times a day but this is controversial and the advice of an ophthalmologist is essential.

- Sicca syndrome and visual impairment due to corneal neovascularization may produce corneal scarring and blindness. Symptoms usually develop several weeks after the onset of TEN.

5 Specific systemic therapy

- There is no controlled evidence that any specific systemic therapy improves prognosis. In particular there is no evidence that systemic steroids are beneficial and adverse effects are numerous. Steroids should NOT be used as a standard therapy for TEN.

- Uncontrolled reports suggest that cyclosporin (3–4mg/kg/day) and cyclophosphamide (150–300mg per day) are beneficial but neither drug is established as a standard therapy in TEN and these drugs should not be prescribed without specialist advice.

- Uncontrolled studies have also suggested a beneficial response to intravenous immunoglobulin therapy and plasmapheresis but the risk of infection and fluid imbalance does not justify regular use.

15 Disorders due to physical agents

Disorders due to heat

- Patients exposed to heat present with a spectrum of disorders, from mild oedema/syncope (vasodilatation), though mild to moderate disorders (cramps and exhaustion) but with intact thermoregulation, to heat stroke where thermoregulation fails.
- *Predisposing factors:* obesity, strenuous exercise, alcohol, old age, anticholinergic drug ingestion, and hot climate.

Heat cramps

- Typically painful spasm of heavily exercising muscles (commonly in calves or feet) thought to be due to salt depletion.
- The diagnosis is clinical and further investigation rarely indicated.

Treatment

- Rest, massage of affected muscle and fluid replacement, either intravenously (N saline 1 litre over 2h repeated if necessary) or orally with 0.1% salt solution.
- Plain salt tablets may be used – take with copious amounts of water; in the stomach they will produce a hypertonic solution and may cause gastric irritation.
- Freshly squeezed orange juice (partly diluted with water) provides a simple way to replace salt, potassium, and water.
- Admission to hospital rarely indicated.

Heat exhaustion

- The symptoms reflect the effects of salt and water depletion, dehydration, and accumulation of metabolites.
- Predominant salt loss presents insidiously over days (cramps, nausea, weakness, postural dizziness, malaise), whereas mainly water loss presents more acutely with headache, nausea, and CNS symptoms (confusion, delirium, incoordination).
- *Examination:* Usually the patient is flushed and sweating with evidence of dehydration. Body temperature may be normal or mildly elevated ($\sim 38°C$).
- *Investigations:* U&E may show hyper- or hypo-natraemia and pre-renal failure. FBC may show haemoconcentration. Mild elevations of CK and LFTs are common. Urine should be examined for myoglobinuria if the serum CK is markedly elevated > 2000U/l (rhabdomyolysis).

Treatment

- Assess fluid deficit and replace with ivi if severe.
- Rest and fluid replacement are the mainstay.
- Young persons may just require aggressive oral rehydration [water, salt, commercially available rehydration preparations (e.g. *Dioralyte®*)] and may require 4–6 litres over 6–8 hours.
- Intravenous therapy should be guided by electrolytes (caution with $\downarrow$ or $\uparrow$ Na^+); a suggested regimen is N saline 1 litre over 30 min followed by another over 1 hour, then alternating bags of 5% dextrose and N saline 2 hourly: be guided by the clinical state and U&E of the patient. The elderly will require more cautious fluid replacement, if indicated, guided by CVP.
- Recovery is usually rapid (12–24 hours).

Disorders due to physical agents

Heat stroke

Excessive exposure to heat or strenuous exercise in a hot environment results in eventual failure of the thermoregulatory mechanisms, with rising body temperature and extensive multisystem damage.

Presentation

- Symptoms include headache, nausea, dizziness, parasthesiae in limbs, piloerection, confusion, delirium, seizures, and coma.
- Examination shows elevated body temperature ($> 40°C$). There is profuse sweating unless the patient is severely dehydrated. Initially there is tachycardia and increased cardiac output which falls as cardiovascular collapse ensues. Neurological findings include muscle rigidity, dystonias, ataxia, seizures, and coma.

Investigations

U&E	$\downarrow$ or $\uparrow$ K^+, dehydration, renal failure from ATN or rhabdomyolysis, $\downarrow$ or $\uparrow$ Na^+
CK, AST and LDH	Raised with rhabdomyolysis
Glucose	Normal or low
Ca^{2+}, PO_4^{3-}, Mg^{2+}	All usually low
Clotting screen	Evidence of DIC
FBC	Haemoconcentration, neutrophilia
ABG	Initial respiratory alkalosis, then metabolic (lactic) acidosis
Urine	Usually small volumes and concentrated. Test for myoglobin, tubular casts, protein
ECG	Commonly shows non-specific ST and T wave changes and / or SVT
AST	If > 1000 IU/litre in the first 24 hours, prognosis is poor with serious brain, kidney, and liver injury

Management

i *Stabilize the patient*

- Ensure adequate airway and ventilation. Give oxygen.
- Start peripheral iv fluids (crystalloid) promptly; insert CVP line ± PA (Swan-Ganz) catheter to guide fluid replacement ± inotropes .
- Insert a urinary catheter and aim for an output of > 30ml/h. If myoglobinuria is present consider alkaline diuresis (p668). Anuria and hyperkalaemia are indications for dialysis (p283).
- Treat seizures with iv diazepam (p370); phenytoin has been reported to be ineffective.
- Exclude hypoglycaemia.

ii *Reduce body temperature promptly*

- Begin external cooling with ice packs (in axillae, groin, and neck), tepid sponging and cooling fans; cold water immersion is inappropriate for unstable patients.
- Violent shivering should be suppressed as it interferes with cooling; give chlorpromazine 10–25mg iv slowly.
- Stop cooling when body temperature reaches 39°C; the temperature will fall further and hypothermia is to be avoided.
- Dantrolene has been effective in some cases but needs further evaluation.

Hypothermia: Assessment

This is defined as a core (rectal) temperature $< 35°C$; it is designated mild $(32–35°C)$, moderate $(26–32°C)$, or severe $(< 26°C)$.

Risk factors

- Increasing age (impaired thermoregulation, reduced metabolism)
- Abnormal mental state
- Immobility (orthopaedic, Parkinsonism)
- Drugs (alcohol, barbiturate, major tranquillizers, antidepressants)
- Endocrine (hypothyroidism, hypoglycaemia, adrenal insufficiency, hypopituitarism)
- Autonomic neuropathy (DM, Parkinsonism)
- Malnutrition
- Renal failure
- Sepsis (excessive heat loss from vasodilatation)
- Exposure (inadequate clothing/heating, near-drowning)

Presentation

- Mild hypothermia presents as shivering which is maximal at $35°C$ and decreases thereafter, being absent at temperatures below $32°C$. Other symptoms include mild confusion, weakness, fatigueability, lethargy, ataxia, and dysarthia.
- Progressive hypothermia is associated with delirium, coma, bradycardia and low respiratory rate, cardiac arrhythmias, dilated unresponsive pupils, and loss of reflexes. The EEG is 'flat' at $< 20°C$. Asystole occurs at $< 15°C$.
- *Complications*: VF atrial tachy- and brady-arrhythmias, ARDS, aspiration pneumonia, pancreatitis, bowel ischaemia, acute renal failure, rhabdomyolysis, DIC.

Investigations

- Check the core temperature with a low reading rectal thermometer.
- Urgent bloods   *U&Es, CK* (dehydration, rhabdomyolysis). *Glucose* (usually high). *Amylase* (pancreatitis 2° to hypothermia).
- Routine bloods   FBC, phosphate ($\downarrow$), magnesium ($\downarrow$) Blood cultures Thyroid function Toxic screen Serum cortisol
- ABG: The values obtained are abnormal – an artefactual lower pH and higher P_aO_2 and P_aCO_2 – as most ABG machines assume the sample was taken at $37°C$. Some machines can be programmed with the patient's temperature to allow correction for the lower temperature before the sample is analysed. Alternatively, to correct pH add 0.015 for every degree the patient's temperature is below $37°C$. The P_aO_2 and P_aCO_2 need to be decreased by 7.2% and 4.4% respectively for every degree below $37°C$.
- ECG: This may show bradycardia, tachycardia, AF and/or prolongation of PR and QTC intervals. 'J'-waves are seen with temperatures $< 30°C$, as a hump in the interval between the QRS and T waves (best seen in V4–V6).
- Urine: MCS, dipstick (blood and protein), ?myoglobinuria.

Hypothermia: Management

1 Stabilize the patient

- Ensure the airway is protected and give oxygen. Avoid hyperventilation as an acute fall in P_aCO_2 may trigger VF.
- If the patient is unconscious, and injury suspected, immobilize the cervical spine until fracture can be excluded.
- Establish venous access; exclude hypoglycaemia.
- Start volume expansion with warm, iv crystalloid infusion if dehydrated (e.g. 5% dextrose 80–100ml/h) (fluid may be warmed in a 'blood-warmer' device). CVP monitoring and PA wedge pressure monitoring may help guide fluid replacement.
- Insert a urinary catheter to monitor urine output (potential rhabdomyolysis).
- Give iv thiamine 250mg if there is an alcohol history.
- Severe metabolic acidosis (pH < 7.1) should be treated with slow iv bicarbonate infusion (see p716) monitoring ABG. Avoid rapid changes in pH. Milder degrees of acidosis are well tolerated and require no specific treatment.
- *Ventricular fibrillation* is common (precipitated by rapid changes in P_aCO_2 or pH, intubation without adequate pre-oxygenation, movement) and should be treated as normal (p6) while active rewarming proceeds (see below). Class 1 agents (lignocaine) may be ineffective at low temperatures; *bretylium tosylate* is more successful in cardioverting intractable VF. Atrial arrhythmias and ventricular ectopics without haemodynamic compromise do not require treatment.
- In the event of cardio-respiratory arrest, resuscitation should be continued until core temperature reaches at least 35°C as the cold temperature may provide a degree of neuroprotection.

2 Rewarming

- Patients with mild hypothermia may be managed with passive external rewarming. Cover the patient, including scalp, in warm, dry blankets ('space blanket' if available). Give warmed iv fluids to correct dehydration. Aim for a rise in temperature of 0.5–1°C/h and monitor closely for complications. Hypotension may be due to rapid vasodilatation; slow the rate of rewarming ± iv fluids.
- Moderate or severe hypothermia may require active re-warming, either external (heated blankets, water-bottles, warm bath) or internal [heated humidified oxygen, peritoneal dialysis with rapid exchange of warm fluids (~ 40°C), extra-corporeal blood warming techniques (e.g. haemodialysis, cardiopulmonary bypass]. This may result in vasodilatation, hypotension, and arrhythmias and should only be used in patients who are unstable or in cardiac arrest. Apply initially only to the trunk to avoid excessive vasodilatation of extremities.

3 Other measures

- If the temperature is slow to correct, consider whether the patient is Addisonian or hypothyroid. If you suspect myxoedema, give liothyronine 20–40µg iv (T3) and hydrocortisone (HC) 200mg iv repeating as necessary (p460 and p468). Always give HC with T3 in case there is underlying hypoadrenalism.
- After septic screen, consider broad spectrum antibiotics for aspiration pneumonia or underlying sepsis as a precipitating factor. Give prophylactic antibiotics to patients with moderate-severe hypothermia (e.g. cefotaxime 1–2g q8h).

Hypothermia: Localized injury

Chilblains (perniosis)

- *Presentation:* Painful, itching, dark red swellings, typically seen on the fingers or toes. Rarely the calves may be affected. Horse-riding in the winter months may result in chilblains on the upper, outer thighs, despite the riding trousers. More common in women.
- *Diagnosis* is easy; all inflammation is warm except chilblains which are cool to touch.
- *Treatment* is symptomatic and warmer covering. The lesions may recur every winter.

Trench foot

- *Presentation:* Usually occurs 12–24 hours after exposure to cold and damp. Initially the foot is cold and pale, with reduced sensation and pulses. This is followed by hyperaemia, painful swelling, sometimes with ulceration or gangrene if severe.
- *Treatment:* Conservative with elevation, rest, and strict attention to asepsis.

Frostbite

Presentation

- This results from freezing of the tissues and ischaemic necrosis due to vasospasm. Symptoms include numbness, stinging, or burning pain.
- Superficial frostbite (skin and sub-cutaneous tissues only) appears pale and has a somewhat soft and 'rubbery' feel.
- Deep frostbite involves deeper tissues, even bone, resulting in a hard, 'woody' feel.

Treatment

- Treat any associated hypothermia (as above).
- If there is any possibility of refreezing, do not thaw (even if it means walking on frozen feet); refreezing increases tissue damage.
- <u>Rapid</u> rewarming is essential to minimize tissue necrosis; immerse in a water bath (40–42°C if tolerated) for several minutes.
- There is often considerable pain that may require iv/im analgesia.
- Clean the affected part and apply topical disinfectants (iodine 5–10%), bed rest, elevation. Debridement should be delayed until the limb has demarcated.
- Give tetanus prophylaxis if necessary.
- There is some evidence for the use prophylactic antibiotics (after appropriate swabs) in patients with deep frostbite (high dose penicillin).
- Heparin has not been shown to be useful.

Disorders due to physical agents

Diving accidents

Decompression illness

Water pressure increases by 1 atmosphere for every 10m (33ft) below the surface. The increased pressure increases the amount of dissolved nitrogen in the plasma. Rapid ascent results in the formation of bubbles as the gas comes out of solution.

Symptoms
- Usually occur within the first hour of surfacing but may be delayed by up to 36 hours.
- 'Deep' muscle aches ('the bends').
- Skin symptoms: pain, parasthesiae, itching, and burning.
- 'The chokes': retrosternal pain, cough, breathlessness.
- Neurological symptoms: paraplegia, urinary retention, patchy spinal cord necrosis due to retrograde venous thombosis. Suspect all neurological symproms are due to decompression illness until proven otherwise.

Air embolism

If the breath is held on ascent (due to breath-holding or laryngospasm) the volume of gas in the lungs expands, and large pressure gradients are generated. Eventually alveoli rupture resulting in pneumothorax, pneumomediastinum, and sub-cutaneous emphysema. Ruptured pulmonary veins allow arterial air embolism (commonly into the carotid circulation).

- Symptoms vary from behaviour changes, confusion, focal neurological defects, seizures, coma, and death. A variety of other symptoms may occur depending on the arterial bed the emboli travel to and due to the free air in the thoracic cavity.

Treatment
- Give oxygen, analgesia, and intravenous fluids if dehydrated. Do not give nitrous oxide (*Entonox®*).
- If there is a possibility of air embolism lie on the left side with head-down tilt to collect air in the right atrium. Occasionally it may be possible to aspirate the air from the right atrium with a venous catheter.
- ***Immediate recompression*** is the only effective treatment. Contact your local poisons unit (see p854 for telephone numbers) who will be able to put you in contact with your nearest recompression chamber to your hospital and arrange urgent transfer.
- Never attempt recompression in water.

Pneumothorax (see p184)

Near-drowning

- When immersed in water, a period of breath-holding is followed by involuntary inspiration. Aspiration of water, bacteria, and other particulate material follows.
- The distinction between fresh-water (hypotonic) and salt-water (hypertonic) drowning is only useful in that fresh-water inhalation results in marked haemolysis, electrolyte disturbances, intravascular volume overload, whereas salt-water ingestion may result in hypovolaemia and haemoconcentration. Their management is identical.
- In practice the volume of water aspirated is small; in 10–15%, laryngospasm results in 'dry drowning' and asphyxia.

Presentation

- Symptoms may range from none, to cough and mild breathlessness, to cardiorespiratory arrest and coma.
- Initial examination, blood gases, and CXR may be normal and do not predict subsequent clinical course.
- Examine specifically for trauma to cervical or thoracic spine.

Prognostic features

Survival is related to duration of submersion, extent and duration of hypoxia, water temperature, extent of hypothermia, presence of aspiration, adequacy of initial resuscitative efforts, age, and presence of co-existing medical conditions.

Management

- Asymptomatic patients should be observed for at least 6–12 hours. If examination, arterial gases, and CXR remain normal, they may be discharged.
- At the scene, manoeuvres to 'drain the lungs' are potentially dangerous and ineffective; aggressive mouth-to-mouth resuscitation and cardiac massage should be started if necessary.
- Give oxygen as soon as available. Intubate and ventilate if there is persistent hypoxia. 5–10 cm H_2O PEEP may improve oxygenation.
- Patients with history of diving or evidence of head or spine trauma should be treated as having head/spine injury until proven otherwise.
- Hypothermia should be treated in the usual manner (p750). The low temperatures may provide a degree of neuro-protection and resuscitative efforts should not be stopped until the core temperature reaches $> 35°C$.
- Metabolic acidosis is invariable; if pH < 7.1, give iv bicarbonate 50ml 8.4% over 15–20 minutes (see lactic acidosis, p224).
- If there is clinical or radiological evidence of chest infection begin treatment with broad spectrum antibiotics (e.g. cefotaxime and metronidazole or amoxycillin, gentamicin and metronidazole).

Electric shock

- Damage is caused by a combination of thermal tissue injury and direct injury from the electric current passing though the tissue.
- The treatment is supportive.

Domestic electric shock

- Skin burns at the site of entry and exit of the current are common. These should be referred to a burns centre for specialist management.
- Cardiac damage may result in ST and T wave changes on ECG, VF, asystole, and other cardiac arrhythmias. Monitor for at least 24 hours, if the ECG is abnormal.
- Rhabdomyolysis with varying degrees of renal failure is common due to tetanic contraction and ischaemic necrosis of skeletal muscle (p294). There may be severe muscle burn injury even when there is minimal skin damage. If suspected, refer to a burns or plastic surgery unit.
- Neurological damage results in altered mental state, confusion, depersonalization, and patchy spinal cord demyelination.
- Heat may also be responsible for intravascular coagulation and ischaemic necrosis of other tissues. This is classically delayed by several hours. Treatment is supportive.
- Exclude co-existent fractures of spine and long bones.

Lightning injuries

- The voltage and current are several orders of magnitude greater than domestic electrical injuries (up to 10^5 A and 10^6 V) but exposure is extremely brief. Most of the current passes over the skin and deep tissue damage is less common.
- Skin entry burns have a 'fern-like' pattern and are mainly superficial or partial thickness burns..
- Most patients survive without any significant arrhythmias. Ventricular fibrillation or asystole are occasionally seen. Myocardial infarction, ECG abnormalities, and late arrhythmias have been reported.
- Dilated pupils may be the result of transient autonomic sympathetic discharge and should not deter active resuscitation.
- Direct injury to abdominal viscera, lungs, spinal cord, and tympanic membrane may be seen. Late complications include optic atrophy and cataracts.

Smoke inhalation

- This causes a combination of thermal and chemical injury to the lungs and varying degrees of systemic toxicity.
- The main cause of death in patients with smoke inhalation is cerebral hypoxia secondary to carbon monoxide exposure.
- Combustion of household materials can also generate a number of other toxic substances such as sulphur dioxide, nitrogen dioxide, acrolein (from wood and petroleum), hydrochloric acid (PVC), toluene diisocyanate (polyurethane), and hydrogen cyanide that may result in direct lung, skin, and conjunctival injury.

Presentation

- Common symptoms include cough, sore thoat, breathlessness, pleuritic retrosternal chest pain, headache, dizziness, nausea.
- Examination: Note the skin colour (normal, cyanotic). Look for perioral and perinasal burns, singeing of nasal hair, burns of oral mucosa (markers of significant, thermal, respiratory-tract injury).
- Note cough and colour of sputum (?black), tachypnoea, wheeze, stridor and/or tachycardia. Assess mental state (?confused).

Initial investigations

- ABG   (Hypoxia, CO_2 retention) – note the <u>calculated</u> O_2 saturation from the machines is overestimated in the presence of significant COHb.
- Carboxy-Hb   (COHb) level from co-oximeter (available in some ITUs or contact duty biochemist). Non-smokers < 1%, smokers 4–6%, > 10% significant CO exposure, > 50% coma, > 70% fatal (see p640).
- CXR   May be normal. Progressive interstitial and alveolar shadowing mimicking cardiogenic pulmonary oedema (upper > lower lobes)
- ECG   Non-specific ST-T wave changes or signs of myocardial ischaemia.
- Pulse oximetry   Inaccurate; may only be normal in the presence of high levels of COHb.

Indications for admission

- History of significant smoke inhalation injury
- Clinical signs of significant lung injury (above)
- Confusion
- COHb level > 15%,
- Hypoxia (P_aO_2 < 10kPa on air)
- Raised P_aCO_2 on air.

Management   *The initial ABG and CXR may be normal and do not predict subsequent clinical course.*

- Resuscitate the patient (Airway, Breathing, Circulation).
- If the initial CXR and ABG are normal, observe the patient for 4–6 hours and if there is no clinical deterioration, discharge with instructions to return if they develop any respiratory symptoms.
- Give supplemental, humidified, cooled oxygen.
- Treat bronchospasm with inhaled and iv bronchodilators (see p167).
- Encourage deep breathing and cough to clear secretions; there may be copious sputum production. Send a specimen for culture.
- Start antibiotics if there is evidence of infection.
- ***Indications for intubation and ventilation*** include falling P_aO_2 despite maximal inspired oxygen, failure to clear secretions, or risk of upper airways obstruction (see ARDS, p188).

Carbon monoxide poisoning see p644.

Acute mountain sickness

- Usually seen within 24–36 hours of ascent.
- Symptoms include headache (most common), lethargy, irritability, difficulty concentrating, nausea, vomiting, palpitations, breathlessness, dizziness, and difficulty sleeping. Symptoms often worsen over the first 2–3 days then resolve completely by day 5–7.
- Examination and investigations are usually normal except for mild dehydration, alkalaemia, and bicarbonate diuresis if acclimatization has begun.
- The most effective treatment is descent to lower altitude and supplemental oxygen. Encourage bed rest and fluid intake. Sedatives may depress respiratory drive, exacerbating hypoxia, and mask signs of altered mental status.
- Dexamethasone is effective in reducing the symptoms of acute mountain sickness but does not reduce the objective manifestations of the illness or retard progression; it is only recommended if descent to lower altitude is not possible or delayed.
- Do not use diuretics acutely.

Acute high-altitude pulmonary oedema (HAPO)

- Non-cardiogenic pulmonary oedema occurs within 12–96 days of ascent.
- Type 1 HAPO is said to occur when an unacclimatized individual ascends to high altitude; Type 2 HAPO is said to occur when a high-altitude resident develops pulmonary oedema after returning from a visit to a lower altitude. The distinction is important as treatment differs (see below).
- Symptoms are as for acute mountain sickness (see above), but in addition there is low-grade fever, cough, and breathlessness at rest. Examination shows pulmonary oedema WITHOUT the usual signs of heart failure (elevated JVP, S3 gallop, cardiac enlargement).
- Investigations: ABG shows respiratory alkalosis and hypoxaemia; ECG may show sinus tachycardia with signs of right-heart strain. CXR may show patchy lung shadowing.

Treatment
- Mild type 1 and 2 HAPO may be treated with oxygen and bed rest; symptoms usually resolve in 1–2 days. Treatment with diuretics, digitalis, and steroids have not been shown to be useful.
- Moderate-severe type 1 HAPO may require intubation and ventilation with PEEP. Type 2 HAPO usually responds to bed rest and supplemental oxygen only.

High-altitude encephalopathy

- Usually occurs within 24 hours of ascent over 12,000 feet (~ 3600m).
- Initial symptoms of acute mountain sickness (see above) progress to papilloedema, retinal haemorrhages, ataxia, and focal neurological defects, seizures, and coma.
- Treatment is with oxygen and immediate descent to lower altitudes. High doses of dexamethasone may be beneficial but mannitol and diuretics are not routinely given.

Prevention
- Gradual ascent, adequate rest and fluids, and avoidance of strenuous exercise reduce the incidence of high-altitude illness.
- Prophylactic acetazolamide (250mg po q8–12h) given the day before and for the first few days of ascent reduces the incidence and severity of acute mountain sickness.

Disorders due to physical agents

High altitude illness
Acute high-altitude pulmonary oedema
High-altitude encephalopathy 763

Teaching points: High altitude illness

- High altitude illness is usually seen when an unacclimatized individual travels to altitudes above ~ 7000 feet (2300m); the incidence and severity increases progressively with higher altitudes and with rapid rates of ascent.

- Acute symptoms occurs within 6–8 hours of ascent with marked individual variation in tolerance to hypoxaemia at altitude.

- Commercial airlines cruising at altitudes of 29,000–37,000 have cabin pressures equivalent to an altitude of 6000–8000 feet; thus travellers may be briefly exposed to conditions that may provoke mild high-altitude sickness !

Stings and insect bites

Acute presentation (within 2–3 hours)

History Ask specifically if reactions have occurred in the past and if there is any past history of angioedema, urticaria, bronchospasm, or anaphylaxis. Most patients developing anaphylaxis have no previous history of significant reaction.

Examine the wound for the 'stinger' and remove carefully. Observe the patient carefully for 1–2 hours for any signs of evolving anaphylaxis (generalized urticaria and pruritus, bronchospasm, or oropharyngeal oedema). If present the patient requires urgent treatment (see below)

Management

1 *Local reactions*
- Clean the wound of any foreign material.
- Apply an ice compress.
- Give tetanus prophylaxis if appropriate.
- Discharge with instructions to return if they develop breathlessness, wheeze, rash, oropharyngeal swelling, or generalized pruritus.
- Some would advocate giving patients who may be potentially immuno-supressed (e.g. diabetes, high-dose steroid therapy) prophylactic anti-biotics (e.g. co-amoxiclav po) but there is little evidence this is of benefit.
- Observe patients with prior history of systemic reactions closely.

2 *Systemic reaction* (see p212, anaphylaxis*)*
- Secure the airway: If respiratory obstruction is imminent, intubate and ventilate or consider emergency cricothyroidotomy (see p810). A 14 or 16G needle and insufflation with 100% O_2 can temporize until the anaesthetist arrives.
- Give oxygen; if there is refractory hypoxia, intubate and ventilate.
- **Give intramuscular adrenaline 0.5–1mg** (0.5–1ml of 1 in 1000 adrenaline injection) and repeat every 10 minutes according to bp and pulse. Administer this *before* searching for intravenous access so as not to waste time.
- Establish venous access and start iv fluids (colloid if hypotensive). Persistent hypotension requires iv inotropes (see p210).
- **Intravenous adrenaline** may be required if the patient is severely ill with poor circulation. Give *slow* injection of 500 micrograms (5ml of the dilute 1 in 10,000 adrenaline injection) at 1ml/minute *stopping* when a response is obtained.
- If the patient continues to deteriorate, start intravenous aminophylline infusion (see p167). Patients on beta-blockers may not respond to adrenaline injection and require iv salbutamol infusion.
- Isolated bronchospasm may be treated with nebulized ß-agonists (salbutamol or adrenaline, p166). If there is prior history of systemic reactions, im adrenaline is the treatment of choice.
- Give iv hydrocortisone 100–300mg and chlorpheniramine 10–20mg .
- Continue H_1 antagonist (e.g. chlorpheniramine 4mg q4–6h) for at least 24–48h; longer if urticaria and pruritus persist.
- Do not forget local wound care as above.

3 *Prevention*
Patients prone to serious reactions from stings should be provided with, and instructed on, the use of commercially available 'bee-sting' kits. [Available freely in the US and on a named-patient basis in the UK from the manufacturers (see BNF.)] These contain pre-filled syringes of adrenaline for im injection and one also contains chewable tablets of chlorpheniramine.

Delayed presentation

- Due to local toxic reaction or infection, and rarely with serum sickness, vasculitis, Henoch-Schönlein purpura, and haemolysis.
- Clean the wound and give tetanus prophylaxis if indicated as above.
- Practically, it is difficult to distinguish a local toxic reaction from infection. Treat with both an oral antihistamine and oral antibiotic (e.g. chlorpheniramine 4mg q4–6h and co-amoxiclav).
- Elevate if there is marked swelling and consider surgical drainage of fluctuant masses.

Snakebite

- The only indigenous venomous snake in the UK is the adder (*Vipera berus*) and acute envenomation is rare.

Presentation

- Local effects include pain, swelling, erythema, bruising, tender regional lymphadenopathy.
- Systemic effects such as hypotension and syncope, angioedema, abdominal colic, diarrhoea and vomiting, coagulopathy and spontaneous haemorrhage, ECG abnormalities, shock, ARDS, rhabdomyolysis, and renal failure are ominous, but *V. berus* bites are seldom fatal in adult humans.

Management

- Identify the snake if at all possible. The instinctive response on being bitten is to give the snake a ritual beating, but this does not help in the identification.
- Non-poisonous bites should be cleaned, anti-tetanus prophylaxis given to the patient if needed, with prophylactic antibiotics as for animal bites (see p250).

Poisonous snake bites

First aid

- Immobilize the bitten part and keep below the level of the heart if possible.
- A veno-occlusive tourniquet should be placed immediately above the bite, taking care not to obstruct the arterial supply.
- Incision and suction of the wound is only indicated if the patient is seen within 15–20 minutes, the snake is large and identified as poisonous, the victim is young or elderly, and the nearest source of anti-venom is more than 2 hours away.
- The patient should be kept calm and quiet to avoid tachycardia and further vasodilatation and venom absorption.

In hospital

- All patients with bites from poisonous snakes should be admitted.
- Establish venous access and send blood for FBC, coagulation profile, U&E, group and X-match. Examine urine for myoglobin or haemoglobin.
- Treat hypotension and shock (p210).
- Watch for evolving compartment syndrome.
- All bites should be cultured and treated with antibiotics (see bites). Some authorities recommend high-dose hydrocortisone and antihistamine to reduce local inflammation and systemic symptoms.
- Indications for anti-venom treatment include systemic features (as above), coagulopathy, neutrophil leukocytosis, and if swelling extends to wrist/ankle within 4 hours of a bite on the hand/foot.
- *Contact your regional centres for details on identification, management and supply of anti-venom for adder and certain foreign snakes (see p854).*
- General measures: All bites should be swabbed for MC&S (see bites).

16 Practical procedures

Central line insertion

You will need the following:

- Sterile dressing pack and gloves
- 10ml and 5ml syringe with green (21G) and orange (25G) needles
- Local anaesthetic (e.g. 2% lignocaine)
- Central line (e.g. 16G long Abbocath® or Seldinger catheter)
- Saline flush
- Silk suture and needle
- No. 11 scalpel blade
- Sterile occlusive dressing (e.g. Tegaderm®)

Risks

- Arterial puncture (remove and apply local pressure)
- Pneumothorax (insert chest drain or aspirate if required)
- Haemothorax
- Chylothorax (mainly left subclavian lines)
- Infection (local, septicaemia, bacterial endocarditis)
- Brachial plexus or cervical root damage (over enthusiastic infiltration with local anaesthetic)
- Arrhythmias

General procedure

- The basic technique is the same whatever vein is cannulated.
- Lie the patient supine ($\pm$ head-down tilt).
- Turn the patient's head away from the side you wish to cannulate.
- Clean the skin with iodine or chlorhexidine: from the angle of the jaw to the clavicle for internal jugular vein (IJV) cannulation and from the mid-line to axilla for the subclavian approach.
- Use the drapes to isolate the sterile field.
- Flush the lumen of the central line with saline.
- Identify your landmarks (see p771 and p772).
- Infiltrate skin and sub-cutaneous tissue with local anaesthetic.
- Have the introducer needle and Seldinger guide-wire within easy reach so that you can reach them with one hand without having to release your other hand. Your fingers may be distorting the anatomy slightly making access to the vein easier and if released it may prove difficult to relocate the vein.
- With the introducer needle in the vein, check that you can aspirate blood freely. Use the hand that was on the pulse to immobilize the needle relative to the skin and mandible or clavicle.
- Remove the syringe and pass the guide wire into the vein; it should pass freely. If there is resistance, remove the wire, check that the needle is still within the lumen, and try again.
- Remove the needle leaving the wire within the vein and use a sterile swab to maintain gentle pressure over the site of venepuncture to prevent excessive bleeding.
- With a No. 11 blade make a nick in the skin where the wire enters, to facilitate dilatation of the sub-cutaneous tissues. Pass the dilator over the wire and remove, leaving the wire *in situ*.
- Pass the central line over the wire into the vein. Remove the guide-wire, flush the lumen with fresh saline, and close off to air.
- Suture the line in place and cover the skin penetration site with a sterile occlusive dressing.

Measuring the CVP – tips and pitfalls

- When asked to see a patient at night on the wards with an abnormal CVP reading, it is a good habit to always re-check the zero and the reading yourself.
- Always do measurements with the mid-axillary point as the zero reference. Sitting the patient up will drop the central filling pressure (pooling in the veins).
- Fill the manometer line, being careful not to soak the cotton ball stop. If this gets wet it limits the free-fall of saline or dextrose in the manometer line.
- Look at the rate and character of the venous pressure. It should fall to its value quickly and swing with respiration.
- If it fails to fall quickly consider whether the line is open (i.e. saline running in), blocked with blood clot, positional (up against vessel wall; ask patient to take some deep breaths), arterial blood (blood tracks back up the line). Raise the whole dripstand (if you are strong), and make sure that the level falls. If it falls when the whole stand is elevated it may be that the CVP is very high.
- It is easier, and safer, to cannulate a central vein with the patient supine or head down. There is an increased risk of air embolus if the patient is semi-recumbent.

Internal jugular vein cannulation

The internal jugular vein (IJV) runs just posterolateral to the carotid artery within the carotid sheath and lies medial to the SCM in the upper part of the neck, between the two heads of SCM in its medial portion and enters the subclavian vein near the medial border of the anterior scalene muscle (see figure). There are three basic approaches to IJV cannulation: medial to sternocleidomastoid (SCM), between the two heads of SCM, or lateral to SCM. The approach used varies and depends on the experience of the operator and the institution.

- Locate the carotid artery between the sternal and clavicular heads of SCM at the level of the thyroid cartilage; the IJV lies just lateral and parallel to it.

- Keeping the fingers of one hand on the carotid pulsation, infiltrate the skin with LA thoroughly, aiming just lateral to this and ensuring that you are not in a vein.

- Ideally, first locate the vein with a blue or green needle. Advance the needle at 45° to the skin, with gentle negative suction on the syringe, aiming for the ipsilateral nipple, lateral to the pulse.

- If you fail to find the vein, withdraw the needle slowly, maintaining negative suction on the syringe (you may have inadvertently transfixed the vein). Aim slightly more medially and try again.

- Once you have identified the position of the vein, change to the syringe with the introducer needle, cannulate the vein, and pass the guide-wire into the vein (see p771).

Tips and pitfalls

- Venous blood is dark, and arterial blood is pulsatile and bright red!

- Once you locate the vein, change to the syringe with the introducer needle, taking care not to release your fingers from the pulse; they may be distorting the anatomy slightly making access to the vein easier and if released it may prove difficult to relocate the vein.

- The guide-wire should pass freely down the needle and into the vein. With the left IJV approach, there are several acute bends that need to be negotiated. If the guide-wire keeps passing down the wrong route, ask your assistant to hold the patient's arms out at 90° to the bed, or even above the patient's head, to coax the guide-wire down the correct path.

- For patients who are intubated or requiring respiratory support it may be difficult to access the head of the bed. The anterior approach may be easier (see figure) and may be done from the side of the bed (the left-side of the bed for right-handed operators, using the left hand to locate the pulse and the right to cannulate the vein).

- The IJV may also be readily cannulated with a long Abbocath®. No guide-wire is necessary, but, as a result, misplacement is commoner than with the Seldinger technique.

- When using an Abbocath®, on cannulating the vein, remember to advance the sheath and needle a few mm to allow the tip of the plastic sheath (~ 1mm behind the tip of the bevelled needle) to enter the vein. Holding the needle stationary, advance the sheath over it into the vein.

- Arrange for a CXR to confirm the position of the line.

Internal jugular vein cannulation

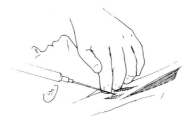

(a) Surface anatomy of external and internal jugular veins

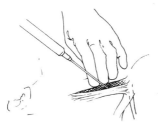

(b) Anterior approach: the chin is in the midline and the skin puncture is over the sternal head of SCM muscle

(c) Central approach: the chin is turned away and the skin puncture is between the two heads of SCM muscle.

Internal jugular vein cannulation

Subclavian vein cannulation

The axillary vein becomes the subclavian vein (SCV) at the lateral border of the 1st rib and extends for 3–4cm just deep to the clavicle. It is joined by the ipsilateral IJV to become the brachiocephalic vein behind the sterno-clavicular joint. The subclavian artery and brachial plexus lie posteriorly, separated from the vein by the scalenus anterior muscle. The phrenic nerve and the internal mammary artery lie behind the medial portion of the SCV and, on the left, lies the thoracic duct.

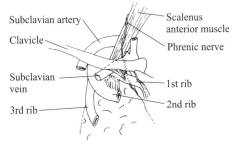

The subclavian vein and surrounding structures

- Select the point 1cm below the junction of the medial third and middle third of the clavicle. If possible place a bag of saline between the scapulae to extend the spine.
- Clean the skin with iodine or chlorhexidine.
- Infiltrate skin and sub-cutaneous tissue and periosteum of the inferior border of the clavicle with local anaesthetic up to the hilt of the green (21G) needle, ensuring that it is not in a vein.
- Insert the introducer needle with a 10ml syringe, guiding gently under the clavicle. It is safest to initially hit the clavicle, and 'walk' the needle under it until the inferior border is just cleared. In this way you keep the needle as superficial to the dome of the pleura as possible. Once it has just skimmed underneath the clavicle, advance it slowly towards the contralateral sternoclavicular joint, aspirating as you advance. Using this technique the risk of pneumothorax is small, and success is high.
- Once the venous blood is obtained, rotate the bevel of the needle towards the heart. This encourages the guide-wire to pass down the brachiocephalic rather than up the IJV.
- The wire should pass easily into the vein. If there is difficulty, try advancing during the inspiratory and expiratory phases of the respiratory cycle.
- Once the guide-wire is in place, remove the introducer needle, and pass the dilator over the wire. When removing the dilator, note the direction that it faces; it should be slightly curved downwards. If it is slightly curved upwards, then it is likely that the wire has passed up into the IJV. The wire may be manipulated into the brachiocephalic vein under fluoroscopic control but if not available it is safer to remove the wire and start again.
- After removing the dilator pass the central venous catheter over the guide-wire, remove the guide-wire, and secure as above.
- A chest X-ray is mandatory after subclavian line insertion to exclude a pneumothorax and to confirm satisfactory placement of the line, especially if fluoroscopy was not employed.

Pulmonary artery catheterization   1.

Indications

PA catheters (Swan-Ganz catheters) allow direct measurement of a number of haemodynamic parameters that aid clinical decision-making in critically ill patients (evaluate right and left ventricular function, guide treatment and provide prognostic information). The catheter itself has no therapeutic benefit and there have been a number of studies showing increased mortality (and morbidity) with their use. Consider inserting a PA catheter in any critically ill patient, after discussion with an experienced physician, if the measurements will influence decisions on therapy (and not just to reassure yourself). Careful and frequent clinical assessment of the patient should always accompany measurements and PA catherization should not delay treatment of the patient.

General indications (not a comprehensive list) include:-

- Management of complicated myocardial infarction.
- Assessment and management of shock.
- Assessment and management of respiratory distress (cardiogenic vs non-cardiogenic pulmonary oedema).
- Evaluating effects of treatment in unstable patients (e.g. inotropes, vasodilators, mechanical ventilation, etc.).
- Delivering therapy (e.g. thrombolysis for pulmonary embolism, prostacyclin for pulmonary hypertension, etc.).
- Assessment of fluid requirements in critically ill patients.

Equipment required

- Full resuscitation facilities should be available and the patient's ECG should be continuously monitored.
- Bag of heparinized saline for flushing the catheter and transducer set for pressure monitoring. (Check that your assistant is experienced in setting up the transducer system BEFORE you start.)
- 8F introducer kit (pre-packaged kits contain the introducer sheath and all the equipment required for central venous cannulation).
- PA catheter: Commonly a triple lumen catheter, that allows simultaneous measurement of RA pressure (proximal port) and PA pressure (distal port)and incorporates a thermistor for measurement of cardiac output by thermodilution. Check your catheter before you start.
- Fluoroscopy is preferable, though not essential.

General technique

- Do not attempt this without supervision if you are inexperienced.
- Observe strict aseptic technique using sterile drapes, etc.
- Insert the introducer sheath (at least 8F in size) into either the internal jugular or subclavian vein in the standard way (pp770–772). Flush the sheath with saline and secure to the skin with sutures.
- Do not attach the plastic sterile expandable sheath to the introducer yet but keep it sterile for use later once the catheter is in position (the catheter is easier to manipulate without the plastic covering).
- Flush all the lumens of the PA catheter and attach the distal lumen to the pressure transducer. Check the transducer is zeroed (conventionally to the mid-axillary point). Check the integrity of the balloon by inflating it with the syringe provided (2ml air) and then deflate the balloon.
- The procedure is detailed on the following pages.

Pulmonary artery catheterization

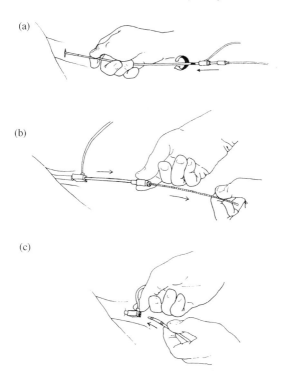

Pulmonary artery catheterization

(a) The sheath and dilator are advanced into the vein over the guide-wire. A twisting motion makes insertion easier.

(b) The guide-wire and dilator are then removed. The sheath has a haemostatic valve at the end preventing leakage of blood.

(c) The PA catheter is then inserted through the introducer sheath into the vein (see p776).

Pulmonary artery catheterization 2.

Insertion technique

- Flush all the lumens of the PA catheter and attach the distal lumen to the pressure transducer. Check the transducer is zeroed (conventionally to the mid-axillary point). Check the integrity of the balloon by inflating it with the syringe provided (~ 2ml air) and then deflate the balloon.

- Pass the tip of the PA catheter through the plastic sheath, keeping the sheath compressed. The catheter is easier to manipulate without the sheath over it; once in position, extend the sheath over the catheter to keep it sterile.

- With the balloon deflated, advance the tip of the catheter to approx 10–15cm from the right IJV or SCV, 15–20cm from the left (the markings on the side of the catheter are at 10cm intervals: 2 lines = 20cm). Check that the pressure tracing is typical of the right atrial pressure (see figure opposite).

- Inflate the balloon and advance the catheter gently. The flow of blood will carry the balloon (and catheter) across the tricuspid valve, through the right ventricle and into the pulmonary artery (see figure p777).

- Watch the ECG tracing closely whilst the catheter is advanced. The catheter commonly triggers runs of VT when crossing the tricuspid valve and through the RV. The VT is usually self-limiting, but should not be ignored. Deflate the balloon, pull back, and try again.

- If more than 15cm of catheter is advanced into the RV without the tip entering the PA, this suggests the catheter is coiling in the RV. Deflate the balloon, withdraw the catheter into the RA, reinflate the balloon and try again using clockwise torque while advancing in the ventricle, or flushing the catheter with cold saline to stiffen the plastic. If this fails repeatedly, try under fluoroscopic guidance.

- As the tip passes into a distal branch of the PA, the balloon will impact and not pass further, the wedge position, and the pressure tracing will change (see figure opposite).

- Deflate the balloon and check that a typical PA tracing is obtained. If not, try flushing the catheter lumen, and, if that fails, withdraw the catheter until the tip is within the PA and begin again.

- Reinflate the balloon slowly. If the PCW pressure is seen before the balloon is fully inflated, it suggests the tip has migrated further into the artery. Deflate the balloon and withdraw the catheter 1–2 cm and try again.

- If the pressure tracing flattens and then continues to rise, you have 'overwedged'. Deflate the balloon, pull back the catheter 1–2 cm, and start again.

- When a stable position has been achieved, extend the plastic sheath over the catheter and secure it to the introducer sheath. Clean any blood from the skin insertion site with antiseptic and secure a coil of the PA catheter to the patient's chest to avoid inadvertent removal.

- Obtain a CXR to check the position of the catheter. The tip of the catheter should ideally be no more than 3–5cm from the mid-line.

Pulmonary artery catheterization

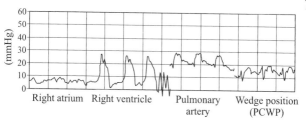

Pressure tracings during pulmonary artery catheterization

Normal values of right heart pressures and flows	
Right atrial pressure	0–8mmHg
Right ventricle	
systolic	15–30mmHg
end diastolic	0–8mmHg
Pulmonary artery	
systolic / diastolic	15–30/4–12mmHg
mean	9–16mmHg
Pulmonary capillary wedge pr.	2–10mmHg
Cardiac index	2.8–4.2l/min/m^2)

(See p226 for haemodynamic formulae.)

Pulmonary artery catheterization 3.

Tips and pitfalls

- Never withdraw the catheter with the balloon inflated.
- Never advance the catheter with the balloon deflated.
- Never inject liquid into the balloon.
- Never leave the catheter with the balloon inflated as pulmonary infarction may occur.
- The plastic of the catheter softens with time at body temperature and the tip of the catheter may migrate further into the PA branch. If the pressure tracing with the balloon deflated is 'partially wedged' (and flushing the catheter does not improve this), withdraw the catheter 1–2 cm and reposition.
- Sometimes it is impossible to obtain a wedged trace. In this situation one has to use the PA diastolic pressure as a guide. In health there is ~ 2–4mmHg difference between PA diastolic pressure and PCWP. Any condition which causes pulmonary hypertension (e.g. severe lung disease, ARDS, long-standing valvular disease) will alter this relationship.
- *Valvular lesions, VSDs, prosthetic valves, and pacemakers:* If these are present then seek advice from a cardiologist. The risk of SBE may be sufficiently great that the placement of a PA catheter may be more detrimental than beneficial.
- PEEP (see p808). Measurement and interpretation if PCWP in patients on PEEP depends on the position of the catheter. Ensure the catheter is below the level of the left atrium on a lateral CXR. Removing PEEP during measurement causes marked fluctuations in haemodynamics and oxygenation and the pressures do not reflect the state once back on the ventilator.

Complications

- *Arrhythmias:* Watch the ECG tracing closely whilst the catheter is advanced. The catheter commonly triggers runs of VT when crossing the tricuspid valve and through the RV. If this happens, deflate the balloon, pull back, and try again. The VT is usually self-limiting, but should not be ignored.
- *Pulmonary artery rupture:* (~ 0.2% in one series). Damage may occur if the balloon is overinflated in a small branch. Risk factors include mitral valve disease (large v wave confused with poor wedging), pulmonary hypertension, multiple inflations, or hyperinflations of balloon. Haemoptysis is an early sign. It is sfaer to follow PA diastolic pressures if these correlate with the PCWP.
- Pulmonary infarction
- *Knots:* Usually occur at the time of initial placement in patients where there has been difficulty in traversing the RV. Signs include loss of pressure tracing, persistent ectopy, resistance to catheter manipulation. If this is suspected or has occurred, stop manipulation and seek expert help.
- *Infection:* Risks increase with length of time the catheter is left *in situ.* Pressure transducer may occasionally be a source of infection. Remove the catheter and introducer and replace only if necessary.
- *Other complications:* Complications associated with central line insertion, thrombosis and embolism, balloon rupture, intracardiac damage.

Indications for temporary pacing

1 Following acute myocardial infarction

- Asystole

- Symptomatic complete heart block (CHB) (any territory).
- Symptomatic 2° heart block (any territory).
- Trifascicular block   – alternating LBBB and RBBB
  - 1° heart block + RBBB + LAD
  - new RBBB and left posterior hemiblock
  - LBBB and long PR interval
- After anterior MI   – asymptomatic CHB
  - asymptomatic 2° (Mobitz II) block
- Symptomatic sinus bradycardia unresponsive to atropine
- Recurrent VT for atrial or ventricular overdrive pacing

2 Unrelated to myocardial infarction

- Symptomatic sinus or junctional bradycardia unresponsive to atropine (e.g. carotid sinus hypersensitivity)
- Symptomatic 2° heart block or sinus arrest
- Symptomatic complete heart block
- Torsades de pointes tachycardia
- Recurrent VT for atrial or ventricular overdrive pacing
- Bradycardia-dependent tachycardia
- Drug overdose (e.g. verapamil, beta-blockers, digoxin)
- Permanent pacemaker box change in a patient who is pacing dependent

3 Before general anaesthesia

- The same principles as for acute MI (see above)
- Sinoatrial disease, 2° (Wenckebach) heart block only need prophylactic pacing if there are symptoms of syncope or pre-syncope.
- Complete heart block

Transvenous temporary pacing

- The technique of temporary wire insertion is described on p782.
- The most commonly used pacing mode and the mode of choice for life-threatening bradyarrhythmias is ventricular demand pacing (VVI) with a single bipolar wire positioned in the right ventricle: (see p784 for an explanation of common pacing modes).
- In critically ill patients with impaired cardiac pump function and symptomatic bradycardia (especially with right ventricular infarction), cardiac output may be increased by up to 20% by maintaining atrio-ventricular synchrony. This requires two pacing leads, one atrial and one ventricular, and a dual pacing box.

Epicardial temporary pacing

- Following cardiac surgery, patients may have *epicardial wires* (attached to the pericardial surface of the heart) left in for up to 1 week in case of post operative heart block or bradyarrhythmia. These may be used in the same way as the more familiar trans-venous pacing wires, but the threshold may be higher.

Atrio-ventricular sequential pacing

In critically ill patients with impaired cardiac pump function and symptomatic bradycardia (especially with right ventricular infarction), cardiac output may be increased by up to 20% by maintaining atrio-ventricular synchrony. This requires two pacing leads, one atrial and one ventricular, and a dual pacing box.

Patients most likely to benefit from AV sequential pacing

- Acute MI (especially RV infarction)
- 'Stiff' left ventricle: (aortic stenosis, HCM, hypertensive heart disease, amyloidosis)
- Low cardiac output states (cardiomyopathy)
- Recurrent atrial arrhythmias

Temporary cardiac pacing 1.

Ventricular pacing

- *Cannulate a central vein*: The wire is easiest to manipulate via the RIJ approach but is more comfortable for the patient via the right sub-clavian (SC) vein. The LIJ approach is best avoided as there are many acute bends to negotiate and a stable position is difficult to achieve. Avoid the left subclavicular area as this is the preferred area for permanent pacemaker insertion and should be kept 'virgin' if possible. The femoral vein may be used but the incidence of DVT and infection is high.

- *Insert a sheath* (similar to that for PA catheterization) through which the pacing wire can be fed. Pacing wires are commonly 5F or 6F and a sheath at least one size larger is necessary. Most commercially available pacing wires are pre-packed with an introducer needle and plastic cannula similar to an Abbocath® which may be used to position the pacing wire. However, the cannula does not have a haemostatic seal. The plastic cannula may be removed from the vein, leaving the bare wire entering the skin, once a stable position has been achieved. This reduces the risk of wire displacement but also makes re-positioning of the wire more difficult should this be necessary, and the infection risk is higher.

- Pass the wire through the sterile plastic cover that accompanies the introducer sheath and advance into the upper right atrium (see figure opposite) but do not unfurl the cover yet. The wire is much easier to manipulate with gloved hands without the additional hindrance of the plastic cover.

- Advance the wire with the tip pointing towards the right ventricle; it may cross the tricuspid valve easily. If it fails to cross, point the tip to the lateral wall of the atrium and form a loop. Rotate the wire and the loop should fall across the tricuspid valve into the ventricle.

- Advance and rotate the wire so that the tip points inferiorly as close to the tip of the right ventricle (laterally) as possible.

- If the wire does not rotate down to the apex easily, it may be because you are in the coronary sinus rather than in the right ventricle. (The tip of the wire points to the left shoulder.) Withdraw the wire and re-cross the tricuspid valve.

- Leave some slack in the wire; the final appearance should be like the outline of a sock with the 'heel' in the right atrium, the 'arch' over the tricuspid and the 'big toe' at the tip of the right ventricle.

- Connect the wire to the pacing box and check the threshold. Ventricular pacing thresholds should be < 1.0 volts, but threshold up to 1.5V is acceptable if another stable position canot be achieved.

- Check for positional stability. With the box pacing at a rate higher than the intrinsic heart rate, ask the patient to take some deep breaths, cough forcefully, and sniff. Watch for failure of capture, and if so reposition the wire.

- Set the output to 3 volts and the box on 'demand'. If the patient is in sinus rhythm and has an adequate blood pressure set the box rate to just below the patient's rate. If there is complete heart block or bradycardia set the rate at 70–80/min.

- Cover the wire with the plastic sheath and suture sheath and wire securely to the skin. Loop the rest of the wire and fix to the patient's skin with adhesive dressing.

- When the patient returns to the ward, obtain a CXR to confirm satisfactory positioning of the wire and to exclude a pneumothorax.

<table>
<tr><td>

Checklist for pacing wire insertion

</td></tr>
</table>

- Check the screening equipment and defibrillator are working.
- Check the type of pacing wire: atrial wires have a pre-formed J that allows easy placement in the atrium or appendage and is very difficult to manipulate into a satisfactory position in the ventricle. Ventricular pacing wires have a more open, gentle 'J'.
- Check the pacing box (single vs dual or sequential pacing box) and leads to attach to the wire(s). Familiarize yourself with the controls on the box: you may need to connect up in a hurry if the patient's intrinsic rhythm slows further.
- Remember to don the lead apron before wearing the sterile gown, mask, and gloves.

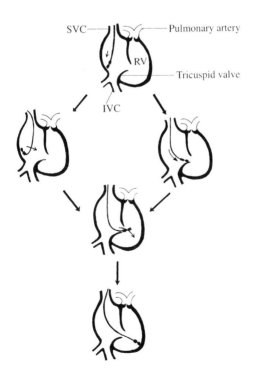

Insertion of a ventricular pacing wire (see text for details)

Temporary cardiac pacing 2.

Atrial pacing

- The technique of inserting an atrial temporary wire is similar to that of ventricular pacing.
- Advance the atrial wire until the 'J' is re-formed in the right atrium.
- Rotate the wire and withdraw slightly to position the tip in the right atrial appendage. Aim for a threshold of < 1.5 volts.
- If atrial wires are not available, a ventricular pacing wire may be manipulated into a similar position or passed into the coronary sinus for left atrial pacing.

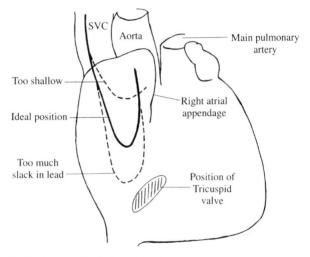

Positioning an atrial wire for atrial pacing

Temporary cardiac pacing   3.

Complications (see table opposite)

1 *Ventricular ectopics or VT*
- Non-sustained VT is common as the wire crosses the tricuspid valve (especially in patients receiving an isoprenaline infusion) and does not require treatment.
- Try to avoid long runs of VT and if necessary withdraw the wire into the atrium and wait until the rhythm has settled.
- If ectopics persist after the wire is positioned, try adjusting the amount of slack in the wire in the region of the tricuspid valve (either more or less).
- Pacing the right ventricular outflow tract can provoke runs of VT.

2 *Failure to pace and/or sense*
- It is difficult to get low pacing thresholds (< 1.0V) in patients with extensive myocardial infarction (especially of the inferior wall), cardiomyopathy, or who have received class I anti-arrhythmic drugs. Accept a slightly higher value if the position is otherwise stable and satisfactory.
- If the position of the wire appears satisfactory and yet the pacing thresholds are high, the wire may be in a left hepatic vein. Pull the wire back into the atrium and try again, looking specifically for the ventricular ectopics as the wire crosses the tricuspid valve.
- The pacing threshold commonly doubles in the first few days due to endocardial oedema.
- If the pacemaker suddenly fails, the most common reason is usually wire displacement.
  - Increase the pacing output of the box.
  - Check all the connections of the wire and the battery of the box.
  - Try moving the patient to the left lateral position until arrangements can be made to reposition the wire.

3 *Perforation*
- A pericardial rub may be present in the absence of perforation (especially post MI).
- *Presentation:* Pericardial chest pain, increasing breathlessness, falling blood pressure, enlarged cardiac silhouette on CXR, signs of cardiac tamponade, left diaphragmatic pacing at low output.
- *Management*
  - If there are signs of cardiac tamponade arrange for urgent ECHO and pericardial drainage (p788).
  - Reposition the wire.
  - Monitor the patient carefully over the next few days with repeat ECHOs to detect incipient cardiac tamponade.

4 *Diaphragmatic pacing*
- High output pacing (10V), even with satisfactory position of the ventricular lead may cause pacing of the left hemidiaphragm. At low voltages this suggests perforation (see above).
- Right hemidiaphragm pacing may be seen with atrial pacing and stimulation of the right phrenic nerve.
- Reposition the wire if symptomatic (painful twitching, dyspnoea).

Complications of temporary pacing

- Complications associated with central line insertion
- Ventricular ectopics
- Non-sustained VT
- Perforation
- Pericarditis
- Diaphragmatic pacing
- Infection
- Pneumothorax
- Cardiac Tamponade

Pericardial aspiration   1.

Equipment

Establish peripheral venous access and check that full facilities for resuscitation are available. Pre-prepared pericardiocentesis sets may be available. You will need:-

- Trolley as for central line insertion, with iodine or chlorhexidine for skin, dressing pack, sterile drapes, local anaesthetic (lignocaine 2%), syringes (including a 50ml), needles (25G and 22G), No. 11 blade, and silk sutures
- Pericardiocentesis needle (15cm, 18G) or similar Wallace cannula.
- J-guide wire ($\geqslant$ 80cm, 0.035 diameter)
- Dilators (up to 7 French)
- Pigtail catheter ($\geqslant$ 60 cm with multiple sideholes, a large Seldinger-type CVP line can be used if no pigtail is available)
- Drainage bag and connectors
- Facilities for fluoroscopy or echocardiographic screening

Technique

- Position the patient at ~ 30°. This allows the effusion to pool inferiorly within the pericardium.
- Sedate the patient lightly with midazolam (2.5–7.5mg iv) and fentanyl (50–200µg iv) if necessary. Use with caution as this may drop the bp in patients already compromised by the effusion.
- Wearing a sterile gown and gloves, clean the skin from mid-chest to mid-abdomen and put the sterile drapes on the patient.
- Infiltrate the skin and sub-cutaneous tissues with local anaesthetic starting 1–1.5cm below the xiphisternum and just to the left of mid-line, aiming for the left shoulder and staying as close to the inferior border of the rib cartilages as possible.
- The pericardiocentesis needle is introduced into the angle between the xiphisternum and the left costal margin angled at ~ 30°. Advance slowly aspirating gently and then injecting more lignocaine every few mm, aiming for the left shoulder.
- As the parietal pericardium is pierced, you may feel a 'give' and fluid will be aspirated. Remove the syringe and introduce the guide-wire through the needle.
- Check the position of the guide-wire by screening. It should loop within the cardiac silhouette only and not advance into the SVC or pulmonary artery.
- Remove the needle leaving the wire in place. Enlarge the skin incision slightly using the blade and dilate the track.
- Insert the pigtail over the wire into the pericardial space and remove the wire.
- Take specimens for microscopy, culture (and inoculate a sample into blood culture bottles), cytology and haematocrit if blood stained (a FBC tube; ask the haematologists to run on the Coulter counter for rapid estimation of Hb).
- Aspirate to dryness watching the patient carefully. Symptoms and haemodynamics (tachycardia) often start to improve with removal of as little as 100ml of pericardial fluid.
- If the fluid is heavily blood stained, withdraw fluid cautiously; if the pigtail is in the right ventricle, withdrawal of blood may cause cardio-vascular collapse. Arrange for urgent Hb/haematocrit.
- Leave on free drainage and attached to the drainage bag.
- Suture the pigtail to the skin securely and cover with a sterile occlusive dressing.

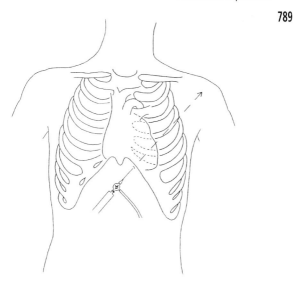

Pericardial aspiration

Pericardial aspiration 2.

Aftercare

- Closely observe the patient for recurrent tamponade (obstruction of drain) and repeat ECHO.
- Discontinue anti-coagulants.
- Remove the drain after 24 hours or when the drainage stops.
- Consider the need for surgery (drainage, biopsy or pericardial window) or specific therapy (chemotherapy if malignant effusion, antimicrobials if bacterial, dialysis if renal failure, etc.).

Tips and pitfalls

1 If the *needle touches the heart's epicardial surface*, you may feel a 'ticking' sensation transmitted down the needle: withdraw the needle a few mm, angulate the needle more superficially and try cautiously again, aspirating as you advance.

2 *If you do not enter the effusion*, and the heart not encountered:

- Withdraw the needle slightly and advance again, aiming slightly deeper, but still towards the left shoulder.
- If this fails, try again aiming more medially (midclavicular point or even suprasternal notch).
- Consider trying the apical approach (starting laterally at cardiac apex and aiming for right shoulder), if echo confirms sufficient fluid at the cardiac apex.

3 If available, *intrathoracic ECG* can be monitored by a lead attached to the needle as it is advanced. This is seldom clinically useful in our experience. Penetration of the myocardium results in ST elevation, suggesting the needle has been advanced to far.

4 *Difficulty in inserting the pigtail*

- This may be because of insufficient dilatation of the tract (use a larger dilator).
- Holding the wire taught (by gentle traction) while pushing the catheter may help; take care not to pull the wire out of the pericardium.

5 *Haemorrhagic effusion vs blood*

- Compare the Hb of the pericardial fluid to the venous blood Hb.
- Place some of the fluid in a clean container; blood will clot whereas haemorrhagic effusion will not as the 'whipping' action of the heart tends to defibrinate it.
- Confirm the position of the needle by first withdrawing some fluid and then injecting 10–20ml of contrast; using fluoroscopy, see if the contrast stays within the cardiac sillhouette.
- Alternatively, if using ECHO guidance, inject 5–10ml saline into the needle looking for 'microbubble contrast' in the cavity containing the needle tip. Injecting 20ml saline rapidly into a peripheral vein will produce 'contrast' in the right atrium and ventricle and may allow them to be distinguised from the pericardial space.
- Connect a pressure line to the needle; a characteristic waveform will confirm penetration of the right ventricle (see figure p777).

Complications of pericardiocentesis

- Penetration of a cardiac chamber (usually right ventricle)
- Laceration of an epicardial vessel
- Arrhythmia (atrial arrhythmias as the wire is advanced, ventricular arrhythmias if the RV is penetrated)
- Pneumothorax
- Perforation of abdominal viscus (liver, stomach, colon)
- Ascending infection

DC cardioversion 1.

Relative contraindications
- Digoxin toxicity
- Electrolyte disturbance ($\downarrow Na^+$, $\downarrow K^+$, $\downarrow Ca^{2+}$, $\downarrow Mg^{2+}$, acidosis)
- Inadequate anti-coagulation and chronic AF

Check list for DC cardioversion

• Defibrillator	Check this is functioning with a fully equipped arrest trolley to hand in case of arrest.
• Informed consent	(Unless life-threatening emergency.)
• 12 lead ECG	AF, flutter, SVT, VT, signs of ischaemia or digoxin. If ventricular rate is slow have an external (transcutaneous) pacing system nearby in case of asystole.
• Nil by mouth	For at least 4 hours.
• Anti-coagulation	Does the patient require anti-coagulants? Is the INR > 2.0? (Has it been so for > 3 wks ?)
• Potassium	Check this is > 3.5mmol/l.
• Digoxin	Check there are no features of digoxin toxicity (see p646). If taking $\geq 250\mu g$/day check that renal function and recent digoxin level are normal. If there are frequent ventricular ectopics, give iv Mg^{2+} 8mmol.
• Thyroid function	Treat thyrotoxicosis or myxoedema first.
• iv access	Peripheral venous cannula.
• Sedation	Short general anaesthesia (propofol) is preferable to sedation with benzodiazepine and fentanyl. Bag the patient with 100% oxygen.
• Select energy	(See table opposite.)
• Synchronization	Check this is selected on the defibrillator for all shocks (unless the patient is in VF or haemo-dynamically unstable). Adjust the ECG gain so that the machine is only sensing QRS complexes and not P or T waves.
• Paddle placement	Conductive gel pads should be placed between the paddles and the skin. Position one just to the right of the sternum and the other to the left of the left nipple (ant.-mid-axillary line), Alternatively, place one anteriorly just left of the sternum, and one posteriorly to the left of mid-line. There is no convincing evidence for superiority of one position over the other.
• Cardioversion	Check no one is in contact with the patient or with the metal bed. Ensure your own legs are clear of the bed! Apply firm pressure on the paddles.
• Unsuccessful	Double the energy level and repeat up to 360J. Consider changing paddle position (see above). If prolonged sinus pause or ventricular arrhythmia during an elective procedure, stop.
• Successful	Repeat ECG. Place in recovery position until awake. Monitor for 2–4h and ensure effects of sedation have passed. Patients should be accompanied home by friend or relative if being discharged.

Complications of DC cardioversion

- Asystole/bradycardias
- Ventricular fibrillation
- Thromboembolism
- Transient hypotension
- Skin burns
- Aspiration pneumonitis

Suggested initial energies for DC shock for elective cardioversion

• Sustained VT	200J.	Synchronized
• Atrial fibrillation	50–100J.	Synchronized
• Atrial flutter	50J.	Synchronized
• Other SVTs	50J.	Synchronized

- If the initial shock is unsuccessful, increase the energy (50, 100, 200, 360J) and repeat.
- If still unsuccessful consider changing paddle position and try 360 Joules again. It is inappropriate to persist further with elective DC cardioversion.

DC cardioversion 2.

Notes

1 Anti-coagulation

The risk of thromboembolism in patients with chronic AF and dilated cardiomyopathy is 0–7% depending on the underlying risk factors.

Increased risk
- Prior embolic event
- Mechanical heart valve
- Mitral stenosis
- Dilated left atrium

Low risk
- Age < 60 years
- No underlying heart disease
- Recent onset AF (< 3 days)

Anti-coagulate patients at risk with warfarin for at least 3–4 weeks. For recent onset AF (1–3 days), anti-coagulate with iv heparin for at least 12–24 hours and, if possible, exclude intracardiac thrombus with a transoesophageal ECHO prior to DC shock. If there is thrombus, anti-coagulate with warfarin as above. For emergency cardioversion of AF (< 24h), heparinize prior to shock.

The risk of systemic embolism with cardioversion of atrial flutter and other tachyarrhythmias is very low, provided there is no ventricular thrombus, since the co-ordinated atrial activity prevents formation of clot. Routine anti-coagulation with warfarin is not necessary but we would recommend heparin before DC shock as the atria are often rendered mechanically stationary for several hours after shock even though there is co-ordinate electrical depolarization.

After successful cardioversion, if the patient is on warfarin, continue anti-coagulation for at least 3–4 weeks. Consider indefinite anti-coagulation if there is intrinsic cardiac disease (e.g. mitral stenosis) or recurrent AF.

2 Special situations

Pregnancy DC shock during pregnancy appears to be safe. Auscultate the fetal heart before and after cardioversion and if possible, fetal ECG should be monitored.

Pacemakers There is a danger of damage to the pacemaker generator box or the junction at the tip of the pacing wire(s) and endocardium. Position the paddles in the anteroposterior position as this is theoretically safer. Facilities for back-up pacing (external or transvenous) should be available. Check the pacemaker post cardioversion – both early and late problems have been reported.

Intra-aortic balloon counterpulsation 1.

Indications
- Cardiogenic shock post MI
- Acute severe mitral regurgitation
- Acute ventricular septal defect
- Pre-operative (ostial left coronary stenosis)
- Weaning from cardiopulmonary bypass

Rarely
- Treatment of ventricular arrhythmias post MI
- Unstable angina (as a bridge to CABG)

Contraindications
- Aortic regurgitation
- Aortic dissection
- Severe aorto-iliac atheroma
- Bleeding diathesis
- Dilated cardiomyopathy (if patient not a candidate for transplantation)

Complications
- Aortic dissection
- Arterial perforation
- Limb ischaemia
- Thrombocytopenia
- Peripheral embolism
- Balloon rupture

Principle

The device consists of a catheter with a balloon (40ml size) at its tip which is positioned in the descending thoracic aorta. The balloon inflation/deflation is synchronized to the ECG. The balloon should inflate just after the dicrotic notch (in diastole), thereby increasing pressure in the aortic root and increasing coronary perfusion. The balloon deflates just before ventricular systole, thereby decreasing afterload and improving left ventricular performance (see below).

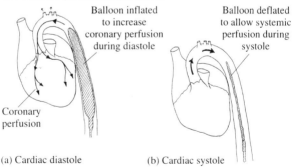

Balloon inflated to increase coronary perfusion during diastole

Balloon deflated to allow systemic perfusion during systole

Coronary perfusion

(a) Cardiac diastole   (b) Cardiac systole

Counterpulsation has a number of beneficial effects on the circulation.
- Increased in coronary perfusion in diastole.
- Reduced LV end diastolic pressure.
- Reduced myocardial oxygen consumption.
- Increased cerebral and peripheral blood flow.

The IAB cannot assist the patient in asystole or VF; it requires a minimum cardiac index of 1.2–1.4l/min/m^2, often necessitating additional inotropes.

Intra-aortic balloon counterpulsation

Intra-aortic balloon counterpulsation   2.

Technique

Balloon insertion

Previous experience is essential. Formerly, a cut-down to the femoral artery was required, but newer balloons come equipped with a sheath which may be introduced percutaneously. Using fluoroscopy, the balloon is positioned in the descending thoracic aorta with the tip just below the origin of the left subclavian artery. Fully anti-coagulate the patient with iv heparin. Some units routinely give iv antibiotics (flucloxacillin) to cover against *Staph.* infection.

Triggering and timing

The balloon pump may be triggered either from the patient's ECG (R wave) or from the arterial pressure waveform. Slide switches on the pump allow precise timing of inflation and deflation during the cardiac cycle. Set the pump to 1:2 to allow you to see the effects of augmentation on alternate beats.

Trouble-shooting

- Seek help from an expert! There is usually an on-call cardiac perfusionist or technician, senior cardiac physician or surgeon.
- Counterpulsation is inefficient with heart rates over 130/min. Consider anti-arrhythmics or 1:2 augmentation instead.
- Triggering and timing: For ECG triggering, select a lead with most pronounced R wave; ensure that the pump is set to trigger from ECG not pressure; permanent pacemakers may interfere with triggering-select lead with negative and smallest pacing artefact. Alternatively, set the pump to be triggered from the external pacing device. A good arterial waveform is required for pressure triggering; the timing will vary slightly depending on the location of the arterial line (slightly earlier for radial artery line, cf. femoral artery line). Be guided by the haemodynamic effects of balloon inflation and deflation rather than the precise value of delay.
- Limb ischaemia: Exacerbated by poor cardiac output, adrenaline, noradrenaline and peripheral vascular disease. Wean off and remove the balloon (see below).
- Thrombocytopenia: Commonly seen; does not require transfusion unless there is overt bleeding and returns to normal once the balloon is removed. Consider prostacyclin infusion if platelet counts fall below 100×10^9/l.

IABP removal

- The patient may be progressively weaned by gradually reducing the counterpulsation ratio (1:2, 1:4, 1:8, etc.) and/or reducing the balloon volume and checking that the patient remains haemodynamically stable.
- Stop the heparin infusion and wait for the ACT (activated clotting time) to fall < 150s (APTT < 1.5 normal).
- Using a 50ml syringe, have an assistant apply negative pressure to the balloon.
- Pull the balloon down until it abuts the sheath; do not attempt to pull the balloon into the sheath.
- Withdraw both balloon and sheath and apply firm pressure on the femoral puncture site for at least 30 minutes or until the bleeding is controlled.

The aim of therapy is to relieve hypoxia and maintain or restore a normal P_aCO_2 for the individual. Relative indications for mechanical ventilation are discussed in the appropriate chapters. This section discusses some of the principles involved.

Oxygen therapy

- Oxygen should be administered by a system that delivers a defined percentage, between 28% and 100% according to the patients requirements (e.g. via fixed percentage delivery masks such as Ventimask Mk iv).
- A Hudson mask or nasal cannulae give very variable F_iO_2 depending upon both flow rate of oxygen and the patients breathing pattern.
- Nasal prongs only deliver at F_iO_2 of 30% at flows of 2 lit/min, and become less efficient at higher flow rates ($\sim$ 35% at 3 lit/min with little further increase with increasing flow). Higher flow rates require humidification.
- A properly positioned, high flow oxygen mask, using oxygen at 6 l/min, can provide an F_iO_2 of 60%.
- Combining nasal prongs and a high flow mask can achieve an F_iO_2 of $\sim$ 80–90%.
- In practice it is rarely possible to consistently deliver $> 60\%$ unless using CPAP or ventilation.
- Where sudden deterioration in oxygenation occurs always check the delivery system for empty cylinders, disconnected tubing, etc.

Indications

- Type I respiratory failure
- Type II respiratory failure (controlled therapy)
- Bronchial asthma
- Acute myocardial infarction
- Sickle cell crisis
- Carbon monoxide poisoning
- Cluster headaches

Complications

- Tracheobronchitis occurs with inhalation of $\geqslant 80\%$ oxygen for over 12 hours and presents as retrosternal pain, cough, and dyspnoea.
- Parenchymal lung damage from oxygen occurs with $F_iO_2 > 60\%$ for more than 48 hours without intermittent periods of breathing air.

Monitoring oxygen therapy

- The results of oxygen therapy should generally be measured by intermittent or continuous oximetry and intermittent arterial blood gases.
- Oximetry is an invaluable aid, but has limitations. In some situations (e.g. Guillain-Barré syndrome) falling oximetry is a very late marker of impending respiratory failure, and CO_2 accumulation (e.g. in COAD) is clearly not monitored by oximetry.
- A S_aO_2 of 93% correlates very approximately with a P_aO_2 of 8kPa, and below 92% the P_aO_2 may fall disproportionately quickly.

Principles of respiratory support 2.

Lung expansion techniques

- Periodic 'sighs' are a normal part of breathing and reverse micro-atelectasis. Lung expansion techniques are indicated for patients who cannot or will not take periodic large breaths (e.g. post abdominal or chest surgery, neuromuscular chest wall weakness).
- Post operative techniques used commonly by physiotherapists include incentive spirometry, coached maximal inspiration with cough, combined with postural drainage and chest percussion.
- Volume generating devices such as **'the BIRD'** are triggered by the patient initiating inspiration, and deliver a pre-set tidal volume to augment the patient's breath. Liaise with your physiotherapist.
- Several other 'volume-generating' devices are available, such as the **'Bromptonpac'**, which trigger via a nasal mask. Contact the chest team or anaesthetisis to set up.
- 'Pressure-generating' techniques (such as CPAP, NIPPV, and BiPAP) have the advantage that even if a leak develops around the mask, the ventilator is able to 'compensate' to provide the patient with the prescribed positive pressure (see below).
- For both volume and pressure generating techniques, the patients must be able to protect their airway and generate enough effort to trigger the machine.

Continuous positive airways pressure (CPAP)

- CPAP provides a constant positive pressure throughout the respiratory cycle.
- It acts to splint open collapsing alveoli which may be full of fluid (or a collapsing upper airway in obstructive sleep apnoea), increases functional residual capacity (FRC) and compliance, such that the work of breathing is reduced and gas exchange is improved.
- It allows a higher F_iO_2 (approaching 80–100%) to be administered, cf. standard oxygen delivery masks.
- CPAP should usually be commenced after liaison with anaesthetists; in a patient for active management it should usually be started on the ITU.
- A standard starting pressure is 5cmH$_2$O; > 10cmH$_2$O pressure is rarely used.

Indications

- Acute respiratory failure (e.g. secondary to infection), where simple face mask oxygen is insufficient at treating hypoxamia.
- Acute resporatory failure where ventilation is either inappropriate or to be avoided if at all possible.
- Weaning from the ventilator.
- Obstructive sleep apnoea (OSA).
- In those for active management it is not a substitute for ventilation, and usually only buys a modest amount of time before intubation is required.
- Patient needs to :
  - be awake and alert
  - be able to protect the airway
  - possess adequate respiratory muscle strength
  - be haemodynamically stable

Mechanical ventilation

Negative pressure ventilation (NPV)

- This works by 'sucking' out the chest wall and is used in chronic hypo-ventilation (e.g. polio, kyphoscoliosis, or muscle disease). Expiration is passive.

- The 'iron lung' or tank ventilator is the most well known; alternatives include thoracic cuirasses with a semi-rigid cage around the chest only and other devices which may be custom built.

- These techniques do not require tracheal intubation. However, access to the patient for nursing care is difficult, and positive pressure ventilation is the modality of choice in the acute setting; the patient may be extubated in a 'tank ventilator' once the acute episode is over.

- Alternative devices such as rocking beds may be considered for stable patients requiring long term-ventilatory assistance.[1]

Intermittent positive pressure ventilation (IPPV)

Indications

Deteriorating gas exchange due to a potentially reversible cause of respiratory failure (p178–182).

- Pneumonia
- Exacerbation of COAD
- Massive atelectasis
- Respiratory muscle weakness
  Myaesthenia gravis
  Acute infective polyneuritis

- Head injury
- Cerebral hypoxia
  (e.g. post cardiac arrest)
- Intracranial bleed
- Raised intracranial pressure
- Major trauma or burns

- Ventilation of the ill patient on the ITU is via either an ET tube or a tracheostomy. If ventilation is anticipated to be needed for > 1 week, consider a tracheostomy.

There are two basic types of ventilator.

- **Pressure cycled ventilators** deliver gas into the lungs until a prescribed pressure is reached, when inspiratory flow stops and, after a short pause, expiration occurs by passive recoil. This has the advantage of reducing the peak airway pressures without impairing cardiac performance in situations such as ARDS. However, if the airway pressures increase or compliance decreases the tidal volume will fall, so patients need to be monitored closely to avoid hypoventilation.

- **Volume cycled ventilators** deliver a preset tidal volume into the lungs over a predetermined inspiratory time (usually ~ 30% of the breathing cycle), hold the breath in the lungs (for ~ 10% of the cycle), and then allow passive expiration as the lungs recoil.

---

[1] Hill NS (1986) *Chest* **90**: 897.

Nasal ventilation

- Nasal intermittent positive pressure ventilation (NIPPV) delivers a positive pressure for a prescribed inspiratory time, when triggered by the patient initiating a breath, allowing the patient to exhale to atmospheric pressure.

- The positive pressure is supplied by a small machine via a tight-fitting nasal mask.

- It is generally used as a method of home nocturnal ventilation for patients with severe musculoskeletal chest wall disease (e.g. kyphoscoliosis) or with obstructive sleep apnoea (OSA).

- It has also been used with modest success as an alternative to formal ventilation via ET tube in patients where positive <u>expiratory</u> pressure is not desirable, e.g. acute asthma, COAD with CO_2 retention, and as a weaning aid in those in whom separation from a ventilator is proving difficult.

- The system is relatively easy to set up by experienced personnel, but some patients take to it better than others. It should not be commenced by inexperienced personnel.

Positive pressure ventilation   1.

CMV (continuous mandatory ventilation)

- CMV acts on a preset cycle to deliver a given number of breaths per minute of a set volume. The duration of the cycle determines the breath frequency.

  The *minute volume* is calculated by (*tidal volume* x *frequency*).

- The relative proportions of time spent in inspiration and expiration (I:E ratio) is normally set at 1:2, but may be altered, e.g. in acute asthma, where air trapping is a problem, a longer expiratory time is needed (p168); in ARDS, where the lung compliance is low, a longer inspiratory time is beneficial (inverse ratio ventilation, see p190)

- The patients should be fully sedated. Patients capable of spontaneous breaths who are ventilated on CMV can get 'stacking' of breaths, where the ventilator working on its preset cycle may give a breath on top of one which the patient has just taken, leading to over-inflation of the lungs, a high peak inspiratory pressure, and the risk of pneumo-thorax.

- Prolonged use of this mode will result in atrophy of the respiratory muscles; this may prove difficult in subsequent 'weaning', especially in combination with a proximal myopathy from steroids, e.g. in acute asthma.

- Ventilation may either be terminated abruptly or by gradual transfer of the ventilatory workload from the machine to the patient ('weaning').

SIMV (synchronized intermittent mandatory ventilation)

- SIMV modes allow the patient to breath spontaneously and be effect-ively ventilated and allows gradual transfer of the work of breathing on to the patient. This may be appropriate when weaning the patient whose respiratory muscles have wasted. It is inappropriate in acutely ill patients (e.g. acute severe asthma, ARDS); CMV with deep sedation reduces oxygen requirement and respiratory drive and allows more effective ventilation.

- Exact details of the methods of synchronization vary between machines, but all act in a similar manner: the patient breathes spontaneously through the ventilator circuit. The ventilator is usually preset to ensure that the patient has a minimum number of breaths per minute, and if the number of spontaneous breaths falls below the preset level then a breath is delivered by the machine.

- Most SIMV modes of ventilation provide some form of positive pressure support to the patient's spontaneous breaths to reduce the work of breathing and ensure effective ventilation (see below).

Pressure support

- Positive pressure is added during inspiration to relieve part or all of the work of breathing.

- This may be done in conjunction with an SIMV mode of ventilation, or as a means of supporting entirely spontaneous patient-triggered ventilation during the process of weaning.

- It allows the patients to determine their own respiratory rate, and should ensure adequate inflation of the lungs and oxygenation. It is, however, only suitable for those whose lung function is reasonably adequate and who are not confused or exhausted.

Positive pressure ventilation 2.

PEEP (positive end expiratory pressure)

- PEEP is a preset pressure added to the end of expiration only, to maintain the lung volume, prevent airway or alveolar collapse, and open up atelectic or fluid-filled lung (e.g. in ARDS or cardiogenic pulmonary oedema).
- It can significantly improve oxygenation by making more of the lung available for gas exchange. However, the trade-off is an increase in intrathoracic pressure which can significantly decrease venous return and hence cardiac output. There is also an increased risk of pneumothorax.
- 'Auto-PEEP' is seen if the patient's lungs do not fully empty before the next inflation (e.g. asthma).
- In general PEEP should be kept at a level of 5–10cmH$_2$O where required, and the level adjusted in 2–3 cmH$_2$O intervals every 20–30 minutes according to a balance between oxygenation and cardiac performance.
- Measurement and interpretation if PCWP in patients on PEEP depends on the position of the catheter. PCWP will always reflect pulmonary venous presures if they are greater than PEEP. If the catheter is in an apical vessel where the PCWP is normally lower due to the effects of gravity, the pressure measured may be the alveolar (PEEP) pressure rather than the true PCWP; in a dependent area the pressures are more accurate. Removing PEEP during measurement causes marked fluctuations in haemodynamics and oxygenation and the pressures do not reflect the state once back on the ventilator.

High-tech alternatives

Where desperate situations arise these are sometimes useful.

High frequency ventilation

- The ventilator delivers either 30–250 breaths/min (high frequency positive pressure ventilation), 60–500 breaths/min (jet ventilation), or 200–2000/min (high frequency oscillation). The tidal volumes are low but turbulence and diffusion in the airways allows CO$_2$ and O$_2$ exchange.
- Rarely used. The main indications are ARDS unresponsive to conventional ventilation techniques (p188–192) or a bronchopleural fistula.

Extracorporeal gas exchange (ECGE)

- ECMO (extra-corporeal membrane oxygenation) is a form of partial cardiopulmonary bypass that may be used for some patients with ARDS. It has no survival advantage over conventional techniques. Extracorporeal CO$_2$ removal is more effective.

IVOX (Intravascular oxygenation)

- The device consists of multiple fine microtubes through which oxygen is passed. It can be inserted percutaneously via the femoral vein into the IVC where gas exchange occurs by passive diffusion.

Cricothyroidotomy

Indications

- To bypass upper airway obstruction (e.g. trauma, infections, neo-plasms, post operative, burns and corrosives) when oral or naso-tracheal intubation is contraindicated.
- In situations when endotracheal intubations fail (e.g. massive naso-pharyngeal haemorrhage, structural deformities, obstruction due to foreign bodies, etc.)
- As an elective procedure in select patients to provide a route for suction of airway secretions (e.g. patients in neuromuscular disease). This should be converted to a tracheotomy if required for prolonged periods or if infection or inflammation occurs.

Procedure

This should **not** be attempted if you have not been taught it by an experienced physician/surgeon. Seek help.

- Locate the thyroid and cricoid cartilages.
- The cricothyoird space is just under 1cm in its vertical dimension. The cricothyroid artery runs across the mid-line in the upper portion.
- Clean the skin with iodine and isolate the area with sterile towels.
- Infiltrate the skin and the area around the cricothyroid space with local anaesthetic.
- Make a 3cm vertical mid-line incision through the skin, taking care not to cut the membrane.
- Palpate the cricothyroid membrane through the incision.
- Stabilize the larynx by holding between the index finger and thumb.
- Make a short transverse incision in the lower third of the cricothyroid membrane, just scraping over the upper part of the cricoid cartilage (preferably using the tip of a No. 11 blade to go through the mem-brane). This minimizes the risk of cutting the cricothyroid artery.
- Dilate the membrane with forceps, insert the tracheotomy tube through the incision into the trachea, and secure.

Percutaneous cricothyrotomy using the Seldinger technique is quicker, may be performed by non-surgeons at the bedside, and is safer. See figure. After anaesthetizing the area, a needle is used to puncture the crico-thyroid membrane and through this a guide-wire is introduced into the trachea. Over this a series of dilators and the tracheostomy tube can be safely positioned.

Complications of cricothyrotomy

- Haemorrhage – usually due to damage to the cricothyroid artery
- Tube misplacement may occur in up to 15% of cases
- Subglottic stenosis
- Hoarseness
- Laryngotracheal-cutaneous fistula

(a)

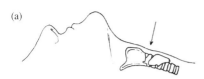

(b)

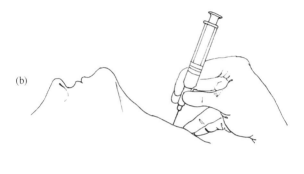

(c)

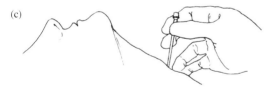

Needle cricothyroidotomy

Endotracheal intubation

This is the best method for providing and maintaining a clear airway for ventilation, protection against aspiration, and suctioning and clearing lower respiratory tract secretions. The most common indication for urgent intubation by a physician is cardiac arrest. This is not a technique for the inexperienced: the description below is not intended as a substitute for practice under supervision of a skilled anaesthetist.

You will need
- Laryngoscope, usually with a curved blade (Macintosh)
- Endotracheal tube (8–9mm internal diameter for men and 7–8mm for women) and appropriate adaptors
- Syringe for cuff inflation and clamp to prevent air escaping from the cuff once inflated
- Scissors and tape or bandage to secure the tube
- Lubricating jelly (e.g. KY jelly ®)
- Suction apparatus with rigid (Yankauer) and long flexible catheters

Potential problems during intubation
- Certain anatomical variations (e.g. receding mandible, short neck, prominent incisors, high arched palate) as well as stiff neck or trismus may make intubation complicated; summon experienced help.
- Vomiting: suction if necessary. Cricoid pressure may be of use.
- Cervical spine injury: immobilize the head and neck in line with the body and try not to extend the head during intubation.
- Facial burns or trauma may make orotracheal intubation impossible. Consider cricothyroidotomy (see p810).

Procedure
- Place the patient with the neck slightly flexed and the head extended. Take care if cervical injury is suspected.
- Cricoid pressure: The oesophagus can be occluded by compressing the cricoid cartilage posteriorly against the body of C6. This prevents passive regurgitation into the trachea but not active vomiting. Ask your assistant to maintain pressure until the tube is in place and the cuff inflated.
- Pre-oxygenate the patient by hyperventilation with ≥ 85% oxygen for 15–30 seconds. Open the mouth and suction to clear the airway.
- With the laryngoscope in your left hand, insert the blade on right side of mouth. Advance to base of tongue, identifying the tonsillar fossa and the uvula. Push the blade to the left moving the tongue over. Advance the blade until the epiglottis comes into view.
- Insert the blade tip between the base of the tongue and the epiglottis (into the vallecula) and pull the whole blade (and larynx) upwards along the line of the handle of the laryngoscope to expose the vocal cords. Brief suction may be necessary to clear the view.
- Insert the ET tube between the vocal cords and advance it until the cuff is just below the cords and no further. Inflate the cuff with air.
- If the cords cannot be seen, do not poke at the epiglottis hoping for success, call for more skilled help and revert to basic airway management.
- Intubation must not take longer than 30 seconds; if there is any doubt about the position, remove the tube, reoxygenate, and try again.
- With the tube in place, listen to the chest during inflation to check that BOTH sides of the chest are ventilated. If the tube is in the oesophagus, chest expansion will be minimal though the stomach may inflate; air entry into the chest will be minimal.
- Tie the ET tube in place and secure to prevent it from slipping up or down the airway. Ventilate with high concentration oxygen.

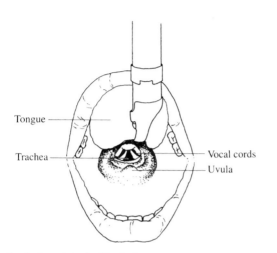

Landmarks for endotracheal intubation

Aspiration of a pneumothorax

If the pneumothorax is < 75% and the patient is haemodynamically stable, it is reasonable to attempt aspiration of the pneumothorax in the first instance (see p186).

You will need the following:

- 10ml and 50ml syringe with green (18G) and orange (25G) needles
- Dressing pack (swabs, sterile drapes, antiseptic) and sterile gloves
- 19G Venflon® or alternative cannula
- Local anaesthetic (e.g. 2% lignocaine)
- Three-way tap

Procedure

- 1 assistant is required.
- Sit patient up, propped against pillows with hand behind his/her head; ensure you are comfortable and on a similar level.
- Select the space to aspirate, the 2nd intercostal space in the mid-clavicular line. Confirm with CXR that you are aspirating the correct side (a surprisingly common cause of disasters is aspirating the normal side).
- Clean the skin and use aseptic technique.
- Connect a 50ml syringe to a three-way tap in readiness, with the line which will be connected to the patient turned 'off' so that no air will enter the pleural cavity on connecting the apparatus.
- Infiltrate 5–10ml of lignocaine from skin to pleura, just above the upper border of the rib in the space you are using. Confirm the presence of air by aspirating approximately 5ml via a green needle.
- Insert a 16G or larger intravenous cannula into the pneumothorax, preferably whilst aspirating the cannula with a syringe, so that entry into the pleural space is confirmed. Allow the tip of the cannula to enter the space by approximately 1cm.
- Ask the patient to hold their breath and remove the needle. Swiftly connect the 3–way tap. Aspirate 50ml of air/ fluid and void it through the other lumen of the tap. Repeat.
- Aspiration should be stopped when resistance to suction is felt, the patient coughs excessively, or ≥ 2.5 litres of air has been aspirated.
- Withdraw the cannula and cover the site with a dressing plaster (e.g. Elastoplast or Band-aid)
- Check post procedure CXR. If there is significant residual pneumothorax insert a chest drain.

Aspiration of a pleural effusion

The basic procedure is similar to that for a pneumothorax – the site is different: one or two intercostal spaces posteriorly below the level at which dullness is detected. Ideally all cases should have an USS first to confirm the level of the effusion and ensure that the diaphragm is not higher than anticipated due to underlying pulmonary collapse.

- Position the patient leaning forward over the back of a chair or table. Clean the skin and infiltrate with local anaesthetic as above.
- Insert the cannula and aspirate the effusion with a 50ml syringe, voiding it through the 3–way tap. Repeat until resistance is felt and the tap is dry.
- Check a post procedure CXR.

Insertion of a chest drain   1.

You will need the following:

- Dressing pack (sterile gauze, gloves, drapes, Betadine®)
- Local anaesthetic (~ 20ml 1% lignocaine), 10ml syringe, green (18G) and orange (25G) needles.
- Scalpel and No. 11 blade for skin incision; 2 packs silk sutures (1–0)
- 2 forceps (Kelly clamps), scissors, needle holder (often pre-packaged as a 'chest drain set')
- Chest tubes – a selection of 24, 28, 32, and 36 Fr
- Chest drainage bottles, with sterile water for underwater seal
- 1 assistant

Procedure

- Position the patient leaning forward over the back of a chair or table. If possible, premedicate the patient with an appropriate amount of opiate ~ 30 minutes before.
- Mark the space to be drained in the mid-axillary line; usually the 5th intercostal space for pneumothorax, below the level of the fluid for an effusion. Clean the skin.
- Select the chest tube: small (24 Fr) for air alone, medium (28 Fr) for serous fluid, or large (32–36 Fr) for blood/pus. Remove the trocar. Check that the underwater seal bottles are ready.
- Infiltrate the skin with 15–20ml of lignocaine 1%. Make a short sub-cutaneous tunnel for the chest tube before it enters the pleural space (see figure). Anaesthetize the periosteum on the top of the rib. Check that you can aspirate air/fluid from the pleural space.
- Make a horizontal 2cm incision in the anaesthetized skin of the rib space. Use the forceps to blunt-dissect through the fat and intercostal muscles to make a track large enough for your gloved finger down to the pleural space. Stay close to the upper border of the rib to avoid the neurovascular bundle.
- Check the length of the tube against the patient's chest to confirm how much needs to be inserted into the patient's chest. Aim to get the tip to the apex for a pneumothorax; keep the lowermost hole as low as possible (~ 2cm into the chest) to drain pleural fluid.
- Insert two sutures across the incision (or a purse-string, see figure opposite). These will gently tighten around the tube once inserted to create an airtight seal but do not knot – these sutures will be used to close the wound after drain removal.
- Remove the trocar. Clamp the end of the tube with the forceps and gently introduce the tube into the pleural space. Rotating the forceps 180° directs the tube to the apex (see figure). Condensation in the tube (or fluid) confirms the tube is within the pleural space. Check that all the holes are within the thorax and connect to the underwater seal. Tape these to the skin
- Gently tighten the skin sutures (see above) but do not knot. The drain should be secured with several other stitches and copious amounts of adhesive tape. They are very vulnerable to accidental traction. Wrap adhesive tape around the join between the drain and the connecting tubing.
- Prescribe adequate analgesia for the patient for when the anaesthetic wears off.
- Arrange for a CXR to check the position of the drain.
- Do not drain off more than 1 litre of pleural fluid/24 hours to avoid re-expansion pulmonary oedema.

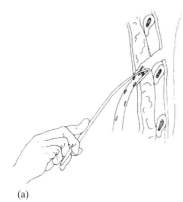

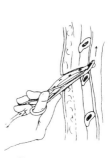

(a)

(b)

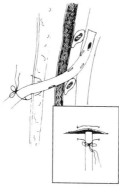

(c)

Insertion of a chest drain   2.

Tips and pitfalls

- The chest drain should only be left in place while air or fluid continue to drain. The risk of ascending infection increases with time. Prophylactic antibiotics are not usually indicated.
- **Malpositioned tube**: Obtain a CXR post procedure (and daily) to check the position of the drain and examine the lung fields
  - If the drain is too far out, there will be an air leak and the patient may develop sub-cutaneous emphysema. Ideally, remove the drain and replace with a new drain at a new site; the risk of ascending infection is high if the 'non-sterile' portion of the tube is just pushed into the chest.
  - If the drain is too far in, it may be uncomfortable for the patient and impinge on vital structures (e.g. thoracic aorta). Pull the tube out the appropriate distance and re-suture.
- **Obstructed tube**: Check the water column in the chest drain bottle swings with respiration. This will stop if the tube is obstructed.
  - Check the drains and tubing are free of bends and kinks.
  - Blood clots or fibrin may block the tube and may be 'milked' cautiously.
  - If the lung is still collapsed on CXR, replace the chest drain with a new tube at a new site.
- **Lung fails to re-expand**: This is either due to an obstructed system or persistent air leak (e.g. tracheobronchial fistula).
  - If the chest drain continues to bubble, apply suction to the drain to help expand the lung. Consider inserting further drains or surgical repair of leak.
  - If the chest drain is obstructed (see above), replace the drain.
- **Removing the chest drain**
  - DO NOT clamp the chest drain.
  - Remove the dressings and release the sutures holding the drain in place. Leave the skin incision sutures (purse-string) in position to close the wound once the drain is removed.
  - Remove the drain in a gentle motion, either in inspiration or in expiration with Valsalva.
  - Tighten the skin sutures. These should be removed after 3–4 days and a fresh dressing applied.
  - Any residual pneumothorax should be treated depending on the patient's symptoms, with a fresh chest drain if necessary.

Complications

- Bleeding (intercostal vessels, laceration of lung, spleen, liver)
- Pulmonary oedema (too rapid lung expansion)
- Empyema
- Sub-cutaneous emphysema
- Residual pneumothorax or effusion (malpositioned or obstructed chest drain)

Ascitic tap

Indications

- Diagnose or exclude spontaneous bacterial peritonitis (SBP)
- Ascitic protein
- Ascitic cytology may require 100ml fluid
- Ascitic amylase (pancreatic ascites)
- Stain and culture for AFBs; lymphocyte count (N < 500 cells/mm^3)
- To drain cirrhotic or malignant ascites for patient comfort or fluid overload

	Transudate	Exudate
Total protein	< 30g/l	$\geqslant$ 30g/l
LDH	< 225IU/l	$\geqslant$ 225IU/l
Ascitic protein : serum protein	< 0.5	> 0.5
Ascitic LDH : serum LDH	< 0.6	> 0.6

Ascitic tap

- Lie patient supine, and tilted slightly to the left or right.
- Select the site (level with umbilicus, and 2–3 cm lateral to a line passing to mid-inguinal point) and clean the area with iodine or equivalent. Ensure the bladder is empty and avoid any scars.
- Use a 20ml syringe with a 18G (green) needle. In obese patients use a longer needle (e.g. 18G Abbocath®). If you plan to use a larger needle, infiltrate the area with local anaesthetic before proceeding.
- Insert the needle slowly into the abdomen whilst aspirating until fluid is obtained. If blood is obtained, remove the needle and apply pressure to the puncture site for 2 minutes, and try at a different site.
- Inoculate 5mls of the fluid into each bottle of a set of blood culture bottles (in cirrhotics for ?bacterial peritonitis) and send some in a sterilin® or plain bottle for microscopy (5ml) and protein (1ml).
- Remove the needle and apply a sterile plaster over the puncture site

Causes of transudative and exudative ascites	
Transudative ascites	*Exudative ascites*
• Cirrhosis	• Cirrhosis (rarely)
• Cardiac failure	• Pancreatic
• Nephrotic syndrome	• Tuberculous peritonitis
	• Budd-Chiari syndrome (hepatic vein thrombosis)
	• Malignancy

N.B. Most causes of transudates can also give rise to exudates and vice versa.

Total paracentesis

Daily small volume paracentesis is time-consuming, unnecessary, and increases the risk of infection and ascitic leakage. It is dangerous to leave a peritoneal tap catheter in place for more than a few hours. The risk of infection in our experience is great. It is safer to drain the ascites to dryness.

The rate of fluid drainage should be as fast as possible. During the first 3–6 hours of paracentesis, there is a significant increase in cardiac output, a decrease in systemic vascular resistance, and a modest fall in mean arterial pressure (by 5–10mmHg). In the presence of tense ascites the right atrial pressure (RAP) may be artificially elevated by transmitted intra-abdominal pressure, and RAP may fall acutely by ~ 3–5cm water. Thus fluid replacement is essentail.

- Use either a Kuss needle (if available), a large 14G long Abbocath® (used for central lines), a peritoneal dialysis catheter or a Swan-Ganz introducer (8.5F and rather large for the purpose).

- To avoid the catheter blocking due to omentum plugging the end, remove the metal introducer under strict aseptic conditions, and carefully make several perforations in the plastic of the catheter using a green or blue needle. Avoid holes close together and re-insert the metal introducer needle very carefully to avoid causing a tear in the cannula (this would increase the risk of the cannula breaking off in the abdomen). Note – the manufacturers do not recommend this; some companies produce special catheters with pre-formed side-holes. Always use these if available.

- Take a 'drip set' (iv fluid 'giving set') and, with a sterile blade, cut off the reservoir, leaving the tubing, luer locking device, and rate control mechanism. If a PD cannula or other device is used then some form of tubing needs to be attached to facilitate drainage.

- Position the patient supine and slightly tilted to one side. Select, clean, and infiltrate the site with 2% lignocaine as for ascitic tap.

- Insert the cannula (attached to a 20ml syringe), aspirating as one advances the cannula. When ascitic fluid is obtained, advance the needle ~ 5mm more, then advance the plastic cannula holding the metal introducer, ready to prevent it going any deeper (as for inserting a Venflon®).

- Remove the metal introducer and attach the drainage tube (modified 'giving set'). Strap the introducer to the abdominal wall with elastoplast. It is not necessary to suture the cannula in place since it will be removed within 3–4 hours.

- Drain the ascites as rapidly as possible into an appropriate receptacle (have bucket to hand for emptying the contents).

- When the ascites stops draining or slows down, move the patient from side to side, and lie towards the drainage site.

- When drainage is complete, remove the catheter, apply plaster, and lie the patient with the drainage site uppermost for at least 4 hours.

Insertion of Sengstaken-Blakemore or Minnesota tube

The Sengstaken-Blakemore or Minnesota tube are inserted to control variceal bleeding when other measures (injection sclerotherapy, intravenous vasopressin, or octreotide) have failed. It should not be used as the primary therapy of bleeding varices since it is unpleasant, and increases the risk of oesophageal ulceration. If placed in the unintubated patient there is a very real risk of aspiration.

Seek experienced or specialist help early. Balloon tamponade is not a definitive procedure: make arrangements for variceal injection or oesophageal transection once the patient is stable. Continue infusions of vasopressin or octreotide (p488–90).

You will need the following:
- Sengstaken or Minnesota tube
- Bladder syringe (for balloons)
- Sphygmomanometer
- X-ray contrast (diluted)

Procedure
- It is assumed that the patient is already being resuscitated, and is receiving intravenous vasopressin or octreotide (p488). The patient should ideally be intubated and ventilated. If not, there is an increased risk of aspiration. This risk may be reduced in the unintubated patient by injecting 10mg metoclopramide immediately before insertion. This can cause temporary cessation of haemorrhage and reduce the aspiration risk. Have a low threshold for sedation, endotracheal intubation, and ventilation.
- The SBT or Minnesota tube should be stored in the fridge (to maximize stiffness) and removed just before use. Familiarize yourself with the various parts before insertion if necessary. Check the integrity of the balloons before you insert the tube.
- Place an endoscope protection mouthguard in place (to prevent biting of the tube). Cover the end of the tube with KY jelly, and, with the patient in the left semi-prone position, push the tube down, asking the patient to swallow (if conscious). If the tube curls up in the mouth, try again or try another cooled tube.
- Insert at least 50cm, and start inflating the gastric balloon with 200ml water containing gastrografin (this enables the balloon to be visualized on a CXR or AXR). Clamp the balloon channel. Then gently pull back on the tube until the gastric balloon abuts the gastro-oesophageal junction (resistance felt), then pull further until the patient is beginning to be tugged by pulling. Note the position at the edge of the mouth piece (mark with pen), and attach with elastoplast to the side of the face. Weight contraptions should not be necessary.
- In general the oesophageal balloon should never be used. Virtually all bleeding varices occur at the oesophagogastric junction and are controlled using this technique.
- If the bleeding continues, inflate the oesophageal balloon. Connect this to a sphygmomanometer via a 3–way tap to monitor the balloon pressure. Inflate to 40mmHg and close the 3–way tap. Check the pressure in this balloon every 1–2 hours. Do not deflate every hour.
- Do NOT leave the balloons inflated for more than 12 hours since this increases the risk of oesophageal ulceration.
- Obtain a CXR to check the position of the tube.
- The gastric channel should be aspirated continuously.
- If facilities for variceal injection are available, remove the SBT or MT immediately prior to endoscopy. If not, discuss the patient with your regional centre and transfer if appropriate.

Insertion of Sengstaken-Blakemore tube

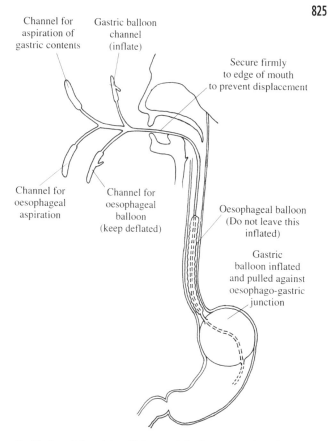

Channel for aspiration of gastric contents

Gastric balloon channel (inflate)

Secure firmly to edge of mouth to prevent displacement

Channel for oesophageal aspiration

Channel for oesophageal balloon (keep deflated)

Oesophageal balloon (Do not leave this inflated)

Gastric balloon inflated and pulled against oesophago-gastric junction

Positioning of Sengstaken-Blakemore tube for compression of oesophageal varicies

Transjugular liver biopsy

Indications

It is not without risk, and should not be applied merely to obtain histology for completeness.

- Bleeding diathesis contraindicating conventional biopsy techniques
- The biopsy will assist diagnosis and subsequent management

Procedure

This is relatively straight-forward, and is based on the assumption that by taking the biopsy through the hepatic vein any bleeding will occur into circulation.

A large introducer is placed into the internal jugular vein or femoral vein. A catheter is introduced through this and manipulated into the hepatic vein. The catheter is removed leaving a guide wire *in situ*. A metal transjugular biopsy needle is passed over the wire and advanced into the hepatic vein. One has to avoid being too peripheral (risk of capsular puncture). The wire is removed, and the needle advanced whilst suction is applied. A biopsy is obtained by the 'Menghini' technique. The biopsies obtained are much poorer than those obtained by conventional techniques.

Transjugular intrahepatic porto-systemic shunt (TIPSS)

Indications

- Uncontrolled or recurrent bleeding of oesophageal or gastric varices
- Diuretic resistant ascites

Principle

To lower the portal pressure acutely, a shunt is placed between a hepatic vein and portal vein tributary. Blood then flows from the high pressure portal system to the lower pressure hepatic venous system which drains into the ivC. The lowered portal pressure then makes bleeding from oesophageal varices less likely.

It is carried out in relatively few specialist centres and is technically quite difficult. Its advantage is that it does not require a general anaesthetic, the risk is lower than for a formal portacaval or mesocaval shunt procedure, and it does not hinder future liver transplantation. The centres carrying out most of these procedures in the UK are The Royal Free Hospital, London, Newcastle RI, Edinburgh RI, and Addenbrookes, Cambridge. Contact your regional centre if you feel this may be appropriate.

Method

The internal jugular vein is catheterized, and a cannula passed through the right atrium into the IVC, and into an hepatic vein. The portal vein is localized by USS, and a metal transjugular biopsy needle advanced through the liver substance into one of the portal vein tributaries (usually right portal vein). A wire is then passed into the portal vein and the metal needle withdrawn, leaving the wire joining the hepatic vein and portal vein. An expandable stent is then passed over the wire, and expanded by balloon inflation. A typical stent size is 8–12mm.

Complications

- The mortality is ~ 3%, usually from a capsular puncture.
- Hepatic encephalopathy occurs in ~ 20%.
- Failure to reduce portal pressure may occur if there are large extra-hepatic shunts. These may need to be embolized.

Percutaneous liver biopsy

Procedure

- Obtain patient consent, warning of risk of bleeding, pneumothorax, gall-bladder puncture, and failed biopsy. Warn about shoulder tip pain, which may last several hours.
- Ensure prothrombin time is < 3 seconds prolonged cf. control, and the platelet count is $> 80 \times 10^9$/l, and that there is no other bleeding diathesis (e.g. severe renal failure in which platelet function is impaired). Other contraindications are ascites, and possibly tumour depending on planned management (risk of tumour seeding).
- If available always use ultrasound guidance, especially if the liver is small and cirrhotic.
- You will need a biopsy needle (Tru-cut or Menghini), 1% lignocaine, an orange (25G) and green (18G) needle, 5ml syringe, a No. 11 scalpel blade, iodine or equivalent, sterile towels, a plaster, sterile gloves, a dressing pack, and a bottle of formalin.
- Pre-medicate the patient with an appropriate amount of analgesia (e.g. 30–60mg dihydrocodeine) 15–30 minutes before the procedure.
- Lie the patient supine with the right hand behind their head. Percuss the upper border of the liver in expiration and mark with a pen. Select a site 2 intercostal space below the upper border, making sure it is not too close to the costal margin (and thence gall-bladder).
- Clean the skin with antiseptic and infiltrate with lignocaine as far as the capsule. Always go just above a rib, and make an incision with the scalpel to facilitate the larger biopsy needle passing through the skin. The capsule is felt as a grating feeling, and if the syringe is allowed to float on the palm of the hand will be seen to move with gentle respiration when the tip of the needle has penetrated the capsule. Do not prevent the needle from moving with respiration as this will increase the risk of capsular tear, and do NOT ask the patient to breathe deeply with the needle in this position.
- Remove the needle. Rehearse the patient asking them to breathe in, then out and stop (in expiration). It is imperative during the actual biopsy that they do not take a sudden gasp of breath. Rehearse it several times. We find it useful to keep saying 'stop, stop' etc. until the biopsy is complete. Avoid saying 'hold' since many patients will then breathe in at the crucial moment.
- Make a small skin incision with the scalpel and insert the biopsy needle when the patient is at end expiration.
- After the biopsy (do not attempt more than 2 passes), place a plaster over the site and ask the patient to lie on their right side for 4 hours.
- Nursing observations are pulse and bp every 15 minutes for 1 hour, every 30 minutes for 2 hours, hourly for 3 hours, 2 hourly for 8 hours. Avoid evening or late afternoon biopsies.

Plugged biopsy technique

This technique is used if there is a mild bleeding diathesis, and can be performed when the prothrombin time is up to 6 seconds prolonged with a platelet count of $> 40,000$mm.[3] The biopsy is done through a sheath and the tract embolized using Gelfoam to try to prevent bleeding. Seek experienced help.

Acute peritoneal dialysis

Does not require vascular access or anti-coagulation. Provides insufficient dialysis for the hypercatabolic patient. (Creatinine clearance rate of ~ 10ml/min may be achieved). This requires:-

- Peritoneal dialysis catheter (may be inserted under LA on the ward)
- Intact peritoneal cavity free of infection, herniae, adhesions

Complications of peritoneal dialysis

Peritonitis The commonest complication of CAPD : 0.8 episode/pt/yr. Infection occurs through the lumen of the catheter, along catheter tract, transmurally from GIT, or haematogenously (rare).

Assessment
- Common features are cloudy PD bag (99%), abdominal pain (95%), and abdominal tenderness (80%).
- Other features include fever (33%), nausea and vomiting (30%), leucocytosis (25%), diarrhoea or constipation (15%).
- Investigations: PD effluent cell count (peritonitis if > 100 neutrophils/mm^3), culture PD fluid (inoculate a blood culture bottle), Gram stain PD fluid, FBC (for leukocytosis), blood cultures.

Management
- All patients require antibiotics, but may not require admission. The antibiotics used depends on Gram stain and culture results. A typical protocol would be ciprofloxacin or vancomycin, plus metronidazole. Patients who have high fever with leukocytosis, and/or who are systemically unwell warrant iv antibiotics.
- Gram-negative infection, in particular *Pseudomonas*, is associated with more severe infection. Severe episodes may be accompanied by ileus, whatever the organism.
- If pain is prominent, give analgesia (opiate) and consider intermittent peritoneal dialysis (IPD) instead of PD.
- Patients may lose up to 25g protein/day in severe cases and should receive adequate nutritional support.
- If the infection is resistant to treatment, consider removal of Tenckhoff catheter and atypical organisms (e.g. fungi).
- Consider underlying gastrointestinal pathology especially if multi-bacterial, Gram-negative organisms, or other symptoms.

Fluid overload

Mild cases may respond to hypertonic exchanges (6.36% or 4.25% dextrose), fluid restriction (1 litre/day), and large doses of diuretics (e.g. frusemide 500mg bd). With pulmonary oedema, fluid removal is best achieved by rapid cycle IPD (4.25% dextrose, 60 min cycle time).

Poor exchanges
- Constipation may cause malposition of catheter
- Malpositioned catheter: The catheter should sit in pelvis, but occasionally flips upwards to lie against the diaphragm, causing shoulder tip pain and poor drainage. If the patient is constipated try laxatives, but may require surgical repositioning.
- Omentum wrapping around tip of catheter can be prevented by omentectomy at time of insertion.
- Fibrin debris blocking catheter seen as white deposits in effluent. Treat by addition of heparin (1000U/litre) to bags.

Hyperglycaemia

A significant amount of the dextrose in peritoneal dialysis solutions is absorbed (especially with 'heavy' 4.26% dextrose bags). Renal failure induces insulin resistance, so an elevated blood glucose may occur, as well as hypercholesterolaemia. Diabetic patients require special attention to insulin therapy.

Intermittent haemodialysis

A blood flow of ~ 250–300ml/min is needed across the dialysis membrane. The equivalent clearance obtained is approximately 20ml/min.

- **Vascular access.** Vascular access may be obtained by fashioning an AV shunt using the radial artery, or more commonly by using a Vascath which uses venous rather than arterial blood. This involves cannulation of the internal jugular, subclavian, or femoral vein.
- **Anti-coagulation.** Heparin is normally used. If contraindicated, e.g. recent haemorrhage, then prostacyclin may be used, but may cause hypotension and abdominal cramps.
- **Haemodynamic stability.** Patients with multi-organ failure commonly develop hypotension during haemodialysis. This may be ameliorated by high sodium dialysate, and priming the circuit with 4.5% human albumin solution.

Complications of haemodialysis

Hypotension Usually occurs within the first 15 minutes of commencing dialysis. It probably involves activation of circulating inflammatory cells by the membrane, osmotic shifts, and possibly loss of fluid. *Treatment:* Cautious fluid replacement and inotropes (watch for pulmonary oedema if over-transfused).

Risk factors or exacerbating factors for hypotension
- Multi-organ failure
- Autonomic neuropathy
- Valvular lesions (e.g. mitral regurgitation, aortic stenosis)
- Arrhythmias
- Pericardial tamponade
- MI or poor LV function
- Sepsis

Line infection Central lines are a common focus of infection. When a dialysis patient develops a fever of > 38°C it should be assumed that the neck line is infected even if an alternative septic focus is known. *Management:* Take blood cultures both peripherally and from the neck line and replace the central line (avoid 'railroading' over the previous line). Treat empirically with vancomycin 750mg-1g iv in 100ml N saline over 1h at end of dialysis. Vancomycin should be given slowly or severe vasodilatation may give rise to the 'red man syndrome'. An alternative is teicoplanin 400mg iv followed by 200mg iv daily. Both drugs are poorly removed by haemodialysis, a single dose will ensure therapeutic levels for several days. 90% will be due to *Staph. aureus* or *epidermidis*. Right-sided endocarditis may occur (p96).

Dialysis disequilibrium This occurs during the initial dialysis especially in patients with marked uraemia, and is more common in paatients with pre-existing neurological disease. *Clinical features:* Headache, nausea and vomiting, fits, cerebral oedema. *Treatment:* Treat cerebral oedema as on p359. Short and slow initial dialyses may prevent this.

Dialyser reaction This is caused by an IgE or complement response against the ethylene oxide (sterilizing agent) or the cellulose component. Use of 'biocompatible' membranes [e.g. polysulfone, polyacrylonitrile (PAN)] or dialysers sterilized by steam or γ-irradiation may prevent further reactions. The circuit should also be rinsed with N saline. *Clinical features* are of allergy: Itching, urticaria, cough and wheeze. Severe reactions may cause anaphylaxis. *Management:* Stop dialysis and treat anaphylaxis (see p212) – antihistamines (chlorpheniramine 10mg iv), hydrocortisone 100mg iv, bronchodilators (salbutamol 5mg by nebulizer), and, if severe, adrenaline (1mg im).

Air embolism Rare, potentially fatal. Symptoms may vary depending on patient's position. If sitting, air may pass directly to the cerebral veins causing coma, fits, death. If lying, air may pass to R ventricle and then to pulmonary vessels causing SOB, cough, and chest tightness. *If suspected:* Clamp dialysis lines, lie patient head-down on left side, administer 100% O_2 by mask. Aspiration of air with an intracardiac needle may be attempted in extreme circumstances.

Complications of haemodialysis	
• Hypotension	• Cramps
• Line infection	• Air embolism
• Dialysis disequilibrium	• Haemorrhage
• Dialysis reaction (allergy)	

Haemofiltration and haemodiafiltation

Continuous arteriovenous haemofiltration (CAVH) implies bulk solute transport across a membrane and replacement. Haemodiafiltration (CAVHD) involves the pumping of dialysate across the other side of the membrane. For both, arterial blood (driven by arterial pressure) is continuously filtered at a relatively low flow rate (50–100ml/min). Continuous venovenous haemofiltration involves pumping blood from a venous access to the dialysis membrane (150–200ml/min) (CVVH or CVVHD). The equivalent GFR obtained by these are approximately 15–30ml/min. These are used most commonly on ITU. Both of these methods cause less haemodynamic instability, and are particularly useful in patients with multi-organ failure.

Plasmapheresis

A therapy directed towards removal of circulating high molecular weight compounds not removed by dialysis. Paticularly used in the removal of antibodies, or lipoproteins.

Indications

- Myasthenia gravis
- Guillain-Barré syndrome
- Goodpasture's syndrome
- Thrombotic thrombocytopenic purpura (TTP)
- Haemolytic uraemic syndrome (HUS)
- Severe hyperlipidaemia
- Multi-system vasculitis
- Hyperviscosity syndrome (e.g. Waldenstrom's macroglobulinaemia)
- HLA antibody removal

Method

Requires central venous access with a large bore, dual lumen cannula. Usually five treatment sessions are given on consecutive days. Plasma is removed and replaced with, typically, 2 units FFP, 3 litres 4.5% albumin. iv calcium (10ml 10% calcium gluconate) should be given with the FFP. Febrile reactions may occur as with other blood products. Plasmapheresis has no effect on the underlying rate of antibody production, but is a useful treatment in acute situations such as Goodpasture's and myasthenia gravis.

- For HUS and TTP one must use fresh frozen plasma ONLY (preferably cryodepleted), usually a minumum of 3l/day (see p564).
- For hyperviscosity syndrome, a centrifugation system is required rather than a plasma filter (see p590).
- For lipopheresis there may be severe reactions if the patient is on an ACE inhibitor.
- An alternative to plasmapharesis is immunoabsorption in which 2 columns are used in parallel. This may be used in the removal of HLA antibodies, anti-GBM disease, or multi-system vasculitis

Renal biopsy

Indications (see table opposite)

Biopsy is now performed using real-time ultrasound guidance.

Contraindications

- Bleeding diathesis – unless correctable prior to biopsy
- Solitary functioning kidney
- Uncontrolled hypertension, i.e. diastolic > 100mmHg
- Urinary tract obstruction
- Small kidneys, since it is unlikely to reveal any treatable condition
- Patient unable to comply with procedure (? biopsy under GA)

Prior to biopsy

- Check Hb, clotting screen, G&S serum.
- Ensure ivU or ultrasound has been carried out to determine presence and size of two kidneys.
- Consent patient quoting ~ 1% risk of bleeding requiring transfusion.
- Do not attempt this if you have not been taught by an expert.

Technique

- You will need a Tru-Cut or other biopsy needle (e.g. Bioptigun®). Ensure you are familiar with the workings of the needle.
- Position patient prone on bed with pillows under abdomen.
- Visualize lower pole of either kidney with ultrasound (right kidney lies more inferiorly and may be easier to image).
- Sterilize skin, drape with towels. Infiltrate local anaesthetic (10mls 2% lignocaine) under skin and to depth of kidney. Make a small skin incision with a scalpel to facilitate entry of biopsy needle.
- Insert biopsy needle as far as the renal capsule under US guidance.
- Ask patient to hold breath in at the end of inspiration (displaces kidney inferiorly) and take biopsy from lower pole.
- Apply sterile dressing.
- Bed rest for 24h to minimize risk of bleeding.
- Monitor bp and pulse half hourly for 2h, 1 hourly for 4h, then 4 hourly for 18h.
- Send renal biopsy tissue for light microscopy, immunofluorescence, and EM. Special stains (e.g. Congo red) if indicated.

Complications

- Bleeding: Microscopic haematuria is usual; macroscopic haematuria in 5–10%; bleeding requiring transfusion in 1%.
- Formation of an intrarenal AV fistula may occur, but is rarely of significance. If bleeding occurs from this, angiography and embolization may be needed.
- Loin pain if severe suggests bleeding.
- Pneumothorax is now rare.
- Ileus rarely.
- Laceration of liver, spleen, bowel rarely.

Renal transplant biopsy

Indications

- Decline in transplant function
- Primary non-function post transplant

Procedure

In principle the technique is similar to native renal biopsy, though the transplanted kidney lies more superficially in the iliac fossa. Ultrasound localization is useful. Biopsy may be taken from either upper or lower pole. Some centres find fine needle aspiration biopsy (FNAB) useful in diagnosis of transplant rejection.

Indications for renal biopsy

- Cause is unknown
- Heavy proteinuria ($> 2g/day$)
- Features of systemic disease
- Active urinary sediment
- Immune-mediated ARF
- Prolonged renal failure (> 2 weeks)
- Suspected interstitial nephritis (drug induced)

pH$_i$ determination (gastric tonometer)

Patients in shock have reduced splanchnic perfusion and oxygen delivery. The resulting mucosal ischaemia may be difficult to diagnose clinically until it presents as GI bleeding or the sepsis syndrome. The earliest change detectable following an ischaemic insult to the gut is a fall in intramucosal pH. Gastric mucosal pH parallels the changes in pH in other portions of the GI tract and monitoring this allows detection of gut ischaemia early.[2]

A tonometer is essentially an NG-tube with a second lumen leading to a balloon which lies within the mucosal folds of the stomach. The balloon is inflated with 0.9% saline for 30–90 minutes. This allows CO_2 from the mucosa to diffuse into the saline and equilibrate. The saline is then removed and analysed for pCO_2 with simultaneous arterial blood $[HCO_3^-]$ measurement. pH$_i$ is then calculated using a modification of the Henderson-Hasselbalch equation.

The correction factors and equations are supplied with the tonometer and you are advised to consult the literature that the tonometer is supplied with.

[2] Fiddian-Green RG, Baker S (1987) *Critical Care Med* **15**: 153–156.

Joint aspiration

Many synovial joints can be safely aspirated by an experienced operator. Knee effusions are common and aseptic aspiration can be safely performed in casualty. The risk of inducing a septic arthritis is less than 1 in 10,000 aspirations, but certain rules should be followed.

- Anatomical landmarks are identified
- The skin is cleaned with alcohol or iodine
- A no touch technique is essential

Indications for synovial fluid aspiration in casualty

- Suspected septic arthritis
- Suspected crystal arthritis
- Suspected haemarthrosis
- Relief of symptoms by removal of effusion in degenerative arthritis.

Contraindications to joint aspiration

- Overlying sepsis
- Bleeding diathesis

Knee joint Patient lies with knee slightly flexed and supported. The joint space behind the patella either medially or laterally is palpated, the skin cleaned, and a needle (18G, green) inserted horizontally between the patella and femur using a no-touch technique. There is a slight resistance as the needle goes through the synovial membrane. Aspirate on the syringe until fluid is obtained.

Elbow joint Flex the elbow to 90° and pass the needle between the proximal head of the radius (locate by rotating patients hand) and the lateral epicondyle; or the needle can be passed posteriorly between the lateral epicondyla and the olecranon.

Ankle joint Plantarflex the foot slightly, palpate the joint margin between extensor hallucis longus (lateral) and tibialis anterior (medial) tendons just above tip of medial malleolus.

When synovial fluid is obtained:-

- Note the colour and assess viscosity
- Microscopy for cell count and crystals
- Gram stain and culture
- Synovial fluid glucose ($\downarrow$ cf. blood glucose in sepsis)

Synovial fluid analysis

Condition	Viscosity	Opacity	Leukocyte count (per mm³)
Normal	High	Clear	< 200
Osteoarthritis	High	Clear	1000 (< 50% PMN)
Rheumatoid	Low	Cloudy	1–50,000 PMN
Crystal	Low	Cloudy	5–50,000 PMN
Sepsis	Low	Cloudy	10–100,000 PMN

(a) Right knee, extended   (b) Right knee, flexed

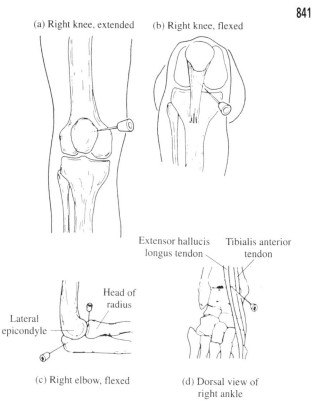

Extensor hallucis   Tibialis anterior
longus tendon   tendon

Lateral
epicondyle

Head of
radius

(c) Right elbow, flexed   (d) Dorsal view of
                           right ankle

Approaches used for joint aspiration (after Crawley M (1974) *Br Hosp Med* **11**: 747–55)

Intracranial pressure monitoring

Indications

- Cerebral trauma (GCS ≤ 8, compression of basal cistern on CT, mid-line shift > 0.5mm on CT, raised ICP not requiring surgery)
- Acute liver failure (Grade 4 coma with signs of ↑ ICP)
- Metabolic diseases with ↑ ICP (e.g. Reye's syndrome)
- Post-operative oedema (after neurosurgery)
- After intracranial haemorrhage (SAH or intracerebral)

ICP monitoring in patients who are at risk of unexpected rises in ICP should ideally be started before secondary brain injury has occurred, and where it would influence management of the patient. As facilities in neurosurgical centres may be limited, it has been suggested that these patients may be effectively managed in District Hospitals.[3]

Contraindications

- Uncorrectable coagulopathy
- Local infection near placement site or meningitis
- Septicaemia

Method

- There are several types of devices available (subdural, extradural, parenchymal, or intraventricular); parenchymal and intraventricular monitors are more accurate but carry a higher risk than extradural monitors. They should be implanted by experienced persons only.
- There are pre-packaged kits available (e.g. the Codman® subdural bolt). This monitor is inserted in the pre-frontal region and the kit contains the necessary screws for creating a burr-hole, spinal needles to perforate the dura, etc.
- The ICP waveform obtained is a dynamic recording that looks superficially very similar to the pulse waveform. It is due to pulsations of the cerebral blood vessels within the confined space of the cranium, with the effects of respiration superimposed.
- Cerebral perfusion pressure = mean arterial pressure – ICP.
- The normal resting mean ICP measured in a supine patient is less than 10mmHg (< 1.3kPa).
- The level which requires treatment depends to some extent on the disease: in benign intracranial hypertension values of ~ 40mmHg may not be associated with neurological symptoms; in patients with cerebral trauma treatment should be initiated with mean ICP > 25mmHg, though this value is debated.
- There are several types of pressure waves described of which the most significant are 'A waves' – sustained increases of the ICP lasting 10–20 minutes up to 50–100mmHg (6–13kPa). These are associated with a poor prognosis.
- The readings of the ICP monitors should always be accompanied by careful neurological examination.
- Treatment of raised ICP is discussed on p350.

Complications

- Infection (up to 5%)
- Bleeding (local, subdural, extradural, or intracerebral)
- CSF leak
- Seizures
- Misreading of ICP pressures

[3] Goodwin J et al (1993) Clin Int Care **4**: 190–192.

Lumbar puncture 1.

Contraindications

- Raised intracranial pressure (falling level of consciousness with falling pulse, rising bp, vomiting, focal signs, papilloedema). In general a CT scan should *always* be carried out prior to LP to exclude an obstructed CSF system or SOL (see p330).
- Coagulopathy or ↓ platelets ($< 50 \times 10^9/l$).

You will need the following:

- Spinal needles.
- Dressing pack (sterile gauze, drapes, antiseptic, gloves, plaster).
- Local anaesthetic (e.g. 2% lignocaine), 5ml syringe, orange (25G) and blue (22G) needles.
- 3 sterile bottles for collecting CSF and glucose bottle.
- Manometer and 3-way tap for measuring the opening CSF pressure.

Procedure

For suspected meningitis, antibiotics should be given first (see p330).

- Explain the procedure to the patient.
- Spend time positioning the patient, this is crucial to success. Lie patient on their left side (or R side if you are left handed), with back on edge of bed, fully flexed (knees to chin), with a folded pillow between their legs, keeping the back perpendicular to the bed. Flexion separates the interspaces between the vertebrae.
- The safest site for LP is the L4–L5 interspace (the spinal cord ends at L1–L2). An imaginary line drawn between the iliac crests intersects the spine at the L4 process or L4–L5 space exactly. Mark the L4,5 intervertebral space (e.g. with a ballpoint pen).
- Clean the skin widely and place the sterile drapes over the patient..
- Inject 0.25–0.5ml 2% lignocaine under skin at pen mark with the 25G needle. Anaesthetize the deeper structures with the 22G needle. Use the anaesthetic sparingly: this may distort the anatomy making the procedure difficult and unnecessarily longer.
- Insert the spinal needle (stilette in place) in the mid-line, aiming slightly cranially (towards umbilicus), horizontal to the bed. Do not advance the needle without the stylet in place.
- With experience, you will feel the resistance of the spinal ligaments, and then the dura, followed by a 'give' as the needle enters the subarachnoid space. Alternatively, periodically remove the stylet and look for escape of CSF. Replace the stylet before advancing.
- Measure CSF pressure with manometer and 3-way tap. Normal opening pressure is 7–20cm CSF with the patient in the lateral position. CSF pressure is increased with anxiety, SAH, infection, space occupying lesion, benign intracranial hypertension, CCF.
- Collect 0.5–1.5ml fluid in 3 serially numbered bottles and remember to fill the glucose bottle.
- Send specimens promptly for microscopy, culture, protein, glucose (with a simultaneous plasma sample for comparison), and where appropriate, virology, syphilis serology, cytology for malignancy, AFB, oligoclonal bands (multiple sclerosis), cryptococcal antigen testing, India ink stains, and fungal culture.
- Remove needle and place a plaster over the site.
- Patient should lie flat for at least 6h and have hourly neurological observation and bp measurement. Encourage fluid intake.

(a)

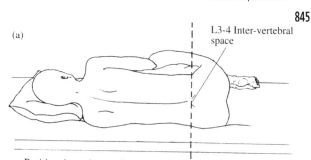

L3-4 Inter-vertebral space

Position the patient so that the line joining the iliac crests is perpendicular to the bed.

(b)

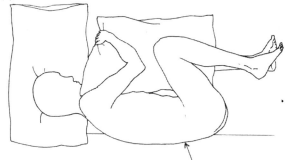

Ask the patient to curl up with a pillow between the knees to open the interspace. Point the needle cranially and advance gently.

Lumbar puncture   2.

Complications of lumbar puncture

- *Headache:* Common (up to 25%). Typically present when the patient is upright and better when supine. May last for days. Thought to be from intracranial traction due to CSF depletion from a persistent leak from the LP site. May be prevented by using finer spinal needles, keeping the patient supine for 6–12 hours post LP, and encouraging fluid intake. Treat with simple analgesia, fluids, and reassurance.
- *Trauma to nerve roots:* Rarer but seen if the needle does not stay in the mid-line. The patient experiences sharp pains or parasthesiae down the leg. Withdraw the needle and if the symptoms persist, stop the procedure and seek expert help.
- *Bleeding:* Minor bleeding may occur with a 'traumatic tap' when a small spinal vein is nicked. The CSF appears bloody (see below) but the bleeding stops spontaneously and does not require specific therapy. Coagulopathy, severe liver disease, or thrombocytopenia carries the risk of subarachnoid/subdural bleeding and paralysis.
- *Coning:* Herniation of cerebellar tonsils with compression of the medulla is very rare unless the patient has raised ICP. Always get a CT brain scan prior to LP and review this yourself if possible. Mortality is high, but the patient may respond to standard measures for treating this (see p424).
- *Infection:* Rare if proper sterile technique used.

CSF analysis

- **Normal values:**   Lymphocytes < 4/mm³; polymorphs 0mm³
  Protein < 0.4g/l
  Glucose > 2.2mmol/l (or > 70% plasma level)
  Opening pressure < 200mm CSF

	Bacterial	Viral	TB meningitis
Appearance	Turbid	Clear	Clear
Cells (mm³)	5–2000	5–500	5–1000
Main cell type	Neutrophil	Lymphocyte	Lymphocyte
Glucose (mM))	Very low	Normal	Low
Protein (g/l)	Often > 1.0	0.5 – 0.9	Often > 1.0
Other tests	Gram stain Bacterial antigen	PCR	Ziehl-Neesen Fluorescent test PCR

- **Bloody tap:** Artefact is indicated by fewer red cells in successive bottles, no yellowing of CSF (xanthochromia). The true WBC count may be estimated by:-

$$\text{True CSF WBC} = \text{CSF WBC} - \frac{\text{Blood WBC} \times \text{CSF RBC}}{\text{blood RBC}}$$

(i.e. if the patient's blood count is normal, subtract approx. one white cell for every 1000 RBC). To estimate the true protein level subtract 10mg/l for every 1000 RBCs/mm³ (be sure to do the count and protein estimation on the same bottle).
- **Subarachnoid haemorrhage:** (see p362) xanthochromia (yellow CSF). Red cells in equal numbers in all bottles. The RBCs will excite an inflammatory response (↑ CSF WCC), most marked after 48h.
- ↑ ↑ **CSF protein:** Acoustic neuroma and spinal tumours; Guillain-Barré syndrome (p408).

Lumbar puncture

Reference intervals: Biochemistry

Substance	Reference interval
Acid phosphatase (total)	1–5 IU/litre
Acid phosphatase (prostatic)	0–1 IU/litre
ACTH	< 80ng/litre
Alanine aminotransferase (ALT)	5–35 IU/litre
Albumin	35–50 g/litre
Aldosterone*	100–500 pmol/litre
Alkaline phosphatase	30–300 IU/litre (adults)
α-fetoprotein	< 10 kU/litre
Amylase	0–180 Somogyi U/dl
Angiotensin II*	5–35 pmol/litre
Antidiuretic hormone (ADH)	0.9–4.6 pmol/litre
Aspartate transaminase (AST)	5–35 IU/litre
Bicarbonate	24–30mmol/litre
Bilirubin	3–17mmol/litre (0.25–1.5 mg/dl)
Calcitonin	< 0.1μg/litre
Calcium (ionized)	1.0–1.25mmol/litre
Calcium (total)	2.12–2.65mmol/litre
Chloride	95–105mmol/litre
†Cholesterol	3.9–5.5mmol/litre
LDL cholesterol	1.55–4.4mmol/litre
HDL cholesterol	0.9–1.93mmol/litre
Cortisol am	450–700nmol/litre
midnight	80–280nmol/litre
Creatine kinase (CK)	Men 25–195 IU/litre
	Women 25–170 IU/litre
Creatinine	70–≤ 130μmol/litre
C-reactive protein (CRP)	0–10
Ferritin	12–200μg/litre
Folate	5–6.3nmol/litre (2.1–2.8μg/l)
γ-glutamyl transpeptidase (γ-GT)	Men 11–51 IU/litre
	Women 7–33 IU/litre
Glucose (fasting)	3.5–5.5mmol/litre
Glycosylated haemoglobin (HbA$_1$C)	5–8%
Growth hormone	< 20m U/litre
Iron	Men 14–31μmol/litre
	Women 7–33 IU/litre
Lactate dehydrogenase (LDH)	70–250 IU/litre
Magnesium	0.75–1.05mmol/litre
Osmolality	278–305mosmol/kg
Parathyroid hormone (PTH)	< 0.8–8.5pmol/litre
Phosphate (inorganic)	0.8–1.45mmol/litre
Potassium (K$^+$)	3.5–5.0mmol/litre
Prolactin	Men < 450 U/l; Women < 600 U/l
Prostate specific antigen (PSA)	0–4ng/ml

Biochemistry – contd.

Substance	Reference interval
Protein (total)	60–80g/litre
Red cell folate	0.36–1.44µmol/l (160–640µg/l)
Renin (erect/recumbent)*	2.8–4.5/1.1–2.7pmol/ml/h
Sodium (Na^+)	135–145mmol/litre
Thyroid stimulating hormone (TSH)	0.3–3.8mU/litre
Thyroxine (T4)	70–140nmol/litre
Thyroxine (free)	10.0–26.0pmol/litre
Total iron binding capacity (TIBC)	54–75µmol/litre
Triglyceride (fasting)	0.55–1.90mmol/litre
Tri-iodothyronine (T3)	1.2–3.0nmol/litre
Urea	2.5–6.7mmol/litre
Urate	Men 0.21–0.48mmol/litre
	Women 0.15–0.39mmol/litre
Vitamin B_{12}	0.13–0.68nmol/litre (> 150ng/litre)

849

* The sample requires special handling: contact the lab.
† The level of cholesterol should be taken in clinical context.
Lowering levels above 5.5mmol/l reduces morbidity and mortality in primary and secondary prevention trials.

Reference intervals: Urine

Substance	Reference interval
Adrenaline	0.03–0.10 µmol/24h
Cortisol (free)	≤ 280nmol/24h
Dopamine	0.65–2.70 µmol/24h
Hydroxyindole acetic acid (HIAA)	16–73µmol/24h
Hydroxymethylmandelic acid (HMMA, VMA)	16–48µmol/24h
Metanephrines	0.03–0.69µmol/mmol creatinine
Noradrenaline	0.12–0.5 µmol/24h
Osmolality	350–1000mosmol/kg
Phosphate (inorganic)	15–50mmol/24h
Potassium	14–120mmol/24h
Sodium	100–250mmol/24h

Reference intervals: Cerebrospinal fluid see p846.

Reference intervals: Ascitic fluid see p820.

Reference intervals: Haematology

Measurement		Reference interval
WBC (white blood cells)		$3.2-11.0 \times 10^9$/l
RBC (red blood cells)	Men	$4.5-6.5 \times 10^{12}$/l
	Women	$3.9-5.6 \times 10^{12}$/l
Haemoglobin (Hb)	Men	13.5–18.0 g/dl
	Women	11.5–16.0 g/dl
Haematocrit (HCT) or packed cell volume (PCV)	Men	0.4–0.54 l/l
	Women	0.37–0.47 l/l
Mean cell volume (MCV)		82–98 fl
Mean cell haemoglobin (MCH)		26.7–33.0 pg
Mean cell hamoglobin concentration (MCHC)		31.4–35.0 g/dl
Platelet count		$120-400 \times 10^9$/l
Neutrophils	%	40–75 %
	Abs. no.	$1.9-7.7 \times 10^9$/l
Monocytes	%	3.0–11.0%
	Abs. no.	$0.1-0.9 \times 10^9$/l
Eosinophils	%	0.0–7.0 %
	Abs. no.	$0.0-0.4 \times 10^9$/l
Basophils	%	0.0–1.0 %
	Abs. no.	$0.2-0.8 \times 10^9$/l
Lymphocytes	%	20–45%
	Abs. no.	$1.3-3.5 \times 10^9$/l
Reticulocyte count*		0.8–2.0% ($25-100 \times 10^9$/l)
Erythrocyte sedimentation rate (ESR)		depends on age (& ↑ in anaemia)
	Men	~ (age in years)-2
	Women	~ (age in years+10) -2
Prothrombin time (PT) – factors II, VII, and X.		10–14 seconds
Activated partial thromboplastin time (APTT) – factors VIII, IX, XI, and XII		35–45 seconds

* Only use percentages if red cell count is normal; otherwise use absolute value.

Guidelines on oral anti-coagulation

International normalized ratio (INR)	Clinical condition
2.0–3.0	Treatment of DVT, PE, TIAs; chronic AF.
3.0–4.5	Recurrent DVTs and PEs; arterial grafts and arterial disease (including MI); prosthetic cardiac valves.

Acid-base balance

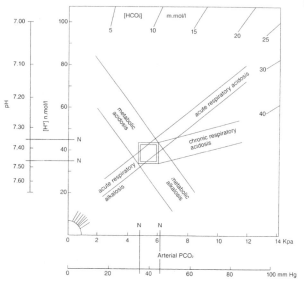

Acid base nomogram in the interpretation of arterial blood-gases (after Flenley DC (1971) *Lancet* **I**: 270–3)

Nomogram for body size

852

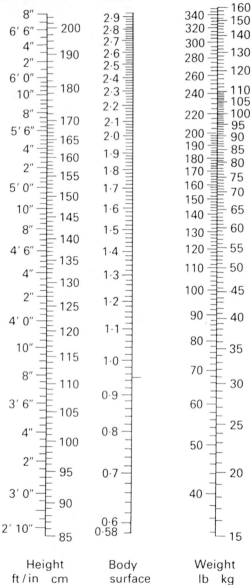

Height
ft / in   cm

Body
surface
m²

Weight
lb   kg

Useful telephone numbers

Liver Units

Royal Free Hospital, London	0171 794 0500
Addenbrookes Hospital, Cambridge	01223 245151
Freemans Hospital, Newcastle	0191 284 3111
Queen Elizabeth Hospital, Birmingham	0121 472 1311
St James Hospital, Leeds	0113 2433144
Edinburgh Royal Infirmary, Edinburgh	0131 5361000
Kings College Hospital, London	0171 737 4000

UKTS

United Kingdom Transplant Service	0117 9757575

Poisons Units

London	0171 635 9191
Newcastle	0191 2325131
Leeds	0113 2430715
Edinburgh	0131 5362300
Birmingham	0121 5075588
Cardiff	01222 709901
Belfast	01232 240503

National Teratology Unit

Drug & Chemical Exposure in Pregnancy	0191 2325131

Tropical & Infectious Diseases

St Pancras, London	0171 387 4411
Northwick Park, London	0181 869 2831 (daytime)
	0181 864 3232 (out of hours)
	(Bleep infectious disease Reg)
Liverpool	0151 7089393
Glasgow	0141 9467120
	Travel line, daytime
	Registrar on call out of hours

Anti-venom kits for snakebites

For information on identification and management contact:-

Oxford	01865 220968
Liverpool	0151 708 9393
Liverpool (supply only)	0151 525 5980
London	0171 635 9191

Virus reference laboratory

Colindale, London	0181 200 4400